Concepts and Activities

Nursing
Pharmacology

Concepts and Activities

Nursing Pharmacology

Mary Jo Gerlach, RN, MSNEd
Assistant Professor, Adult Nursing, Medical College of Georgia
The Health Sciences University of the State of Georgia
School of Nursing
Athens, Georgia

Springhouse Corporation
Springhouse, Pennsylvania

Staff

Executive Director, Editorial
Stanley Loeb

enior Publisher, Trade and tbooks
M. ie B. Rose, RN,BSN,MEd

Art D. tor
John H. ard

Drug Infor. tion Editor
George J. Bl. , RPh,MS

Editors
Diane Labus, Dav. Moreau, Nancy Priff

Copy Editors
Diane M. Armento, Pam. Wingrod

Clinical Consultant
Marlene Ciranowicz, RN,MSN,CDE

Designers
Stephanie Peters (associate art director), Mary Stangl (book designer), Donald G. Knauss, Laurie Mirijanian, Janice Nawn, Susan Hopkins Rodzewich

Manufacturing
Deborah Meiris (director), Anna Brindisi, Kate Davis, T.A. Landis

Editorial Assistants
Caroline Lemoine, Louise Quinn, Betsy K. Snyder

©1994 by Springhouse Corporation. All rights reserved. No part of this book may be used or reproduced in any manner whatsoever without written permission except for brief quotations embodied in critical articles and reviews. Some material in this book was adapted from *Clinical Pharmacology and Nursing,* 2nd ed. ©1992, Springhouse Corporation. Printed in the United States of America. For information, write Springhouse Corporation, 1111 Bethlehem Pike, P.O. Box 908, Springhouse, PA 19477-0908.

CANP-020895

R A member of the Reed Elsevier plc group

Library of Congress Cataloging-in-Publication Data

Nursing pharmacology / [edited by] Mary Jo Gerlach.
  p.   cm. — (Concepts and activities)
  Includes bibliographical references and index.
  1. Pharmacology. 2. Nursing. I. Gerlach, Mary Jo. II. Series.
  [DNLM: 1. Drugs—nurses' instruction. 2. Drugs—programmed instruction. 3. Drug Therapy—nurses' instruction. 4. Drug Therapy—programmed instruction. 5. Pharmacology—nurses' instruction. 6. Pharmacology—programmed instruction. QV 18 N974 1994]
RM301.N87 1994
615'.1—dc20
DNLM/DLC   93-37149
ISBN 0-87434-579-0   CIP

Contents

Contributors

Mary Qualey Bear, RN,EdD, RN-BSN Weekend Coordinator, Brenau Hall School of Nursing, Atlanta

Julia Lowe Behr, RN,MSN, Instructor, Parent-Child Nursing, Medical College of Georgia, The Health Sciences University of the State of Georgia, School of Nursing, Augusta

Carol Ann Burnes, RN,MSN, Nurse Practitioner, Northeast Health District, Athens, Ga.

Sharon W. Butler, RN,MSN, Assistant Professor, Medical College of Georgia, The Health Sciences University of the State of Georgia, School of Nursing, Augusta

Emily Ann Cook, RN,CS,PhD, Assistant Professor, Medical College of Georgia, The Health Sciences University of the State of Georgia, School of Nursing, Athens

Patricia R. Cook, RN,MSN, Assistant Professor, ADN Program Director, University of South Carolina–Aiken, Aiken

Benna E. Cunningham, RN,MSN, Instructor, Psychiatric/Mental Health Nursing, Medical College of Georgia, The Health Sciences University of the State of Georgia, School of Nursing, Augusta

Anne M. Desmond, RN,MN,CPN, Assistant Professor, Parent-Child Nursing, Medical College of Georgia, The Health Sciences University of the State of Georgia, School of Nursing, Athens

Caroline diDonato-Gonzalez, RN,MSN,CEN, Assistant Professor, Adult Nursing, Medical College of Georgia, The Health Sciences University of the State of Georgia, School of Nursing, Augusta

Linda Dufour, RN,MSN, Assistant Professor, Department of Nursing, West Georgia College, Dalton

Mary Jo Gerlach, RN,MSNEd, Assistant Professor, Adult Nursing, Medical College of Georgia, The Health Sciences University of the State of Georgia, School of Nursing, Athens

Gertrude G. Groves, RN,EdD, Head, School of Nursing, University of South Carolina-Aiken, Aiken

Joyce A. Guillory, RN,PhD, Assistant Professor, Morris Brown College, Atlanta

Linda W. Johnston, RN,MSN,PhD,CBF Assistant Professor, Associate Nursing Degree Program, University of South Carolina–Aiken, Aiken

Victoria J. Moody, BS,LD, Principal Nutritionist, Northeast Health District, Athens, Ga.

Donna R. Meirath Moriarity, RN,MSN,CDE, Assistant Professor, Medical College of Georgia, The Health Sciences University of the State of Georgia, School of Nursing, Athens

Patricia F. Schlotzhauer, RN,BSN, Charge Nurse, Orthopedics and Neurology, St. Mary's Hospital, Athens, Ga.

Janet C. Sims, RN,MSN, Unit Director, Cardiology, Athens Regional Medical Center, Athens, Ga.

Paula B. Spruill, RN,MSN, Instructor, Adult Nursing, Medical College of Georgia, The Health Sciences University of the State of Georgia, School of Nursing, Athens

Melissa Spurr, RN,MSN, Assistant Professor, Adult Nursing, Medical College of Georgia, The Health Sciences University of the State of Georgia, School of Nursing, Augusta

Caroline B. Wach, RN,MSN, Director of Nursing, King Springs Village, Smyrna, Ga.

Carolyn E. Wright, RN,MSN, Nursing Unit Coordinator, CVT Surgical Services, Crawford Long Hospital, Atlanta

Acknowledgments

A number of people provided support, encouragement, and patience throughout the preparation of this material. Special thanks to:
• students for continually seeking knowledge
• the contributors for sharing their expertise
• my husband, Fred, for his support and encouragement
• my son, Fred, for his support and computer expertise.

Preface

As the first book in the new *Concepts and Activities* series, *Nursing Pharmacology* delivers a unique way for readers to study an important core subject. Each chapter offers key concepts that crystallize important information and then provides numerous study activities designed to challenge the reader and boost information retention.

Organized into ten units, this book provides a conceptual framework for organizing pharmacologic information for clinical application. Unit One builds a foundation for the rest of the book. It covers the fundamentals of pharmacology, the nursing process related to drug therapy, and the vital aspects of drug administration, including dosage calculations. Units Two through Nine present individual drug classes and related nursing care. The final unit discusses drugs that require advanced preparation for administration, such as antineoplastic and anesthetic agents; those used infrequently, such as antitubercular and antileprotic agents; or those used only in certain circumstances, such as cation-exchange resins and ammonia-detoxicating agents.

Like all titles in the *Concepts and Activities* series, *Nursing Pharmacology* follows an easy-to-use, highly effective format. Each chapter begins with objectives that focus the reader's attention. They are followed by an overview of concepts that clearly presents core information and establishes the data base from which the reader can complete the study activities. In Units Two through Nine, the overview follows a consistent structure to enhance learning. For each drug class, it addresses pharmacokinetics, pharmacodynamics, pharmacotherapeutics, drug interactions, adverse drug reactions, and nursing implications.

The second half of every chapter features study activities that reflect the overview and accurately measure student learning. Activities may include multiple-choice questions based on clinical simulations, true-or-false statements, carefully selected fill-in-the-blank statements, matching exercises, and short-answer questions. Each chapter concludes with study activity answers and, where appropriate, rationales.

To highlight important information and make it easy to access and use, the book includes the following recurring features:

- *Selected major drugs,* a ready-reference chart that presents the major indications and usual adult dosages for each major drug in clinical use.
- *Drug interactions,* an easy-to-read chart presenting drugs that may interact with the prescribed medication and the possible effects of that interaction.

• *Sample nursing diagnoses,* an alphabetized list of appropriate nursing diagnoses based on the chapter's content and the North American Nursing Diagnosis Association (NANDA) taxonomic classification.

The book concludes with additional useful information. Appendices include commonly used abbreviations in drug therapy, which are vital to students and practitioners alike, and the NANDA taxonomy of nursing diagnoses. Selected references lead the reader to more detailed sources of pharmacologic information. A comprehensive index quickly directs the reader to the desired information.

To provide the most current, accurate, and clinically appropriate information, *Nursing Pharmacology* was prepared by practicing clinicians and academicians and reviewed extensively by nurses and pharmacists from appropriate specialty areas. Their combined efforts have produced a valuable source of information for years to come.

CHAPTER 1

Fundamentals of pharmacology

OBJECTIVES

After studying this chapter, the reader should be able to:

1. Differentiate among the branches of pharmacology: pharmacokinetics, pharmacodynamics, pharmacotherapeutics, toxicology, and pharmacognosy.

2. Briefly define prescription, nonprescription, and recreational drugs.

3. Explain the differences among a drug's chemical, generic, official, and trade names.

4. Define the five schedules of controlled drugs.

5. List several sources of relevant drug information for nurses.

6. Describe how drug dosage forms affect drug absorption.

7. Discuss how decreased binding between plasma proteins and an active drug can cause an excess of free active drug in the body.

8. Explain the significance of a drug's half-life in terms of the frequency of dosing and the patient's clinical responses.

9. Describe the significance of a drug's onset of action, peak concentration, and duration of action.

10. Differentiate between drug action and drug effect.

11. Differentiate between drug tolerance and dependence.

12. Discuss three kinds of drug interactions and their effects on the patient.

13. Define adverse drug reaction.

14. Differentiate between dose-related and patient sensitivity-related adverse reactions.

OVERVIEW OF CONCEPTS

Pharmacology is the scientific study of the origin, nature, chemistry, effects, and uses of drugs. The science is made up of five branches: pharmacokinetics, pharmacodynamics, pharmacotherapeutics, toxicology, and pharmacognosy.

Pharmacokinetics refers to the absorption, distribution, metabolism, and excretion of a drug in a living organism. *Pharmacodynamics* is the study of the biochemical and physical effects of drugs and the mechanisms of drug actions in living organisms. *Pharmacotherapeutics* (clinical pharmacology) is the use of drugs (clinical indications) in the prevention or treatment of disease. *Toxicology* represents the study of poisons, including the adverse effects of drugs on living organisms. *Pharmacognosy* refers to the study of natural drug sources, such as plants, animals, or minerals and their products.

Pharmacology   Pharmacology is an interdisciplinary science. The nurse must use information from physical, biological, and social sciences to ensure that drug therapy helps the patient achieve and maintain optimum health without causing toxicity or drug dependence. Pharmacokinetics, pharmacodynamics, pharmacotherapeutics, and adverse drug reactions will be discussed in more detail later in this chapter.

Terminology
The nurse must know the following terms to understand and interpret drug-related information for patients.
- A *drug* (medication) is a pharmacologic agent that interacts with living organisms to produce biological effects.
- A *prescription drug* is used under the supervision of a health care professional who is licensed to prescribe or dispense drugs according to state laws.
- A *nonprescription drug* (over-the-counter, or OTC, drug) can be used by consumers safely without the supervision of a licensed health care practitioner, provided consumers follow the manufacturer's directions.
- A *controlled drug* may lead to drug abuse or dependence; therefore, its use is controlled by federal, state, and local laws.
- *Drug abuse* describes the self-directed use of drugs for nontherapeutic purposes, a practice that does not comply with the sociocultural norms of a given culture.
- *Drug dependence* results when a person cannot control drug intake. This dependence may be physiologic, psychological, or both.
- *Drug misuse*, the improper use of common drugs, can lead to acute and chronic toxicity with such problems as gastrointestinal (GI) bleeding, kidney damage, or liver damage.
- A *recreational drug* is one used for its pleasant psychological or physical effects with no therapeutic intent.

Drug nomenclature
The *chemical name* of a drug precisely describes the drug's anatomic and molecular structure. When the manufacturer wishes to market a new drug, the United States Adopted Names (USAN) Council selects a *generic name*. In most cases, the generic name is derived from the chemical name but abbreviated for simplicity. The drug company selling the product selects the *trade name* (brand name or proprietary name); trade names are protected by copyright. In 1962, the federal government mandated the use of *official names* so that only one official name would represent each drug. The official names (generic names) are listed in the United States Pharmacopeia (USP) and National Formulary (NF).

Legal regulations and standards

As a society develops and uses drugs, it needs to establish controls regulating the manufacture, distribution, and use of those drugs. The Food and Drug Administration (FDA) monitors new drug development. Religious and social mores may provide informal controls on drug use. In most cases, a society's attitudes and values more strictly determine the acceptable limits of drug use than formal controls. Formal controls range from individual institutional policies to governmental legislation. Control of international drug trade depends largely on the voluntary cooperation of nations; no administrative or judicial structure exists to enforce control of international drug trade.

Legislative drug control in the United States began in 1906 with the passage of the Federal Food, Drug, and Cosmetic Act (FFDCA). While the FFDCA primarily addressed the issue of food purity, it also designated the USP and NF as the official standards for drugs. (For a summary of selected laws and amendments adopted since 1906, see *Federal drug legislation*, page 4.)

The Comprehensive Drug Abuse Prevention and Control Act (CSA or Controlled Substances Act of 1970) strengthened drug enforcement authority. The Act designated five categories, or schedules, that classified drugs according to their abuse potential.

- *Schedule I* drugs have a high abuse potential, are used only for research in the United States, or pose unacceptable dangers. The patient needs FDA clearance to obtain Schedule I drugs, which include narcotics, such as heroin; hallucinogens, such as LSD; and depressants, such as methaqualone.
- *Schedule II* drugs have a high abuse potential and accepted therapeutic uses. Physical or psychological dependence may result from their use. Schedule II drugs include narcotics, such as morphine, codeine, and meperidine; stimulants, such as amphetamines; and depressants, such as secobarbital.
- *Schedule III* drugs have a lower abuse potential than those in Schedule I and II, and have accepted therapeutic uses. They may cause moderate-to-low physical or psychological dependence. These drugs include stimulants, such as benzphetamine; depressants, such as butabarbital; and anabolic steroids, such as ethylestrenol and methyltestosterone.
- *Schedule IV* drugs have a lower abuse potential than Schedule III drugs and are therapeutically useful. They include narcotics, such as pentazocine; stimulants, such as fenfluramine; and depressants, such as chloral hydrate.
- *Schedule V* drugs have a lower abuse potential and varied therapeutic uses. Most are dispensed like other nonnarcotic prescription drugs, but some may be dispensed without a prescription, depending on state regulations. Schedule V includes drugs that contain small amounts of narcotics, such as codeine, dihydrocodeine, and

Federal drug legislation

The federal government has legislated drug manufacture, sales, and use since the passage of the Federal Food, Drug, and Cosmetic Act (FFDCA) in 1906. The following list gives the major legislative acts and their significance.

YEAR	LEGISLATION	SIGNIFICANCE
1906	FFDCA	Designated official standards for drugs (United States Pharmacopeia and National Formulary)
1912	FFDCA—Sherley Amendment	Prohibited drug companies from making fraudulent claims about their products
1914	Harrison Narcotic Act	Classified certain habit-forming drugs as narcotics and regulated their importation, manufacture, sale, and use
1938	FFDCA—Amendment	Provided for governmental approval of new drugs before they enter interstate commerce; defined labeling requirements
1945	FFDCA—Amendment	Provided for certification of certain drugs through testing by the Food and Drug Administration
1952	FFDCA—Durham-Humphrey Amendment	Distinguished between prescription and over-the-counter drugs; specified procedures for the distribution of prescription drugs
1962	FFDCA—Kefauver-Harris Amendment	Provided assurance of the safety and effectiveness of drugs and improved communication about drugs
1970	Comprehensive Drug Abuse Prevention and Control Act (Controlled Substance Act)	Outlined controls on habit-forming drugs; established governmental programs to prevent and treat drug abuse; assisted with the campaign against drug abuse by developing a classification that categorized drugs according to their abuse liability
1983	Orphan Drug Act	Offered substantial tax credits to companies to develop drugs that are used to treat rare diseases or that have a limited market.

diphenoxylate, when used as antitussives or antidiarrheals in combination products.

Although state drug controls must conform to federal laws, states usually impose additional regulations, such as determining the legal age for drinking alcohol. Local drug regulations imposed by counties or municipalities usually involve restriction on the sale or use of alcohol or tobacco. Institutional drug controls must conform to federal, state, and local regulations. Public and private institutions adopt and impose drug controls primarily to prevent health problems and legal violations by people within the institution.

The federal government also establishes and enforces drug standards to ensure the uniform quality of drugs. The standards pertain to such factors as drug purity, potency, and effectiveness.

Sources of drug information

Sources of drug information for physicians, nurses, and pharmacists who need current data include pharmacopeias (official), compendia (nonofficial), printed matter from pharmaceutical firms, drug handbooks, and journals. Research constantly adds to the body of drug information.

Pharmacokinetics

Pharmacokinetics deals with a drug's actions in a human body as it is absorbed, distributed, metabolized, and excreted. Many variables affect the method and rate of absorption, onset of action, time of peak action, duration of action, ability to maintain an effective blood concentration level, and dosage schedule.

Drug absorption

Drug absorption is affected by the route of administration and other variables, such as the absorptive surface area and blood flow.

Oral drug absorption

The oral route of drug administration remains the preferred route for drug therapy, especially because it promotes patient comfort, safety, and ease of use. Orally administered drugs include compressed tablets, sustained-release formulations, and other formulations. A compressed tablet provides a readily administered, standard dosage form. Sustained-release formulations release the drug in a controlled, predictable manner, providing safe and effective drug absorption in the GI tract. The nurse should avoid breaking or dividing an unscored compressed tablet or a sustained-release preparation to provide a lower dose for a patient because these actions may cause too-rapid release of the drug.

Manufacturers use several processes to produce sustained-release formulations. The oldest process involves applying an enteric coating, which creates a barrier between the drug and the acids in the stomach or intestinal mucosa. This coating allows the tablet to pass undisturbed through the stomach to the lower small intestine, where a more basic pH safely dissolves it. Another process uses beads or granules with varying thicknesses of protective coatings on them. The various coatings dissolve at different times, thereby releasing the drug at different rates over an extended time. Capsules containing coated granules should not be opened or chewed, because doing so immediately releases active drug into the body.

The newest sustained-release formulation, the osmotic pump, provides controlled release of a drug over several hours. Osmotic pumps usually are tablets with special semipermeable membrane coverings. The tablet's covering allows water to enter. The drug in solution can then leave the tablet but only through a single small hole made by a laser beam during formulation.

Chewable tablets were developed to simplify drug administration for children. Sublingual or buccal tablets are useful for administering drugs that require rapid patient response. They dissolve quickly in the mouth and pass through the oral mucosa into the bloodstream, thereby avoiding the destructive effects of stomach acid.

Parenteral drug absorption

Absorption of parenteral drugs depends primarily on the selected route of administration. Intravenous (I.V.) administration requires no absorption time; intramuscular (I.M.) and subcutaneous (S.C.) administration require varying amounts of time.

I.M. injections with a long-acting effect may be formulated in an oil or as microfine crystals. The nurse should never administer either formulation into a vein or artery because the crystals or oil may create emboli. The general rule regarding formulations is: *If the formulation looks cloudy or thick, do not inject it into a vein or an artery.*

Other variables

Many variables besides drug formulation affect drug absorption.
Surface area. Most absorption of orally administered drugs occurs in the small intestine, where the mucosal villi provide extensive surface area. If large sections of the small intestine have been surgically removed, drug absorption is decreased because of the reduced surface area. In some cases, the shortened length of the intestine also reduces intestinal transit time, which decreases the time that a drug is exposed to the intestinal lining for absorption.
Blood flow. Drug absorption also depends on blood flow to the absorption site. Food stimulates blood flow to the GI viscera and may enhance drug absorption. Strenuous physical exercise, however, may divert the blood to the skeletal muscles and slow drug absorption.
Pain and stress. Pain and stress can decrease the total amount of drug absorbed, possibly by decreasing blood flow, reducing GI motility, or triggering pyloric sphincter contraction, which causes gastric retention.
First-pass effect. Normally, orally administered drugs do not go directly into the systemic circulation after absorption. They move from the intestinal lumen to the mesenteric vascular system to the portal vein, and into the liver before passing into the general circulation. During this passage, part of a drug dose may be metabolized. Enzymes in the intestinal wall, liver, and terminal portal vein may metabolize a significant portion of the drug to an inactive form before it passes into the circulatory system and the site of action. This metabolic change of a drug before it reaches the systemic circulation is referred to as the first-pass effect.

For drugs that undergo a significant first-pass effect, the orally administered dose required for a therapeutic response is much greater than the dose for a route that bypasses the portal circulation (such as the vaginal, parenteral, or sublingual route). Although such routes avoid the first-pass effect, they are not always preferred. Orally administered drugs that are susceptible to the first-pass effect (and reach the circulatory system in reduced amounts) include dopamine, lidocaine, propranolol, morphine, reserpine, nitroglycerin, and warfarin.

Solubility. The solubility of the administered drug must match the cellular constituents of the absorption site. Lipid-soluble (fat-soluble) drugs can penetrate lipoid (fat) cells; water-soluble drugs cannot. For example, a water-soluble drug, such as penicillin, cannot penetrate the highly lipoid cells of the blood-brain barrier. However, a highly lipid-soluble drug, such as thiopental, can penetrate the lipoid cells, cross the blood-brain barrier, and induce an effect, such as anesthesia.

GI motility. High-fat meals and solid food affect GI transit time by delaying gastric emptying, which in turn delays initial drug delivery to intestinal absorption surfaces. Administration of such drugs as atropine, scopolamine, and belladonna alkaloids may slow intestinal motility and prolong intestinal transit time. Laxatives and diarrhea shorten the drug's contact time with the intestinal mucosa, thereby decreasing drug absorption.

Dosage form. The dosage form also affects the drug absorption rate and the time needed to reach peak effect. For example, the time needed for sublingual tablets to reach peak effect is less than the time needed for compressed tablets and sustained-release preparations.

Drug interactions. Combining one drug with another drug or with food can cause interactions that affect drug absorption. To avoid drug-drug or drug-food interactions, the nurse should consult the appropriate current compendia or a pharmacist before administering a new drug or teaching the patient about a drug.

Routes for drug absorption

The three routes of drug administration discussed here are the enteral, parenteral, and topical. The enteral route is used when drugs are administered by mouth or rectum or directly into the intestinal system (such as by a gastrostomy tube). The parenteral route is used for drugs administered as injections into a vein, artery, muscle, joint, skin layer, or spinal column. The topical route is any administration to the skin or mucous membranes.

Enteral route. Drug absorption after enteral administration can occur in the oral mucosa, gastric mucosa, small and large intestine, or rectum. Absorption through the oral mucosa usually is restricted to small quantities of sublingual and buccal preparations. The gastric mucosa usually is not used for drug absorption because of the small gastric surface area. Two substances that are absorbed directly from the gastric mucosa, however, are alcohol and aspirin. The gastric region is an important site for disintegrating and dissolving tablets or capsules in preparation for absorption in the small intestine.

The major site of absorption for drugs administered by the enteral route is the small intestine. The relatively large surface area, alkaline secretions, and rapid capillary blood flow of the small intestine facilitate absorption of most drugs.

Rectal drug absorption circumvents the first-pass effect, but only if the drug is administered in the lower rectum. Drug absorption by this route may be erratic. The lack of fluid, as well as the presence of stool in the rectum, can inhibit drug dissolution and delay absorption by the intestinal mucosa.

Parenteral route. Parenteral drugs may be administered by intradermal, S.C, I.M, I.V., intrathecal, or intra-articular routes. However, nurses usually do not administer drugs by intra-articular and intrathecal routes.

Use of the intradermal route requires parenteral drug administration between the skin layers just below the surface (stratum corneum). The drug then diffuses slowly from the injection site into the microcapillary circulation. In most cases, the intradermal route is limited to allergens of various strengths used in diagnostic allergy testing. A faster introduction of an allergen into a sensitive person could cause a life-threatening allergic reaction.

Use of the subcutaneous route involves administering drugs in the region below the epidermis. This promotes drug diffusion to the capillary vascular system at a much faster rate than that achieved by the intradermal route.

Parenteral drug absorption from I.M. sites depends on whether an I.M. solution, suspension, or emulsion is used. Solutions, which are clear preparations that contain one or more substances dissolved in a fluid, provide an immediate therapeutic effect. Suspensions, which contain crystalline particles and look cloudy, and emulsions, which have an oil-like base, prolong drug activity by slowing active drug absorption from the I.M. injection site. The muscle area selected for I.M. administration also may make a difference in the absorption rate. For example, blood flows faster through the deltoid muscle than through the gluteal muscle; however, the gluteal muscle can accommodate a larger volume of drug (up to 5 ml) than the deltoid muscle (up to 2 ml).

Administering drugs by the I.V. route bypasses absorption barriers and provides an immediate systemic response. The nurse always should read the product brochure before administering an I.V. drug to determine the method and diluent for reconstitution, the administration rate, and any restrictions. I.V. drugs should be administered slowly so that the sensitive target tissues do not absorb excessive amounts of the drug, which could cause such effects as fatal heart block.

Intrathecal administration places the parenteral drug directly into the cerebrospinal fluid, thereby avoiding the absorption barrier between the blood and brain. During intrathecal administration, physicians use only those drugs clearly labeled "For Intrathecal Use Only."

Intra-articular drug administration involves placing the solution directly into the synovial joint fluid to provide a local effect. Systemic drug absorption after intra-articular drug administration usually is negligible.

Topical route. Using topical routes of drug administration involves applying drugs to various body surfaces. The transdermal drug delivery system (TDDS) involves application of a protective film to an unshaven, preferably hairless skin area. The TDDS provides continuous drug delivery to achieve a constant, steady concentration of drug in the blood. The nurse should review the manufacturer's recommendations before applying the transdermal patch because different areas of the skin have different permeabilities. The nurse also should rotate application sites to prevent tissue irritation.

Topical ointments, creams, and gels typically provide local rather than systemic effects. Because drug absorption of topical preparations is unreliable, physicians seldom use or encourage the use of the topical route.

Rapid local drug absorption usually occurs with use of ophthalmic preparations because the drug typically is administered in solution. Ophthalmic drugs can be administered to the eyes as solutions, ointments, or ophthalmic inserts (small elliptic disks placed directly on the eyeball behind the lower eyelid). Because of the eye's ability to remove foreign substances rapidly, ophthalmic solutions and ointments usually require reapplication every 2 to 4 hours. Ophthalmic inserts provide a sustained-release preparation for drug administration.

Drugs applied to the ears usually result in negligible drug absorption. An otic preparation primarily is used for its local effect, to soften and loosen earwax and ease its removal or to treat a superficial ear canal rash or infection. The skin behind the ear (postauricular skin) provides an area for rapid drug absorption. A scopolamine patch for transdermal administration is an example of a drug that is administered in the postauricular area.

Drug absorption from local nasal instillation may cause local or systemic effects. Although nasal decongestant drops and sprays act locally to induce vasoconstriction, excessive use or abuse may result in systemic absorption. For example, nasal products that contain vasoconstrictors, such phenylephrine or pseudoephedrine, can increase blood pressure.

Drug administration by the inhalation route demands the delivery of micron-size particles that can move through the bronchial tree and reach the affected parts of the lung. Drug administration by this route can provide a local effect (such as isoproterenol to treat asthma) or a systemic effect (such as vasopressin to treat diabetes insipidus).

Drug distribution

Drug distribution refers to the process by which a drug is carried from its site of absorption to its site of action. Several factors affect drug distribution: blood flow, the drug's affinity for lipid or aqueous tissue, and protein binding.

During drug distribution through the vascular or lymphatic system, the drug comes in contact with various proteins and remains free or binds to plasma carrier protein, storage tissue, or receptor protein. As soon as a drug binds to a plasma carrier protein (such as albumin) or storage tissue protein, it becomes inactive. This renders it unavailable for binding to a receptor protein and incapable of exerting therapeutic activity. However, a bound drug can free itself rapidly to maintain a balance between the amounts of free and bound drug. Only the free, or unbound, drug remains active.

The percentage of free drug usually is constant for a particular drug, but can be affected by a patient's medical condition. For example, malnutrition, which directly affects the liver, deprives the body of protein building blocks and decreases plasma albumin production. This decrease in plasma albumin leads to a decrease in protein-binding sites and boosts the amount of free drug in the plasma, which may be undesirable.

Drug metabolism

Drug metabolism, or biotransformation, refers to the body's ability to change a drug biologically from its dosage or parent form to a more water-soluble form called a metabolite. This process varies for different types of drugs and can create active or inactive metabolites. Metabolism transforms a drug so that the renal and biliary systems can excrete it more readily. Illness can alter drug metabolism. For example, cirrhosis can damage the liver, hampering its ability to remove drugs and allowing the drugs to remain in the blood for a prolonged time.

Drug excretion

The body eliminates drugs by metabolism (usually hepatic) and excretion (usually renal). It also can eliminate drugs via the lungs, exocrine glands, liver, skin, and GI tract. Medical interventions, such as peritoneal dialysis or hemodialysis, also can remove drugs.

The physician must determine how long a drug will remain in the body to predict the frequency of the drug dosage schedule. Usually, the rate of drug excretion from the body can be estimated by determining the drug's half-life. Drug half-life represents the time required for the total amount of a drug in the body to diminish by one-half. (For an illustration, see *Determining drug half-life*.)

Drug half-life also is a useful tool when assessing drug accumulation. A drug that is not readministered is eliminated almost completely after five half-lives, but a regularly administered drug reaches a "constant" total body amount, or steady state, after five half-lives. After reaching the steady state, blood concentration levels of the drug will fluctuate above and below the "average" concentration level, but will remain within a constant range.

For some drugs, the time required to reach therapeutic blood concentration levels may be too long. For example, the half-life of digoxin is 1.6 days; however, the physician would not be able to wait 8 days (1.6 days times 5 half-lives) to achieve steady-state blood concentration levels to control a life-threatening arrhythmia. Therefore, an initial large dose, called a loading dose, would be rapidly administered to

Determining drug half-life

Drug half-life can be determined from a drug concentration-time curve by measuring the time required for a drug blood concentration level to decrease by one-half. For example, this graph shows a drug's concentration of 100 mcg/ml at 2 hours and a concentration of 50 mcg/ml at 4 hours (a half-life of 2 hours).

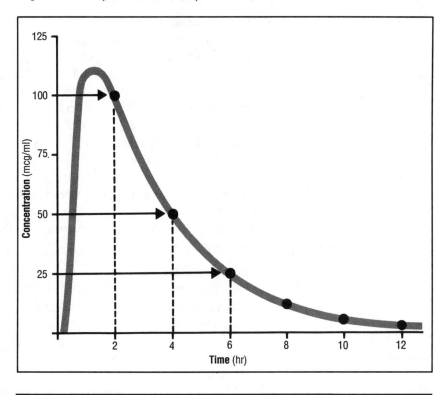

reach the desired therapeutic blood concentration level. Subsequently, smaller "maintenance doses" would be given daily to replace the amount of drug eliminated since the last dose. These doses maintain therapeutic blood concentration levels in the body at all times.

Drug clearance refers to removal of a drug from the body. A drug with a low clearance rate is removed from the body slowly; one with a high clearance rate is removed rapidly. A drug with a high clearance rate may require more frequent administration and higher doses than a comparable drug with a low clearance rate. Drugs with a low clearance can accumulate to toxic concentrations in the body unless they are administered less frequently or at lower doses.

Blood concentration levels

The concentration level of a drug in the blood helps determine whether the therapeutic goals have been reached with the drug regimen. Drug concentration levels usually are measured by the amount of the drug in plasma or serum; however, samples also can be taken from any other fluid, such as cerebrospinal fluid or saliva.

Pharmacodynamics

Pharmacodynamics is the study of the mechanisms by which drugs produce biochemical or physiologic changes in the body. A drug's pharmacodynamic phase occurs during pharmacokinetic phases of drug absorption, distribution, metabolism, and excretion.

Mechanisms of action

To understand pharmacodynamics, the nurse must differentiate between drug action and drug effect. *Drug action* refers to the interaction at the cellular level between a drug and cellular components, such as the complex proteins that make up the cell membrane, enzymes, or target receptors. *Drug effect* is the response that results from drug action, which may affect total body function. For example, when insulin is administered, the expected drug action is glucose transport across the cell membrane. Reduction of the blood glucose level represents the expected drug effect.

A drug may modify cell function or the rate of function, but *a drug cannot impart a new function to a cell or target tissue.* Therefore, the drug effect, or response, depends on what the cell should be capable of accomplishing.

Drug receptors

A receptor is a specialized reactive substance or macromolecule (large groups of molecules, such as a cell membrane, protein, or enzyme). Drugs interact with receptors like keys in locks. A drug that displays an affinity for a receptor and enhances or stimulates its functioning is an *agonist*. A drug that occupies a receptor site and prevents the agonist from acting is an *antagonist*.

Two types of antagonists—competitive and noncompetitive—exist. In the presence of an agonist, a competitive antagonist will respond only if its concentration is higher than that of the agonist. A noncompetitive antagonist inhibits agonist response regardless of agonist concentration.

Drug receptors usually are classified by the effects they produce. However, a nonselective drug may interact with more than one receptor, causing multiple effects. Also, some receptors are classified further by their specific effects. For example, beta receptors usually produce increased heart rate and bronchial relaxation, besides other systemic effects. They can be further subdivided into $beta_1$ receptors, which act primarily on the cardiac tissue, and $beta_2$ receptors, which act primarily on smooth muscles and gland cells. Administration of a nonselective beta antagonist or beta blocker, such as propranolol, to a patient with tachycardia will decrease the heart rate. Unfortunately, the nonselective properties also will block $beta_2$ receptors, which could precipitate an asthmatic attack in a susceptible patient.

The major factors determining the outcome of drug action include the location and function of the receptors with which the drug interacts and the drug concentration at the receptor site. If the drug interacts with common receptors located throughout the body, the drug effects will be widespread. Drugs that exhibit a widespread response may cause toxicity that affects many organ systems; these drugs have a narrow margin of safety. For example, chemotherapeutic drugs that destroy rapidly reproducing cancer cells may also destroy skin, hair, and blood cells.

If a drug interacts with specific receptors that are unique to highly differentiated cells, the response should be quite predictable. For instance, controlled doses of radioactive iodine, which has a strong affinity for receptor sites in the thyroid gland, effectively treat hyperthyroidism.

Therapeutic index

Because most drugs produce multiple effects, the relationship between a drug's desired therapeutic effects and its adverse effects is termed the drug's *therapeutic index,* or its margin of safety. The human therapeutic index usually represents a measure of the difference between an effective dose for 50% of the patients treated and the minimal dose at which adverse reactions occur. All drugs with a narrow therapeutic index should be monitored routinely and thoroughly.

Pharmacotherapeutics

Pharmacotherapeutics refers to the use of drugs to prevent or treat disease. The steps of therapeutics include assessing the problem, assessing the options, selecting the therapy, implementing the therapy, monitoring the therapy, and reassessing the problem. During the assessment phase, the nurse may take the patient's history and review the results of diagnostic studies. During treatment, the nurse monitors the patient for therapeutic—and adverse—effects, recording expected and unexpected reactions. The physician may adjust the therapy if the patient's problem resolves or progresses, if adverse effects occur, or if the therapy proves unsuccessful.

The physician may elect acute, empiric, supportive, palliative, maintenance, supplemental, or replacement therapy, depending on the severity, urgency, and prognosis of the patient's condition.

Acute therapy is used for critically ill patients, such as a trauma patient who requires volume expanders to treat blood loss and pressor agents to treat hypotension.

Empiric therapy is based on practical experience rather than pure scientific data. Physicians frequently treat fever spikes in hospitalized patients initially with empiric antibiotic therapy. They select the antibiotic by deducing which microorganisms the patient is most susceptible to (based on the patient's general health, hospital stay, or chronic diseases) instead of waiting for the results of culture and sensitivity tests.

Factors affecting patient response

Because no two people possess identical physiologic or psychological compositions, drug response varies greatly, depending on the following factors:
- age
- sex
- genetic makeup
- diet, especially inadequate food intake, intake that alters albumin concentration, and alcohol intake
- exercise
- stress
- smoking
- pregnancy and lactation
- circadian variations
- environmental factors, such as sunlight exposure, barometric pressure, and occupational exposure to toxins
- drug interactions, drug hypersensitivity, and immunizations
- acute or chronic diseases
- infection, fever, trauma
- body system (especially cardiovascular, gastrointestinal, hepatic, renal, and immune) function

Supportive therapy does not treat the cause of the disease but maintains other threatened body systems until the patient's condition resolves. For example, no antiviral agents are available to treat acute viral gastroenteritis, which causes nausea, vomiting, and diarrhea. An affected patient typically receives fluid and electrolyte replacements to prevent dehydration until the condition resolves.

Palliative therapy is used for patients with end-stage or terminal diseases to make them as comfortable as possible. For example, continuous infusions of high-dose narcotic analgesics may be used to manage pain in a patient with terminal cancer, or home oxygen may be supplied for a patient with end-stage pulmonary disease.

Maintenance therapy is used for patients with chronic conditions that do not resolve. This therapy seeks to maintain the patient's level of well-being while preventing further disease progression, if possible. As an example, maintenance therapy for hypertension can help prevent decreased renal function, impaired vision, or cerebrovascular accident.

Supplemental or replacement therapy may be short- or long-term. A patient with iron-deficiency anemia, for example, may receive iron supplements for 6 months until the hemoglobin level and hematocrit are corrected and the body's stores of iron are replenished. However, a patient with diabetes mellitus who cannot produce sufficient insulin may require lifelong injections that substitute for the missing hormone.

A physician considers many factors when selecting a drug for a patient, including the drug's potential risks and benefits, therapeutic index, and cost as well as the likelihood of patient compliance with the regimen.

Clinical response to drugs

Patient and treatment factors can affect any patient's response to drugs, which may include adverse and cumulative drug reactions. *Patient-related factors* include certain diseases that can alter the drug's absorption, distribution, metabolism, and excretion, thereby requiring dosage adjustments. Age, genetics, sex, body build, and circadian variations also affect drug response. Very young and very old patients are most susceptible to compromising alterations. (For more information, see *Factors affecting patient response.*)

Two *treatment-related factors*—the route and timing of drug administration—can affect drug activity and patient response. To help ensure that treatment-related factors do not have a negative effect on patient response, the nurse should store the drug according to the manufacturer's suggestions and should check the expiration date before administering it.

Tolerance and dependence are common responses to certain drugs. *Tolerance* refers to a patient's decreased response to a repeated drug dose: the patient needs more drug to produce the same effect. *Dependence* refers to a physical or psychological need for a drug. A cancer patient using a narcotic analgesic for severe pain can display tolerance and dependence. However, the psychological needs of the cancer patient who wants to maintain a reasonable level of pain relief differ from those of a substance abuser who desires a drug's euphoric effects.

The nurse can maintain an effective therapeutic drug regimen by understanding the prescribed drug and closely monitoring the patient's clinical response. Knowledge of the half-life of a drug and the physiological factors that may alter the half-life enables the nurse to understand the appropriate dosing interval for a patient. Knowledge of drug interactions and adverse reactions also helps ensure accurate patient monitoring and effective patient education.

Drug interactions

Interactions may occur between drugs or between food and drugs. They may involve prescription or OTC drugs. When obtaining a patient history, the nurse always should ask specifically about the use of OTC products.

Interactions involving two drugs usually produce a combined effect equal to the single most active component of the mixture. Such an interaction, called *indifference,* does not alter the therapeutic effects of either drug, nor does it produce any unpredictable adverse reactions.

Two or more drugs administered to a patient also can produce *additive effects* that usually are equivalent to the sum of the effects of either drug administered alone in higher doses. For example, acetaminophen 325 mg and codeine 30 mg are equal in analgesic effect. When combined, as in Codeine #3, their analgesic effect is equal to acetaminophen 650 mg or codeine 60 mg.

A *synergistic effect* occurs when two drugs producing the same qualitative effect are combined to produce a greater response than either drug alone. For example, if a central nervous system (CNS) depressant, such as ethanol, is combined with other drugs that have CNS depressant effects (drowsiness or sedation), these effects are enhanced and psychomotor skills are impaired.

An *antagonistic drug interaction* occurs when the combined response of two drugs is less than the response produced by either drug when given alone.

Adverse drug reactions

An adverse drug reaction (side effect) is a harmful, undesirable patient response to a specific drug therapy. These reactions may result from any clinically useful drug and may be dose-related or patient sensitivity-related. Some dose-related reactions are anticipated and preventable with careful prescription and administration. Others are unavoidable if primary therapeutic effects are to be achieved. Patient sensitivity-related reactions may not be predictable, because they stem from a drug allergy or idiosyncratic response.

Drug allergies are categorized into four basic groups: Types I, II, III, and IV. Type I reactions, which are immediate responses to stings and drugs, include anaphylaxis, urticaria, and angioedema. Type II reactions, which are drug-induced autoimmune disorders, include granulocytopenia induced by sulfonamide drugs. Type III reactions are responses to penicillins, sulfonamides, and iodides in which an antibody is targeted against tissue antigens. They include urticarial skin eruptions, arthralgia, lymphadenopathy, and fever. Type IV reactions, which are caused by reexposure to an antigen, include the contact dermatitis caused by poison ivy.

Patient sensitivity–related adverse reactions that do not result from known pharmacologic properties of a drug or from patient allergy but that are peculiar to the patient are idiosyncratic responses. This type of response sometimes is of genetic origin and may be manifested, for example, by nervousness and excitability after ingestion of a tranquilizing agent, such as phenobarbital.

Age-related considerations

A child's age, physiologic state, body composition, immature organ function, and other factors can affect pharmacokinetics. For example, an infant's gastric pH is higher (less acidic) than an adult's. Therefore, a child under age 1 will absorb more of a drug. Because the percentage of body fat is lower in children than in adults, the distribution of fat-soluble drugs is limited. As the percentage of fat increases with age, so does the distribution of fat-soluble drugs. An infant's immature liver may metabolize drugs inefficiently and immature kidneys may slow renal excretion of drugs. Also, target organ immaturity and altered recep-

Physiologic effects of aging on pharmacokinetics

Various age-related changes can affect drug absorption, distribution, metabolism, and excretion in geriatric patients, as described in the table below.

PHYSIOLOGIC CHANGE	EFFECT ON PHARMACOKINETICS
Absorption	
Decreased gastric acidity	Altered drug solubility and absorption
Reduced blood flow to gastrointestinal (GI) tract and decreased number of cells in GI tract available for absorption	Delayed drug absorption
Decreased GI motility	Increased transit time and drug absorption
Distribution	
Relative increase in body fat and decrease in total body water	Increased volume of distribution and prolonged half-life and duration of action for highly fat-soluble drugs; decreased volume of distribution for highly water-soluble drugs
Reduced plasma levels of albumin	Decreased predictability of drug distribution, and reduced number of receptor sites available for protein-bound drugs
Decreased size and weight, resulting in smaller overall volume	Increased blood concentrations of a drug
Metabolism	
Decreased liver mass and functioning	Reduced ability to metabolize drugs
Decreased blood flow to the liver	Delivery of less drug for metabolism to active compounds
Excretion	
Decreased glomerular filtration and tubular secretion, and smaller renal reserve	Decreased creatinine production, which may mask a sign of renal dysfunction (increased serum creatinine levels) until dysfunction is severe
Dehydration	Impaired renal function

tor sensitivity may affect a pediatric patient's response to a drug and may require a dosage adjustment.

Because of these age-related variations, a pediatric patient may require repeated doses at different intervals to achieve therapeutic effects. Dehydration and acid-base or electrolyte imbalances also can alter the therapeutic and toxic effects of a medication. The nurse must monitor a child with these disorders closely for adverse drug reactions.

In a geriatric patient, many physiologic changes of aging affect pharmacokinetic properties. (For details, see *Physiologic effects of aging on pharmacokinetics*.) Pharmacodynamic changes in geriatric patients result from the aging organ system and its role in drug-receptor or drug-organ interactions. For example, aging causes many receptors to function less efficiently and reduces the density of beta-adrenergic receptors, thereby reducing geriatric patients' responses to such drugs as isoproterenol and increasing the risk of toxicity with beta-blocker therapy. Aging also reduces the number of neurotransmitters, making geriatric patients more susceptible to the adverse extrapyramidal effects of neuroleptics and other drugs. Age-related changes in the CNS and cardiovascular and endocrine systems also may affect a drug's pharmacodynamic properties in a geriatric patient.

In geriatric patients, age-related changes can cause drugs to have unusual effects in various body systems. For example, aging of the liver can lead to increased therapeutic and toxic effects or more rapid drug metabolism. Age-related cardiovascular and renal changes also may alter drug metabolism and excretion. In patients with renal disease, the kidneys produce renal prostaglandins to help maintain renal perfusion. To help prevent toxicity, the nurse should administer reduced dosages of drugs that are excreted primarily by the kidneys.

Certain factors place the geriatric patient at increased risk of adverse drug reactions. These include advanced age, small physique, multiple illnesses, use of multiple medications, types of drugs prescribed (such as CNS depressants), previous adverse drug reactions, living alone, and malnutrition. Identification of high-risk geriatric patients can allow the nurse to protect them from many drug-related problems.

STUDY ACTIVITIES

Fill in the blank

1. The scientific study of the origin, nature, chemical effects, and uses of drugs is known as _____.

2. _____ is the study of the biochemical and physical effects of drugs.

3. Consumers can use _____ drugs safely without the supervision of licensed health care practitioners.

4. Drug _____ represents the time required for the total amount of a drug to be reduced by one-half.

5. The relationship between a drug's desired therapeutic effects and its adverse effects is called the _____.

True or false

6. Water-soluble drugs readily cross the blood-brain barrier.
   ☐ True   ☐ False

7. Strenuous physical exercise is likely to slow drug absorption from the GI tract.
   ☐ True   ☐ False

8. Drugs that have a narrow therapeutic index need routine and thorough monitoring.
   ☐ True   ☐ False

9. The gastric pH is lower in an infant than in an adult.
☐ True   ☐ False

10. In geriatric patients, a relative decrease in body fat and an increase in body water alter drug distribution.
☐ True   ☐ False

Multiple choice

11. Which branch of pharmacology deals with drug absorption, distribution, metabolism, and excretion?
   A. Pharmacokinetics
   B. Pharmacodynamics
   C. Pharmacotherapeutics
   D. Pharmacognosy

12. Which drug is included in Schedule II of the Controlled Substances Act?
   A. Heroin
   B. Benzphetamine
   C. Chloral hydrate
   D. Morphine

13. What is the major site of absorption for orally administered drugs?
   A. Buccal cavity
   B. Stomach
   C. Small intestine
   D. Large intestine

Matching related elements

Match the type of therapy on the left with its description on the right.

14. ___ Replacement therapy   **A.** Is based on practical experience rather than pure scientific data

15. ___ Empiric therapy   **B.** Provides supplemental, short- or long-term therapy

16. ___ Palliative therapy   **C.** Involves intensive therapy for critically ill patients

17. ___ Maintenance therapy   **D.** Maintains patient well-being while preventing further disease progression

18. ___ Acute therapy   **E.** Makes the patient with a terminal disease as comfortable as possible

ANSWERS **Fill in the blank**
   1. Pharmacology
   2. Pharmacodynamics
   3. Over-the-counter
   4. Half-life
   5. Therapeutic index

True or false

6. False. Water-soluble drugs cannot penetrate the highly lipoid cells of the blood-brain barrier; lipid-soluble drugs readily cross this barrier.

7. True.

8. True.

9. False. An infant's gastric pH is higher (less acidic) than an adult's. Therefore, a child under age 1 will absorb more of a drug.

10. False. Geriatric patients usually develop a relative increase in body fat and a decrease in body water, which alters drug distribution.

Multiple choice

11. A. Pharmacokinetics refers to drug absorption, distribution, metabolism, and excretion; pharmacodynamics, the study of mechanisms of drug action; pharmacotherapeutics, the use of drugs to prevent and treat disease; and pharmacognosy, the study of natural drug sources.

12. D. Morphine is a Schedule II drug. Heroin belongs to Schedule I; benzphetamine, to Schedule III; and chloral hydrate, to Schedule IV.

13. C. Most absorption of such drugs occurs in the small intestine, where the mucosal villi provide the most extensive surface area.

Matching related elements

14. B

15. A

16. E

17. D

18. C

CHAPTER 2

The nursing process and drug therapy

OBJECTIVES
After studying this chapter, the reader should be able to:
1. Explain the steps of the nursing process as they relate to drug therapy.
2. Identify the critical components of a drug history.
3. Identify the components of a teaching plan.
4. Explain how patient characteristics, the nurse-patient relationship, and the therapeutic regimen affect patient compliance.
5. Describe how the nurse uses outcome criteria during evaluation.
6. Explain how to evaluate therapeutic effects, adverse drug reactions, drug interactions, patient teaching, and patient compliance.
7. Explain the importance of documenting nursing care and patient response to nursing care.

OVERVIEW OF CONCEPTS
The nursing process is a framework that aids in the development, implementation, and evaluation of patient care. It consists of five essential steps: assessment, formulation of a nursing diagnosis, planning, implementation of the nursing care plan, and evaluation. Because the nursing process is dynamic, it lets the nurse develop and modify a total plan of care in a logical sequence for a particular patient.

Assessment related to drug therapy
During assessment, the nurse gathers information that helps guide the patient's drug therapy. Important sources of information include the patient's drug history (obtained from the patient, parent, spouse or partner, or others who know the patient well), the patient's previous medical record, physical assessment of the patient, and laboratory or diagnostic test results. Assessment occurs continually. Therefore, the nurse must update assessment data as new information becomes available.

As part of the assessment, the nurse must obtain a comprehensive drug history. This is particularly important because many patients have more than one physician, which increases the risk of having conflicting or incompatible drug regimens. The drug history should include questions that cover general information about the patient, such as aller-

Components of a drug history

When obtaining a drug history, the nurse can use the following list as a guide.

General information
- Allergies
- Drugs
- Food
- Medical history
- Associated acute or chronic illnesses and diseases
- Habits
- Dietary
- Use of recreational drugs such as alcohol, tobacco, and stimulants (including caffeine)
- Socioeconomic status
- Age
- Educational level
- Occupation
- Income level
- Health insurance coverage
- Life-style and beliefs
- Support systems
- Marital status
- Childbearing status
- Attitudes toward health and health care
- Use of the health care system
- Daily activities pattern
- Sensory deficits

Prescription and over-the-counter drugs
- Reason for use
- Knowledge of drugs
- Frequency or dosage
- Effectiveness
- Adverse reactions
- Pattern or routine

gies, medical history, habits, socioeconomic status, lifestyle and beliefs, and sensory deficits. It also should assess the patient's history of drug use, including the use of prescription and over-the-counter (OTC) drugs and home remedies. (For details, see *Components of a drug history.*)

When obtaining information about a patient's history of drug use, the nurse should explore the following: the reason for using the drug; the patient's knowledge of when the drug should be taken, the dosage, and its efficacy; and the route of administration. This information is especially important because it may provide insight into reasons why a particular drug regimen succeeds or fails.

Besides obtaining a drug history during assessment, the nurse needs to consider the patient's cognitive abilities and the body systems that may be affected by the prescribed drugs. A patient with intact cognitive abilities should be able to understand and implement the actions needed to comply with a drug regimen. If a patient's cognitive abilities are impaired, the nurse may need to teach a family member or friend to administer the drug, refer the patient to a home health care professional, recommend a day-care setting, or consider admitting the patient to an extended-care facility.

After completing the drug history, the nurse needs to assess the body systems that may be affected by the patient's prescribed drug regimen. Every drug produces a particular effect on a specific body system or systems. Some of the effects may represent the desired action of the drug. However, every drug can affect other body systems in adverse ways. For example, chemotherapeutic agents kill cancer cells, yet they also destroy other rapidly reproducing cells, causing nausea, hair loss, and anemia). The nurse must closely monitor a drug's adverse effects to ensure that the patient's health does not become seriously compromised.

Nursing diagnoses related to drug therapy

Analysis of assessment data helps the nurse develop a particular nursing diagnosis. The North American Nursing Diagnosis Association (NANDA) has developed a list of approved nursing diagnoses, which are arranged in groups of diagnostic categories and provide standardized terminology for discussing patient problems and care.

The two most common diagnoses related to drug therapy are *knowledge deficit* and *noncompliance*. A *knowledge deficit* can occur for various reasons. For example, it may be related to a new drug regimen, a prescribed diet, or self-management of a chronic disease, such as congestive heart failure. Its defining characteristics include statement of misconception, verbalization of the problem, request for information, inaccurate follow-up on instructions, inadequate test performance, and inappropriate or exaggerated behaviors.

Defining characteristics of *noncompliance* include behavior indicating failure to follow a regimen, supported by direct observation or statement by the patient or an informed observer; failure on objective tests; evidence of complications; exacerbations of symptoms; failure to keep appointments; failure to progress; and inability to set or maintain mutual goals. To assess the potential for *noncompliance,* the nurse must consider all factors related to the patient's lifestyle and beliefs. To increase the potential for compliance, the nurse may help the patient decrease the regimen's complexity or perform other interventions.

Planning related to drug therapy

The planning step of the nursing process consists of two major components: outcome criteria (patient goals) and nursing interventions.

Writing outcome criteria

This list describes the essential components of outcome criteria and provides examples of those components.

Content area
Describes the subject that the patient will focus on or the response to be elicited
- action of digoxin
- taking pulse

Action verb
Describes how the patient will achieve the objective
- *verbalize* the action of digoxin
- *demonstrate* pulse taking and recording

Time frame
Gives a target date for completion of the outcome criteria
- verbalize the action of digoxin *after the initial teaching session*
- demonstrate pulse taking and recording *before discharge*

Criterion modifiers
Add specificity to the subject, action, or time frame
- *correctly* verbalizes the *major* action of digoxin after the initial teaching session
- demonstrate *proper* pulse taking and recording before discharge *with a degree of accuracy within 4 beats of the pulse the nurse takes*

Outcome criteria state the desired patient behaviors or responses that should result from nursing care. Each criterion should be measurable and objective, concise, realistic for the patient, and attainable by nursing management. Also, each criterion should include only one behavior, expressed in terms of patient expectations, and should indicate a time frame. (For details, see *Writing outcome criteria*.)

After developing the outcome criteria, the nurse determines the interventions needed to help the patient reach the desired behavior or response goals. Interventions are the actions that the nurse implements to help the patient meet the identified outcome criteria. Interventions for effective drug therapy typically include patient teaching to educate the patient about the prescribed drug regimen and enhance compliance.

Developing a teaching plan is an essential part of patient teaching. Each teaching plan should include outcome criteria, a content outline that identifies the information to be covered in each patient-teaching session, teaching methods to be used (such as lecture, discussion, demonstration, or simulation), and evaluation criteria. (For more information, see *Basic learning and teaching principles*.)

Basic learning and teaching principles

The following list summarizes basic learning and teaching principles that the nurse can use when teaching about drug therapy.

Learning principles
- The patient must be motivated to learn, physically and emotionally ready, and actively involved in the process.
- Learning should be based on prior knowledge and experiences.
- Learning is more effective when knowledge can be applied immediately.
- Information must be compatible with the patient's expectations and goals.
- Repetition can reinforce learning.

Teaching principles
- Nurse-patient rapport aids patient teaching.
- Effective communication is essential.
- Environmental control can influence teaching effectiveness.
- Behavioral objectives can guide the teaching session and aid in evaluation.
- Cultural, ethnic, and religious beliefs must be considered when planning teaching sessions.
- Evaluation is an essential part of teaching.

Patient compliance

To achieve the optimal effects from drug therapy, the patient must comply with the prescribed regimen. However, patient characteristics and clinical characteristics can affect patient compliance.

Patient characteristics include demographic, physiologic, and psychosocial factors and drug knowledge. Their effects on compliance vary. For example, the nurse should consider demographic factors, including the patient's educational level, when planning patient teaching. This enables the nurse to develop and present information at the level appropriate for the patient. Physiologic factors, such as a chronic disease or lack of knowledge about it, may cause the patient to stop taking medication if the disease appears to improve.

Clinical characteristics include the nurse-patient relationship and the therapeutic regimen, which also may have diverse effects on compliance. For example, a nurse-patient relationship that is trusting and informative promotes patient satisfaction and compliance. A therapeutic regimen that is complex, is costly, produces adverse effects, or alters the patient's lifestyle or routines may lead to noncompliance. To avoid interfering with the patient's routines when establishing a drug regimen, the nurse should discuss the times most convenient for the patient to take the medication.

Implementation related to drug therapy

During the implementation step of the nursing process, the nurse puts interventions into action and provides care as described in the nursing care plan. By following the care plan and gearing actions toward the outcome criteria, the nurse can implement proposed interventions effectively.

Implementation of drug therapy typically includes working with the physician, administering drugs as prescribed, calculating dosages, preparing drugs, staying alert for medication errors, documenting drugs given, and teaching patients about drugs.

Evaluation related to drug therapy

Evaluation is a systematic procedure for determining the effectiveness of the nursing care. The nurse may evaluate drug effects and interactions, patient teaching, and patient compliance. Evaluation of drug effects and interactions requires that the nurse continually monitor for therapeutic effects, adverse drug reactions, and drug interactions and modify care accordingly.

Evaluation of patient teaching is based on outcome criteria or behavioral objectives. For patient teaching, the nurse may use two types of evaluation: formative (or concurrent) and summative (at the conclusion of the teaching learning session or retrospective). Formative evaluation offers the advantage of allowing for feedback during the teaching session.

Evaluation of patient compliance to the prescribed drug regimen may involve physiologic assessment, ratings by health care professionals, patient self-reporting, pill counts, and direct observation. Combining two or more of these methods produces more accurate evaluation of patient compliance.

If evaluation reveals that the outcome criteria have not been met or have been met only partially, the nurse may need to revise the plan of care. The nurse should reevaluate and revise care until each nursing diagnosis resolves.

Documentation related to drug therapy

Although documentation is not a step in the nursing process, the law requires the nurse to document activities related to drug therapy, including the time of administration, the quantity administered, and the patient's reaction to the drug. Documentation also serves as a way to communicate the plan of care to other health care professionals and as a guide to future drug therapy.

STUDY ACTIVITIES

Fill in the blank

1. The nursing process is a framework that aids in the _____, _____ , and _____ of patient care.

2. The five essential steps of the nursing process are _____, _____, _____, _____, and _____.

3. When obtaining a patient's drug history, the nurse must gather specific information about prescription and OTC drugs and general

information about _____, _____, _____,

_____, _____, and _____.

4. The two major components of the planning step of the nursing

process are _____ and _____.

5. The nurse may perform a _____ evaluation at the conclusion
of a patient-teaching session.

True or false

6. The nursing process is dynamic in that it allows the nurse to develop and modify a total plan of care for a patient.
□ True □ False

7. The two most common nursing diagnoses related to drug therapy are *knowledge deficit* and *altered nutrition.*
□ True □ False

8. It is unethical for the nurse to obtain information about the patient's drug history from previous medical records.
□ True □ False

9. The evaluation step of the nursing process is continuous.
□ True □ False

10. Learning is more effective when knowledge can be applied some time in the future.
□ True □ False

Multiple choice

11. Which of the following does the nurse use to formulate nursing diagnoses for a patient?
A. Outcome criteria
B. Evaluation data
C. Intervention criteria
D. Assessment data

12. When determining the patient's potential for incompatible drug regimens, the nurse is using which step of the nursing process?
A. Assessment
B. Planning
C. Implementation
D. Documentation

13. By law, the nurse must document drug therapy. However, the nurse may omit which of the following facts in documentation?
A. Time of drug administration
B. Time of peak drug concentration
C. Quantity of drug administered
D. Patient's reaction to the drug

14. For a patient, the nurse writes this outcome criterion: *The patient accurately demonstrates the steps of I.V. administration of penicillin by the time of discharge.* In this criterion, the phrase *I.V. administration of penicillin* is an example of:
 A. A content area
 B. An action verb
 C. A time frame
 D. A criterion modifier

15. In this outcome criterion, the phrase *by the time of discharge* is an example of:
 A. A content area
 B. An action verb
 C. A time frame
 D. A criterion modifier

ANSWERS   **Fill in the blank**
 1. Development, implementation, evaluation
 2. Assessment, formulation of a nursing diagnosis, planning, implementation of the nursing plan of care, evaluation
 3. Allergies, medical history, habits, socioeconomic status, lifestyle and beliefs, sensory deficits
 4. Outcome criteria, nursing interventions
 5. Summative (or retrospective)

True or false
 6. True.
 7. False. The two most common nursing diagnoses related to drug therapy are *knowledge deficit* and *noncompliance*.
 8. False. Important sources of assessment data include the patient's drug history, the patient's previous medical record, physical assessment of the patient, and laboratory or diagnostic test results.
 9. True.
 10. False. Learning is more effective when knowledge can be applied immediately.

Multiple choice
 11. D. Analysis of assessment data helps the nurse formulate particular nursing diagnoses, which become the basis for care.
 12. A. During the assessment step, the nurse gathers data that helps guide the patient's drug therapy.
 13. B. The law requires the nurse to document activities related to drug therapy, including the time of administration, the quantity administered, and the patient's reaction to the drug.
 14. A. The content area of an outcome criterion describes the subject that the patient will focus on or the response to be elicited.
 15. C. The time frame *(by the time of discharge)* gives a target date for completion of the outcome criteria.

CHAPTER 3

Principles of drug administration

OBJECTIVES   After studying this chapter, the reader should be able to:

   1. Recognize the essential components of a properly written medication order.

   2. Differentiate among types of medication orders.

   3. Identify the five "rights" of drug administration.

   4. Compare the oral, sublingual, and buccal routes of administration.

   5. Explain the purpose of rectal administration of drugs.

   6. Differentiate among the techniques for administering medications via these parenteral routes: intradermal, subcutaneous, intramuscular, and intravenous.

   7. Discuss other common routes of medication administration, including the dermal, ophthalmic, otic, and respiratory routes.

OVERVIEW OF CONCEPTS   Drug administration is a fundamental nursing responsibility. To help prevent errors when administering drugs, the nurse must understand medication orders, apply the five "rights" of medication administration, and use the appropriate routes of medication administration.

Medication orders   In most cases, physicians write medication orders, pharmacists dispense the ordered drugs, and nurses administer them to patients. In some circumstances, other health care professionals legally may prescribe and dispense medications, as outlined in the state's medical practice act.

   No matter who prescribes the medication, the medication order must be written clearly and completely. It must include the patient's full name, the generic or trade name of the drug, its dosage form and route (if more than one form of the drug is available), the dose to be given at each administration, and the frequency of administration (time schedule). The prescriber should date, time, and sign the order and should include any specific instructions for the nurse to follow. (For an example, see *Components of a medication order,* page 30.)

Components of a medication order

The prescriber writes medication orders for hospitalized patients on the order sheet in the patient's chart. As shown in the sample below, the medication order should give the patient's full name, the name of the drug, the dosage form, the dose amount, the administration route, the time schedule, the prescriber's signature, and the date and time of the order. (<u>Note</u>: Prescriber's order sheets vary from one health care facility to another.)

PRESCRIBER'S ORDER SHEET		William R. Weaver ——— Patient's full name Room 541 Hosp. No. 12-38-62-1 Date of Birth 12/17/42 Date of Admission 3/2/93
DATE AND TIME	**ORDER**	
Date and time — 3/2/93 10 AM	Admit to medical unit Regular diet A. P and lateral chest X-ray type & cross-match — unit whole blood	
Name of drug —	Synthroid 0.2 mg P.O. daily	— Route of administration — Time schedule
Dosage amount —	Ferrous sulfate 325 mg. P.O. t.i.d. p.c.	
	John Jackson, M.D.	— Prescriber's signature

These types of medication orders are routine in the hospital:

- *Standard written orders* apply until the prescriber writes another order to alter or discontinue the first one. Some written orders may include a specific termination date. Many hospitals have policies that indicate how long standard written orders remain valid. For example, a hospital may require that narcotic orders be terminated after 72 hours and that the prescriber must rewrite the order if the patient still needs the drug after the termination date.
- *Single orders* are written for drugs that are given only once. For example, diazepam (Valium) may be administered once before surgery to help reduce anxiety.

- *Stat or ASAP orders* require drug administration immediately (stat) or as soon as possible (ASAP) for an urgent patient problem.
- *P.R.N. orders* prescribe drug administration as needed or as applicable. In a p.r.n. order, the prescriber should indicate the specific reasons or conditions for which the nurse should administer the drug. When the patient receives a p.r.n. medication, the nurse must chart all appropriate information on the patient's record, including the reason for administering the drug and the degree of drug effectiveness.
- *Standing orders* establish guidelines for treating a particular disease or set of symptoms. Nursing units typically have a list of approved standing orders for each physician. When administering any medication by standing order, the nurse must rely on personal expertise and judgment. For example, the nurse must assess the patient's need for the medication and the patient's history of drug allergies before executing a standing order.
- *Verbal or telephone orders* may be required in urgent situations. Some occasions require the nurse to write the order as dictated by the prescriber. To help avoid errors, the nurse writing the verbal order should repeat the order aloud for verification. Telephone orders should be avoided whenever possible because of the risk of miscommunication. Ideally, a second nurse should monitor the call to confirm the order. The nurse should verify the telephone order with the prescriber by spelling the drug name and repeating the dosage, in digits. The prescriber must cosign all verbal and telephone orders within the time period established by institutional policy.

Five "rights" of medication administration

To help ensure accurate drug administration, health care professionals observe the five "rights" of medication administration, which include the right drug, dose, patient, time, and route.

Because of the vast number of drugs available today, the nurse must discriminate among similar-sounding drug names, such as digoxin (Lanoxin) and digitoxin (Crystodigin) or lorazepam (Ativan) and diazepam (Valium). The nurse always should compare the name of the drug on the medication order with the name on the container label.

In determining that the patient receives the right dose, the nurse should mentally calculate the approximate dose and then calculate the actual dose in writing, using the correct formula. Many hospitals require double checks of dosage calculations (or calculation checks by another nurse or the pharmacist) for children's medications and drugs with narrow safety margins, such as insulin. In determining the appropriate dosage for a patient, the prescriber considers many factors, including the patient's age, size or body surface area, and previous experience with the drug as well as the integrity and functioning of the patient's body systems.

To ensure that the right patient receives the medication, the nurse should compare the patient's identification bracelet carefully against the medication administration record. As a further check, the nurse should ask the patient to state his or her name.

Many hospitals establish routine times for drug administration. For example, the hospital may require that all drugs given three times daily (t.i.d.) are administered at 8 a.m., 2 p.m., and 8 p.m. In other cases, the right time for drug administration may depend on assessment findings, such as vital signs, or specific conditions, such as the presence of food in the stomach, specific intervals between doses, and use of other drugs that may interact with the drug to be administered.

The nurse must pay close attention to the administration route specified in the medication order and on the product label. The rate of drug absorption and prescribed dose depend on the administration route. Drugs that require rapid absorption may be given directly into the bloodstream (intravenously). Drugs that require slower absorption may be administered, for example, as an enteric-coated preparation.

Routes of drug administration

Drugs are manufactured and ordered in many different forms and may be administered by various routes. (However, some drugs can be administered only by one particular route.) The administration route helps determine the absorption rate and effectiveness of the medication.

Gastrointestinal routes

The gastrointestinal (GI) tract provides a fairly safe but relatively slow-acting site for drug absorption. Oral, sublingual, buccal, and rectal preparations are given via the GI tract.

Oral

Orally routed drug forms include tablets, capsules, and liquids. As long as the patient is alert and can swallow, oral administration is relatively simple and safe.

After being swallowed by the patient, most tablets and capsules dissolve in the stomach and are absorbed in the small intestine. For the patient who has difficulty swallowing, some tablets are available in chewable form. Drugs that are irritating to the stomach commonly are manufactured as enteric-coated tablets. These unscored tablets should never be divided, crushed, or given with food or milk. Capsules seal the medication in a gelatinous shell. Some capsules and tablets contain sustained-release drugs, which dissolve over an extended period of time.

Oral forms of liquid medications contain the drug mixed in a syrup or elixir. These drug forms are absorbed more readily than tablets and capsules and may be used for patients who have difficulty swallowing tablets and for pediatric patients.

Sublingual and buccal

Uncoated tablets are used for the sublingual and buccal routes. The tablets disintegrate and dissolve in the mouth, under the tongue (sublingual) or between the cheek and gum (buccal). Sublingual and buccal drugs are absorbed directly into the bloodstream from the oral mucosa. This allows the drugs to produce therapeutic actions rapidly—in some cases, within a few seconds. Because the drugs do not enter the GI tract, they bypass the liver—and the breakdown that otherwise would reduce the percentage of the drug available. (For more information, see Chapter 1, Fundamentals of Pharmacology.)

Rectal

A drug administered via the rectal route can provide local or systemic effects. Rectal administration may be used for a patient who cannot take oral medications, such as an unconscious patient or one with a nasogastric tube connected to continuous suction.

A drug may be administered in the form of a suppository or an enema. Upon insertion, a suppository will melt at body temperature. It should be retained for 20 minutes to achieve its desired effect. A retention enema, which usually must be retained for at least 30 minutes, may be used to administer medication. A nonretention enema (medicated or unmedicated) is given to evacuate the lower bowel.

Parenteral routes

Parenteral routes provide a rapid onset of drug action and help ensure high blood levels of the drug. Common routes for parenteral drugs include the intradermal, subcutaneous (S.C.), intramuscular (I.M.), and intravenous (I.V.) routes. The time needed for a drug's onset of action to occur for these routes decreases with the order in which they are listed. Because all parenteral routes disrupt skin integrity, the nurse must be alert for signs of infection related to parenteral drug administration.

Intradermal

The intradermal route is used for skin tests, such as tuberculin and allergy tests, and for administration of local anesthetics, such as xylocaine and lidocaine. The nurse gives intradermal injections in the area of the scapula, dorsal upper arm, or ventral forearm (the site of choice), using a 1-ml syringe with a 25G needle that is $\frac{1}{2}$" to $\frac{5}{8}$" long. To ensure wheal formation in the upper layers of the skin, the nurse should hold the needle at no more than a 15-degree angle. Then the nurse should inject the medication slowly and should not aspirate or massage the site. Finally, the nurse should record the location of the injection.

Subcutaneous

The S.C. route provides a slow, sustained release of medication and a longer duration of action. It is used when the total volume injected is no more than 1 ml of liquid. Many medications, such as insulin, heparin, and epinephrine, are given by the S.C. route.

Common S.C. injection sites include the abdomen, lateral aspects of the upper arm and thigh, and the area over the scapula. To administer an S.C. injection, the nurse needs a syringe with a 23G to 25G needle that is ½″ to ⅝″, depending on the angle of the injection (a ⅝″ needle is used for a 45-degree angle; a ½″ needle is used for a 90-degree angle). The nurse should rotate injection sites to ensure proper drug absorption and minimize tissue damage.

Intramuscular

Because muscles have a rich blood supply, the I.M. route provides rapid drug absorption. Intramuscular injections are used to administer drugs that are irritating to subcutaneous tissue (such as penicillin) or to give more than 1 ml of a drug. However, the recommended maximum volume for a single I.M. injection for an adult is 5 ml.

Commonly used I.M. injection sites include the dorsogluteal, ventrogluteal, vastus lateralis, rectus femoris, and deltoid muscles. The nurse must identify the site accurately because major blood vessels and nerves cross these areas and an injection given at an inappropriate site could damage them. The nurse also should rotate injection sites to avoid damaging a muscle. The size of the syringe and needle vary with the age and size of the patient, amount of adipose tissue present, site used, and the type and amount of medication to be given.

When administering a medication that is extremely caustic to subcutaneous tissue, the nurse may use the air-bubble or Z-track method of administration. With the air-bubble method, the nurse withdraws 0.2 cc of air after drawing the correct dose of a medication into the syringe. This forms a bubble that helps clear all of the drug out of the needle, which prevents the drug from leaking into the subcutaneous tissue.

The Z-track method involves pulling the skin to one side and holding it there while giving the injection and then returning the skin to its normal position upon removal of the needle. This technique interrupts the path made by the needle and prevents the backflow of medication into the subcutaneous tissue.

Intravenous

Medications are administered intravenously to obtain an immediate onset of action, to attain the highest possible blood concentration level of a drug (such as in life-threatening emergencies), to treat conditions that require constant drug titration, or to treat a patient who cannot tolerate drug administration by another route.

Common sites for indwelling I.V. catheters or intermittent devices include the veins on the hand and wrist, the forearm veins in the antecubital fossa, the scalp veins (in infants), the subclavian and jugular veins (for long-term administration), and the superficial veins of the leg and foot (when other sites cannot be used). The nurse should insert the I.V. infusion device as distal as possible to maintain future sites.

Because I.V. administration produces a rapid onset of action, the nurse must be especially cautious when administering a drug that can cause systemic reactions or affect major organs. For example, the nurse should be extremely careful when giving narcotics to relieve pain because respiratory failure may occur if they are given in too large a dose or too quickly.

Other routes of administration

The dermal or topical route may be used with creams, lotions, ointments, powders, and patches. Most topical drugs are applied for their local effects. However, some drugs, such as the nitroglycerin ointment or patch, are given by this route to ensure slow systemic absorption. The absorption rate depends on the vascularity of the region and the skin condition at the site. When a transdermal patch must be reapplied, the nurse should rotate the site to avoid irritation.

Medications are administered by the ophthalmic and otic routes for their local effects. When instilling a medication into the eyes or ears, the nurse should use good administration techniques to avoid infection. The nurse also should review the prescription to verify the strength, frequency, and location of the medication administration (O.D., right eye; O.S., left eye; O.U., both eyes).

Common methods for administering drugs by the respiratory route include the use of nebulizers, aerosols, inhalers, and vaporizers. The respiratory route is used to treat such conditions as asthma and to administer some forms of anesthesia. Respiratory drugs (inhalants) require careful administration because they are absorbed rapidly due to the rich blood supply of the lungs and because they produce systemic effects.

Pediatric administration techniques

When administering medication to a pediatric patient, the nurse must pay special attention to the five rights and be particularly observant for adverse reactions and drug interactions. To help ensure safe, effective drug therapy, the nurse must administer drugs by the appropriate route and try to elicit the child's cooperation.

Oral route. Because the oral route usually is the least traumatic, it commonly is used to administer drugs to children. Many pediatric medications come in palatable and colorful preparations, but others do not. Although the child willingly may swallow a drug at first, the child may spit, drool, or choke after realizing a drug tastes unpleasant. Therefore, the nurse should camouflage the taste, as needed.

Intramuscular and subcutaneous routes. For an I.M. injection, the nurse should use the smallest gauge needle appropriate for the drug. The recommended injection sites vary with the child's age. (For details, see *Pediatric I.M. injection sites,* page 36.)

Pediatric I.M. injection sites

The nurse can use several landmarks to identify I.M. injection sites for pediatric patients. The vastus lateralis and rectus femoris muscles are the recommended sites for an infant or toddler. The dorsogluteal and ventrogluteal sites can be used only after the toddler has been walking for about 1 year.

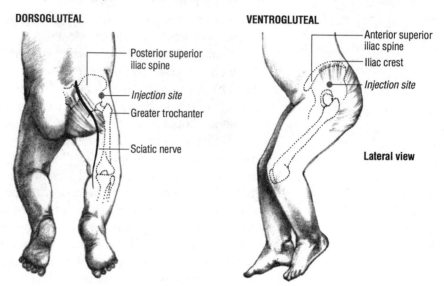

DORSOGLUTEAL

- Posterior superior iliac spine
- *Injection site*
- Greater trochanter
- Sciatic nerve

VENTROGLUTEAL

- Anterior superior iliac spine
- Iliac crest
- *Injection site*

Lateral view

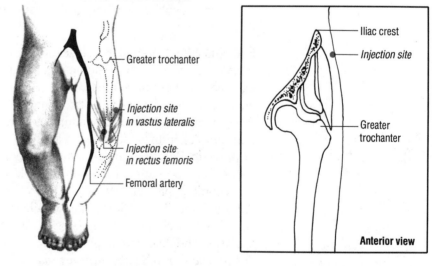

VASTUS LATERALIS AND RECTUS FEMORIS

- Greater trochanter
- *Injection site in vastus lateralis*
- *Injection site in rectus femoris*
- Femoral artery

- Iliac crest
- *Injection site*
- Greater trochanter

Anterior view

Subcutaneous administration is the same in a child as in an adult. The nurse should remember to provide an age-appropriate explanation and position the child properly.

Intravenous route. The I.V. route for drug administration commonly is used for pediatric patients. Silastic catheters are preferred because they are less irritating to the vein. When selecting a site for I.V. catheter insertion, the nurse should consider the veins of the hand and lower arm before considering more proximal areas. Then if infiltration occurs, the nurse can use proximal veins, such as those of the wrist and forearm. The same rule applies to selecting an I.V. site in a lower extremity. In an infant, the nurse may use a head vein for I.V. access. The nurse should secure the I.V. catheter in a way that allows frequent observation of the site to detect signs of complications.

Intraosseous route. For a critically ill child under age 3, drugs may be administered by the intraosseous route. This temporary route is used in emergencies, when I.V. access is unavailable.

Topical route. In an infant or small child, thin epidermis and large body surface area allow for increased absorption of—and increased severity of adverse reactions to—topical drugs. To reduce the risk of toxic effects, the nurse should apply a topical medication as thinly as possible and to as small a body surface area as possible.

Rectal route. Drug absorption from the rectum may be unpredictable. Nevertheless, rectal administration may be required if the oral route is contraindicated. After inserting the lubricated suppository past the rectal sphincter with a gloved hand, the nurse must hold the buttocks together to prevent expulsion of the drug.

Other routes. For drops that are administered by the ophthalmic, otic, or nasal routes, the nurse must be aware of certain special considerations. For all three routes, the major challenge is to gain the child's cooperation or restrain the child, which may require coworker's assistance.

To administer eye drops, the nurse may place the hand that holds the dropper on the child's forehead so that it will move as the child's head moves and decrease the risk of injury.

Before instilling ear drops, the nurse should warm the solution to body temperature. Then the nurse should position the child with the affected ear up. When administering drops to a child under age 3, the nurse should pull the pinna down and back; to one over age 3, up and back.

When instilling nose drops, the nurse should position the child with the head tipped back to prevent the medication from entering the throat rather than the nasal passages.

STUDY ACTIVITIES **Multiple choice**

1. The physician writes a prescription for digoxin (Lanoxin) 0.25 mg P.O. daily. This prescription is an example of a:
    A. Single order
    B. Stat order
    C. Standing order
    D. Standard written order

2. Which of the following is a parenteral administration route?
    A. Subcutaneous
    B. Respiratory
    C. Dermal
    D. Buccal

3. Anne Burns, age 76, is admitted to the unit after surgery. Her physician writes several medication orders. Which one is incomplete?
    A. Morphine sulfate 10 mg I.M. q 3 to 4 hours p.r.n. for severe pain
    B. Promethazine hydrochloride (Phenergan) 25 mg q 3 to 4 hours p.r.n. for nausea
    C. Artificial tears 1 to 2 drops O.U. q.i.d. and p.r.n. for eye dryness
    D. Tylenol #3 1 tablet q 3 to 4 hours P.O. p.r.n. for mild to moderate pain

4. What is the maximum volume of drug that may be administered to an adult in a single I.M. injection?
    A. 1 ml
    B. 2 ml
    C. 5 ml
    D. 10 ml

5. Which site commonly is used to give an I.M. injection to an adult?
    A. Jugular vein
    B. Vastus lateralis
    C. Rectus abdominis
    D. Subclavian vein

True or false

6. The route of administration has no effect on drug absorption.
    ☐ True   ☐ False

7. The nurse should give p.r.n. medications as needed.
    ☐ True   ☐ False

8. Respiratory drugs are absorbed rapidly because of the rich blood supply of the lungs.
    ☐ True   ☐ False

9. State medical practice acts empower specific health care professionals to prescribe drugs.
☐ True   ☐ False

10. The nurse should use the same site every time a transdermal patch is reapplied.
☐ True   ☐ False

Matching related elements
Match the medication orders on the left with the appropriate description on the right.

11. ___ Single orders   **A.** Require drugs to be administered only once

12. ___ Stat orders   **B.** Provide guidelines for treating a particular disease or set of symptoms

13. ___ Verbal orders   **C.** Are dictated to and written by the nurse, but should be avoided

14. ___ Standard written orders   **D.** Apply until another order alters or discontinues them

15. ___ Standing orders   **E.** Must be carried out immediately

Fill in the blank

16. The nurse may give _____ injections in the area of the scapula, dorsal upper arm, or ventral forearm.

17. Because parenteral drug administration disrupts skin integrity, the nurse should be alert for signs of _____.

18. To minimize tissue damage, the nurse should _____ S.C. injection sites.

19. When medication is caustic to subcutaneous tissue, the nurse may administer an I.M. injection via the _____ method, which displaces the skin to interrupt the path of the needle.

20. The _____ route is used during life-threatening situations to ensure that medication is absorbed quickly.

21. The nurse should give an intradermal injection at no more than a _____-degree angle.

22. The _____ and _____ muscles are the preferred sites for administering an I.M. injection to an infant.

23. The nurse should insert an I.V. infusion device as _____ as possible to maintain future sites.

24. The five "rights" of medication administration are the right

_____, _____, _____, _____, and _____.

ANSWERS

Multiple choice

1. D. Standard written orders apply until the prescriber writes another order to alter or discontinue the first one. Single orders are used for drugs given only once; stat orders, for drugs given immediately; standing orders, for drugs administered according to institutional protocols for treating a particular disease or set of symptoms.

2. A. Parenteral routes include the intradermal, subcutaneous, intramuscular, and intravenous routes.

3. B. All medication orders should include the drug name, dosage form, dose amount, administration route, and time schedule. This order does not indicate the administration route.

4. C. The recommended maximum volume for a single I.M. injection for an adult is 5 ml.

5. B. Common sites for I.M. administration include the dorsogluteal, ventrogluteal, vastus lateralis, rectus femoris, and deltoid muscles. Subclavian and jugular veins may be used for I.V. administration.

True or false

6. False. The rate of drug absorption and prescribed dose depend on the administration route. Drugs that require rapid absorption usually are administered intravenously.

7. True.

8. True.

9. True.

10. False. When a transdermal patch must be reapplied, the nurse should rotate the site to avoid irritation.

Matching related elements

11. A

12. E

13. C

14. D

15. B

Fill in the blank

16. Intradermal

17. Infection

18. Rotate

19. Z-track

20. Intravenous

21. 15

22. Vastus lateralis, rectus femoris

23. Distal

24. Drug, dose, patient, time, route

CHAPTER 4

Dosage measurements and calculations

OBJECTIVES   After studying this chapter, the reader should be able to:
1. Convert between different systems of measurement.
2. Compute drug dosages, using the fraction, ratio, and "desired-available" methods.
3. Reconstitute drugs and calculate their dosage.
4. Calculate dosages for percentage and ratio solutions.
5. Determine intravenous (I.V.) drip rates.

OVERVIEW OF CONCEPTS   Most health care facilities now use the unit-dose system of drug delivery. In this system, the pharmacist dispenses a supply of single doses, wrapped and labeled, of all drugs. At times, however, the nurse must calculate the correct dose for the patient. To prepare the nurse to fulfill this responsibility, this chapter presents information on systems of measurement, conversions among systems of measurement, calculations of drug dosages (including reconstituted drugs and drugs in percentage and ratio solutions) and I.V. drip rates.

Systems of measurement   The physician may use several systems of measurement when ordering drugs. The three systems of measurement most commonly used in clinical settings are the metric, apothecaries', and household systems. Other systems are used for specific drugs. The nurse should understand all of these systems thoroughly.

Metric system
The metric system, which is used by the U.S. Pharmacopoeia, is the most widely used because of its accuracy and international acceptance. In this system, the liter is the basic unit of measure for liquids; the gram, for solids. Smaller and larger units of measure reflect the basic units of measure, such as the milliliter (ml), which equals one one-thousandth of a liter, and the kilogram (kg), which equals 1,000 grams.

Apothecaries' system

The apothecaries' system is the oldest system of measure. It uses Roman numerals and special symbols to represent units of measure. Its basic unit of measure for liquids is the minim (𝕄), which is about the size of a water drop; for solids and weights, the grain (gr).

Household system

In the United States, most people use the household system of measurement for recipes, over-the-counter drugs, and home remedies. Although this system is the most familiar, it is not the most accurate because of discrepancies in the size of measuring tools, such as spoons. In this system, the teaspoon and tablespoon are the most commonly used liquid measurements in the clinical setting. Therefore, their size has been standardized to 5 ml and 15 ml respectively.

Other systems of measurement

Some drugs require special systems of measurement. For example, insulin is measured in units (U). The international standard of U-100 insulin means that 1 milliliter of insulin solution contains 100 units of insulin, regardless of type. To avoid errors, the nurse should draw up insulin only in an insulin syringe measured in units. Other drugs measured in units include antibiotics, vitamins, hormones, and heparin.

Electrolytes, such as potassium chloride, may be measured in milliequivalents (mEq). Drug manufacturers indicate the number of metric units required to provide the prescribed number of milliequivalents. For example, a manufacturer's information may state that 1 ml equals 4 Meq.

Conversions between systems of measurement

When a drug is ordered in one system of drug measurement but is supplied in another, the nurse must make a conversion between the two systems, using the appropriate equivalents. (For key equivalents, see *Units of exchange among systems of measurement*.)

Fraction method for conversions

A simple conversion technique, the fraction method uses an equation that consists of two fractions. The first fraction places the ordered dosage (to be converted) over X units of available dosage. The second fraction consists of the standard equivalents between the ordered and available measures.

For example, the physician orders 300 mg of aspirin. The bottle is labeled *aspirin gr v per tablet.* The milligram dosage represents the ordered dosage, and the grain dosage represents the available dosage. Because the amount of the available dosage is unknown, it is represented by an *X.* The first fraction of the equation appears as:

$$\frac{300 \text{ mg}}{X \text{ gr}}$$

Units of exchange among systems of measurement

The following shows some approximate liquid equivalents among the household, apothecaries', and metric systems.

HOUSEHOLD	APOTHECARIES'	METRIC
1 teaspoonful (tsp)	1 fluidram (f℥)	5 ml
1 tablespoonful (tbs)	1/2 fluidounce (f℥)	15 ml
2 tbs (1 ounce [1 oz])	1 (f℥)	30 ml
1 measuring cupful	8 (f℥)	240 ml
1 pint (pt)	16 (f℥)	473 ml
1 quart (qt)	32 (f℥)	946 ml (1 liter)
1 gallon (gal)	128 (f℥)	3,785 ml

The following shows some approximate solid equivalents between the apothecaries' system and the metric system.

APOTHECARIES'	METRIC
15 grains (gr)	1 gram (g) (1,000 mg)
10 gr	0.6 g (600 mg)
7 1/2 gr	0.5 g (500 mg)
5 gr	0.3 g (300 mg)
3 gr	0.2 g (200 mg)
1 1/2 gr	0.1 g (100 mg)
1 gr	0.06 g (60 mg) or 0.065 g (65 mg)
3/4 gr	0.05 g (50 mg)
1/2 gr	0.03 g (30 mg)
1/4 gr	0.015 g (15 mg)
1/60 gr	0.001 g (1 mg)
1/100 gr	0.6 mg
1/120 gr	0.5 mg
1/150 gr	0.4 mg

(continued)

Units of exchange among systems of measurement *(continued)*

The following lists some approximate solid equivalents among the avoirdupois, apothecaries', and metric systems.

AVOIRDUPOIS	APOTHECARIES'	METRIC
1 gr	1 gr	0.065 g
15.4 gr	15 gr	1 g
1 ounce (oz)	480 gr	28.35 g
437.5 gr	1 oz	31 g
1 pound (lb)	1.33 lb	454 g
0.75 lb	1 lb	373 g
2.2 lb	2.7 lb	1 kilogram (kg)

Using the standard equivalent (60 mg equal 1 gr) to convert milligrams to grains, the second fraction appears as:

$$\frac{60 \text{ mg}}{1 \text{ gr}}$$

In both fractions, the same unit of measure must appear in the numerators, and the same unit of measure should appear in the denominators. So the entire equation should appear as:

$$\frac{300 \text{ mg}}{X \text{ gr}} = \frac{60 \text{ mg}}{1 \text{ gr}}$$

To solve for X, cross multiply:

$$300 \text{ mg} \times 1 \text{ gr} = 60 \text{ mg} \times X \text{ gr}$$

$$300 = 60 \text{ X}$$

$$\frac{300}{60} = \frac{60 \text{ X}}{60}$$

$$5 \text{ gr} = X$$

The patient should receive 5 gr (gr v) of aspirin, which in this case equal 1 tablet.

Ratio method for conversions

Like the fraction method for conversions, the ratio method provides a way to express proportions and convert between systems of drug measurement.

In the ratio method, the left half of the equation expresses the ordered dosage and available dosage as a ratio. For example, the physician prescribes $\frac{1}{2}$ ounce of a drug that is dispensed in milliliters. As a result, the first ratio appears as 0.5 oz : X ml. The X represents the unknown dosage in milliliters. The right half of the equation expresses the standard equivalents between the ordered and available measures as a ratio. Because 1 oz equals 30 ml, the second ratio appears as 1 oz : 30 ml. The same unit of measure (oz) must appear in the first half of each ratio, and the same unit (ml) must appear in the second half. The equation should appear as:

$$0.5 \text{ oz} : X \text{ ml} :: 1 \text{ oz} : 30 \text{ ml}$$

To solve for X, multiply the extremes (outer portions) of the ratio and the means (inner portions) of the ratio:

$$0.5 \text{ oz} \times 30 \text{ ml} = X \text{ ml} \times 1 \text{ oz}$$

$$15 \text{ ml} = X$$

Fifteen milliliters equal $\frac{1}{2}$ ounce. Therefore, the patient should receive 15 ml.

The nurse may use the fraction or ratio method for conversions; both yield the same degree of accuracy. Because the fraction method is simpler, however, the remainder of this chapter will present calculations using the fraction method.

Computation of drug dosages

The nurse computes drug dosages in two steps. First, the nurse checks the physician's order and the drug supply. If the ordered drug is available only in another system of measurement, the nurse performs a conversion between the two systems, as described above. If the drug is ordered in units that are available, the nurse proceeds to the next step.

Second, the nurse calculates the quantity of a particular dosage form to be administered. For example, if the order calls for a dose of 250 mg, the nurse must determine the quantity of tablets, powder, or liquid equal to 250 mg. To compute this or any other drug dosage, the nurse may use the fraction (or ratio) or "desired-available" method.

Fraction method

This method uses an equation that consists of two fractions. The first fraction shows the number of units to be given over X, which represents the quantity of the dosage form (usually the number of tablets or milliliters). The second fraction shows the number of units of drug in its dosage form over the quantity of dosage form that contains the measure stated in the numerator. The nurse obtains this information from the drug label. For example, the physician orders 500 mg of ampicillin. Therefore, the first fraction in the equation is:

$$\frac{500 \text{ mg}}{X \text{ tablet}}$$

The drug label states that each tablet contains 250 mg. Therefore, the second fraction is:

$$\frac{250 \text{ mg}}{1 \text{ tablet}}$$

The same units of measure must appear in the numerator of each fractions. The same units must appear in each denominator, but should be different from those in the numerators. The equation should appear as:

$$\frac{500 \text{ mg}}{X \text{ tablet}} = \frac{250 \text{ mg}}{1 \text{ tablet}}$$

Cross multiplying and solving for X determines the quantity of the dosage form to administer:

$$500 \text{ mg} \times 1 \text{ tablet} = 250 \text{ mg} \times X \text{ tablet}$$

$$500 = 250 \text{ X}$$

$$\frac{500}{250} = \frac{250 \text{ X}}{250}$$

$$2 = X$$

In this case, the patient should receive 2 tablets (500 mg) of ampicillin.

In the next example, the nurse must convert between two systems of measurement before calculating the quantity of the dosage form to be administered. The physician orders aspirin 600 mg q 4 to 6 hours p.r.n. for headache. The pharmacy stocks aspirin as gr v per tablet. How many tablets should be administered? To compute this dosage, first the nurse must make the conversion. The milligram dosage represents the ordered dosage and the grain dosage represents the available dosage. Because the amount of the available dosage is unknown, it is represented by an X. The first fraction is:

$$\frac{600 \text{ mg}}{X}$$

The second fraction consists of the standard equivalents between the ordered and available measures. Because milligrams must be converted to grains, the second fraction appears as:

$$\frac{60 \text{ mg}}{1 \text{ gr}}$$

The first equation should appear as:

$$\frac{600 \text{ mg}}{X} = \frac{60 \text{ mg}}{1 \text{ gr}}$$

To solve for X, cross multiply:

$$600 \text{ mg} \times 1 \text{ gr} = X \times 60 \text{ mg}$$

$$600 = 60 \text{ X}$$

$$\frac{600}{60} = \frac{60 \text{ X}}{60}$$

$$10 = X$$

In this example, 600 mg equals 10 grains. The nurse then uses this information to compute the dosage, using the fraction method. The first fraction shows the number of units to be given over X, which represents the quantity of the dosage form (the number of tablets).

$$\frac{10 \text{ gr}}{X}$$

The second fraction shows the number of units of drug in its dosage form over the quantity of dosage form that contains the measure stated in the numerator (as described on the drug label).

$$\frac{5 \text{ gr}}{1 \text{ tablet}}$$

The entire equation should appear as:

$$\frac{10 \text{ gr}}{X} = \frac{5 \text{ gr}}{1 \text{ tablet}}$$

To solve for X and determine the quantity of tables to give the patient, the nurse cross multiplies and completes the equation:

$$10 \text{ gr} \times 1 \text{ tablet} = 5 \text{ gr} \times X$$

$$10 = 5 \text{ X}$$

$$\frac{10}{5} = \frac{5 \text{ X}}{5}$$

$$2 = X$$

In this case, the patient should receive 2 tablets.

"Desired-available" method

The "desired (ordered)-available" method combines the conversion of ordered units into available units and the computation of drug dosage into one step, using the following equation:

$$\frac{\text{ordered}}{\text{units}} \times \frac{\text{conversion}}{\text{fraction}} \times \frac{\text{dosage form}}{\text{stated quantity of drug within each dosage form}} = X \text{ quantity to give}$$

The following example demonstrates how this equation works. The physician prescribes phenobarbital 15 mg P.O. Yet the drug is

for the first element of the equation. Then the nurse uses the conversion fraction

$$\frac{1 \text{ gr}}{60 \text{ mg}}$$

as the second portion of the formula. The measure in the denominator of the conversion fraction must be the same as the measure in the ordered unit. The third element of the equation shows the dosage form over the stated drug quantity within each dosage form:

$$\frac{1 \text{ tablet}}{0.5 \text{ gr}}$$

The completed equation is:

$$15 \text{ mg} \times \frac{1 \text{ gr}}{60 \text{ mg}} \times \frac{1 \text{ tablet}}{0.5 \text{ gr}} = X$$

The nurse then solves the equation for X:

$$15 \times \frac{1}{60} \times \frac{1}{0.5} = X$$

$$\frac{15}{60 \times 0.5} = X$$

$$\frac{15}{30} = X$$

$$0.5 \text{ tablet} = X$$

Solving for X shows that the patient should receive ½ tablet of phenobarbital.

Methods for drug dosage computations in special systems The nurse may use the fraction or ratio method to calculate dosages of drugs measured in special units. For example, the physician orders 2,000 units of heparin S.C. The heparin is available in a vial of 10,000 units per 2 milliliters. Using the fraction method, the equation is:

$$\frac{2,000 \text{ U}}{X \text{ ml}} = \frac{10,000 \text{ U}}{2 \text{ ml}}$$

To solve for X, the nurse cross multiplies and completes the arithmetic:

$$2,000 \text{ U} \times 2 \text{ ml} = 10,000 \text{ U} \times X \text{ ml}$$

$$4,000 = 10,000 \text{ X}$$

$$\frac{4,000}{10,000} = \frac{10,000 \text{ X}}{10,000}$$

$$0.4 = X$$

To receive 2,000 U of heparin, the patient must receive 0.4 ml of fluid from this vial.

When the physician prescribes insulin for a patient, the nurse simply uses an insulin syringe to draw up the number of units ordered. If an insulin syringe is not available, the nurse must calculate the dose. For example, the physician orders 30 units of U-100 regular insulin S.C. stat. (U-100 insulin contains 100 units of insulin per milliliter.) Using the process described earlier, the nurse sets up an equation with two fractions:

$$\frac{30 \text{ U}}{X \text{ ml}} = \frac{100 \text{ U}}{1 \text{ ml}}$$

Cross multiplying and solving for X determines the quantity of insulin to be administered:

$$30 \text{ U} \times 1 \text{ ml} = 100 \text{ U} \times X \text{ ml}$$

$$30 = 100 \text{ X}$$

$$\frac{30}{100} = \frac{100 \text{ X}}{100}$$

$$0.30 = X$$

The nurse should administer 0.30 ml of U-100 insulin to deliver the prescribed dose of 30 units.

Reconstitution of medications

In most cases, the pharmacist reconstitutes drugs for parenteral use. However, the nurse must be able to perform this function, if needed. To reconstitute a powder, the nurse should consult the drug label to determine the type and amount of diluent to add. When diluent is added to a powder, the powder increases the total volume of the prepared solution. Therefore, the label calls for less diluent than the total volume of the prepared solution.

Here is an example that shows how the nurse may use the fraction method when reconstituting a powder. (The ratio method also may be used.) The physician orders oxacillin 500 mg for a patient. The label on a 1-g vial of powdered oxacillin states, "Add 9.2 ml of sterile saline to yield 100 mg/1 ml."

First, the nurse dilutes the powder with 9.2 ml of diluent as instructed on the label. Then the nurse sets up the equation, beginning with the number of units to be given over X (representing number of milliliters):

$$\frac{500 \text{ mg}}{X \text{ ml}}$$

The concentration listed on the label provides the second fraction of the equation:

$$\frac{100 \text{ mg}}{1 \text{ ml}}$$

The entire equation appears as:

$$\frac{500 \text{ mg}}{X \text{ ml}} = \frac{100 \text{ mg}}{1 \text{ ml}}$$

Cross multiplying and solving for X provides the answer:

$$500 \text{ mg} \times 1 \text{ ml} = 100 \text{ mg} \times X \text{ ml}$$

$$500 = 100 \text{ X}$$

$$\frac{500}{100} = \frac{100 \text{ X}}{100}$$

$$5 = X$$

The patient should receive 5 ml to obtain 500 mg of oxacillin.

Dosage calculations for percentage and ratio solutions

At times, the nurse may need to administer a special solution. The physician may order the solution as a percentage, such as a 10% solution, or as a ratio, such as a 3:1,000 solution. A percentage solution has X g per 100 ml. For example, a 10% solution contains 10 g/100 ml. A ratio solution has X g in 1,000 ml of solution. For example, a 3:1,000 solution contains 3 g/1,000 ml.

To determine the appropriate dosage, the nurse may use the fraction or ratio method. As an example, the nurse must prepare 500 ml of a 0.5% lidocaine (Xylocaine) solution and finds on hand a 2% Xylocaine solution and dextrose 5% in water (D_5W), which is the diluent. The nurse must determine the number of milliliters of Xylocaine solution to use, and the number of milliliters of D_5W to use. Using the fraction method, the nurse sets up the following equation:

$$\frac{0.5\%}{X \text{ ml}} = \frac{2\%}{500 \text{ ml}}$$

To determine the dosage, the nurse cross multiplies and solves for X:

$$0.5\% \times 500 \text{ ml} = 2\% \times X \text{ ml}$$

$$250 = 2 \text{ X}$$

$$\frac{250}{2} = X$$

$$125 = X$$

Because the nurse wants a total volume of 500 ml and must use 125 ml of Xylocaine solution the nurse next must determine the amount of D_5W to use as the diluent. Subtracting 125 ml from 500 ml yields the amount of D_5W solution to use (375 ml).

Here is another example. The physician prescribes 1 mg epinephrine S.C. stat. The drug is available in a 1:1,000 solution, which means that it contains 1 g (or 1,000 mg) in 1,000 ml of solution. Based on this information, the nurse sets up the equation as:

$$\frac{1 \text{ mg}}{X \text{ ml}} = \frac{1{,}000 \text{ mg}}{1{,}000 \text{ ml}}$$

To determine the dosage, the nurse cross multiplies and solves for X:

$$1 \text{ mg} \times 1{,}000 \text{ ml} = 1{,}000 \text{ mg} \times X \text{ ml}$$

$$1{,}000 = 1{,}000 \text{ X}$$

$$\frac{1{,}000}{1{,}000} = \frac{1{,}000 \text{ X}}{1{,}000}$$

$$1 = X$$

The nurse should give the patient 1 ml of the 1:1000 solution to administer the ordered 1 mg of epinephrine.

I.V. drip rate calculations

To determine the rate of infusion for an I.V. solution, the nurse needs to know the:
- drip factor (the number of drops, or gtt, contained in 1 ml), which is based on the type of I.V. set used
- amount of fluid (in milliliters) to be infused
- infusion time (in minutes).

Then the nurse can determine the drip rate (the number of drops/minute to be infused) of an l.V. solution, using following equation:

$$\frac{\text{Total number of ml}}{\text{Total number of minutes}} \times \text{drip factor } ^{(gtt/ml)} = \text{drip rate } ^{(gtt/min)}$$

The following example shows how to use this equation. The physician's order calls for 1,000 ml of D5W infused over 8 hours using IVAC tubing, which has a drip factor of 20 drops per milliliter. The nurse uses this data in the standard equation:

$$\frac{1{,}000 \text{ ml}}{8 \text{ hours} \times 60 \text{ }^{min}/_{hour}} \times 20 \text{ }^{gtt}/_{ml} = X \text{ }^{(gtt/min)}$$

After multiplying the number of hours by 60 minutes/hour in the denominator of the fraction, the equation is:

$$\frac{1{,}000 \text{ ml}}{480 \text{min}} \times 20 \text{ }^{gtt}/_{ml} = X \text{ }^{(gtt/min)}$$

After dividing the fraction, the equation is:

$$2.083 \times 20 \text{ }^{gtt}/_{ml} = X \text{ }^{(gtt/min)}$$

The final answer in 41.6 gtt/min, which can be rounded to 42 gtt/min. The nurse should infuse the I.V. solution at 42 drops/minute.

Pediatric dosage calculations

To determine the correct pediatric drug dosage, health care professionals commonly use two computation methods. One is based on the child's weight in kilograms; the other uses the child's body surface area.

Dosage range per kilogram of body weight

Most pharmaceutical companies provide information on safe dosage ranges (in milligrams per kilogram of body weight) for drugs given to children. The following examples shows how to use this information.

The physician orders 150 mg of a drug to be given every 6 hours to an 18-kg child. (Remember that 1 kg equals 2.2 lb). The literature provided by the manufacturer indicates that the safe dosage range for the drug is 30 mg/kg to 35 mg/kg per day, to be given in divided doses. Can the nurse safely administer the ordered dosage?

Using the ratio method to determine the lower limit of the safe dosage range, the nurse sets up the following:

$$30 \text{ mg} : X \text{ mg} :: 1 \text{ kg} : 18 \text{ kg}$$

After cross multiplying the means and the extremes, the nurse finds that X = 540 mg; thus, 540 mg represents the low dosage.

Using the same method, the nurse then calculates the upper limit of the safe dosage range:

$$35 \text{ mg} : X \text{ mg} :: 1 \text{ kg} : 18 \text{ kg}$$

After cross multiplying the means and the extremes, the nurse finds that X = 630 mg, the high dosage.

The safe dosage range for the child is 540 to 630 mg per day. Because the physician ordered 150 mg to be given every 6 hours, the child would receive four doses per day, or a total daily dosage of 150 mg x four doses per day = 600 mg per day. This daily dosage falls within the safe range, so the nurse can safely administer 150 mg every 6 hours.

Body surface area

This method of pediatric dosage calculation may be the most accurate because the child's body surface area is thought to parallel organ growth and maturation and metabolic rate. (For details, see *Calculating pediatric dosages by body surface area*.)

Other rules

The nurse may use three other rules for calculating and verifying pediatric doses:

• Clark's rule. Used for children over age 2, this rule is based on body weight only:

$$\frac{\text{child's weight (pounds)}}{150 \text{ lb (average adult weight)}} \times \text{average adult dose} = \text{child's dose}$$

Calculating pediatric dosages by body surface area

The nurse can determine a correct pediatric dosage by estimating the child's body surface area. If the child is of average size, find the child's weight and corresponding surface area on the first, boxed scale. Otherwise, use the nomogram to the right. To do this, mark the child's height in the first column and weight in the third column; then draw a line between the two marks. Where the line intersects the scale in the second column indicates the child's estimated body surface area in square meters.

To calculate the child's dosage, complete this equation:

$$\frac{\text{body surface area of child}}{\text{average adult body surface area } (1.73m^2)} \times \text{average adult dose} = \text{child's dose}$$

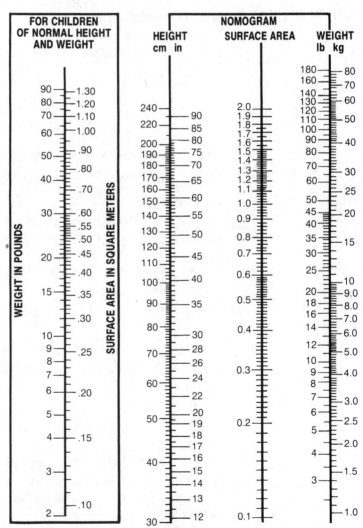

Reprinted with permission from Richard E. Behrman (Ed.). (1992). Nelson textbook of pediatrics (14th ed.). Philadelphia: W.B. Saunders Co.

• Fried's rule. Used for infants under age 1, this rule is based on the child's age only:

$$\frac{\text{child's age (months)}}{\text{150 months (age at which an adult dose would be appropriate)}} \times \text{average adult dose} = \text{child's dose}$$

• Young's rule. Used for children ages 2 to 12, this rule also is based on the child's age only:

$$\frac{\text{child's age (years)}}{\text{child's age (year)} + 12} \times \text{average adult dose} = \text{child's dose}$$

STUDY ACTIVITIES

Matching related elements

Match the metric units of measure on the left with their household or apothecaries' equivalents on the right.

1. ___ 1 gram	**A.** 1 tablespoon
2. ___ 1 liter	**B.** 1 fluidounce
3. ___ 15 milliliters	**C.** 15 grains
4. ___ 30 milliliters	**D.** 1 quart
5. ___ 5 milliliters	**E.** 1 fluidram

Multiple choice

6. The operating room physician prescribes meperidine hydrochloride (Demerol) 50 mg I.M. The nurse finds that the drug is available as 100 mg/ml. What is the correct dose?

    A. 2.0 ml
    B. 1.5 ml
    C. 1.0 ml
    D. 0.5 ml

7. A drug order states, "Maalox 2 oz P.O. a.c. and h.s." How many milliliters should the nurse administer?

    A. 40 ml
    B. 50 ml
    C. 60 ml
    D. 80 ml

8. For Albert Thomas, who has a blood sugar level of 36, the physician orders 2 g of dextrose I.V. stat. The nurse finds that a 20% dextrose solution is available. How much of this solution should the patient receive?

    A. 10 ml
    B. 50 ml
    C. 100 ml
    D. 200 ml

9. The physician orders 600,000 units of penicillin G aqueous I.M. q 6 hours. The pharmacy stocks this penicillin in a 5-ml vial that contains 1,000,000 units. How many milliliters should the nurse administer?

    A. 6.0 ml
    B. 5.0 ml
    C. 4.5 ml
    D. 3.0 ml

10. The nurse prepares to give 3-year-old David Wilson his medication. Which technique for pediatric dosage calculation is most accurate?

    A. Body surface area
    B. Young's rule
    C. Fried's rule
    D. Clark's rule

11. The nurse must administer 1,000 ml of dextrose 5% in 0.45% sodium chloride solution infused over 12 hours. The hospital uses Baxter tubing, which has a drip factor of 10 gtt/ml. Which drip rate should the nurse use?

    A. 14 gtt/min
    B. 20 gtt/min
    C. 21 gtt/min
    D. 40 gtt/min

True or false

12. The three systems of drug measurement most commonly used in clinical settings are the metric, avoirdupois, and household systems.
    ☐ True   ☐ False

13. In the metric system, the gram is the basic unit of measure for liquids, and the liter is the basic unit of measure for solids.
    ☐ True   ☐ False

14. In the household system, the teaspoon and tablespoon are the most commonly used liquid measurements in the clinical setting.
    ☐ True   ☐ False

15. Dextrose is an example of a drug that is measured in units.
    ☐ True   ☐ False

16. Potassium chloride is an example of a drug that is measured in milliequivalents (mEq).
    ☐ True   ☐ False

Fill in the blank

17. To compute drug dosages, the nurse may use the _____,

_____, or _____ methods.

18. A 7% solution contains _____ in _____ of liquid.

19. A 10:1,000 solution contains _____ in _____ of liquid.

20. The physician order acetaminophen (Tylenol) elixir for Donna Berenborn, age 1, who has a fever of 102É F. Donna weighs 8 kg. The safe dosage range for acetaminophen is 8 mg/kg to 10 mg/kg per dose. The maximum safe dose for Donna is _____ mg.

ANSWERS **Matching related elements**
  1. C
  2. D
  3. A
  4. B
  5. E

Multiple choice
  6. D.

$$\frac{50 \text{ mg}}{X \text{ ml}} = \frac{100 \text{ mg}}{1 \text{ ml}}$$

$$50 \text{ mg} \times 1 \text{ ml} = 100 \text{ mg} \times X \text{ ml}$$

$$50 = 100 \text{ X}$$

$$\frac{50}{100} = \frac{100 \text{ X}}{100}$$

$$0.5 \text{ ml} = X$$

  7. C.

$$\frac{2 \text{ oz}}{X \text{ ml}} = \frac{1 \text{ oz}}{30 \text{ ml}}$$

$$2 \text{ oz} \times 30 \text{ ml} = 1 \text{ oz} \times X \text{ ml}$$

$$60 = 1 \text{ X}$$

$$60 \text{ ml} = X$$

  8. A. A 20% solution contains 20 grams/100 ml.

$$\frac{2 \text{ g}}{X \text{ ml}} = \frac{20 \text{ g}}{100 \text{ ml}}$$

$$2 \text{ g} \times 100 \text{ ml} = 20 \text{ g} \times X \text{ ml}$$

$$200 = 20 \text{ X}$$

$$\frac{200}{20} = \frac{20 \text{ X}}{20}$$

$$10 \text{ ml} = X$$

9. D.

$$\frac{600,000 \text{ U}}{\text{X ml}} = \frac{1,000,000 \text{ U}}{5 \text{ ml}}$$

$$600,000 \text{ U} \times 5 \text{ ml} = 1,000,000 \text{ U} \times \text{X ml}$$

$$3,000,000 = 1,000,000 \text{ X}$$

$$\frac{3,000,000}{1,000,000} = \frac{1,000,000 \text{ X}}{1,000,000}$$

$$3 \text{ ml} = \text{X}$$

10. A. The body surface area method may be the most accurate because the child's body surface area is thought to parallel organ growth and maturation and metabolic rate.

11. A.

$$\frac{1,000 \text{ ml}}{12 \text{ hours} \times 60 \text{ }^{\text{min}}\!/_{\text{hour}}} \times 10 \text{ }^{\text{gtt}}\!/_{\text{ml}} = \text{X (drip rate)}$$

$$\frac{1,000 \text{ ml}}{720 \text{ min}} \times 10 \text{ }^{\text{gtt}}\!/_{\text{ml}} = \text{X}$$

$$1.38 \times 10 = \text{X}$$

$$1.38 \text{ (rounded off to 14) }^{\text{gtt}}\!/_{\text{ml}} = \text{X}$$

True or false

12. False. The three systems of measurement most commonly used in clinical settings are the metric, apothecaries', and household systems.

13. False. In the metric system, the liter is the basic unit of measure for liquids; the gram, for solids.

14. True.

15. False. Drugs that are measured in units include insulin, antibiotics, vitamins, hormones, epinephrine, and heparin.

16. True.

Fill in the blank

17. fraction, ratio, "desired-available"

18. 7 grams, 100 milliliters

19. 10 grams, 1,000 milliliters

20. 80.

CHAPTER 5

Autonomic agents

OBJECTIVES

After studying this chapter, the reader should be able to:
1. Describe the functions of the autonomic nervous system.
2. Differentiate among the cholinergic, cholinergic blocking, adrenergic, and adrenergic blocking agents.
3. Contrast the mechanisms of action for the autonomic agents.
4. Discuss the major clinical indications for each class of autonomic agent.
5. Identify drugs that may interact with each class of autonomic agent.
6. Identify significant adverse reactions to the autonomic agents.
7. Describe the nursing implications of autonomic agent therapy.

OVERVIEW OF CONCEPTS

The autonomic nervous system (ANS) is composed of two divisions with opposing actions: the sympathetic and parasympathetic nervous systems. Together, these systems control the activity of glands, involuntary muscles, and other viscera. (For an illustration, see *Autonomic nervous system function.*)

Sympathetic nervous system (SNS)

In the SNS, short preganglionic and long postganglionic neurons transmit nerve impulses to effector (target) organs. These neurons originate from the thoracolumbar region in the spinal cord.

Most of the preganglionic neurons terminate in ganglia near the spinal cord. Those that innervate the adrenal medulla without synapsing at a ganglion cause norepinephrine and epinephrine release. Postganglionic neurons transmit impulses to distant effector organs. Chemical neurotransmitters (norepinephrine, epinephrine, dopamine, and acetylcholine [ACh]) transmit neuron information between adjacent cells.

SNS stimulation produces "fight-or-flight" responses—responses that prepare the individual to cope with stress. These responses include:
• vasoconstriction
• increased heart rate and contractility
• smooth muscle relaxation
• pupillary dilation and decreased accommodation
• bronchial dilation and decreased secretion

Autonomic nervous system function

Through the opposing actions of its sympathetic and parasympathetic divisions, the autonomic nervous system controls the involuntary actions of cardiac muscles, smooth muscles, and glands. It also controls ocular muscles; salivary, lacrimal, and sweat glands; erector pili muscles; and blood vessels.

The sympathetic division prepares the body to expend energy, especially in stressful situations, by releasing the adrenergic catecholamine norepinephrine. Sympathetic stimulation produces such responses as elevated heart rate and blood pressure, cessation of peristalsis, bronchial dilation, hyperglycemia, pupillary dilation, and peripheral cutaneous vasodilation.

The parasympathetic division helps the body conserve energy through release of the cholinergic substance acetylcholine (ACh). Parasympathetic responses include lowered heat rate and blood pressure, increased peristalsis, salivation, diaphoresis, and peripheral cutaneous vasodilation.

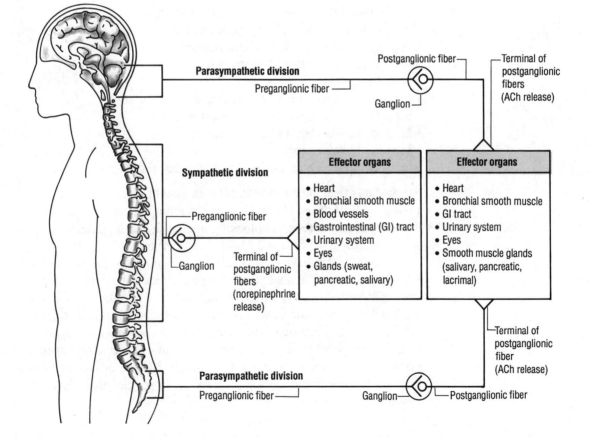

- decreased gastrointestinal (GI) secretions and peristalsis
- urine retention
- increased sweat gland secretion
- decreased pancreatic secretion
- thickened salivary secretions.

Parasympathetic nervous system (PNS)

In the PNS, long preganglionic and short postganglionic neurons convey nerve impulses to effector organs. These neurons originate in the cranial and sacral regions of the central nervous system (CNS). Most preganglionic neurons travel to ganglia in or near effector organ walls. The postganglionic neurons complete the nerve impulse transmission. These neurons are cholinergic; that is, they synthesize and secrete ACh. ACh's action lasts for only a few seconds because most of it is quickly destroyed by the enzyme acetylcholinesterase. However, ACh lasts long enough to stimulate the effector organ.

PNS stimulation typically produces rest and relaxation responses, opposing those of the SNS. These responses include:
- decreased heart rate and contractility
- smooth muscle constriction
- pupillary constriction and increased accommodation
- bronchial constriction and increased secretion
- increased peristalsis and GI secretions
- increased bladder tone
- increased pancreatic, salivary, and lacrimal secretions.

Agents that affect the autonomic nervous system

Four groups of drugs affect the ANS: cholinergic, cholinergic blocking, adrenergic, and adrenergic blocking agents. (For a summary of representative drugs, see Selected Major Drugs: *Autonomic agents.*)

Cholinergic agents directly or indirectly promote the function of ACh. They also are called parasympathomimetics because they produce effects that imitate parasympathetic nerve stimulation. Cholinergic blocking agents interrupt parasympathetic nerve impulses in the CNS and ANS. Because of this, they also are known as parasympatholytics, anticholinergic agents, or antimuscarinics. Adrenergic agents, or sympathomimetics, cause responses similar to those produced by SNS activation. Adrenergic blocking agents, or sympatholytics, disrupt SNS function.

Cholinergic agents   Cholinergic agents fall into two main classes: cholinergic agonists and anticholinesterase agents. Cholinergic agonists include synthetic acetylcholine (ACh); choline esters, such as bethanechol chloride (Duvoid, Myotonachol, Urecholine) and carbachol (Carbacel, Isopto Carbachol, Miostat); and naturally occurring cholinomimetic alkaloids, such as pilocarpine hydrochloride (Adsorbocarpine, Isopto Carpine, Pilocar).

SELECTED MAJOR DRUGS

Autonomic agents

This chart summarizes the major autonomic agents currently in clinical use.

DRUG	MAJOR INDICATIONS	USUAL ADULT DOSAGES
Cholinergic agents		
bethanechol chloride	Urine retention	10 to 50 mg P.O. b.i.d. to q.i.d. or 5 mg S.C. t.i.d. or q.i.d.
edrophonium chloride	Differential diagnosis of cholinergic toxicity and myasthenic crisis	1 mg I.V. followed by an additional 1 mg if patient is not impaired further
neostigmine	Myasthenia gravis	15 mg P.O. every 3 to 4 hours or 0.5 to 2 mg I.V. every 1 to 3 hours
	Postoperative abdominal distention, urine retention	0.5 mg I.M. or S.C. every 4 to 6 hours
Cholinergic blocking agents		
atropine	Reversal of arrhythmias, bradycardia, and sinus arrest	0.4 to 1 mg I.V. every 2 hours, as needed, up to a maximum of 2 mg
	Preanesthesia medication	0.2 to 0.6 mg I.M. 30 to 60 minutes before surgery
	Reversal of neuromuscular blockade caused by cholinergic drugs	0.6 to 1.2 mg I.V. before or concurrently with 2 to 2.5 mg of neostigmine in a separate syringe
	Dyskinesia in parkinsonism	0.1 to 0.2 mg P.O. q.i.d.
dicyclomine	Irritable bowel syndrome	20 mg P.O. q.i.d., up to a maximum of 160 mg daily, or 20 mg I.M. daily in 4 doses
propantheline	Peptic ulcer, spastic bladder	15 mg q.i.d., 30 minutes before meals and h.s.
scopolamine	Preanesthesia medication	0.3 to 0.6 mg I.M., I.V., or S.C. 30 to 60 minutes before surgery
	Motion sickness	0.5 mg topically to postauricular skin (lasts for 3 days) or 0.25 to 0.75 mg P.O. 1 hour before effect is desired
Adrenergic agents: Catecholamines		
dobutamine	Acute congestive heart failure, cardiopulmonary bypass surgery	2.5 to 10 mcg/kg/minute I.V. of a 250-mcg/ml, 500-mcg/ml, or 1,000-mcg/ml solution in dextrose 5% in water (D_5W) or 0.9% sodium chloride solution; rates up to 40 mcg/kg/minute may be required
epinephrine	Bronchospasm, asthma, nasal and ophthalmic congestion, simple open-angle glaucoma, allergic conditions, hypotension, cardiac arrest, superficial bleeding control	Cardiac arrest: 1 to 10 ml of a 1:10,000 solution I.V., repeated at 5-minute intervals; 10 ml of 1:10,000 solution via endotracheal tube Bronchospasm: 0.1 to 0.5 ml of a 1:1,000 solution S.C. or I.M.; 0.1 to 0.3 ml of a 1:200 solution S.C.; or one inhalation, repeat once after at least 1 minute, if needed Hemostasis: 1:50,000 to 1:1,000 applied topically Local anesthetic adjunct: 1:200,000 to 1:20,000 mixed with local anesthetic

(continued)

SELECTED MAJOR DRUGS

Autonomic agents *(continued)*

DRUG	MAJOR INDICATIONS	USUAL ADULT DOSAGES
Adrenergic agents: Catecholamines *(continued)*		
isoproterenol	Asthma, bronchospasm, shock, cardiac arrest, selected arrhythmias	Bronchospasm: 10 to 20 mg sublingually or rectally t.i.d. or q.i.d. up to a maximum of 60 mg daily; 120 to 262 mcg 4 to 6 times/day by hand-held nebulizer; 80 to 160 mcg 4 to 6 times/day by aerosol nebulizer
norepinephrine	Acute hypotension, shock, cardiac arrest, myocardial infarction, anaphylaxis	Initially, 2 to 3 ml/minute I.V. of a 4-mg norepinephrine:1,000 ml D_5W solution; for maintenance, 0.5 to 1 ml/minute I.V.
Adrenergic agents: Noncatecholamines		
albuterol	Bronchospasm	One to two inhalations every 4 to 6 hours; or 2 to 4 mg P.O. t.i.d. or q.i.d. up to a maximum of 32 mg daily
metaproterenol	Bronchodilation	Initially, 20 mg P.O. t.i.d. to q.i.d.; ten inhalations of a 5% solution by hand-held nebulizer; or 2 to 3 sprays by aerosol nebulizer every 3 to 4 hours up to a maximum of 12 sprays daily
terbutaline	Bronchodilation, preterm labor	10 mcg/minute I.V. infusion up to a maximum of 80 mcg/minute for 4 hours, then oral therapy until term; 2.5 to 5 mg P.O. t.i.d.; 0.25 mg S.C., repeated in 15 to 30 minutes if needed; or two inhalations separated by 1 minute no more often than every 6 hours
Adrenergic blocking agents: Alpha-adrenergic blockers		
phentolamine	Hypertension associated with pheochromocytoma	5 mg I.M. or I.V. before surgery; 5 mg I.V., if needed, during surgery
	Prevention of necrosis related to extravasation	5 to 10 mg in 10 ml 0.9% sodium chloride solution injected into the area of extravasation
Adrenergic blocking agents: Beta-adrenergic blockers		
atenolol	Hypertension, angina	Initially, 50 mg P.O. once daily; increased to 100 mg daily after 1 to 2 weeks if needed; reduced to 50 mg every other day for patients with renal failure
metoprolol	Hypertension	100 mg daily P.O., increased weekly to achieve desired effects (usual range, 100 to 450 mg daily)
	Myocardial infarction	5 mg I.V. every 2 minutes for three doses; then 50 mg P.O. every 6 hours for 48 hours; then 100 mg P.O. every 12 hours
propranolol	Hypertension	40 mg P.O. b.i.d.; increased to achieve desired effects up to a maximum of 640 mg daily (usual range, 120 to 240 mg in two or three divided doses, or 120 to 160 mg of sustained-release capsules once daily)
	Angina	10 to 20 mg P.O. t.i.d. or q.i.d.; increased every 3 to 7 days to achieve desired effects up to a maximum of 320 mg daily (usual dosage, 160 mg daily in divided doses)

Autonomic agents *(continued)*

DRUG	MAJOR INDICATIONS	USUAL ADULT DOSAGES
Adrenergic blocking agents: Beta-adrenergic blockers *(continued)*		
propranolol *(continued)*	Arrhythmias	10 to 30 mg P.O. t.i.d. or q.i.d.; for emergencies, 1 to 3 mg I.V. push (1 mg/minute) repeated in 2 to 3 minutes
	Hypertrophic subaortic stenosis	20 to 40 mg P.O. t.i.d. or q.i.d., or 80 to 160 mg sustained-release capsules P.O. once daily
	Myocardial infarction	180 to 240 mg P.O. daily in three or four divided doses up to a maximum of 240 mg daily
	Migraine	80 mg P.O. daily in divided doses, increased as needed (usual range, 160 to 249 mg daily)
Adrenergic blocking agents: Autonomic ganglionic blockers		
trimethaphan	Hypertension, controlled hypotension in surgery	3 to 4 ml/minute I.V. of a 1 mg/ml solution (500 mg or 10 ml of drug in 500 ml D_5W); adjusted to individual's need (within range of 0.3 to 6 mg/minute)

Acetylcholine rarely is used clinically because it can cause unpredictable effects and is destroyed rapidly by acetylcholinesterase.

Anticholinesterase agents are reversible (having a duration of action of minutes to hours) or irreversible (having a duration of action of days or weeks). Reversible agents include ambenonium (Mytelase), edrophonium chloride (Tensilon), neostigmine (Prostigmin), physostigmine salicylate (Antilirium), and pyridostigmine (Mestinon, Regonol). Irreversible agents include echothiophate and isoflurophate, which are used to treat glaucoma and esotropia. (For more information, see Chapter 33, Other major drugs.)

Pharmacokinetics

Usually, cholinergic agonists are administered intraocularly, orally, or subcutaneously to minimize adverse effects. All cholinergic agonists are metabolized by cholinesterases at muscarinic and nicotinic receptor sites, in the plasma, and in the liver. They all are excreted by the kidneys.

Most anticholinesterase agents are absorbed readily from the GI tract, subcutaneous tissue, and mucous membranes. Only physostigmine readily penetrates the blood-brain barrier. Most anticholinesterase agents are metabolized by plasma esterases and are excreted in the urine.

Pharmacodynamics

Cholinergic agonists work by mimicking the action of ACh at the autonomic effector site. Anticholinesterase agents inhibit the action of acetylcholinesterase, the enzyme that ordinarily inactivates ACh. By doing this, they increase the amount of ACh at receptor sites and prolong its effects.

Pharmacotherapeutics

Common clinical indications for cholinergic agents include treatment of atonic bladder conditions (such as urine retention) and reduction of intraocular pressure in the anterior chamber of the eye. The latter indication is useful in patients with glaucoma and in those undergoing ocular surgery. (For information about ophthalmic uses, see Chapter 33, Other major drugs.)

In addition to these indications, anticholinesterase agents are used to treat GI tract atony, promote muscle contraction in patients with myasthenia gravis, and diagnose myasthenia gravis. In fact, edrophonium chloride is the drug of choice for diagnosing myasthenia gravis. Some of these drugs also are used as antidotes to neuromuscular blocking agents, tricyclic antidepressants, belladonna alkaloids, and narcotics.

Drug interactions

Autonomic agents interact with a wide variety of drugs. (For details, see Drug Interactions: *Autonomic agents.*)

Adverse drug reactions

Adverse reactions to cholinergic agonists are common and typically result from their nonspecific effects on the PNS. Usually, the greater the dose, the greater the generalized parasympathomimetic effect.

For example, the use of bethanechol to reduce urine retention also increases GI motility, which may cause nausea, belching, vomiting, cramps, and diarrhea. Its other effects may include blurred vision and, with high doses, vasodilation, decreased heart rate, decreased force of cardiac contraction, and hypotension. Salivation or sweating may increase, and bronchial constriction may produce shortness of breath. Cholinergic overstimulation can result from hypersensitivity, drug overdose, or, rarely, from subcutaneous (S.C.) administration. Overstimulation may cause circulatory collapse, resulting in hypotension, shock, and cardiac arrest.

Adverse reactions to anticholinesterase agents are similar. However, they are difficult to predict in a patient with myasthenia gravis. The therapeutic dose varies from day to day, and muscle weakness may result from underdosage, resistance, or overdosage. Differentiating between a toxic response and myasthenic crisis may be difficult. A physician who uses edrophonium to distinguish between the two must have respiratory support equipment and emergency drugs, such as atropine or pralidoxime, available to counteract a cholinergic crisis.

Cholinergic blocking agents

Cholinergic blockers block the action of ACh at muscarinic receptors in the PNS. They are divided into two classes: ganglionic blockers and antimuscarinic drugs. Although the former block the transmission of

DRUG INTERACTIONS

Autonomic agents

Drug interactions involving autonomic agonists usually occur with drugs that also act on the autonomic nervous system.

DRUG	INTERACTING DRUGS	POSSIBLE EFFECTS
Cholinergic agents		
cholinergic agonists (bethanechol, carbachol, pilocarpine)	other cholinergic agents, particularly anticholinesterase agents	Increased risk of cholinergic toxicity
	cholinergic blockers	Decreased acetylcholine effects
	quinidine	Decreased effects of cholinergic agonist
anticholinesterase agents (ambenonium, edrophonium, neostigmine, physostigmine, pyridostigmine)	other cholinergic agents, particularly cholinergic agonists	Increased acetylcholine effects at the neuromuscular junction
	cholinergic blockers	Decreased effects of anticholinesterase agents; masking of early signs of cholinergic crisis
	neuromuscular blockers (atracurium, gallamine, metocurine, pancuronium, tubocurarine, vecuronium)	Decreased acetylcholine effects at the neuromuscular junction
	ester anesthetics	Increased risk of anticholinesterase agent toxicity
Cholinergic blocking agents		
atropine, belladonna, clidinium, dicyclomine, glycopyrrolate, hyoscyamine, oxybutynin, propantheline, scopolamine	disopyramide, tricyclic and tetracyclic antidepressants, antidyskinetics (including amantadine), antiemetics and antivertigo agents (including buclizine, cyclizine, meclizine, and diphenhydramine), antipsychotics (including haloperidol, phenothiazines, thioxanthenes, cyclobenzaprine, and orphenadrine)	Increased anticholinergic effects
	cholinergic agonists (bethanechol), anticholinesterase agents (neostigmine, pyridostigmine)	Decreased antimuscarinic effects
	digoxin	Increased serum concentration level of digoxin
	opiate-like analgesics	Decreased gastrointestinal (GI) motility
	nitroglycerin	Delayed sublingual absorption of nitroglycerin
Adrenergic agents		
catecholamines (dobutamine, dopamine, epinephrine, isoproterenol, norepinephrine)	alpha blockers (phentolamine)	Hypotension
	oral hypoglycemic agents	Decreased insulin effects, hyperglycemia
	beta blockers (propranolol)	Decreased effects of both drugs, hypertension, bronchial constriction, asthma

(continued)

DRUG INTERACTIONS

Autonomic agents *(continued)*

DRUG	INTERACTING DRUGS	POSSIBLE EFFECTS
Adrenergic agents *(continued)*		
catecholamines *(continued)*	sympathomimetics	Additive effects (hypertension, arrhythmias), increased adverse effects
noncatecholamines (albuterol, ephedrine, isoetharine, mephentermine, metaproterenol, metaraminol, methoxamine, nylidrin, phenylephrine, ritodrine, terbutaline)	general anesthetics, cyclopropane, halogenated hydrocarbons	Arrhythmias, increased hypotension if used with agents having predominant beta$_2$ activity (ritodrine, terbutaline)
	monoamine oxidase (MAO) inhibitors	Severe hypertension
	oxytocics	Counteraction of oxytocic effects (ritodrine, terbutaline), hypertensive crisis, cerebrovascular accident
	tricyclic antidepressants	Increased pressor effects, increased hypertension, arrhythmias
	urinary alkalinizers (acetazolamide, sodium bicarbonate)	Decreased excretion, prolonged action
Adrenergic blocking agents: Alpha-adrenergic blockers		
ergoloid mesylates, ergotamine	alcohol	Hypotension
	caffeine	Increased ergotamine effects
	dopamine	Increased pressor effects
	nitroglycerin	Hypotension
	sympathomimetics, including many over-the-counter medications	Increased cardiac stimulation; hypotension with rebound hypertension
Adrenergic blocking agents: Beta-adrenergic blockers		
acebutolol, atenolol, labetalol, metoprolol, nadolol, pindolol, propranolol, timolol	antacids	Delayed drug absorption from GI tract
	lidocaine	Increased plasma level of lidocaine and possible toxicity; additive cardiac depressant effects
	insulin and oral hypoglycemic agents	Hypoglycemia or hyperglycemia; masking of tachycardia as a sign of hypoglycemia (diaphoresis and agitation still present)
	anti-inflammatory drugs (indomethacin, salicylates)	Decreased hypotensive effects of beta-adrenergic blockers
	barbiturates	Increased metabolism of beta-adrenergic blockers that are metabolized extensively
	cardiac glycosides	Additive bradycardia, depressed atrioventricular conduction
	calcium channel blockers (primarily verapamil)	Increased pharmacologic and toxicologic effects of both agents

DRUG INTERACTIONS

Autonomic agents *(continued)*

DRUG	INTERACTING DRUGS	POSSIBLE EFFECTS
Adrenergic blocking agents: Beta-adrenergic blockers *(continued)*		
acebutolol, atenolol, labetalol, metoprolol, nadolol, pindolol, propranolol, timolol *(continued)*	sympathomimetics (epinephrine, dobutamine, dopamine, isoproterenol, terbutaline, metaproterenol, albuterol, ritodrine)	Hypertension, reflex bradycardia
	cimetidine	Decreased metabolism of beta-adrenergic blockers; decreased pulse rate
	rifampin	Reduced therapeutic response to metoprolol and propranolol
	theophyllines	Impaired bronchodilating effects of theophyllines by nonselective beta-adrenergic blockers
	clonidine	Unopposed alpha effects when clonidine is discontinued, leading to a life-threatening increase in blood pressure
labetalol	halothane anesthetics	Increased hypotension
Adrenergic blocking agents: Autonomic ganglionic blockers		
mecamylamine, trimethaphan	anesthetics	Increased hypotensive effects
	depolarizing muscle relaxants, nondepolarizing muscle relaxants	Increased neuromuscular blocking effects with prolonged respiratory depression

adrenergic and cholinergic stimuli, their clinical use is limited to their adrenergic effects. Therefore, they are discussed later in the section on "Adrenergic blocking agents." The antimuscarinic drugs, of which atropine sulfate is the prototype, exert their blocking effect at postganglionic cholinergic nerve endings at muscarinic receptor sites. They are the focus of this section.

Drugs in this class include the belladonna alkaloids (atropine sulfate, homatropine hydrobromide, hyoscyamine sulfate, and scopolamine hydrobromide), their synthetic derivatives (the quaternary ammonium agents clidinium bromide, glycopyrrolate, and propantheline bromide), and the tertiary amines (benztropine mesylate, dicyclomine hydrochloride, ethopropazine hydrochloride, oxybutynin chloride, and trihexyphenidyl hydrochloride). Because the tertiary amines are used almost exclusively to treat parkinsonism, these agents are discussed in Chapter 7, Antiparkinsonian agents.

Pharmacokinetics

The belladonna alkaloids are absorbed more readily and distributed more widely than their derivatives. They readily cross the blood-brain barrier; other drugs in this class do not. Scopolamine has a greater effect in the CNS than does atropine, and strongly affects the eye and its secretory glands. Atropine has a greater effect on the heart, intestine, urinary tract, and the bronchi.

The belladonna alkaloids are metabolized in the liver and excreted by the kidneys as unchanged drug and metabolites. The quaternary derivatives and tertiary amines are hydrolyzed in the GI tract and liver and are excreted in the feces and the urine.

The administration route helps determine how quickly the cholinergic blockers take effect. Via the intravenous (I.V.) route, most have an onset of 1 minute; by the intramuscular (I.M.) or S.C. route, onset takes about 30 minutes; by the oral route, about 30 to 60 minutes. The duration of action of these drugs is up to 6 hours.

Pharmacodynamics

Cholinergic blockers compete in a dose-dependent manner with ACh (and cholinergic agonists) at muscarinic receptor sites in the CNS, autonomic ganglia, and organs innervated by parasympathetic nerves. The higher the drug dose, the greater the competition with ACh.

The cholinergic blockers usually block the effects of the parasympathetic nerves, allowing the adrenergic SNS to predominate. Some cholinergic blockers can cross the blood-brain barrier, further affecting the CNS. In low or moderate doses, cholinergic blockers stimulate the CNS, causing excitation; in higher doses, they depress the CNS.

Muscarinic receptors also exist in the heart at the sinoatrial node and atrioventricular (AV) node. Vagal stimulation results in a slowing of the heart rate and decreased AV conduction. The cholinergic blocker atropine blocks the influence of vagal stimulation on the heart, resulting in increased heart rate.

The cholinergic blockade produced by these drugs may be overcome by increasing the ACh concentration at receptor sites. This can be accomplished by administering the anticholinesterase agent physostigmine (the antidote for cholinergic blocker overdose), which blocks the enzyme that destroys ACh.

Pharmacotherapeutics

The primary clinical indications for the cholinergic blockers include spastic conditions of the GI and urinary tracts, arrhythmias, motion sickness, parkinsonism, and chronic asthma. For example, parenteral atropine is the drug of choice to treat sinus bradycardia, and scopolamine is the drug of choice to treat motion sickness. (For more information, see Chapter 22, Adsorbent, antiflatulent, digestive, antiemetic, and emetic agents.)

These agents also are used as preanesthesia medications to reduce excitement, salivation, and gastric secretions, to depress the respiratory system, and to block vagal stimulation during anesthesia. They are used as relaxants for the GI tract during such diagnostic procedures as endoscopy or sigmoidoscopy. They also may be used as cycloplegics and mydriatics during ophthalmologic surgery and examinations. They serve as antidotes to cholinergic agents and certain organophosphate pesticides.

Drug interactions
Cholinergic blockers may interact with various drugs. (For details, see Drug Interactions: *Autonomic agents,* pages 65 to 67.)

Adverse drug reactions
The cholinergic blockers' widespread action may produce numerous adverse reactions. Dosage is particularly crucial; the difference between a therapeutic and toxic dosage is small. Also, the following people are more susceptible than others to adverse effects: infants, elderly patients, fair-skinned children with Down's syndrome, and children with spastic paralysis or brain damage.

Adverse reactions increase in severity as dosage increases. Low doses decrease salivation, bronchial secretions, and sweating. As the dosage increases, pupils dilate, visual accommodation decreases, and heart rate increases. Higher doses inhibit urination and intestinal motility and decrease gastric secretions.

With drug overdose, all effects are exaggerated. Patients who experience cholinergic blocker toxicity are described as "Hot as a hare, blind as a bat, dry as a bone, and mad as a hatter." CNS excitation is prominent at toxic levels. Patients become restless, irritable, disoriented, and even hallucinatory or delirious. If the process is not reversed (physostigmine is the antidote), the excitatory phase is followed by CNS depression, unconsciousness, medullary paralysis, and death.

Cholinergic blockers may precipitate problems in patients with some underlying diseases. They can cause a dangerous rise in intraocular pressure in a patient with unrecognized acute angle-closure glaucoma, tachycardia and circulatory failure in one with coronary artery disease, or urine retention in one with benign prostatic hypertrophy. These drugs also can lead to heat stroke, especially in an elderly patient with cardiovascular disease.

Adrenergic agents
Adrenergic agents include endogenous substances (such as epinephrine, norepinephrine, and dopamine) and synthetic drugs (such as isoproterenol and dobutamine) that may be classified as catecholamines or noncatecholamines. Adrenergics may be divided further by their method of action. They may be direct-acting (acting on the sympathetically innervated organ or tissue), indirect-acting (triggering the

release of a neurotransmitter, usually norepinephrine), or dual-acting (combining direct and indirect actions).

Catecholamines include dobutamine hydrochloride (Dobutrex), dopamine hydrochloride (Intropin), epinephrine (Inhalation: Bronkaid Mist, Primatene Mist), epinephrine hydrochloride and epinephrine bitartrate (Parenteral: Adrenalin Chloride, Sus-Phrine; Inhalation: AsthmaHaler, Medihaler-Epi), isoproterenol hydrochloride (Oral: Isuprel; Inhalation: Vapo-Iso), isoproterenol sulfate (Inhalation: Medihaler-Iso), and norepinephrine (Levophed, Noradrenaline).

Noncatecholamines include albuterol (Proventil), ephedrine sulfate (Efedron Nasal Jelly, Va-tro-nol Nose Drops), isoetharine hydrochloride (Arm-a-Med, Beta-2, Bronkosol, Dey-Lute, Dispos-a-Med), isoetharine mesylate (Bronkometer), mephentermine sulfate (Wyamine), metaproterenol sulfate (Alupent, Metaprel), metaraminol bitartrate (Aramine), methoxamine hydrochloride (Vasoxyl), nylidrin hydrochloride (Arlidin), phenylephrine hydrochloride (Neo-Synephrine), ritodrine hydrochloride (Yutopar), and terbutaline sulfate (Brethaire, Brethine, Bricanyl).

Pharmacokinetics

Catecholamines are destroyed by digestive enzymes, but are absorbed rapidly from mucous membranes. I.M. absorption is more rapid than S.C. absorption because this route results in less local vasoconstriction. These drugs are distributed widely in the body, metabolized in the liver and other tissues, and excreted primarily in the urine.

Unlike catecholamines, most noncatecholamines are effective orally. (Isoetharine, however, is degraded if swallowed). Drugs administered by inhalation, such as albuterol, are absorbed gradually from the bronchi. Oral drugs are absorbed well from the GI tract and are distributed widely in body fluids and tissues. Metabolism occurs in the liver, lungs, GI tract, and other tissues. Excretion occurs primarily in the urine. Acidic urine increases excretion of many noncatecholamines; alkaline urine slows their excretion.

The administration route largely determines the onset of action, peak concentration level, and duration of action of the catecholamines and noncatecholamines. However, noncatecholamines usually have a longer duration of action than catecholamines.

Pharmacodynamics

Most adrenergic agents stimulate alpha or beta receptors to produce their pharmacologic effects, thus mimicking the action of norepinephrine or epinephrine. Other adrenergic agents, called dopaminergic agents, act primarily on SNS receptors stimulated by dopamine.

Agents that act on alpha receptors are called alphamimetics or alpha agonists. Their most important therapeutic effects involve vasoconstriction of arterioles in the skin, kidneys, mesentery area, and splanchnic area. Agents that act on beta receptors are known as betamimetics or beta agonists. Their most important therapeutic effects are cardiac stimulation, smooth muscle relaxation, and vasodilation of blood vessels in the brain, heart, and skeletal muscle. Agents that act on dopamine receptors are called dopaminergic agents or agonists. Dopamine receptors exist primarily in the CNS. However, dopamine also stimulates $beta_1$ receptors in the heart, increasing the force of myocardial contraction. Through its indirect activity, dopamine also stimulates norepinephrine release. (For more information, see *Adrenergic agents: Receptor activity, drug action, and uses,* page 72.)

The clinical effects of catecholamines depend on the dosage, administration route, and (in the cardiovascular system) the vascular bed. They produce positive inotropic effects (marked increase in cardiac contraction strength) and positive chronotropic effects (increased heart rate). Catecholamines may precipitate spontaneous firing in the Purkinje fibers, producing pacemaker activity and possibly producing premature ventricular contractions and fibrillation. Other clinical effects of catecholamines may include CNS stimulation, increased systemic blood flow, bronchodilation, decreased bronchial secretions, decreased GI peristalsis, relaxation of the urinary bladder sphincter, increased urine output, and decreased glandular secretions.

Noncatecholamines may be direct-acting, indirect-acting, or dual-acting. Direct-acting noncatecholamines achieve their effects by occupying receptor sites on organs and structures innervated by the SNS. Drugs that exhibit primarily alpha activity include methoxamine and phenylephrine; those that selectively exert $beta_2$ activity include albuterol, isoetharine, metaproterenol, nylidrin, ritodrine, and terbutaline. Indirect-acting noncatecholamines exert their effects by stimulating norepinephrine release from its storage sites. Dual-acting noncatecholamines combine both actions, and include ephedrine, mephentermine, and metaraminol.

Pharmacotherapeutics

The particular receptor activity that exists alone or predominates if more than one receptor type is activated determines how the drug is used therapeutically. Drugs with predominant alpha activity cause vasoconstriction and other effects, and are used to relieve hypotension. Drugs with $beta_1$ activity primarily cause cardiac stimulation; so they are used to treat such disorders as bradycardia, heart block, and insufficient cardiac output. Catecholamines with $beta_2$ activity produce bronchodilation and related effects, and are used to treat acute and chronic bronchial asthma, emphysema, bronchitis, and acute hypersensitivity reactions. Drugs with dopaminergic receptor activity tend cause vasodilation. They may be used, for example, to dilate renal arteries, thereby preventing renal shutdown in cardiogenic or septic shock.

Of the catecholamines, norepinephrine has the most nearly pure alpha activity; dobutamine and isoproterenol, beta activity. Epinephrine

Adrenergic agents: Receptor activity, drug action, and uses

This chart summarizes the receptor activity of the major catecholamines and noncatecholamines, the physical effects they produce, and their clinical uses. This information forms an important knowledge base for the nurse administering these drugs.

DRUG	RECEPTOR ACTIVITY	ACTION	USES
Catecholamines			
Direct-acting			
dobutamine	Beta$_1$	Cardiac stimulation	Inotropic drug
dopamine	Dopaminergic, alpha (only at high doses), beta$_1$	Vasoconstriction at high doses Renal vessel dilation at low doses	Shock, hypotension, inotropic drug
epinephrine	Alpha, beta$_1$, beta$_2$	Cardiac stimulation Vasoconstriction Bronchodilation	Anaphylaxis, acute hypotension, cardiac arrest, topical vasoconstriction, glaucoma
isoproterenol	Beta$_1$, beta$_2$	Cardiac stimulation Bronchodilation	Shock, digitalis toxicity, asthma
norepinephrine or levarterenol	Alpha, beta$_1$	Vasoconstriction	Shock, hypotension
Noncatecholamines			
Direct-acting			
albuterol	Beta$_1$ < beta$_2$	Bronchodilation	Asthma, bronchitis, emphysema
isoetharine	Beta$_1$ < beta$_2$	Bronchodilation	Inhalation therapy
metaproterenol	Beta$_1$ < beta$_2$	Bronchodilation	Inhalation therapy
methoxamine	Alpha	Vasoconstriction	Hypotension, termination of paroxysmal atrial tachycardia
nylidrin	Beta$_1$, beta$_2$	Vasodilation	Peripheral vascular disorders
phenylephrine	Alpha, beta (weak)	Vasoconstriction	Shock, hypotension, nasal congestion, termination of paroxysmal atrial tachycardia
ritodrine	Beta$_1$ < beta$_2$	Smooth muscle relaxation	Uterine relaxation in preterm labor
terbutaline	Beta$_1$ < beta$_2$	Bronchodilation	Uterine relaxation, emphysema, asthma, preterm labor
Dual-acting			
ephedrine	Alpha, beta, central nervous system	Bronchodilation Vasoconstriction	Nasal congestion, hypotension, narcolepsy
mephentermine	Alpha < beta	Vasoconstriction Appetite suppression	Hypotension, appetite suppression
metaraminol	Alpha > beta	Vasoconstriction	Shock, hypotension

stimulates alpha and beta receptors. Dopamine primarily exhibits dopaminergic, alpha-agonist, and beta$_1$ receptor activity.

The therapeutic uses of catecholamines also are related to their local effects. Their local vasoconstrictive actions make them useful as nasal decongestants to treat inflammatory and allergic conditions; as ophthalmic decongestants to treat conjunctivitis and ocular congestion; as adjuncts to topical miotics and other drugs to treat simple open-angle glaucoma; as topical hemostatics to control superficial bleeding; as local anesthetic adjuncts to prolong action by retarding absorption; and as antiallergens to treat hypersensitivity and anaphylaxis.

Because noncatecholamines stimulate the SNS and produce varied physiologic effects, they are used widely to correct hypotension and relax bronchial, uterine, and vascular smooth muscles. The drugs exhibit many differences, making general statements difficult. They are more or less effective, depending on the administration route, dose, desired therapeutic effect, and patient tolerance.

Drug interactions
Catecholamine and noncatecholamine adrenergic agents can cause serious drug interactions. (For details, see Drug Interactions: *Autonomic agents,* pages 65 to 67.)

Adverse drug reactions
Because of the widespread actions of adrenergic agents, adverse reactions can occur in almost all body systems. For example, catecholamines and noncatecholamines may cause adverse CNS reactions, such as restlessness, nervousness, anxiety, headache, dizziness, and insomnia. They also may produce adverse cardiovascular reactions, such as palpitations, bradycardia or tachycardia, arrhythmias, and hypotension or hypertension. Their adverse musculoskeletal reactions may be weakness or tremors; GI reactions may include nausea and vomiting.

Other adverse reactions may occur and vary with the drug and its class. For example, extravasation of an I.V. catecholamine can cause local vasoconstriction that leads to necrosis and tissue sloughing. In patients with diabetes, noncatecholamines can cause transient elevations in blood glucose level, increase insulin requirements, and may aggravate the already compromised microcirculation.

Adrenergic blocking agents
Adrenergic blockers are classified according to their site of action as alpha-adrenergic blockers, beta-adrenergic blockers, or autonomic ganglionic blockers. Alpha-adrenergic blockers include ergoloid mesylates (Hydergine), ergotamine tartrate (Ergomar, Ergostat, Medihaler-Ergotamine), phenoxybenzamine hydrochloride (Dibenzyline), phentolamine mesylate (Regitine), and prazosin hydrochloride. (For information on prazosin, see Chapter 16, Antihypertensive agents.)

Nonselective beta-adrenergic blockers include carteolol (an antihypertensive agent discussed in Chapter 16, Antihypertensive agents), labetalol hydrochloride (Normodyne, Trandate), nadolol (Corgard), propranolol hydrochloride (Inderal), and timolol maleate (Blocadren). These agents affect beta$_1$-receptor sites (mainly in the heart) and beta$_2$-receptor sites (in bronchi, blood vessels, and the uterus). Selective beta blockers include acebutolol hydrochloride (Sectral), atenolol (Tenormin), betaxolol hydrochloride (discussed in Chapter 33, Other major drugs), esmolol hydrochloride (discussed in Chapter 14, Antiarrhythmic agents), and metoprolol tartrate (Lopressor). They primarily affect beta$_1$-receptor sites. Some beta-blockers, such as pindolol (Visken) and acebutolol (Sectral), are classified as partial agonists because they also exhibit intrinsic sympathetic activity. The clinically useful autonomic ganglionic blockers are mecamylamine hydrochloride (Inversine) and trimethaphan camsylate (Arfonad).

Pharmacokinetics
The pharmacokinetics of alpha-adrenergic blockers is not understood well. Most are absorbed erratically when administered orally and more rapidly and completely when administered sublingually or by inhalation. The various alpha-adrenergic blockers vary considerably in their onset of action, peak concentration level, and duration of action.

Beta-adrenergic blockers usually are absorbed rapidly and well from the GI tract and are protein-bound. They are distributed widely in body tissues, with the highest concentrations found in the heart, liver, lungs, and saliva. Most beta blockers are metabolized in the liver and excreted primarily in the urine. The onset of action is primarily dose- and drug-dependent; peak concentration level is route-dependent. The duration of action is dose-dependent and ranges from 4 hours for oral timolol to 24 hours for oral atenolol.

After oral administration, autonomic ganglionic blockers are absorbed well from the GI tract. However, higher doses are required at night, and lower doses in warm weather. The drugs are distributed widely, may be metabolized by pseudocholinesterase, and are excreted primarily by the kidneys. Their onset of action is route-dependent, beginning immediately after I.V. administration and within 30 minutes to 2 hours after oral administration. With oral therapy, the peak concentration level occurs in 3 to 5 hours, and the duration of action is 6 to 12 hours. With I.V. therapy, the duration is 10 to 30 minutes.

Pharmacodynamics
Adrenergic blockers block impulse transmission at adrenergic neurons or adrenergic receptor sites, thereby blocking SNS stimulation. They may do this by interrupting the action of sympathomimetic (adrenergic) agents, reducing available norepinephrine, or preventing the action of cholinergic agents.

Alpha-adrenergic blockers interrupt the actions of sympathomimetic agents at alpha-adrenergic receptor sites, relaxing vascular smooth muscle, increasing peripheral vasodilation, and decreasing blood pressure. They also may cause reflex tachycardia because the decrease in systemic blood pressure activates baroceptor reflexes that increase impulse activity in sympathetic cardiac nerves. If severe, this tachycardia may precipitate coronary insufficiency, angina, or even heart failure.

The alpha-adrenergic blocker ergotamine not only acts on receptors, but also stimulates smooth muscle directly, producing vasoconstriction primarily in the uterus and blood vessels. This action produces decreased cerebral blood flow and a decline in arterial pressure, which makes it effective in treating vascular (migraine) headaches.

Beta-adrenergic blockers prevent SNS stimulation by inhibiting the action of catecholamines and other sympathomimetic agents at beta-adrenergic receptor sites. Beta-adrenergic blockers produce a competitive blocking action at adrenergic nerve endings and in the adrenal medulla; this accounts for their widespread effects. These agents can reduce or block myocardial stimulation, vasodilation, bronchodilation, glycogenolysis, and lipolysis. The effects of this blockade include increased peripheral vascular resistance, decreased systemic blood pressure, decreased contractile force, decreased myocardial oxygen consumption, slowed AV node conduction, and decreased cardiac output. Pulmonary manifestations include increased bronchial smooth muscle tone; metabolic manifestations include inhibition of the sympathetic response to hypoglycemia. CNS manifestations include weakness, lethargy, and fatigue. Other manifestations include decreased plasma resin activity and decreased production of aqueous humor in the eye.

Selective beta-adrenergic blockers, which preferentially block $beta_1$-receptor sites, produce effects related to prevention of cardiac excitation. Nonselective beta blockers, which block $beta_1$- and $beta_2$-receptor sites, prevent not only cardiac excitement, but also bronchiolar dilation.

Besides blocking sympathetic stimulation of the adrenal medulla to prevent epinephrine and norepinephrine secretion into the systemic circulation, autonomic ganglionic blockers prevent nerve impulse transmission by competing with ACh at postganglionic synapses in the ANS. This blockade causes primarily sympatholytic effects: vasodilation and decreased blood pressure. Like the other adrenergic blockers, these drugs exert potent hypotensive effects. However, they also produce undesirable effects, such as inhibited diaphoresis, loss of body heat, and lowered body temperature.

Pharmacotherapeutics

The adrenergic blockers are used therapeutically to disrupt SNS function. The most important therapeutic effects of alpha-adrenergic blockers are smooth muscle relaxation, vasodilation, increased blood flow to the skin and other organs, and decreased blood pressure. These effects prove beneficial in hypertension and peripheral vascular disorders, including vascular headaches, Raynaud's disease, acrocyanosis, and frost-bite.

Phenoxybenzamine and phentolamine rarely are used to treat primary (essential) hypertension because of the risk of rebound tachycardia. However, they are important in treating secondary hypertension caused by pheochromocytoma, an adrenal gland tumor that secretes excessive epinephrine and norepinephrine. Phentolamine also is used to prevent tissue necrosis and sloughing related to extravasation of I.V. vasopressor drugs, such as norepinephrine or dopamine.

The most widely used adrenergic blocking agents, beta-adrenergic blockers are used extensively to treat hypertension, arrhythmias, and angina as well as hyperthyroidism and related disorders. Their clinical usefulness is based largely on their cardiovascular effects. Cardiovascular indications for beta blockers include hypertension, angina pectoris, prevention of reinfarction after myocardial infarction (MI), supraventricular arrhythmias, and hypertrophic cardiomyopathy. Other uses include the treatment of migraine headaches, anxiety, open-angle glaucoma, pheochromocytoma, and the cardiovascular symptoms associated with thyrotoxicosis. These agents also are used for ophthalmic indications. (For details, see Chapter 33, Other major drugs.)

The autonomic ganglionic blockers are not used widely because of their adverse effects. However, they are used selectively to treat hypertensive emergencies, pulmonary edema, and uncomplicated malignant hypertension. They also are used to predict effects of a sympathectomy and to provide controlled hypotension during surgery, such as for brain tumors, cerebral aneurysms, AV fistulas, aortic grafts, transplants, and coarctation.

Drug interactions
Adrenergic blockers may interact with various drugs. (For details, see Drug Interactions: *Autonomic agents,* pages 65 to 67.)

Adverse drug reactions
Adverse reactions to alpha-adrenergic blockers are related primarily to their vasodilating effects. However, many other adverse reactions can occur. Cardiovascular manifestations may include orthostatic hypotension or severe hypertensive episodes, bradycardia or tachycardia, edema, dyspnea, light-headedness, flushing, arrhythmias, angina, MI, cerebrovascular spasm, or a shocklike state.

Adverse CNS reactions may include paresthesia, muscle weakness, fatigue, nervousness, depression, insomnia, drowsiness, lethargy, vertigo, syncope, confusion, sedation, headache, or CNS stimulation. Adverse GI effects are common and may include sublingual irritation, nausea, vomiting, diarrhea, heartburn, abdominal pain, or exacerbation of peptic ulcer disease. Other effects may occur, such as eye, ear, nose, and throat problems; dermatologic reactions; and genitourinary reactions, including urinary frequency, impotence, incontinence, and pria-pism.

Overuse of ergotamine may produce ergotism, which is charac-terized by cold, pale, numb extremities (caused by prolonged vasocon-striction) and diminished or absent arterial pulses. Ergotism also may produce muscle pain, confusion, vomiting, seizures, or vision loss. Treatment requires immediate discontinuation of the drug and symp-tomatic therapy.

Generally, beta-adrenergic blockers cause few adverse reactions. Most reactions are drug- or dose-dependent and commonly result from I.V. administration or from administration to geriatric patients or those with impaired renal or hepatic function. Although most patients toler-ate beta-adrenergic blockers fairly well, patients with arteriosclerosis, bronchospastic disease, congestive heart failure (CHF), diabetes melli-tus, or thyrotoxicosis are at special risk for adverse reactions.

Beta-adrenergic blocker toxicity is marked primarily by cardiovas-cular reactions, CNS disturbances, and GI distress similar to the ad-verse reactions caused by alpha-adrenergic blockers. In addition, respi-ratory distress (bronchospasm) may occur, especially in patients with bronchial asthma, bronchitis, or emphysema.

Adverse reactions to autonomic ganglionic blockers are related to their broad, nonspecific blocking effects on the PNS and SNS. Mild ad-verse reactions commonly affect many body systems and resemble those caused by the alpha-adrenergic blockers. Other reactions may in-clude suppression of diaphoresis and respiratory depression.

Severe—often dose-related—adverse reactions to ganglionic block-ers can include extreme hypotension, rapid pulse, cyanosis, angina-like pain, vascular collapse, abdominal distention, paralytic ileus, urine re-tention, dizziness, syncope, tremors, mental disturbances, paresthesia, and impaired sexual function. Allergic reactions may include urticaria, pruritus, and a histamine-like reaction to I.V. administration.

Nursing implications   When caring for a patient who is receiving an autonomic agent, the nurse should be aware of the following implications.
- Develop appropriate nursing diagnoses for the patient. (For exam-ples, see Sample Nursing Diagnoses: *Autonomic agents,* page 78.)
- Do not administer an autonomic agent to a patient with a condition that contraindicates its use.
- Administer an autonomic agent cautiously to a patient at risk because of a preexisting condition.
- Advise the physician if the patient has been taking an agent that may interact with the prescribed autonomic agent.
- Monitor the patient for adverse reactions and signs of drug interac-tions.
- Notify the physician if adverse reactions or drug interactions occur.
- Monitor for signs of effectiveness of the prescribed agent.

SAMPLE NURSING DIAGNOSES

Autonomic agents

The following nursing diagnoses address representative problems and etiologies that a nurse may encounter when caring for a patient receiving an autonomic agent.
- Activity intolerance related to skeletal muscle weakness caused by an anticholinesterase, adrenergic, or adrenergic blocking agent
- Altered cardiopulmonary tissue perfusion related to drug interaction between a beta-adrenergic blocker and another prescribed drug
- Altered nutrition: less than body requirements, related to the adverse gastrointestinal (GI) effects of an adrenergic blocker
- Altered peripheral tissue perfusion related to the adverse cardiovascular effects of a non-catecholamine
- Altered urinary elimination related to the adverse genitourinary effects of an alpha-adrenergic blocker, cholinergic agonist, or noncatecholamine
- Decreased cardiac output related to the adverse cardiovascular effects of a cholinergic, cholinergic blocking, or adrenergic agent
- Diarrhea related to the adverse GI effects of a cholinergic agent, catecholamine, or adrenergic blocker
- Fluid volume deficit related to catecholamine-induced nausea and severe vomiting
- High risk for altered body temperature related to risk of heat stroke caused by a cholinergic blocker
- High risk for injury related to adverse drug reactions
- High risk for injury related to a preexisting condition that contraindicates the use of an autonomic agent
- High risk for injury related to a preexisting condition that requires cautious use of an autonomic agent
- High risk for injury related to drug interactions
- High risk for trauma related to the adverse central nervous system effects of an adrenergic agent or alpha-adrenergic blocker
- Impaired gas exchange related to paradoxical bronchospasm caused by a noncatecholamine
- Impaired tissue integrity related to tissue necrosis resulting from extravasation of a parenterally administered catecholamine
- Ineffective breathing pattern related to bronchoconstriction caused by the cholinergic agent
- Ineffective breathing pattern related to respiratory depression caused by an autonomic ganglionic blocker
- Knowledge deficit related to the prescribed autonomic agent
- Pain related to anginal pain caused by an adrenergic agent
- Pain related to headache caused by an adrenergic agent or alpha-adrenergic blocker
- Sensory or perceptual alterations (visual) related to the adverse effects of a cholinergic blocker in a patient with undiagnosed glaucoma
- Sleep pattern disturbance related to insomnia caused by an adrenergic agent
- Sexual dysfunction related to impotence caused by an adrenergic blocker

---

- Teach the patient and family the name, dose, frequency, action, and adverse effects of the prescribed autonomic agent.
- Help the patient and family develop a system for keeping track of each dose and its effect.
- Instruct the patient to notify the physician if the drug is ineffective or if adverse reactions occur.

Cholinergic agents

- Have respiratory support equipment available. Keep suction equipment, oxygen, and a mechanical ventilator on hand if edrophonium is used.
- Monitor vital signs and auscultate breath sounds at least once every 4 hours. (Assess the patient for 30 minutes to 1 hour after S.C. administration of bethanechol.)
- Monitor closely for signs of a toxic response: circulatory collapse (with a cholinergic agonist) or generalized weakness, fasciculations, dysphagia, and respiratory weakness (with an anticholinesterase agent).
- Keep atropine (0.6 mg) readily available in a syringe as an antidote.
- Monitor visual acuity closely if patient displays decreased effectiveness of prescribed cholinergic agent. Advise the patient that vision may blur during therapy.
- Take safety precautions if the patient develops vision disturbances. For example, move the call bell close to the patient and supervise ambulation.
- Administer the cholinergic agent when the patient's stomach is empty to minimize adverse reactions.
- Apply pressure to the inner canthus to prevent systemic absorption from ocular administration of a cholinergic agent.
- Assist the patient with frequent oral hygiene, if increased salivation occurs.
- Change bed linens and clothing as needed to prevent skin breakdown in a patient with diaphoresis.
- Monitor urine output in a patient who is receiving a cholinergic agonist for acute urine retention. Urination should occur within 1 hour. If not, notify the physician and expect to perform urinary catheterization.
- Monitor and record changes in muscle strength daily for a patient with myasthenia gravis who is receiving an anticholinesterase agent.
- Expect to administer a higher dosage of the anticholinesterase agent if the patient demonstrates decreased muscle strength.
- Take seizure precautions for a patient receiving an anticholinesterase agent.
- Show the patient how to assess and record changes in muscle strength during anticholinesterase therapy.
- Reassure the patient and family that anxiety is an adverse reaction to an anticholinesterase agent.
- Describe ways to manage common adverse reactions. For example, tell the patient to take the drug with food or milk if nausea occurs after an oral dose of an anticholinesterase agent.

Cholinergic blocking agents

- Closely monitor any patient who is at increased risk for adverse reactions (an infant, elderly patient, fair-skinned child with Down's syndrome, or a child with spastic paralysis or brain damage).
- Monitor vital signs at least every 4 hours.
- Administer an analgesic, as prescribed, to a patient who is in pain and is receiving a cholinergic blocker. This helps reduce the risk of CNS excitation.
- Administer a cholinergic blocker 30 minutes before meals and at bedtime when used to reduce GI motility. Advise the patient to limit milk and bedtime snacks because they increase gastric secretions.
- Monitor the patient for signs of heat stroke, such as dehydration, flushing, and decreased level of consciousness. Be aware that cholinergic blocker-induced heat stroke is more common during strenuous activity, in hot weather, and in elderly patients with cardiovascular disease.
- Encourage the patient to drink additional fluids (unless contraindicated) when engaging in strenuous activity or when the weather is hot.
- Advise the patient to keep the room temperature cool (by using fans or air conditioners) and to stay out of the sun.
- Monitor the patient for signs and symptoms of urine retention, such as urinary frequency and voiding of small amounts. Record fluid intake and output for patients with benign prostatic hypertrophy. Notify the physician, if necessary.
- Teach the patient to prevent drug toxicity by taking only the amount of medicine ordered. If a dose is missed, advise the patient to take the missed dose as soon as possible or wait until the time of the next dose and take a single dose only. Stress that the patient should not to double the dose without consulting the physician.
- Teach the patient to eat a high-fiber diet and drink plenty of fluids to prevent constipation.
- Advise the patient to wear dark glasses and not to drive if mydriasis or cycloplegia occurs.
- Teach the patient about the need for scrupulous oral hygiene to decrease caries and periodontal disease; recommend sugarless gum, hard candy, or ice chips to reduce dry mouth.

Adrenergic agents

- Check the prescription carefully, particularly noting the concentration, dosage, and rate.
- Show the patient and family how to use an inhalation device correctly.
- Teach the patient to blow the nose gently, with both nostrils open to clear nasal passages before administering a nasal medication and to wait for the prescribed interval between inhalations.
- Emphasize using the lowest number of inhalations possible.

he patient with diabetes to notify the physician if glucose test
change or if signs and symptoms of hyperglycemia occur.
xygen and emergency respiratory equipment readily available
catecholamine administration.
administer isoproterenol and inhaled epinephrine concurrent-
e them 4 hours apart.
r the patient's respiratory rate when administering isoproter-
detect rebound bronchospasm.
t hypovolemia, as prescribed, before beginning catecholamine
r.
the patient using an intranasal drug that rebound nasal con-
and hyperemia commonly occur with too frequent use of epi-
ie.
r vital signs, mental status, and muscle strength at least every
s during noncatecholamine therapy.
r the serum potassium level closely to detect hypokalemia in a
receiving prolonged infusion of ritodrine or terbutaline.
r the patient for 12 hours after terbutaline is discontinued
e cardiovascular symptoms may recur.

- Place the patient in a left lateral recumbent position to prevent hypotension during I.V. infusion of ritodrine or terbutaline.
- Infuse I.V. ritodrine or terbutaline into a large vein to avoid extravasation. If extravasation occurs, inject the area within 12 hours with 10
to 15 ml of 0.9% sodium chloride solution containing phentolamine
(Regitine), as prescribed.
- Discontinue ephedrine and notify the physician if wheezing or bronchospasm occurs.
- Teach the patient not to use another aerosol bronchodilator during
terbutaline inhalation therapy.
- Teach the patient to protect the noncatecholamine from light, excessive heat or cold, and moisture, and not to use discolored drugs.

Adrenergic blocking agents
- Measure the patient's vital signs frequently. Be alert for changes in
blood pressure, breath sounds, fluid intake and output, daily weight,
and peripheral circulation.
- Teach the patient to minimize orthostatic hypotension by arising
slowly and dangling the legs before standing.
- Instruct the patient to lie down if light-headedness, weakness, or faint-
ness occurs.
- Notify the physician immediately if the patient develops chest pain
during alpha-adrenergic blocker therapy. Obtain an electrocardiogram and treat the patient as prescribed.
- Monitor for signs of vascular insufficiency (numbness, coldness, and
tingling or weakness in the extremities) in a patient receiving ergotamine.

- Administer an oral alpha-adrenergic blocker with milk to reduce GI distress.
- Administer ergotamine in the early stage of a migraine attack to maximize its effectiveness. Also, have the patient lie quietly in a darkened room after taking ergotamine.
- Teach the patient to avoid alcohol consumption during alpha-adrenergic blocker therapy. Also instruct the patient to avoid over-the-counter cough, cold, allergy, or weight-loss medications that contain alcohol or caffeine unless directed by the physician.
- Obtain blood glucose levels frequently for a patient with diabetes because beta-adrenergic blockers can potentiate hypoglycemia and mask its signs and symptoms.
- Keep the following emergency drugs on hand when giving a beta-adrenergic blocker intravenously: atropine for bradycardia, epinephrine for hypotension, and isoproterenol and aminophylline for bronchospasm.
- Notify the physician immediately if the patient experiences cardiac or respiratory depression, arrhythmias, severe bronchospasm, or severe hypotension during beta-adrenergic blocker therapy. Institute emergency care.
- Check the patient's apical pulse rate before administering the beta-adrenergic blocker (especially if the patient also is taking a cardiac glycoside). Withhold the drug if the patient has a pulse rate below 60 or exhibits adverse reactions to the drug. Teach the patient to measure the pulse rate and report slowing or irregularity to the physician.
- Administer antacids several hours before or after an oral beta-adrenergic blocker.
- Advise the patient not to stop taking the beta-adrenergic blocker abruptly or alter the prescribed dosage, unless ordered. Explain that abrupt withdrawal can cause MI, arrhythmias, or other serious complications.
- Teach the patient with impaired renal function to report a weight gain of 3 to 4 lb (1.4 to 1.8 kg) per day, cough, orthopnea, dyspnea, edema, or anxiety during beta-adrenergic blocker therapy.
- Teach the patient to store the beta-adrenergic blocker at room temperature and to protect it from moisture, light, and air.
- Administer an autonomic ganglionic blocker cautiously to a patient with a history of allergies because it may cause histamine release.
- Have oxygen and a vasopressor available to treat a hypotensive reaction to an autonomic ganglionic blocker. Also keep resuscitation and ventilation equipment nearby.
- Dilute trimethaphan before administering (with 1 mg/ml of dextrose 5% in water) and do not mix it with any other drug for I.V. use. Administer the drug with the patient in a supine, head-down, or Trendelenburg position. Discontinue the drug gradually.

• Monitor the patient for rebound hypertension during withdrawal of the autonomic ganglionic blocker.
• Give lower doses of an autonomic ganglionic blocker in the morning, when the patient's response usually is greater.

STUDY ACTIVITIES

True or false

1. Patients receiving cholinergic agents need little monitoring because these drugs produce few adverse reactions.
 ☐ True ☐ False

2. Cholinergic agents can be used to treat glaucoma.
 ☐ True ☐ False

3. Bethanechol may be used to treat urine retention.
 ☐ True ☐ False

4. Adrenergic agents also are called sympathomimetics.
 ☐ True ☐ False

5. Most adrenergic agents mimic norepinephrine or epinephrine and stimulate alpha or beta receptors to produce their effects.
 ☐ True ☐ False

6. Rebound nasal congestion and hyperemia rarely result from use of intranasal preparations that contain epinephrine.
 ☐ True ☐ False

Multiple choice

7. Which anticholinesterase agent is used primarily to diagnose myasthenia gravis?
 A. Ambenonium
 B. Physostigmine
 C. Pyridostigmine
 D. Edrophonium chloride

8. Anna Baxter, age 42, is scheduled for surgery at 8 a.m. Preoperative preparation includes meperidine hydrochloride and scopolamine hydrobromide. Why is scopolamine used as a preanesthetic agent?
 A. To reduce salivaation and gastric secretions
 B. To reduce postoperative constipation
 C. To reduce the risk of regurgitation
 D. To prevent urine retention

9. How do cholinergic blockers, such as scopolamine, produce their therapeutic effects?
 A. They mimic the action of ACh at muscarinic receptor sites.
 B. They block the action of ACh at nicotinic receptor sites.
 C. They metabolize ACh at the postjunctional membrane.
 D. They compete with ACh at muscarinic receptor sites.

10. Albert Kemlen, age 70, has GI tract spasms, for which his physician prescribes propantheline (Pro-Banthine) 15 mg P.O. q.i.d. During this therapy, which adverse reaction is likely to occur?
A. Dry mouth
B. Bradycardia
C. Urinary frequency
D. Pupillary constriction

11. Sean Knox, age 27, is undergoing I.V. pyelography. Five minutes after the dye is injected, he develops an anaphylactic reaction. The radiologist administers epinephrine 0.5 ml of a 1:1,000 solution S.C. Epinephrine's action on alpha and beta receptors produces which effects?
A. Vasoconstriction, coronary artery dilation, and bronchoconstriction
B. Vasoconstriction, cardiac stimulation, and bronchodilation
C. Vasodilation, cardiac stimulation, and bronchodilation
D. Vasodilation, cardiac relaxation, bronchoconstriction

12. To maintain Mr. Knox's blood pressure, the physician prescribes dopamine, 1 mcg/kg/minute. While receiving dopamine, Mr. Knox develops a headache. What does this symptom suggest?
A. Catecholamine toxicity
B. Inadequate drug dosage
C. Catecholamine hypersensitivity
D. Adverse reaction to the catecholamine

13. Sara Mills, age 46, has just received a prescription for the noncatecholamine metaproterenol (Alupent) to treat bronchial asthma. Before Ms. Mills leaves the office, the nurse double-checks her drug history. The use of which drug may interact with the noncatecholamine, causing severe hypertension?
A. Alpha-adrenergic blocker
B. Monoamine oxidase (MAO) inhibitor
C. Neuromuscular blocker
D. Anticholinesterase agent

14. Olivia Brady, age 62, is admitted to the hospital for treatment of uncontrolled hypertension. The physician prescribes the beta-adrenergic blocker propranolol hydrochloride (Inderal) 40 mg P.O. b.i.d. How does propranolol produce its therapeutic effects?
A. It inhibits neurotransmitter production.
B. It stimulates neurotransmitter metabolism.
C. It chemically inactivates neurotransmitters at receptor sites.
D. It acts as a competitive adrenergic antagonist at beta-adrenergic receptor sites.

15. Penny Linden, age 22, has just received a prescription for ergotamine tartrate (Ergostat) 2 mg P.O. to treat migraine headaches. How does ergotamine relieve headaches?
   A. By binding with opiate receptors
   B. By decreasing peripheral resistance
   C. By decreasing cerebral blood flow
   D. By increasing baroceptor stimulation

Fill in the blank

16. Cholinergic agents achieve their effects by mimicking the action

of _____ or by inhibiting the action of _____ at autonomic effector sites.

17. Like the alpha-adrenergic and beta-adrenergic blockers, autonomic ganglionic blockers exert potent _____ effects.

18. Although the use of ganglionic blocking agents is limited, these

drugs are used selectively to treat _____ emergencies,

_____ edema, and uncomplicated _____.

Matching related elements

Match the adrenergic agent on the left with its major indication(s) on the right.

19. ___ Dobutamine   **A.** Acute CHF and cardiopulmonary bypass surgery

20. ___ Epinephrine   **B.** Asthma, bronchospasm, shock, cardiac arrest, and selected arrhythmias

21. ___ Isoproterenol   **C.** Bronchodilation and preterm labor

22. ___ Norepinephrine   **D.** Acute hypotension, shock, cardiac arrest, myocardial infarction, and anaphylaxis

23. ___ Metaproterenol   **E.** Bronchospasm, asthma, nasal and ophthalmic congestion, open-angle glaucoma, and allergic conditions

24. ___ Terbutaline   **F.** Bronchodilation

ANSWERS   **True or false**
   1. False. Adverse reactions to cholinergic agonists are common and usually result from their nonspecific effects on the PNS.
   2. True.
   3. True.
   4. True.
   5. True.

6. False. Rebound nasal congestion and hyperemia commonly occur with too frequent use of intranasal preparations that contain epinephrine.

Multiple choice

7. D. Edrophonium chloride is the drug of choice for diagnosing myasthenia gravis.

8. A. As preanesthesia drugs, cholinergic blockers reduce excitement, salivation, and gastric secretions, to depress the respiratory system, and to block vagal inhibition during anesthesia.

9. D. Cholinergic blockers, such as scopolamine, act by competing with acetylcholine and cholinergic agonists at muscarinic receptor sites in the CNS.

10. A. Cholinergic blockers decrease GI secretions, including saliva; they also cause increased heart rate, pupillary dilation, decreased accommodation, and urine retention (at higher doses).

11. B. Epinephrine acts on alpha, $beta_1$, and $beta_2$ receptors, causing vasoconstriction, cardiac stimulation, and bronchodilation, respectively. No adrenergic agents cause bronchoconstriction.

12. D. Adverse CNS reactions to catecholamines may include restlessness, nervousness, anxiety, dizziness, headache, and insomnia.

13. B. Concurrent use of a noncatecholamine with an MAO inhibitor may cause severe hypertension. Alpha-adrenergic blockers, neuromuscular blockers, and anticholinesterase agents do not interact with noncatecholamines.

14. D. Beta-adrenergic blockers produce a competitive blocking action at beta-adrenergic receptor sites, at adrenergic nerve endings, and in the adrenal medulla.

15. C. Ergotamine produces vasoconstriction primarily in the uterus and blood vessels. This action decreases cerebral blood flow and arterial pressure.

Fill in the blank

16. Acetylcholine, acetylcholinesterase
17. Hypotensive
18. Hypertensive, pulmonary, malignant hypertension

Matching related elements

19. A
20. E
21. B
22. D
23. F
24. C

CHAPTER 6

Skeletal muscle relaxing agents

OBJECTIVES

After studying this chapter, the reader should be able to:

1. Discuss the physiology of skeletal muscle contraction.
2. Differentiate between spasm and spasticity.
3. Differentiate among the skeletal muscle relaxing agents that act centrally and those that act peripherally.
4. List the therapeutic uses for the various groups of skeletal muscle relaxing agents.
5. Describe the adverse reactions that occur when these agents are given with central nervous system depressants.
6. Describe the nursing implications of skeletal muscle relaxant therapy.

OVERVIEW OF CONCEPTS

Skeletal muscle relaxing agents are used to treat painful musculoskeletal spasms and spasticity. Centrally acting agents may act by depressing the central nervous system (CNS). Peripherally acting agents may act directly on the muscle contractile system. (For a summary of representative drugs, see Selected Major Drugs: *Skeletal muscle relaxing agents*, page 88.)

Skeletal muscle contraction

The CNS and muscles must work together closely to produce normal skeletal muscle function. Skeletal muscles are striated and composed of muscle fibers. Each muscle fiber is innervated by a nerve fiber that contains a motor neuron. The neurons originate in the anterior horn cells of the spinal cord. Neurotransmitters relay excitatory or inhibitory signals to these motor neurons from the spinal cord.

Skeletal muscle fibers are composed of filaments of the proteins actin and myosin. The filaments are embedded in the sarcoplasm, which also contains a network of tubules known as the sarcoplasmic reticulum. When an excitatory or inhibitory signal reaches the neuromuscular junction, sodium rushes into the muscle fiber, releasing calcium ions from the sarcoplasmic reticulum. The calcium ions allow the proteins actin and myosin to move, resulting in muscle contraction.

SELECTED MAJOR DRUGS

Skeletal muscle relaxing agents

This table summarizes the major skeletal muscle relaxants currently in clinical use. (Diazepam is discussed in detail in Chapter 8, Anticonvulsant agents.)

DRUG	MAJOR INDICATIONS	USUAL ADULT DOSAGE
Central acting agents		
carisoprodol	Acute muscle spasms	350 mg P.O. t.i.d. and h.s.
Peripherally acting agents		
dantrolene	Spasticity	25 mg P.O. once daily to 100 mg P.O. q.i.d.
	Prevention of malignant hyperthermic crisis	4 to 8 mg/kg P.O. daily for 1 to 2 days before surgery or for 3 days after crisis
	Treatment of malignant hyperthermic crisis	1 mg/kg I.V. up to a cumulative total of 10 mg/kg
Other agents		
baclofen	Spasticity	40 to 80 mg P.O. daily in three or four divided doses

Musculoskeletal spasms and spasticity

Severe cold, lack of blood flow to a muscle, or overexertion can elicit pain or other sensory impulses that are transmitted by the posterior sensory nerve fibers to the spinal cord and higher levels of the CNS. These impulses may cause a reflex (involuntary) muscle contraction, or spasm. The spasm stimulates the sensory receptors, resulting in a more intense contraction and establishing a cycle. Centrally acting muscle relaxants are believed to break this cycle by acting as a CNS depressant.

Spasticity is a motor disorder characterized by increased muscle tone resulting from hyperexcitability of the anterior motor neurons. This hyperexcitability may arise from lack of inhibition or from excess stimulation produced by signals transmitted from the brain through the interneurons in the spinal cord to the anterior motor neurons. Spasticity is associated with various upper motor neuron disorders, such as multiple sclerosis, cerebral palsy, cerebrovascular accident, and spinal cord injuries. Although skeletal muscle relaxants vary in their efficacy, they reduce spasticity by reducing hyperexcitability.

Centrally acting skeletal muscle relaxants

Trauma, inflammation, anxiety, and pain can cause acute muscle spasms. The following drugs may be used to treat such spasms: carisoprodol (Soma), chlorphenesin carbamate (Maolate), chlorzoxazone (Paraflex), cyclobenzaprine hydrochloride (Flexeril), metaxalone (Skelaxin), methocarbamol (Robaxin), and orphenadrine citrate (Norflex, Norgesic Forte).

Pharmacokinetics

All centrally acting muscle relaxants can be administered orally. Methocarbamol and orphenadrine also can be administered by the intramuscular (I.M.) and intravenous (I.V.) routes. In general, these drugs are absorbed from the gastrointestinal (GI) tract, widely distributed in the body, metabolized by the liver, and excreted by the kidneys. Their onset of action ranges from 30 to 60 minutes; duration of action, from 3 to 24 hours.

Pharmacodynamics

These drugs do not relax skeletal muscles directly or depress neuronal conduction, neuromuscular transmission, or muscle excitability. However, they are known to be CNS depressants.

Pharmacotherapeutics

The centrally acting skeletal muscle relaxants are used as adjuncts to rest and physical therapy in treating acute, painful musculoskeletal conditions. They are ineffective in treating spasticity caused by chronic neurologic disorders, such as cerebral palsy.

Drug interactions

Central acting agents interact with few drugs, but all interact with other CNS depressants (including alcohol), causing additive CNS depression. (For details, see Drug Interactions: *Skeletal muscle relaxing agents,* page 90.)

Adverse drug reactions

The most common adverse reactions to centrally acting skeletal muscle relaxants are extensions of their therapeutic effects on the CNS. Adverse CNS reactions include drowsiness, dizziness, weakness, headache, insomnia, nightmares, paresthesia, depression, vertigo, and ataxia. In addition, methocarbamol may precipitate seizures.

Adverse GI reactions may include nausea, vomiting, diarrhea or constipation, heartburn, and abdominal distress. Other adverse reactions may include tachycardia (with cyclobenzaprine and orphenadrine) or bradycardia, syncope, hypotension, flushing, blurred vision, asthenia, and incoordination. Because of its anticholinergic effect, orphenadrine also may cause dry mouth, urine retention, and urinary hesitancy. Chlorzoxazone may harmlessly discolor the urine an orange or purple-red; methocarbamol, green, black, or brown.

Physical and psychological dependence may result from long-term use of these agents; abrupt cessation of the drug may cause severe withdrawal symptoms.

Peripherally acting skeletal muscle relaxants

Dantrolene sodium (Dantrium) is the only peripherally acting skeletal muscle relaxant. It has a lower incidence of adverse CNS reactions, but high therapeutic doses are hepatotoxic. Dantrolene is most effective for spasticity of cerebral origin, but also is used to prevent and treat malignant hyperthermic crisis.

DRUG INTERACTIONS

Skeletal muscle relaxing agents

Drug interactions involving skeletal muscle relaxants are infrequent. They usually result from simultaneous administration of a central nervous system (CNS) depressant.

DRUG	INTERACTING DRUGS	POSSIBLE EFFECTS
Centrally acting agents		
carisoprodol, chlorphenesin, chlorzoxazone, cyclobenzaprine, metaxalone, methocarbamol, orphenadrine	CNS depressants (alcohol, narcotics, barbiturates, anticonvulsants, tricyclic antidepressants, antianxiety agents)	Increased sedative and other CNS effects, including motor skill impairment and respiratory depression
cyclobenzaprine	monoamine oxidase (MAO) inhibitors	Hyperpyrexia, excitation, seizures
cyclobenzaprine, orphenadrine	cholinergic blockers	Increased anticholinergic effects, including confusion and hallucinations
Peripherally acting agents		
dantrolene	CNS depressants	Increased CNS depression, which may lead to sedation, motor skill impairment, and respiratory depression
Other agents		
baclofen	CNS depressants	Increased CNS depression
	fentanyl	Prolonged analgesia
	lithium carbonate	Increased hyperkinesia
	tricyclic antidepressants	Increased muscle relaxation

Pharmacokinetics

Dantrolene is absorbed poorly from the GI tract. It is highly plasma protein-bound, metabolized in the liver, and excreted in the urine. Although the peak concentration of a single dose of dantrolene occurs about 5 hours after ingestion, the drug's therapeutic benefit may not be evident for a week or more. Because dantrolene undergoes significant hepatic metabolism, its half-life may be prolonged in a patient with impaired liver function.

Pharmacodynamics

Dantrolene is chemically and pharmacologically unrelated to the other skeletal muscle relaxants. It probably acts directly on the muscle contractile mechanism, possibly by inhibiting calcium release from the sarcoplasmic reticulum.

Pharmacotherapeutics

Dantrolene helps manage all types of spasticity, regardless of lesion location, but is most effective when the lesion is cerebral. It is used to treat patients with multiple sclerosis, cerebral palsy, spinal cord injury, or cerebrovascular accident. It is particularly useful for reducing spasticity in patients whose nursing care is impeded by severe muscle contractions. Dantrolene also is the drug of choice to prevent or treat malignant hyperthermic crisis.

Dosages must be titrated to the individual patient's response, always using the lowest dosage possible. Each dosage level should be maintained for 4 to 7 days to determine the patient's response. If benefits are not evident in 45 days, the drug is discontinued to avoid liver damage.

Drug interactions

Dantrolene may interact with CNS depressants. (For details, see Drug Interactions: *Skeletal muscle relaxing agents*.)

Adverse drug reactions

The most common adverse reaction to dantrolene is muscle weakness. The drug also may depress liver function or cause idiosyncratic hepatitis, which can be fatal.

Other common reactions include drowsiness, dizziness, light-headedness, diarrhea, nausea, malaise, and fatigue. If weakness or diarrhea is severe, the dosage may be decreased or the drug discontinued. Other adverse GI reactions that may respond to a dosage decrease include anorexia, vomiting, gastric irritation, abdominal cramps, constipation, difficulty swallowing, and GI bleeding. (Constipation may be severe enough to resemble bowel obstruction.) Adverse neurologic, genitourinary, and cardiovascular reactions also may appear.

Other skeletal muscle relaxants

Two other drugs, baclofen (Lioresal) and diazepam (Valium), are used as skeletal muscle relaxants. Baclofen is the drug of choice in treating spasticity and probably acts in the spinal cord. It is the focus of this section.

Diazepam is a benzodiazepine with antianxiety, hypnotic, and anticonvulsant actions. It also is an effective antispasmodic and may be used alone or with other agents to treat patients with spinal cord injury and cerebral palsy. Diazepam's use is limited by its CNS depressant effects and the tolerance that develops with prolonged use. (For more information on diazepam, see Chapter 8, Anticonvulsant agents).

Pharmacokinetics

Baclofen is absorbed rapidly from the GI tract. It is distributed widely, undergoes minimal liver metabolism, and is excreted primarily in the urine. Although the blood concentration of baclofen peaks in 2 to 3 hours, the drug's onset of therapeutic effect ranges from hours to weeks. Its elimination half-life is 2.5 to 4 hours.

Pharmacodynamics

Biochemically, baclofen resembles an inhibitory neurotransmitter. It works in the spinal cord, where it seems to depress neuron activity, decrease the degree and frequency of muscle spasms, and reduce muscle tone. However, its exact mechanism of action has not been established.

Pharmacotherapeutics

Baclofen's principal clinical indication is for the paraplegic or quadriplegic patient with spinal cord lesions, most commonly caused by multiple sclerosis or trauma. Baclofen reduces the number and severity of painful flexor spasms, but does not improve stiff gait, increase manual dexterity, or improve residual muscle function. Although baclofen and diazepam have comparable antispasmodic effects, baclofen is preferred because it is less sedating.

Drug interactions

Baclofen may interact with other CNS depressants, fentanyl, lithium, and tricyclic antidepressants. (For details, see Drug Interactions: *Skeletal muscle relaxing agents,* page 90.)

Adverse drug reactions

The most common adverse reaction to baclofen is transient drowsiness. Less common adverse reactions include nausea, fatigue, vertigo, hypotonia, muscle weakness, depression, and headache. These can be avoided by a slow titration of the dose.

Geriatric patients and patients with brain disorders may experience psychiatric disturbances, such as hallucinations, euphoria, depression, confusion, and anxiety. Slow titration of the dose also may prevent these adverse reactions.

Adverse GI reactions may include nausea, vomiting, constipation, and, rarely, dry mouth, anorexia, taste disorders, and diarrhea. Cardiovascular reactions include hypotension and, rarely, dyspnea, chest pain, and syncope. Baclofen rarely causes neurologic disturbances, such as insomnia and paresthesia, and genitourinary reactions. Rash, allergic skin disorders, and pruritus may occur with baclofen, as may ankle edema, weight gain, and excessive diaphoresis.

Abrupt withdrawal of the drug may precipitate hallucinations, seizures, and acute exacerbations of spasticity.

Nursing implications

When caring for a patient who is receiving a skeletal muscle relaxing agent, the nurse should be aware of the following implications.
- Develop appropriate nursing diagnoses for the patient. (For examples, see Sample Nursing Diagnoses: *Skeletal muscle relaxing agents.*)
- Do not administer a skeletal muscle relaxant to a patient with a condition that contraindicates its use.
- Administer a skeletal muscle relaxant cautiously to a patient at risk because of a preexisting condition.
- Monitor the patient periodically for adverse reactions to the prescribed skeletal muscle relaxant.
- Take safety precautions if the patient develops sedation or motor skill impairment.

SAMPLE NURSING DIAGNOSES

Skeletal muscle relaxing agents

The following nursing diagnoses address representative problems and etiologies that a nurse may encounter when caring for a patient who is receiving a skeletal muscle relaxing agent.

- Altered thought processes related to psychiatric disturbances caused by a skeletal muscle relaxant
- Constipation related to the adverse gastrointestinal (GI) effects of a skeletal muscle relaxant
- Diarrhea related to the adverse GI effects of a skeletal muscle relaxant
- Fluid volume deficit related to nausea, vomiting, or diarrhea caused by a skeletal muscle relaxant
- High risk for activity intolerance related to possible ineffectiveness of a skeletal muscle relaxant
- High risk for injury related to adverse drug reactions
- High risk for injury related to a preexisting condition that contraindicates the use of a skeletal muscle relaxant
- High risk for injury related to a preexisting condition that requires cautious use of a skeletal muscle relaxant
- High risk for injury related to drug interactions with the prescribed skeletal muscle relaxant
- High risk for trauma related to drowsiness or dizziness caused by a skeletal muscle relaxant
- Impaired adjustment related to physical and psychological dependence on a centrally acting skeletal muscle relaxant
- Impaired physical mobility related to ineffectiveness of dantrolene
- Knowledge deficit related to the prescribed skeletal muscle relaxant
- Pain related to ineffectiveness of a centrally acting skeletal muscle relaxant
- Sensory or perceptual alterations (visual, gustatory, auditory) related to the adverse effects of a skeletal muscle relaxant
- Urinary retention related to the anticholinergic effects of a skeletal muscle relaxant

---

- Monitor for signs of drug interactions. For a patient who must simultaneously receive a CNS depressant, particularly note respiratory status and level of consciousness. Keep emergency equipment available and take safety precautions, as needed.
- Notify the physician if adverse reactions or drug interactions occur.
- Monitor the patient's response to skeletal muscle relaxant therapy. For example, monitor the number and severity of painful flexor spasms or assess the level of spasticity. Notify the physician if the patient's condition does not improve during drug therapy.
- Teach the patient and family the name, dose, frequency, action, and adverse effects of the prescribed skeletal muscle relaxant.
- Inform the patient that the skeletal muscle relaxant may impair mental alertness or physical coordination, increasing the risks associated with operating machinery or driving a motor vehicle.
- Advise the patient to avoid alcohol and other CNS depressants while taking a skeletal muscle relaxant.
- Instruct the patient to take an oral skeletal muscle relaxant with meals or milk to prevent GI distress.

• Teach the patient to notify the physician if adverse reactions occur.

Centrally acting skeletal muscle relaxants
• Avoid abrupt discontinuation of a centrally acting agent.
• Administer I.V. medications over 5 minutes with the patient in the supine position; keep the patient supine for 5 to 10 more minutes. Then help the patient to a sitting position and supervise ambulation.
• Administer I.M. medications deeply and slowly, only in the gluteal muscle, with a maximum of 5 ml in each buttock.

Peripherally acting skeletal muscle relaxants
• Monitor the patient's liver function before and during dantrolene therapy.
• Empty dantrolene capsules into fruit juice or another liquid immediately before administering to a patient who has difficulty swallowing.
• Reconstitute dantrolene with 60 ml of sterile, not bacteriostatic, water for I.V. administration.
• Encourage the patient to increase fluid and high-fiber food intake during therapy. Auscultate bowel sounds every 8 hours during therapy.

Other skeletal muscle relaxants
• Monitor renal function by documenting the patient's fluid intake and output and body weight daily. Patients with impaired renal function may require a dosage reduction because baclofen is excreted primarily by the kidneys.

STUDY ACTIVITIES

Fill in the blank

1. Muscle contraction occurs when a nervous system signal reaches the neuromuscular junction. The stimulus causes _____ to enter the muscle fiber. This releases _____ from the sarcoplasmic reticulum, which allows movement of the proteins _____ and _____.

2. Skeletal muscle relaxing agents are used to treat _____ and _____.

3. Centrally acting skeletal muscle relaxants do not act on skeletal muscles directly, but depress the _____.

4. The peripherally acting skeletal muscle relaxant dantrolene interacts only with _____ drugs.

Matching related elements

Match the drug on the left with its clinical use on the right.

5. Dantrolene   **A.** Acute muscle spasm

6. Carisoprodol   **B.** Malignant hyperthermic crisis

7. Diazepam   **C.** Spasticity in a paraplegic patient

8. Baclofen   **D.** Anxiety and seizures

Short answer

9. Differentiate between a muscle spasm and spasticity.

_____

_____

_____

10. Identify four possible causes of muscle spasm.

_____

11. List four disorders that are associated with spasticity.

_____

Multiple choice

12. Sally Albright, age 35, undergoes a lumbar laminectomy for recurrent disc problems. Two days after surgery, Ms. Albright reports severe muscle cramps and pain. The physician orders chlorzoxazone (Paraflex) 500 mg P.O. t.i.d. How does this agent produce its therapeutic effect?

    A. It depresses neuromuscular transmission.
    B. It depresses the CNS.
    C. It reduces muscle excitability.
    D. It relaxes skeletal muscles.

13. Three days later, Ms. Albright reports that her urine "looks funny." After assessing the urine, what should the nurse do?

    A. Encourage the patient to drink more water.
    B. Withhold chlorzoxazone and notify the physician.
    C. Reassure the patient that the discoloration is harmless.
    D. Monitor the patient's fluid intake and output continuously.

14. Glenn James, age 24, has been a paraplegic since age 18, when he was injured in a diving accident. His physician has just prescribed baclofen (Lioresal) 5 mg P.O. t.i.d. Where is this drug's site of action?

    A. Muscle
    B. Brain
    C. Spinal cord
    D. Myoneural junction

15. On the third day of baclofen therapy, Mr. James is drowsier than usual. What should the nurse do?
   A. Stop the medication and notify the physician.
   B. Inform the physician that the drug is ineffective.
   C. Instruct the staff to rouse the patient every 30 minutes.
   D. Take safety precautions and continue to assess the patient.

16. The nurse assesses Mr. James to evaluate the effectiveness of baclofen therapy. Which finding suggest therapeutic effectiveness?
   A. Decreased flexor spasms
   B. Increased manual dexterity
   C. Decreased stiffness of gait
   D. Improved residual muscle function

17. To prevent GI distress, the nurse should teach Mr. James to take baclofen:
   A. On an empty stomach
   B. Before meals
   C. With milk or meals
   D. At bedtime

18. Marian Mitchell, age 45, has had multiple sclerosis for two years, but only recently has experienced episodes of severe muscle spasticity. Her physician prescribes dantrolene sodium (Dantrium), 25 mg P.O. daily. Before and during dantrolene therapy, the nurse should expect to monitor which laboratory studies?
   A. Liver function
   B. Creatinine clearance
   C. Red blood count and hemoglobin
   D. White blood count and differential

19. Because Ms. Mitchell has difficulty swallowing, the nurse plans to dissolve the dantrolene in juice. How should the nurse prepare the dantrolene–juice mixture?
   A. Mix the drug with juice at least 1 hour before administration and keep the labeled container in the refrigerator.
   B. Substitute sterile water for juice, because oral dantrolene is unstable when mixed with juice.
   C. Request that the pharmacy send the prescribed drug–juice mixture to the nursing unit.
   D. Mix the drug and juice at the patient's bedside, then administer it immediately.

20. To prevent drug interactions with dantrolene, Ms. Mitchell should avoid which substances?
   A. Alcoholic beverages
   B. Juices that contain acid
   C. Caffeine-rich foods and beverages
   D. Cold preparations that contain antihistamines

21. The physician is likely to discontinue dantrolene therapy if Ms. Mitchell experiences no significant relief of spasticity within which period of time?

    A. 24 hours
    B. 1 to 2 days
    C. 14 to 21 days
    D. 45 days

ANSWERS

Fill in the blank

1. Sodium, calcium, actin, myosin
2. Painful musculoskeletal spasms, spasticity
3. Central nervous system
4. CNS depressants

Matching related elements

5. B
6. A
7. D
8. C

Short answer

9. A spasm is an involuntary muscle contraction that results from a sensory stimulus, such as pain. Spasticity is a motor disorder characterized by increased muscle tone resulting from hyperexcitability of the anterior motor neurons.
10. Trauma, inflammation, anxiety, pain
11. Multiple sclerosis, cerebral palsy, cerebrovascular accident, spinal cord injuries

Multiple choice

12. B. Like the other centrally acting skeletal muscle relaxants, chlorzoxazone acts by CNS depression. These drugs do not relax skeletal muscle directly or depress neuronal conduction, neuromuscular transmission, or muscle excitability.
13. C. Chlorzoxazone may harmlessly discolor urine an orange or purple-red. No special intervention is necessary.
14. C. Baclofen acts in the spinal cord, where it seems to depress neuron activity, decrease the degree and frequency of muscle spasms, and reduce muscle tone.
15. D. The most common adverse reaction to baclofen is transient drowsiness. The nurse should take safety precautions and continue to monitor the patient for any change in level of consciousness.
16. A. Baclofen significantly reduces the number and severity of painful flexor spasms, but does not improve stiff gait, increase manual dexterity, or improve residual muscle function.
17. C. To prevent adverse GI reactions such as nausea, vomiting, and constipation, the patient should take baclofen with meals or milk.

18. A. Because dantrolene may depress liver function or cause idiosyncratic hepatitis (which can be fatal), the nurse should monitor the patient's liver function before and during therapy.

19. D. The nurse should dissolve dantrolene in fruit juice or another liquid immediately before administration. Dantrolene should be reconstituted with sterile water for I.V. administration.

20. A. Dantrolene interacts with CNS depressants, including alcohol, causing increased CNS depression.

21. D. If benefits are not evident in 45 days, dantrolene is discontinued to avoid liver damage.

CHAPTER 7

Antiparkinsonian agents

OBJECTIVES
After studying this chapter, the reader should be able to:
1. Describe the signs, symptoms, and effects of Parkinson's disease.
2. Describe the pharmacokinetics and pharmacodynamics of the antiparkinsonian agents.
3. Identify the major adverse effects of the antiparkinsonian agents.
4. Compare the uses of anticholinergic and dopaminergic agents in treating parkinsonism.
5. Describe the nursing implications of antiparkinsonian agent therapy.

OVERVIEW OF CONCEPTS
Drug therapy is an important part of the treatment for Parkinson's disease, also known as paralysis agitans. Parkinson's disease is a progressive, idiopathic neurologic disorder caused by depletion, degeneration, or destruction of dopamine in the neurons of the brain's basal ganglia. It produces parkinsonism, an involuntary movement disorder characterized by four cardinal features: tremors at rest, akinesia (complete or partial loss of muscle movement), rigidity (increased muscle tone), and disturbances of posture and equilibrium. Parkinsonism also can result from drugs, encephalitis, neurotoxins, trauma, arteriosclerosis, or other neurologic disorders.

Two types of drugs are used to treat parkinsonism: synthetic anticholinergic and dopaminergic agents. (For a summary of representative drugs, see Selected Major Drugs: *Antiparkinsonian agents,* page 100.)

Anticholinergic agents
Anticholinergic agents that are used to treat parkinsonism are classified in three chemical categories: synthetic tertiary amines, phenothiazine derivatives, and antihistamines. The synthetic tertiary amines constitute the largest group, including benztropine mesylate (Cogentin), biperiden hydrochloride (Akineton), biperiden lactate (Akineton Lactate), procyclidine hydrochloride (Kemadrin), and trihexyphenidyl hydrochloride (Artane, Trihexane). The antihistamines diphenhydramine hydrochloride (Benadryl) and orphenadrine citrate (Norflex) constitute the remainder of these anticholinergic agents.

SELECTED MAJOR DRUGS

Antiparkinsonian agents

This chart summarizes the major antiparkinsonian agents currently in clinical use.

DRUG	MAJOR INDICATIONS	USUAL ADULT DOSAGE
Anticholinergic agents		
benztropine mesylate	All forms of parkinsonism, especially in the early stages (alone or with other agents)	0.5 to 1 mg P.O. daily for the first few days, increased by 0.5 mg every few days up to the maintenance dosage of 1 to 2 mg P.O., I.V., or I.M. daily
diphenhydramine hydrochloride	All forms of parkinsonism, especially in the early stages (alone or with other agents)	25 mg P.O. t.i.d., increased gradually to 25 to 50 mg P.O. t.i.d. or q.i.d.; or 10 to 100 mg I.M. or I.V. t.i.d. or q.i.d.
trihexyphenidyl hydrochloride	All forms of parkinsonism, especially in the early stages (alone or with other agents)	1 mg P.O. daily, increased by 2 mg every 3 to 5 days up to 3 to 15 mg t.i.d.
Dopaminergic agents		
levodopa	Parkinsonism, especially control of moderate to severe symptoms in Parkinson's disease (timing of initiation of levodopa therapy is controversial)	0.5 to 1 g P.O. b.i.d., t.i.d., or q.i.d., increased by 100 to 750 mg every 3 to 7 days up to 3 to 6 daily in three or more divided doses
carbidopa-levodopa	Parkinsonism, especially control of moderate to severe symptoms in Parkinson's disease	25 mg carbidopa/250 mg levodopa P.O. t.i.d., increased up to 75/300 to 200/2,000 mg daily in divided doses
pergolide mesylate	Adjunct therapy with levodopa or carbidopa-levodopa to treat Parkinson's disease	Initially, 0.05 mg P.O. daily for 2 days, increased by 0.1 to 0.15 mg daily
selegiline	Adjunct therapy with levodopa or carbidopa-levodopa to treat Parkinson's disease	5 to 10 mg P.O. daily every third day for 12 days, then increased by 0.25 mg daily every third day until therapeutic dosage is reached

Pharmacokinetics

After oral administration, the anticholinergic agents are absorbed almost completely in the gastrointestinal (GI) tract. Although the exact distribution of these drugs is unknown, researchers believe that they cross the blood-brain barrier and penetrate brain tissue because they affect the central nervous system (CNS). Most of these agents are metabolized in the liver and excreted by the kidneys.

For most anticholinergic agents, onset of action occurs within 1 hour, peak concentration is reached in 2 to 4 hours, and duration of action is up to 6 hours. Benztropine is longer acting and has a duration of up to 24 hours.

Pharmacodynamics

Anticholinergic agents sometimes are called parasympatholytics because they antagonize functions that are controlled primarily by the parasympathetic nervous system. In the brain, they counteract the cholinergic activity associated with Parkinson's disease. Their exact mechanism of action is not known, but they probably inhibit cerebral motor centers.

Pharmacotherapeutics

Anticholinergic agents are used to treat all forms of parkinsonism but most commonly are used in the early stages of Parkinson's disease when symptoms are mild and do not have a major impact on the patient's life-style. These agents effectively control sialorrhea (excessive saliva flow) and are about 20% effective in reducing the incidence and severity of akinesia and rigidity.

In the early stages of Parkinson's disease, anticholinergic agents may be used alone or with amantadine; during later stages, with levodopa. No single anticholinergic drug is consistently superior, but a patient may respond more favorably to one agent than to another. Trihexyphenidyl is the most widely used drug of this group, followed by benztropine and diphenhydramine.

Most anticholinergic agents maintain their effectiveness with long-term administration and rarely require dosage adjustment after the proper dosage is reached. However, as the disease advances, anticholinergic agents alone are not effective enough. If any antiparkinsonian agent must be discontinued and replaced with another drug, dosage should be reduced gradually. Abrupt withdrawal of anticholinergic agents can produce confusion, exhaustion, and exacerbation of parkinsonian symptoms.

Drug interactions

A few drugs, such as amantadine, levodopa, and antipsychotic agents, produce significant interactions when used with anticholinergic agents. (For details, see Drug Interactions: *Antiparkinsonian agents,* page 102.)

Adverse drug reactions

Adverse reactions to anticholinergic agents usually are dose-limiting; that is, they increase with the dosage and may limit the amount the patient can take. Most adverse reactions are an extension of the drug's pharmacologic effects. They affect various body systems and structures. (For details, see *Dose-related adverse reactions to the anticholinergics,* page 103.)

Anticholinergic agents also can produce various patient-sensitivity-related adverse reactions, including urticaria and allergic skin rashes that may lead to exfoliation. Diphenhydramine also can produce a photosensitivity reaction, causing burning and redness with minimal exposure.

DRUG INTERACTIONS

Antiparkinsonian agents

The most common interactions occur between anticholinergic agents and drugs that have anticholinergic properties. Other interactions involving antipsychotic drugs may produce serious problems. Among the dopaminergic agents, levodopa, selegiline, and meperidine cause the most serious drug interactions. Other dopaminergic agents are responsible for less serious drug interactions, producing additive toxicities or decreasing the effectiveness of the dopaminergic agent.

DRUG	INTERACTING DRUGS	POSSIBLE EFFECTS
Anticholinergic agents		
benztropine, biperiden, procyclidine, trihexyphenidyl, ethopropazine, diphenhydramine, orphenadrine	amantadine	Increased severity of anticholinergic adverse reactions
	levodopa	Decreased levodopa absorption, possibly leading to worsening of parkinsonian signs and symptoms
	antipsychotic agents (phenothiazines, thiothixene, haloperidol, loxapine)	Decreased anticholinergic effects; decreased antipsychotic effects; increased risk of anticholinergic adverse reactions
	over-the-counter cough or cold preparations, diet aids, or analeptics	Increased anticholinergic effects
	alcohol	Increased central nervous system depression
Dopaminergic agents		
levodopa	pyridoxine (vitamin B_6)	Decreased levodopa effects
	type A monoamine oxidase (MAO) inhibitors, furazolidone	Hypertensive crisis; increased toxic effects of levodopa
	phenytoin, benzodiazepines, papaverine	Decreased levodopa effects
	reserpine	Decreased therapeutic response to levodopa
levodopa, pergolide	antipsychotic agents	Decreased levodopa or pergolide effects
levodopa, amantadine	anticholinergic agents	Increased severity of anticholinergic adverse reactions with amantadine, including adverse effects on mental function; decreased levodopa absorption, possibly leading to worsening of parkinsonian signs and symptoms
selegiline	meperidine	Hypertensive crisis

Dopaminergic agents   Dopaminergic agents include six chemically unrelated drugs: levodopa (Dopar, Larodopa, Levopa), the metabolic precursor to dopamine; carbidopa-levodopa (Sinemet), a combination drug composed of carbidopa and levodopa; amantadine hydrochloride (Symmetrel), an antiviral agent; bromocriptine mesylate (Parlodel), a semisynthetic ergot alkaloid; pergolide mesylate (Permax), a dopamine agonist; and selegiline (Eldepryl), a type B monamine oxidase (MAO) inhibitor.

Pharmacokinetics
After oral administration, dopaminergic agents are absorbed from the GI tract into the bloodstream and are delivered to their site of action in

Dose-related adverse reactions to the anticholinergics

Common dose-related adverse reactions to anticholinergic agents are described below. The nurse may use this as a guide when assessing the patient.

Central nervous system
- Confusion
- Restlessness
- Agitation
- Excitement
- Drowsiness
- Dizziness
- Insomnia

Ocular
- Mydriasis (pupillary dilation)
- Blurred vision
- Photophobia
- Increased intraocular pressure

Oral
- Xerostomia (dry mouth)
- Loss of taste
- Speech difficulty

Cardiovascular
- Tachycardia
- Palpitations

Pulmonary
- Drying of bronchial secretions
- Possible dyspnea

Skin
- Decreased sweating

Gastrointestinal
- Constipation
- Nausea
- Vomiting
- Bloated feeling

Genitourinary
- Urinary hesitancy
- Urine retention

the brain. They are metabolized extensively in various areas of the body and are eliminated by the liver, kidneys, or both.

The onset, peak, and duration of the dopaminergic agents vary widely. So do their therapeutic effects. For example, levodopa produces a short-term improvement that subsides 5 hours after a dose and a long-term improvement with prolonged therapy. Amantadine usually produces therapeutic effects within 2 weeks; if it does not, it should be discontinued. Bromocriptine improves parkinsonian signs 30 to 90 minutes after a single dose.

Pharmacodynamics
Dopaminergic agents act in the brain. They improve motor function by increasing the dopamine concentration or enhancing the neurotransmission of dopamine.

Pharmacotherapeutics
Dopaminergic agents commonly are used to treat patients with severe parkinsonism or those who do not respond to anticholinergic agents. The most effective drug for parkinsonism, levodopa can be given alone or with other drugs. In carbidopa-levodopa, the carbidopa allows more levodopa to be converted to dopamine in the brain. Amantadine may be used alone in the early stages of parkinsonism or with other drugs in

the advanced stages. Bromocriptine is used primarily as an adjunct to levodopa in the later stages of parkinsonism. Pergolide and selegiline also are used as adjuncts to levodopa or carbidopa-levodopa therapy.

Drug interactions

Levodopa is responsible for the most serious interactions with other drugs. Concomitant use of levodopa and a type A MAO inhibitor can cause hypertensive crisis; use of levodopa with meperidine can result in death. Other drugs may decrease the effectiveness of a dopaminergic agent. (For details, see Drug Interactions: *Antiparkinsonian agents,* page 102.)

Dietary amino acids can decrease levodopa's effectiveness by competing with it for absorption from the intestine and slowing its transport to the brain. To prevent this interaction, the patient may need to reduce protein intake or avoid taking levodopa with meals.

Adverse drug reactions

Most adverse reactions to dopaminergic agents are dose-related and occur peripherally or in the CNS. When administered in usual dosages, amantadine and selegiline produce the fewest adverse reactions.

Levodopa commonly produces adverse GI reactions, such as nausea, vomiting, and anorexia. It also can cause orthostatic hypotension and less common cardiovascular effects, such as palpitations, tachycardia, arrhythmias, flushing, and hypertension. When given with levodopa, carbidopa decreases the levodopa dosage, which decreases its adverse GI and cardiovascular reactions. However, carbidopa does not reduce levodopa's CNS effects, which include irritability, confusion, and hallucinations. Other adverse reactions to levodopa include dark-colored urine and sweat, urinary frequency or urine retention, and vision disturbances.

Levodopa withdrawal may cause potentially fatal hyperpyrexia and neuroleptic malignant syndrome. It also may cause hematologic effects, such as leukopenia and granulocytopenia.

The main problem with levodopa is its loss of effectiveness after 3 to 5 years of therapy. The problem takes one of two forms: the on-off phenomenon, characterized by sharp fluctuations in mobility and immobility; or the end-of-dose deterioration, a progressive decrease in the duration of beneficial effects from each dose. The use of smaller, more frequent doses of levodopa and the addition of bromocriptine to the regimen can reduce either problem.

Long-term amantadine therapy may cause skin mottling and ankle edema. It also can produce urine retention, orthostatic hypotension, anorexia, nausea, constipation, and adverse CNS reactions, such as lightheadedness, anxiety, and insomnia.

Bromocriptine may cause nausea, vomiting, orthostatic hypotension, anxiety, dizziness, sedation, and skin changes, especially at the start of therapy or when the dosage exceeds 20 mg/day. It also may cause cardiovascular reactions, such as ankle edema and palpitations, and CNS reactions, such as confusion and hallucinations.

Pergolide commonly produces adverse CNS, GI, and cardiovascular reactions. Selegiline causes relatively mild adverse reactions, primarily in the CNS, GI tract, and musculoskeletal system.

Nursing implications   When caring for a patient receiving an antiparkinsonian agent, the nurse should be aware of the following implications.

- Develop appropriate nursing diagnoses for the patient. (For examples, see Sample Nursing Diagnoses: *Antiparkinsonian agents,* page 106.)
- Do not administer an antiparkinsonian agent to a patient with a condition that contraindicates its use.
- Administer an antiparkinsonian agent cautiously to a patient at risk because of a preexisting condition.
- Monitor the patient closely for adverse reactions to the prescribed antiparkinsonian agent. For example, assess regularly for tachycardia and confusion.
- Notify the physician if the patient experiences adverse reactions.
- Monitor the patient's degree of parkinsonian signs and symptoms, such as akinesia, rigidity, and sialorrhea.
- Notify the physician if the patient experiences any change in parkinsonian signs and symptoms.
- Review the patient's medication history periodically to identify new use of a drug that may interact with the antiparkinsonian agent.
- Teach the patient and family the name, dose, frequency, action, and adverse effects of the prescribed antiparkinsonian agent.
- Advise the patient and family to inform the physician of improvement or worsening of parkinsonian signs and symptoms.
- Advise the patient to notify the physician of adverse reactions.
- Instruct family members to report confusion or mental changes in the patient. Also teach them how to maintain a safe environment to prevent patient injury during periods of confusion.
- Teach the patient not to discontinue long-term antiparkinsonian therapy before consulting the physician.
- Give the patient written instructions about the prescribed antiparkinsonian agent.

Anticholinergic agents
- Auscultate breath sounds at least every 8 hours in a patient with chronic pulmonary disease because secretions may thicken and cause dyspnea during anticholinergic therapy.
- Administer an anticholinergic agent during or shortly after meals to prevent adverse GI reactions.
- Record the patient's fluid intake and output during anticholinergic therapy. Observe for decreased output.

SAMPLE NURSING DIAGNOSES

Antiparkinsonian agents

The following nursing diagnoses address representative problems and etiologies that a nurse may encounter when caring for a patient receiving an antiparkinsonian agent.

- Altered health maintenance related to ineffectiveness of the prescribed antiparkinsonian agent
- Altered protection related to the adverse hematologic effects of an antiparkinsonian agent
- Altered thought processes related to the adverse central nervous system effects of an antiparkinsonian agent
- Altered urinary elimination related to the adverse genitourinary effects of an antiparkinsonian agent
- Constipation related to the adverse gastrointestinal effects of an anticholinergic agent
- High risk for injury related to adverse drug reactions
- High risk for injury related to an interaction between levodopa and food
- High risk for injury related to a preexisting condition that contraindicates the use of an antiparkinsonian agent
- High risk for injury related to a preexisting condition that requires cautious use of an antiparkinsonian agent
- High risk for injury related to drug interactions
- Hyperthermia related to levodopa withdrawal
- Impaired physical mobility related to ineffectiveness of the prescribed antiparkinsonian agent (particularly levodopa)
- Knowledge deficit related to the prescribed antiparkinsonian agent
- Noncompliance related to long-term use of an antiparkinsonian agent
- Urinary retention related to use of an antiparkinsonian agent

---

- Encourage a patient with constipation to ambulate and increase fluid and dietary fiber intake, if possible. Administer a bulk-forming laxative or stool softener, as prescribed. Auscultate the patient's bowel sounds at least every 8 hours to detect signs of GI obstruction.
- Teach the patient to relieve dry mouth by drinking cold beverages, sucking on hard candy, or using a nonprescription saliva substitute. Encourage proper oral hygiene.
- Instruct the patient to use caution when performing tasks that require alertness because adverse reactions, such as drowsiness or blurred vision, may occur. Advise the patient that alcohol may increase the drowsiness.
- Advise the patient to avoid prolonged exposure to high temperatures because an anticholinergic agent increases the risk of heat stroke by reducing sweating.
- Instruct the patient not to take over-the-counter (OTC) cough or cold preparations, diet aids, or analeptics (agents used to stay awake) without consulting the physician because of potential interactions with the prescribed anticholinergic agent.

Dopaminergic agents

- Monitor the patient's blood pressure for orthostatic hypotension or, if the patient is taking an MAO inhibitor, hypertension.
- Expect to reduce the bromocriptine dosage for a patient with hepatic dysfunction because bromocriptine undergoes significant first-pass metabolism in the liver.
- Avoid administering levodopa with meals to prevent a drug-food interaction that may decrease drug absorption.
- Give the second daily dose of amantadine earlier in the evening if the patient experiences insomnia.
- Elevate the patient's legs to help relieve drug-induced edema.
- Advise the patient not to exceed the prescribed daily dose because serious adverse reactions could result.
- Explain the importance of frequent blood pressure measurements, and teach the patient to recognize the symptoms of hypotension (dizziness and light-headedness) and hypertension (headache and vision changes).
- Inform the patient that levodopa may cause harmless discoloration of urine and sweat.
- Instruct the patient who is beginning levodopa therapy that the drug may take several weeks or months to reach its maximum effectiveness.
- Teach the patient taking levodopa about the on-off phenomenon and end-of-dose deterioration.
- Instruct the female patient to notify the physician if she becomes pregnant or breast-feeds during dopaminergic therapy.

STUDY ACTIVITIES

Fill in the blank

1. Parkinson's disease also is known as _____.

2. Parkinson's disease is a progressive, idiopathic neurologic disorder

caused by depletion, degeneration, or destruction of _____ in the neurons of the brain's basal ganglia.

3. Parkinsonism is characterized by four cardinal features:

_____, _____, _____, and _____.

True or false

4. Anticholinergic agents do not cross the blood-brain barrier.
   ☐ True   ☐ False

5. Anticholinergic agents usually are used to treat the late stages of Parkinson's disease.
   ☐ True   ☐ False

6. Abrupt withdrawal of an anticholinergic agent can produce confusion, exhaustion, and exacerbation of parkinsonian symptoms.
□ True □ False

7. Adverse reactions to anticholinergic agents usually are dose-related.
□ True □ False

8. To relieve xerostomia associated with anticholinergic therapy, the nurse should encourage the patient to drink hot liquids.
□ True □ False

9. Of the dopaminergic agents, levodopa is responsible for the most serious interactions with other drugs.
□ True □ False

10. Levodopa should be administered with meals to avoid GI distress.
□ True □ False

11. Most adverse reactions to dopaminergic agents are dose-related.
□ True □ False

Multiple choice

12. Loretta Baxter, age 62, recently was diagnosed with early stage Parkinson's disease, for which she will take trihexyphenidyl hydrochloride (Artane) 3 mg P.O. t.i.d., as prescribed. During the patient-teaching session, the nurse encourages Ms. Baxter to consult her physician before taking which drugs?
   A. OTC cough or cold preparations
   B. Multiple vitamin preparations
   C. Acetaminophen
   D. Antacids

13. The nurse also teaches Ms. Baxter about adverse reactions that are likely to occur during anticholinergic therapy. Which reaction would be omitted from this discussion?
   A. Urinary hesitancy
   B. Blurred vision
   C. Loss of taste
   D. Diarrhea

14. Which statement by Ms. Baxter should alert the nurse to the need for more instruction about trihexyphenidyl therapy?
   A. "Because I want to lose 10 pounds, I'll talk with the doctor before I begin taking a diet aid."
   B. "While at the beach, I'll spend several hours a day sunbathing."
   C. "I'll avoid drinking alcohol because it can cause increased drowsiness."
   D. "I'll brush and floss my teeth several times a day."

15. When Ms. Baxter's disease progresses, trihexyphenidyl no longer effectively manages her signs and symptoms. The physician prescribes levodopa (Dopar) 1 g P.O. t.i.d. How should the nurse expect to begin this new drug regimen?

    A. Begin levodopa therapy and discontinue trihexyphenidyl therapy immediately.

    B. Administer equal doses of each agent for one week and then discontinue trihexyphenidyl.

    C. Begin levodopa therapy while gradually discontinuing trihexyphenidyl therapy.

    D. Provide a loading dose of levodopa, then discontinue trihexyphenidyl.

16. Joseph Small, age 68, takes levodopa (Larodopa) 2 g P.O. t.i.d. for Parkinson's disease. Where does levodopa exerts its action?

    A. Brain

    B. Stomach

    C. Small intestine

    D. Circulatory system

17. When should Mr. Small take the levodopa?

    A. With meals

    B. Just before meals

    C. On an empty stomach

    D. Anytime, but with milk

18. While obtaining a drug history, the nurse discovers that Mr. Small takes an MAO inhibitor. If levodopa is taken with a type A MAO inhibitor, their interaction may cause which effect?

    A. Tachycardia

    B. Hypertensive crisis

    C. Nausea and vomiting

    D. Decreased levodopa effectiveness

19. After 4 years of levodopa therapy, Mr. Small's symptoms worsen as he enters the advanced stage of Parkinson's disease. What is the physician most likely to do?

    A. Maintain the current levodopa regimen.

    B. Substitute diphenhydramine for levodopa.

    C. Discontinue drug therapy because it is ineffective.

    D. Add bromocriptine mesylate as an adjunct to levodopa.

20. Jolene Carter, age 61, takes amantadine hydrochloride (Symmetrel) 100 mg P.O. b.i.d. for Parkinson's disease. During a follow-up visit, she reports difficulty sleeping. What should the nurse advise her to do?

    A. Omit the second daily dose.
    B. Take both daily doses with food.
    C. Take the second dose earlier in the evening.
    D. Ask the physician to change her drug therapy.

ANSWERS

Fill in the blank

1. Paralysis agitans
2. Dopamine
3. Tremors at rest, akinesia, rigidity, disturbances of posture and equilibrium

True or false

4. False. Researchers believe that anticholinergic agents cross the blood-brain barrier and penetrate brain tissue because they affect the CNS.
5. False. Anticholinergics most commonly are used in the early stages of Parkinson's disease when symptoms are mild and do not have a major effect on the patient's lifestyle.
6. True.
7. True.
8. False. To relieve xerostomia (dry mouth), the patient may drink cold beverages, suck on hard candy, or use a nonprescription saliva substitute.
9. True.
10. False. The patient should avoid taking levodopa with meals to prevent a drug-food interaction that may decrease drug absorption.
11. True.

Multiple choice

12. A. When taken with an anticholinergic agent, an OTC cough or cold preparation may increase anticholinergic effects. Anticholinergic agents are not known to interact with vitamins, acetaminophen, or antacids.
13. D. Adverse reactions to anticholinergic agents include urinary hesitancy, blurred vision, loss of taste, and constipation.
14. B. Trihexyphenidyl causes decreased sweating and can increase the patient's risk of heat stroke with prolonged exposure to high temperature. The other responses indicate accurate understanding of possible drug interactions and adverse reactions.
15. C. If any antiparkinsonian agent must be discontinued and replaced with another drug, the dosage should be reduced gradually to avoid withdrawal symptoms. Also, levodopa may take several weeks or months to reach its maximum effectiveness.

16. A. After levodopa is absorbed from the GI tract into the bloodstream, it acts in the brain. There it improves motor function by increasing the dopamine concentration or enhancing dopamine neurotransmission.

17. C. Levodopa competes with dietary amino acids for absorption. Therefore, the patient should avoid taking it with meals to prevent a drug-food interaction that decreases drug absorption.

18. B. Type A MAO inhibitors and furazolidone may cause hypertensive crisis and increase the toxic effects of levodopa. Phenytoin, papaverine, and other drugs may decrease levodopa's effectiveness. Tachycardia, orthostatic hypotension, and nausea and vomiting are possible adverse reactions to levodopa.

19. D. Bromocriptine is used primarily as an adjunct to levodopa in the later stages of parkinsonism. Diphenhydramine usually is used in the early stages. Levodopa therapy alone would not be continued because levodopa loses effectiveness after 3 to 5 years.

20. C. If amantadine causes insomnia, the patient may take the second daily dose earlier in the evening. Other changes in drug therapy are not needed.

CHAPTER 8

Anticonvulsant agents

OBJECTIVES   After studying this chapter, the reader should be able to:

  1. Identify the four factors that physicians consider when choosing a specific anticonvulsant agent for a patient.

  2. Describe the mechanisms of action and the types of seizures treated by hydantoins, barbiturates, iminostilbenes, benzodiazepines, succinimides, and valproic acid.

  3. Describe the important adverse actions associated with each of the six major classes of anticonvulsants.

  4. Describe the nursing implications of anticonvulsant therapy.

OVERVIEW OF CONCEPTS   Anticonvulsant agents are prescribed for long-term management of chronic epilepsy (recurrent seizures) and for short-term management of acute isolated seizures unrelated to epilepsy. Anticonvulsants also are used to prevent seizures after trauma or craniotomy. Selected anticonvulsants are used in the emergency treatment of status epilepticus (a series of rapidly recurring seizures without intervening periods of consciousness).

  Accurate diagnosis of a seizure requires a reliable patient history, careful patient observations, an electroencephalogram, and possibly a computed tomography scan or magnetic resonance imaging. To classify a seizure, health care professionals usually refer to the International Classification of Epileptic Seizures.

  The goal of anticonvulsant therapy is to prevent or control seizures. The agent selected depends on the type of seizure. For many patients, anticonvulsant therapy is lifelong.

  Anticonvulsants fall into six major classes: hydantoins, barbiturates, iminostilbenes, benzodiazepines, succinimides, and valproic acid. (For a summary of representative drugs, see Selected Major Drugs: *Anticonvulsant agents.*)

Hydantoins   Phenytoin (Dilantin), the most commonly prescribed anticonvulsant agent, belongs to the hydantoin class of drugs. Ethotoin (Peganone) and mephenytoin (Mesantoin) also are hydantoin anticonvulsants.

SELECTED MAJOR DRUGS

Anticonvulsant agents

This chart summarizes the major anticonvulsant agents currently in clinical use.

DRUG	MAJOR INDICATIONS	USUAL ADULT DOSAGES
Hydantoins		
phenytoin	Complex partial seizures, tonic-clonic seizures	300 to 400 mg P.O. daily in divided doses if a prompt-acting preparation is used, or in a single dose if a sustained-release preparation is used
Barbiturates		
phenobarbital	Partial seizures, tonic-clonic seizures	100 to 300 mg P.O. daily in divided doses
Iminostilbenes		
carbamazepine	Partial seizures, tonic-clonic seizures	Initially, 200 mg P.O. b.i.d.; gradually increased in small increments up to 400 mg t.i.d. until desired response is obtained
Benzodiazepines		
clonazepam	Absence (petit mal) seizures; atypical absence, atonic, and myoclonic seizures	Initially, 1.5 mg P.O. daily in three divided doses, increased by 0.5- to 1-mg increments every 3 days, as needed, up to a maximum of 20 mg. daily
Succinimides		
ethosuximide	Absence seizures	Initially, 250 mg P.O. b.i.d.; for maintenance, 20 to 40 mg/kg P.O. daily; highly individualized
Valproic acid		
valproate sodium, divalproex sodium	Absence, myoclonic, and tonic-clonic seizures	15 mg/kg P.O. daily, up to a maximum of 60 mg/kg daily; dosages are highly individualized and should be divided if they exceed 250 mg daily

Pharmacokinetics

Phenytoin is absorbed slowly, distributed rapidly, and highly protein-bound. It is metabolized by hepatic microsomal enzymes and is excreted as metabolites in the urine, breast milk, and tears. Mephenytoin is absorbed rapidly after oral administration. Mephenytoin and ethotoin are protein-bound, metabolized by the liver, and excreted in the urine.

Phenytoin metabolism is dose-dependent, and displays saturation kinetics. At a certain drug concentration, the hepatic enzymes that metabolize phenytoin become saturated. When this occurs, further increases in drug concentration demonstrate disproportionate increases in plasma concentration. Therefore, incremental dosage increases must be made cautiously.

After oral administration, phenytoin has a variable onset of action that ranges from 30 minutes to 2 hours. Its peak concentration and duration of action also vary greatly. Mephenytoin and ethotoin have a rapid onset of action and achieve peak concentration levels in 2 to 4 hours. Of the hydantoins, mephenytoin has the longest duration of action.

Pharmacodynamics

Hydantoins appear to act in the motor cortex, where they stabilize nerve cells against hyperexcitability and inhibit the spread of seizure activity. Phenytoin also exerts significant effects on excitable tissues outside the central nervous system (CNS) and exhibits antiarrhythmic properties. It decreases the force of myocardial contractions, suppresses ectopic pacemaker activity, improves atrioventricular conduction depressed by digitalis glycosides, and increases the effective refractory period. It also may inhibit effective insulin release.

Pharmacotherapeutics

Phenytoin is the most commonly prescribed anticonvulsant because of its clinical efficacy and relatively low toxicity. It is one of the drugs of choice to treat complex partial and tonic-clonic seizures. Mephenytoin and ethotoin sometimes are prescribed as adjunct therapy for patients who are refractory to, or intolerant of, other anticonvulsants. Mephenytoin is used primarily for partial and tonic-clonic seizures; ethotoin, for complex partial and tonic-clonic seizures.

Drug interactions

All three hydantoins can interact with a wide variety of drugs. (For details, see Drug Interactions: *Anticonvulsant agents.*)

Adverse drug reactions

The adverse effects of hydantoins involve the central nervous, cardiovascular, gastrointestinal (GI), and hematopoietic systems as well as cosmetic effects. The adverse reactions presented here relate to phenytoin and ethotoin; mephenytoin may produce more serious blood dyscrasias, including aplastic anemia.

In the CNS, adverse reactions reflect the drug's concentration in the blood. At concentrations of 25 to 30 mcg/ml, reactions include drowsiness, dizziness irritability, headache, restlessness, nystagmus, and diplopia; at 30 to 40 mcg/ml, ataxia, lethargy, and asterixis; and at 40 to 50 mcg/ml, decreased consciousness and coma.

The major adverse GI reactions include nausea, vomiting, epigastric pain, and anorexia. Adverse cardiovascular reactions are depressed atrial and ventricular conduction and, in toxic states, ventricular fibrillation. With intravenous (I.V.) administration, cardiovascular effects include bradycardia, hypotension, and potential cardiac arrest. The primary hematopoietic reaction is a folic acid deficiency that can cause microcytic anemia.

Cosmetic toxicity includes gingival hyperplasia, hirsutism, and facial coarsening. Other adverse reactions include hyperglycemia, glycosuria, and osteomalacia. Hypersensitivity reactions typically are manifested as pruritus, fever, arthralgia, and a measles-like rash.

DRUG INTERACTIONS

Anticonvulsant agents

The following chart lists drug interactions that may occur with anticonvulsant agents. (*Note:* Because the hydantoins interact with many drugs, this chart lists only the interactions that have major to moderate clinical significance.)

DRUG	INTERACTING DRUGS	POSSIBLE EFFECTS
Hydantoins		
phenytoin, ethotoin, mephenytoin	cimetidine, disulfiram, isoniazid, sulfonamides	Increased toxic effects of phenytoin
	oral anticoagulants	Increased serum phenytoin concentration if phenytoin therapy begins first; transient increase in anticoagulant effects, followed by decreased anticoagulant effects if oral anticoagulant therapy begins first
	phenobarbital	Decreased phenytoin concentration or increased phenytoin concentration (less common)
	diazoxide	Decreased phenytoin effects
	levodopa	Decreased levodopa effects
	chloramphenicol	Increased toxic effects of phenytoin; decreased chloramphenicol effect
	amiodarone	Increased phenytoin concentration; decreased efficacy of amiodarone
	corticosteroids, doxycycline, methadone, metyrapone, oral contraceptives, quinidine, mexiletine	Decreased efficacy of both drugs
	theophylline	Decreased efficacy of phenytoin and theophylline
	thyroid hormone	Increased metabolism of thyroid hormone
	valproic acid	Transient decrease in phenytoin concentration or increased phenytoin concentration
	cyclosporine	Decreased cyclosporine absorption; decreased serum concentration of cyclosporine
	digitoxin	Decreased digitoxin effects
Barbiturates		
phenobarbital, mephobarbital, primidone	hydantoins	Increased toxic effects of barbiturates
	beta blockers (metoprolol, propranolol), corticosteroids, doxycycline, oral anticoagulants, oral contraceptives, quinidine, phenothiazines, tricyclic antidepressants	Decreased effects of both drugs
	chloramphenicol	Decreased chloramphenicol effects; decreased phenobarbital metabolism

continued

DRUG INTERACTIONS

Anticonvulsant agents *(continued)*

DRUG	INTERACTING DRUGS	POSSIBLE EFFECTS
Barbiturates *(continued)*		
phenobarbital, mepho-barbital, primidone *(continued)*	methoxyflurane	Increased methoxyflurane metabolism
	central nervous system (CNS) depressants (antianxiety agents, sedative-hypnotics, most narcotic analgesics, and alcohol)	Additive effects, resulting in increased sedative toxicity
	valproic acid	Decreased hepatic metabolism of phenobarbital
	metronidazole	Increased metronidazole metabolism
	digitoxin	Decreased digitoxin effects
	theophylline	Increased theophylline metabolism, resulting in decreased serum theophylline concentration
	cyclosporine	Decreased plasma cyclosporine concentration
Iminostilbenes		
carbamazepine	erythromycin, isoniazid, propoxyphene, troleandomycin, cimetidine	Increased toxic effects of carbamazepine
	doxycycline, theophylline, warfarin	Decreased efficacy of doxycycline, theophylline, and warfarin through increased breakdown by the liver
	lithium	Neurotoxicity
	oral contraceptives	Decreased efficacy of oral contraceptives
Benzodiazepines		
clonazepam, clorazep-ate, diazepam	CNS depressants	Increased sedative and other CNS effects, possibly causing motor skill impairment and respiratory depression; possible lethal effect, especially with high doses; changes in seizures, especially in frequency or severity
	cimetidine	Increased sedation, increased CNS depression
	oral contraceptives	Decreased benzodiazepine metabolism
Succinimides		
ethosuximide, methsuximide, phensuximide	hydantoins	Decreased hydantoin metabolism
	carbamazepine	Decreased succinimide concentration
Valproic acid		
valproate sodium, divalproex sodium	anticoagulants	Decreased platelet aggregation, causing prolonged bleeding
	phenobarbital	Decreased phenobarbital metabolism

Barbiturates The long-acting barbiturate phenobarbital (Luminal) is used widely in the long-term treatment of epilepsy and selectively in the treatment of status epilepticus. Mephobarbital (Mebaral), also a long-acting agent, is used occasionally as an anticonvulsant. Primidone (Mysoline), a drug that is chemically related to the barbiturates, also is used to treat chronic epilepsy.

Pharmacokinetics
Barbiturates are absorbed slowly but well from the GI tract. They are protein-bound to varying degrees and are distributed well throughout the body. After metabolism in the liver, metabolites and unchanged drug are excreted in the urine. Phenobarbital and primidone also are excreted in breast milk.

Pharmacodynamics
Barbiturates limit seizure activity by increasing the threshold for motor cortex stimuli. They exhibit this anticonvulsant action at subhypnotic doses. Therefore, they usually do not produce addiction when used to treat epilepsy.

Pharmacotherapeutics
These anticonvulsants are effective in treating partial, tonic-clonic, and febrile seizures when used alone or with other anticonvulsants. Although I.V. phenobarbital is used to treat status epilepticus, it exhibits a delayed onset of action. Mephobarbital is used when a patient cannot tolerate the adverse effects of phenobarbital. Primidone is used primarily with other anticonvulsants but may be considered the drug of choice for complex partial seizures. As controlled substances, phenobarbital and mephobarbital are Schedule IV drugs.

Drug interactions
Phenobarbital interacts with many drugs, usually altering their metabolic rate. Mephobarbital and primidone produce similar interactions because they are metabolized to phenobarbital. (For details, see Drug Interactions: *Anticonvulsant agents,* pages 115 and 116.)

Adverse drug reactions
Barbiturate anticonvulsants cause many adverse reactions, ranging from minor to serious. Barbiturate toxicity results primarily in adverse CNS reactions. Significant GI reactions, blood dyscrasias, and emotional or psychiatric reactions also may occur.

The most common dose-related CNS effects include drowsiness, lethargy, and dizziness; nystagmus, confusion, and ataxia occur with large doses. Adverse GI reactions include nausea and vomiting. Folate deficiencies and osteomalacia secondary to the induction of vitamin D metabolism also may occur.

I.V. phenobarbital can cause laryngospasm, respiratory depression, and hypotension secondary to decreased cardiac output. Signs of overdose include respiratory depression, pupillary constriction, oliguria, hypothermia, circulatory collapse, and pulmonary edema. Primidone also may cause acute psychoses, alopecia, impotence, and osteomalacia.

All three barbiturates can produce a hypersensitivity rash. Paradoxical excitement in geriatric patients and children and hyperkinetic behavior in children may occur.

Iminostilbenes

The iminostilbene derivative carbamazepine (Tegretol) acts as an anticonvulsant for partial and generalized tonic-clonic seizures and mixed seizure types. It also exhibits sedative, anticholinergic, antidepressant, muscle relaxant, antiarrhythmic, antidiuretic, and neuromuscular transmission-inhibiting actions.

Pharmacokinetics
Carbamazepine is absorbed slowly and erratically from the GI tract and distributed rapidly to all tissues. Metabolism occurs in the liver, and the drug is excreted in the urine. A small amount crosses the placenta and some is excreted in breast milk. Onset of action varies, with peak serum concentration level occurring after 2 to 8 hours.

Pharmacodynamics
Carbamazepine's anticonvulsant action may occur because it inhibits the spread of seizure activity or neuromuscular transmission in general and because it increases the discharge of noradrenergic neurons.

Pharmacotherapeutics
Carbamazepine is used to treat generalized tonic-clonic seizures and simple and complex partial seizures in adults and children. Its efficacy makes carbamazepine a drug of choice for treating these seizures. Use of the drug also relieves pain of trigeminal neuralgia (tic douloureux).

Drug interactions
Interactions between carbamazepine and other drugs may decrease the steady-state levels of either drug. (For details, see: Drug Interactions: *Anticonvulsant agents,* pages 115 and 116.)

Adverse drug reactions
Dose-related adverse reactions to carbamazepine include drowsiness, diplopia, ataxia, vertigo, nystagmus, headaches, tremors, and dry mouth. Because carbamazepine is related to the tricyclic antidepressants, it can produce many of the same adverse reactions, including heart failure, hypertension or hypotension, syncope, arrhythmias, and myocardial infarction. The drug's mild anticholinergic action may result in urine retention, constipation, and increased intraocular pressure. Long-term use can cause water intoxication.

Occasionally, the drug may cause urticaria, Stevens-Johnson syndrome, aplastic anemia (rare), granulocytopenia, thrombocytopenia, or leukopenia.

Benzodiazepines

The three benzodiazepines that provide anticonvulsant effects are clonazepam (Klonopin), clorazepate dipotassium (Tranxene), and parenteral diazepam (Valium). Only clonazepam is recommended for long-term treatment of epilepsy. Diazepam is used to treat acute status epilepticus; clorazepate, partial seizures as an adjunct. (For the major discussion of benzodiazepines, see Chapter 10, Antianxiety, sedative, and hypnotic agents.)

Pharmacokinetics

The benzodiazepines are absorbed rapidly and almost completely from the GI tract, but are distributed at different rates and can cross the placenta. They are metabolized in the liver and excreted as metabolites primarily in the urine, but also in breast milk. Based on the rate of excretion, benzodiazepines are classified as long-acting, intermediate-acting, or short-acting. The onset of action for benzodiazepines is 5 to 10 minutes, with peak concentration level occurring after 60 to 90 minutes.

Pharmacodynamics

The benzodiazepines provide anticonvulsant, antianxiety, sedative-hypnotic and muscle relaxant effects. They may produce their anticonvulsant effects by increasing the availability of the inhibitory neurotransmitter gamma-aminobutyric acid (GABA) to brain neurons.

Pharmacotherapeutics

Clonazepam is used to treat absence (petit mal), atypical absence, atonic, and myoclonic seizures. Clorazepate is used with other drugs to treat partial seizures. I.V. diazepam is used routinely as the initial control for status epilepticus. Because it is distributed so rapidly, diazepam provides only short-term effects of less than 1 hour. Consequently, a long-acting anticonvulsant, such as phenytoin or phenobarbital, also must be given during diazepam therapy. All three benzodiazepine anticonvulsants are Schedule IV drugs.

Drug interactions

Benzodiazepines can interact with CNS depressants, cimetidine, and oral contraceptives. (For details, see Drug Interactions: *Anticonvulsant agents,* pages 115 and 116.)

Adverse drug reactions

The dose-related adverse reactions to benzodiazepine are primarily neurologic and include drowsiness, confusion, ataxia, weakness, dizziness, nystagmus, vertigo, syncope, dysarthria, headache, tremors, and a glassy-eyed appearance. These reactions diminish as therapy continues. Cardiorespiratory depression may occur with high doses and with I.V. diazepam. Geriatric patients are particularly susceptible to confusion, ataxia, and paradoxical excitement. Idiosyncratic reactions to benzodiazepines include a rash and acute hypersensitivity reactions.

Succinimides

Three drugs from the succinimide class are used to treat absence (petit mal) seizures: ethosuximide (Zarontin), methsuximide (Celontin), and phensuximide (Milontin).

Pharmacokinetics

The succinimides are absorbed well from the GI tract and distributed widely throughout the body. They are metabolized by the liver and excreted in the urine. Their onset of action occurs rapidly, and the peak concentration occurs within 4 hours.

Pharmacodynamics

The succinimides reduce the frequency of absence seizures by depressing nerve transmission in the motor cortex and increasing the seizure threshold.

Pharmacotherapeutics

Ethosuximide is the drug of choice for treating absence seizures, but the dosage needed to control seizures is highly individualized. Methsuximide is prescribed less frequently because of its high incidence of toxicity. However, it is used alone for absence seizures and with other anticonvulsants for complex partial seizures. Phensuximide rarely is used because it is less effective. If used alone for mixed types of seizures, any succinimide may increase the frequency of tonic-clonic seizures.

Drug interactions

The succinimides may interact with hydantoins and carbamazepine. (For details, see Drug Interactions: *Anticonvulsant agents,* pages 115 and 116.)

Adverse drug reactions

The succinimides produce adverse GI, neurologic, hematologic, and genitourinary reactions. In the GI tract, adverse reactions include nausea, vomiting, weight loss, abdominal pain, constipation, and diarrhea. The neurologic complaints are ataxia, dizziness, drowsiness, headache, euphoria, restlessness, irritability, lethargy, and confusion. Psychosis and suicidal ideation occur rarely. Hematologic effects may include eosinophilia, leukopenia, thrombocytopenia, granulocytopenia, and aplastic anemia. Adverse genitourinary reactions are urinary frequency, hematuria, and albuminuria. Hypersensitivity reactions to succinimides also can occur.

Valproic acid

Valproic acid is unrelated structurally to the other anticonvulsants. The two major drugs in the valproic acid class are valproate sodium (Depakene) and divalproex sodium (Depakote).

Pharmacokinetics

The absorption rate of valproic acid depends on the dosage form. Valproate sodium is converted rapidly to valproic acid in the stomach. After absorption, valproic acid is highly protein-bound, metabolized in the liver, and excreted in urine. It readily crosses the placental barrier and also appears in breast milk.

The onset of action of valproic acid occurs in 20 to 30 minutes. The peak serum concentration level of valproate sodium occurs in 1 to 4 hours; of divalproex sodium, in 3 to 5 hours. The time needed to reach peak concentration is longer if the patient has a full stomach or receives enteric-coated tablets.

Pharmacodynamics

The mechanism of action for valproic acid remains unknown, but it may be related to the increased availability of the inhibitory neurotransmitter GABA to brain neurons.

Pharmacotherapeutics

Valproic acid is prescribed for long-term treatment of absence, myoclonic, and tonic-clonic seizures. It also is administered rectally for status epilepticus refractory to other anticonvulsants. Valproic acid must be used cautiously in a young child or a patient receiving multiple anticonvulsants because of possible fatal hepatotoxicity. This risk limits the use of valproic acid as a drug of choice for seizure disorders.

Drug interactions

Valproic acid can interact with anticoagulants and phenobarbital. It also can produce a false-positive result on urine ketone tests. (For details, see Drug Interactions: *Anticonvulsant agents,* pages 115 and 116.)

Adverse drug reactions

Most adverse reactions associated with valproic acid are tolerable and dose-related; however, rare fatal hepatotoxicity has occurred. The drug is not prescribed routinely because of the possibility of hepatotoxicity.

Dose-related reactions affect the CNS and GI tract. Adverse CNS reactions include sedation, drowsiness, dizziness, ataxia, headache, decreased alertness, and muscle weakness. Adverse GI reactions include nausea, vomiting, appetite changes, and diarrhea or constipation.

Adverse hematologic reactions include inhibited platelet aggregation and prolonged bleeding time. A drug rash may occur, as may hyperammonemia in a patient with normal liver function. The use of valproic acid also may produce blood dyscrasias, such as anemia, leukopenia, and thrombocytopenia.

Other anticonvulsants   Three other drugs are used less commonly to treat seizure disorders.

Acetazolamide (Diamox) sometimes is used as adjunct or intermittent therapy in absence, partial, and generalized tonic-clonic seizures. The mechanism of action is unknown, but the drug may suppress the spread of paroxysmal discharges. Hypokalemia and metabolic acidosis represent potentially serious effects associated with its use. The nurse should caution a patient receiving this drug to visit the physician frequently for electrolyte studies.

Trimethadione (Tridione) and paramethadione (Paradione) are used only occasionally as sole or adjunct treatment for refractory absence seizures. They cause significant GI and CNS toxicity and are less effective than the succinimides.

Magnesium sulfate prevents or controls seizures by blocking neuromuscular transmission. The drug is used primarily as an anticonvulsant in preeclampsia or eclampsia. It also is used to treat hypomagnesemic seizures.

Nursing implications

When caring for a patient who is receiving an anticonvulsant agent, the nurse should be aware of the following implications.
- Develop appropriate nursing diagnoses for the patient. (For examples, see Sample Nursing Diagnoses: *Anticonvulsant agents.*)
- Do not administer an anticonvulsant to a patient with a condition that contraindicates its use.
- Administer an anticonvulsant cautiously to a patient at risk because of a preexisting condition.
- Keep oxygen, suction, and resuscitation equipment nearby when administering an I.V. anticonvulsant.
- Monitor the patient for adverse reactions and notify the physician as needed.
- Monitor the frequency of seizure activity and notify the physician if the patient displays continued seizure activity.
- Monitor the serum concentration of the anticonvulsant.
- Take safety precautions if the patient exhibits adverse CNS reactions.
- Teach the patient and family the name, dose, frequency, action, and adverse effects of the prescribed anticonvulsant.
- Instruct the patient not to alter the prescribed drug regimen and to notify the physician if seizure control deteriorates.
- Alert the patient that abrupt discontinuation of the prescribed drug could precipitate seizures or status epilepticus.
- Advise the patient to check all prescription refills to ensure that the drug preparation is the same brand as the previous preparation.
- Advise the patient to avoid hazardous activities until the dosage and adverse reactions become stabilized.
- Teach the family how to care for the patient during a seizure.
- Emphasize the importance of frequent follow-up care and offer information about voluntary community organizations that provide information and support.

Hydantoins
- Administer I.V. phenytoin at a rate not to exceed 50 mg/minute (or 50 mg/3 minutes in a geriatric patient with heart disease) because of its cardiotoxicity. Monitor blood pressure, pulse, and respirations every 5 minutes during administration and every 15 minutes thereafter until the patient is stable. If blood pressure decreases during drug administration, reduce the infusion rate.

SAMPLE NURSING DIAGNOSES

Anticonvulsant agents

The following nursing diagnoses address representative problems and etiologies that a nurse may encounter when caring for a patient who is receiving an anticonvulsant agent.

- Activity intolerance related to anticonvulsant-induced weakness
- Altered health maintenance related to hydantoin-induced hyperglycemia
- Altered health maintenance related to ineffectiveness of the prescribed anticonvulsant
- Altered nutrition; less than body requirements, related to weight loss resulting from succinimide therapy
- Altered oral mucous membrane related to hydantoin-induced gingival hyperplasia
- Altered protection related to anticonvulsant-induced hematologic dysfunction
- Altered protection related to drowsiness, dizziness, and other adverse CNS effects of an anticonvulsant
- Altered thought processes related to the adverse central nervous system (CNS) effects of an anticonvulsant
- Altered urinary elimination related to the adverse genitourinary effects of a succinimide
- Body image disturbance related to cosmetic toxicity resulting from hydantoin use
- Constipation related to the adverse gastrointestinal (GI) effects of an anticonvulsant
- Decreased cardiac output related to anticonvulsant-induced arrhythmias
- Diarrhea related to the adverse GI effects of a succinimide
- Fluid volume deficit related to the adverse GI effects of an anticonvulsant
- Fluid volume excess related to water intoxication with long-term use of carbamazepine
- Health-seeking behaviors related to possible interaction between an anticonvulsant and an oral contraceptive
- High risk for injury related to adverse drug reactions
- High risk for injury related to a preexisting condition that contraindicates the use of an anticonvulsant
- High risk for injury related to a preexisting condition that requires cautious use of an anticonvulsant
- Impaired gas exchange related to barbiturate-induced respiratory depression or laryngospasm
- Impaired physical mobility related to the sedative effects of an anticonvulsant
- Knowledge deficit related to the prescribed anticonvulsant
- Noncompliance related to long-term use of the prescribed anticonvulsant
- Sensory or perceptual alterations (visual) related to the adverse CNS effects of an anticonvulsant
- Sexual dysfunction related to primidone-induced impotence
- Urinary retention related to the adverse genitourinary effects of carbamazepine

---

- Infuse 0.9% sodium chloride solution after I.V. phenytoin, as prescribed, to minimize vein irritation.
- Do not mix I.V. phenytoin with any other drug.
- Avoid intramuscular (I.M.) injections because phenytoin precipitates in muscle tissue.
- Administer an oral hydantoin with meals to minimize GI distress.
- Use only sustained-release capsules for once-daily dosing of phenytoin. Do not exchange these capsules with chewable tablets

because the capsules and tablets provide different strengths of phenytoin.

- Shake suspension preparations well before pouring to ensure exact drug measurement.
- Discontinue phenytoin immediately and notify the physician if a skin rash develops.
- Expect to administer vitamin K to a neonate whose mother received a hydantoin during pregnancy.
- Monitor the patient regularly for signs and symptoms of hyperglycemia and obtain blood glucose levels at least once daily.
- Encourage the patient to express feelings about body image if adverse cosmetic reactions occur. Also explore ways to mask undesired cosmetic changes.
- Recommend use of an additional or different contraceptive method to the female patient who is taking an oral contraceptive and a hydantoin.
- Encourage meticulous tooth brushing and daily flossing.
- Remind the patient to notify the dentist about hydantoin therapy.
- Inform the patient that phenytoin may cause harmless pink, red, or red-brown discoloration of urine.

Barbiturates

- Do not exceed a rate of 60 mg/minute when giving an I.V. barbiturate.
- Do not use a cloudy solution when giving an I.V. barbiturate.
- Administer a reconstituted solution within 30 minutes of preparation.
- Monitor respirations and blood pressure frequently when administering an I.V. barbiturate.
- Be sure the patient actually swallows an oral barbiturate.
- Reassure the patient that the prescribed barbiturate is not addictive when used in subhypnotic doses for seizures.
- Advise the patient to keep the drug in a secure place to prevent others from taking the drug.
- Inform the male patient that impotence may occur.

Iminostilbenes

- Obtain complete blood cell counts with differential, as prescribed.
- Take bleeding and infection precautions if the patient develops thrombocytopenia or leukopenia.
- Check for early signs of urine retention.
- Monitor for signs of fluid excess: auscultate breath sounds every 4 hours, assess for dependent edema, and weigh the patient daily. Also limit the patient's fluid and salt intake. Notify the physician if the patient develops signs of fluid excess, such as shortness of breath.
- Instruct the patient to take carbamazepine with meals to decrease GI distress and enhance absorption.

Benzodiazepines

- Monitor the patient's vital signs during I.V. administration of diazepam.
- Administer I.V. diazepam no faster than 5 mg/minute in adults and over at least 3 minutes in children.
- Do not mix I.V. diazepam with other drugs in the same syringe. Give direct I.V. push only.
- Verify compliance in a patient taking an oral benzodiazepine to detect hoarding.
- Store an oral benzodiazepine in a light-resistant container at room temperature.

Succinimides

- Note that methsuximide contains FD&C Yellow Dye No. 5, which can cause allergic reactions in a patient with asthma or allergies to aspirin or other nonsteroidal anti-inflammatory drugs.
- Administer a succinimide with meals to prevent adverse GI reactions.
- Store the succinimide away from heat. Shake all suspensions well before administration.
- Take bleeding precautions if thrombocytopenia occurs and infection precautions if leukopenia occurs.
- Weigh the patient daily and monitor for nutritional deficiencies. Notify the physician if weight loss exceeds 5 lb (2.2 kg).
- Encourage the patient to eat a well-balanced diet. Administer nutritional supplements as prescribed.
- Inform the patient that phensuximide may cause harmless pink, red, or red-brown discoloration of urine.

Valproic acid

- Monitor liver function and coagulation studies periodically.
- Take bleeding precautions, such as avoiding I.M. and subcutaneous (S.C.) injections if possible and having the patient use a soft-bristle toothbrush and an electric razor.
- Administer valproic acid with meals to minimize adverse GI reactions.
- Advise the patient to keep the flavorful red syrup out of the reach of children.
- Instruct the patient to swallow each capsule whole because the free drug can irritate the GI mucosa.
- Alert the patient with diabetes that the drug may produce a false-positive result on a urine ketone test.
- Remind the patient to report immediately any signs of bleeding so that platelet function can be assessed.
- Teach the patient to recognize the signs and symptoms of hepatotoxicity and to contact the physician immediately if any occur.
- Instruct the patient to inform the physician of valproic acid therapy before any surgery, including dental surgery.

STUDY ACTIVITIES

Matching related elements

Match the anticonvulsant on the left with its description on the right.

1. ___ Phenytoin   **A.** Drug that may cause hepatotoxicity

2. ___ Phenobarbital   **B.** Agent related to tricyclic antidepressants

3. ___ Carbamazepine   **C.** Drug used to treat status epilepticus only

4. ___ Diazepam   **D.** Most commonly used anticonvulsant

5. ___ Ethosuximide   **E.** Drug with delayed onset that is used in status epilepticus

6. ___ Valproic acid   **F.** Drug of choice for treating absence seizures

Multiple choice

7. Sally Reese, age 24, has just received a prescription for phenytoin 300 mg P.O. q.i.d. to treat tonic-clonic seizures. Her medication history reveals that she currently takes an oral contraceptive. When teaching Ms. Reese about her drug therapy, what should the nurse do?
   A. Discuss the signs and symptoms of hypoglycemia.
   B. Teach the patient how to check her blood pressure at home.
   C. Recommend the use of an additional or different contraceptive method.
   D. Advise her to take phenytoin on an empty stomach to enhance absorption.

8. The nurse also teaches Ms. Reese about adverse drug reactions. Which of the following are common adverse reactions to phenytoin?
   A. Alopecia and skin wrinkling
   B. Tachycardia and hypertension
   C. Vitamin and mineral deficiencies
   D. Drowsiness and gingival hyperplasia

9. In the future, if Ms. Reese needs a higher phenytoin dosage, the drug should be increased gradually in increments. Why?
   A. Phenytoin has a variable onset of action.
   B. Phenytoin is excreted in urine as a metabolite.
   C. Phenytoin metabolism displays saturation kinetics.
   D. Phenytoin stabilizes nerve cells against hyperexcitability.

10. Libby Bates, age 29, takes phenobarbital for long-term treatment of tonic-clonic seizures. When caring for Ms. Bates, the nurse should give which of these nursing diagnoses top priority?
    A. Body image disturbance related to barbiturate-induced cosmetic toxicity
    B. High risk for injury related to barbiturate-induced sedation
    C. High risk for infection related to bone marrow depression
    D. Constipation related to barbiturate use

11. The nurse also should teach Ms. Bates to avoid which substance?
   A. Alcohol
   B. Shellfish
   C. Artificial sweeteners
   D. Nitrate-containing foods

12. Bob Peebles, age 48, is admitted to the emergency department with status epilepticus. The nurse can expect the physician to order which I.V. drug first?
   A. Diazepam (Valium)
   B. Phenytoin (Dilantin)
   C. Clonazepam (Klonopin)
   D. Carbamazepine (Tegretol)

13. What is the drug of choice for treating absence seizures?
   A. Magnesium sulfate
   B. Valproic acid
   C. Acetazolamide
   D. Ethosuximide

14. Sam Watson, age 63, takes valproic acid 30 mg/kg P.O. daily. Which assessments should the nurse perform regularly for Mr. Watson?
   A. Blood pressure measurements
   B. Blood sugar and urine ketone testing
   C. Liver function and coagulation studies
   D. Neurologic checks and electrocardiograms (ECGs)

15. Which statement by Mr. Watson should alert the nurse to the need for further patient teaching?
   A. "I'll check to see that my prescriptions are refilled with the same drug."
   B. "I'll notify the physician if my seizure control gets worse."
   C. "I plan to follow the prescribed drug regimen."
   D. "I plan to avoid taking milk in any form."

True or false

16. Phenytoin is the most commonly prescribed anticonvulsant because of its clinical efficacy and relatively low toxicity.
   ☐ True   ☐ False

17. Hydantoin use may cause facial coarsening.
   ☐ True   ☐ False

18. Barbiturates produce their anticonvulsant effects by increasing the availability of GABA to brain neurons.
   ☐ True   ☐ False

19. Phenobarbital, mephobarbital, and clonazepam are Schedule IV drugs.
   ☐ True   ☐ False

20. An I.V. barbiturate should be used within 30 minutes of reconstitution.
☐ True   ☐ False

21. Carbamazepine generally increases the effects of other drugs the patient may be receiving.
☐ True   ☐ False

22. The usual adult dosage of phenytoin is 10 to 20 mg I.V. push.
☐ True   ☐ False

23. Benzodiazepines do not interact with CNS depressants.
☐ True   ☐ False

24. Methsuximide contains FD&C Yellow Dye No. 5, which can cause allergic reactions in a patient who is allergic to aspirin.
☐ True   ☐ False

ANSWERS

Matching related elements

1. D
2. E
3. B
4. C
5. F
6. A

Multiple choice

7. C. Phenytoin can interact with oral contraceptives, decreasing their efficacy. It also may cause hyperglycemia and GI distress, which can be relieved by taking the drug with meals.

8. D. Phenytoin commonly causes adverse CNS reactions, such as drowsiness; cosmetic effects, such as gingival hyperplasia, hirsutism, and facial coarsening; adverse cardiovascular reactions, such as bradycardia and hypotension; and folic acid deficiency.

9. C. When hepatic enzymes become saturated, increases in drug concentration produce disproportionate increases in plasma phenytoin concentration. Although phenytoin has a variable onset of action, undergoes excretion in urine as a metabolite, and stabilizes nerve cells against hyperexcitability, these characteristics do not explain the need for cautious dosage increases.

10. B. The most common dose-related CNS effects of barbiturates include drowsiness, lethargy, and dizziness, which can make the patient susceptible to injury. Barbiturates do not cause cosmetic toxicity, bone marrow depression, or constipation.

11. A. Phenobarbital can interact with alcohol and other CNS depressants, producing increased sedative toxicity.

12. A. I.V. diazepam is used routinely as the initial control for status epilepticus. Carbamazepine, phenytoin, and clonazepam are used to treat different types of seizures.

13. D. Although acetazolamide and valproic acid may be used in patients with absence seizures, ethosuximide is the drug of choice for this indication. Magnesium sulfate is used primarily for seizures in preeclampsia and eclampsia.

14. C. Adverse reactions to valproic acid include fatal hepatotoxicity and hematologic effects, such as inhibited platelet aggregation and prolonged bleeding time. Valproic acid does not affect blood pressure, blood sugar, urine ketones, or ECG readings.

15. D. Milk or milk products have no effect on the action of anticonvulsants. The patient should check prescription refills carefully, notify the physician if seizure control deteriorates, and follow the drug regimen exactly as prescribed.

True or false

16. True.

17. True.

18. False. Barbiturates limit seizure activity by increasing the threshold for motor cortex stimuli.

19. True.

20. True.

21. False. Carbamazepine generally decreases the steady-state levels of other drugs.

22. False. The usual dosage of phenytoin is 300 to 400 mg P.O. daily in divided doses.

23. False. CNS depressants interact with benzodiazepines, enhancing sedative and other CNS depressant effects.

24. True.

CHAPTER 9

Nonnarcotic analgesic, antipyretic, and nonsteroidal anti-inflammatory agents

OBJECTIVES After studying this chapter, the reader should be able to:

1. Describe the pharmacodynamics of the salicylates, acetaminophen, and nonsteroidal anti-inflammatory drugs (NSAIDs).

2. Compare the therapeutic uses of the salicylates, acetaminophen, and NSAIDs.

3. Contrast the drug interactions associated with the salicylates, acetaminophen, and NSAIDs.

4. Compare the adverse reactions to salicylates, acetaminophen, and NSAIDs.

5. Describe the nursing implications of therapy with salicylates, acetaminophen, or NSAIDs.

OVERVIEW OF CONCEPTS This chapter discusses drugs used to control pain, decrease inflammation, and reduce body temperature. These drugs include salicylates (the most widely used), the para-aminophenol derivative acetaminophen, NSAIDs, and the urinary tract analgesic phenazopyridine hydrochloride. (For a summary of representative drugs, see Selected Major Drugs: *Nonnarcotic analgesic agents, antipyretic agents, and NSAIDs.*)

Salicylates Salicylates possess analgesic, antipyretic, and anti-inflammatory properties. They usually cost less than other analgesics and most are readily available without a prescription. In fact, many over-the-counter (OTC) medications for pain, colds, and influenza contain salicylates along with other agents.

Salicylates include aspirin (ASA, Bayer Timed-Release, Empirin), choline magnesium trisalicylate (Trilisate), choline salicylate (Arthropan), diflunisal (Dolobid), salsalate (Disalcid, Mono-Gesic), and sodium salicylate (Pabalate). Despite the recent development of new

SELECTED MAJOR DRUGS

Nonnarcotic analgesic agents, antipyretic agents, and NSAIDs

The following chart features the major salicylates, para-aminophenol derivatives, and nonsteroidal anti-inflammatory drugs (NSAIDs) currently in clinical use.

DRUG	MAJOR INDICATIONS	USUAL ADULT DOSAGES
Salicylates		
aspirin	Mild to moderate pain, fever	325 to 650 mg P.O. every 3 to 4 hours
	Dysmenorrhea	650 mg P.O. every 4 to 6 hours, beginning 1 or 2 days before the onset of menses and continuing until the second or third day of menses
	Rheumatic fever	975 to 1,300 mg P.O. four to six times daily until fever and inflammation subside
	Rheumatoid arthritis	3.6 to 5.4 g P.O. daily in divided doses
	Transient ischemic attacks	325 mg P.O. q.i.d. or 650 mg P.O. b.i.d.
diflunisal	Mild to moderate musculoskeletal pain	Initially, 500 to 1,000 mg P.O., followed by 250 to 500 mg every 8 to 12 hours, not to exceed 1,500 mg daily
	Osteoarthritis	500 to 1,000 mg P.O. daily in two divided doses
Para-aminophenol derivatives		
acetaminophen	Headache, mild to moderate pain, fever, osteoarthritis	325 to 650 mg P.O. or rectally every 3 to 4 hours, as needed, not to exceed 4 g daily
NSAIDs		
diclofenac	Ankylosing spondylitis	100 to 125 mg P.O. daily in 25-mg doses q.i.d. with an additional 25 mg P.O. h.s. as needed
	Osteoarthritis	100 to 150 mg P.O. daily in two or three divided doses
	Rheumatoid arthritis	150 to 200 mg P.O. daily in two to four divided doses
ibuprofen	Mild to moderate pain	200 to 400 mg P.O. every 4 to 6 hours
	Dysmenorrhea	400 mg P.O. every 4 hours, as needed, as soon as pain begins
	Osteoarthritis, rheumatoid arthritis	400 to 800 mg P.O. t.i.d. or q.i.d.
indomethacin	Rheumatoid arthritis, osteoarthritis, ankylosing spondylitis	25 to 50 mg P.O. t.i.d., increased to a maximum of 200 mg daily
	Acute gouty arthritis	50 mg P.O. t.i.d.
	Bursitis, tendinitis	75 to 150 mg P.O. in three or four divided doses
naproxen	Osteoarthritis, rheumatoid arthritis, ankylosing spondylitis	250 to 375 mg P.O., in morning and evening, increased to a maximum of 1,000 mg daily, as needed
	Tendinitis, bursitis, dysmenorrhea, mild to moderate pain	Initially, 500 mg P.O., then 250 mg P.O. every 6 to 8 hours, as needed
tolmetin	Osteoarthritis, rheumatoid arthritis	Initially, 400 mg P.O. t.i.d. (including a dose upon arising and at bedtime), increased as needed, up to a maximum of 1,800 mg daily given in four divided doses

products, aspirin remains the cornerstone of anti-inflammatory drug therapy.

Pharmacokinetics

Absorption of salicylates occurs partly in the stomach but primarily in the upper part of the small intestine. Although absorption usually occurs within 30 minutes, the rate depends on the dosage form, gastric and intestinal pH, presence of food or antacids in the stomach, and gastric emptying time. Salicylates are distributed widely throughout the body.

The liver metabolizes salicylates into several metabolites. As the salicylate dose increases, some metabolic pathways become saturated and cannot metabolize the drug completely. When this happens, metabolism shifts to alternate pathways, resulting in increased formation of toxic metabolites. Decreasing the salicylate dose, even slightly, usually decreases the toxic metabolite formation. The kidneys excrete salicylate metabolites and some unchanged drug.

Pharmacodynamics

Salicylates produce analgesia and reduce inflammation by inhibiting prostaglandin synthesis. (The inflammatory process stimulates prostaglandin formation and release.) They produce their antipyretic effect by stimulating the hypothalamus, which leads to vasodilation and increased diaphoresis. Aspirin inhibits platelet aggregation by interfering with the production of thromboxane A_2, which is necessary for platelet clumping.

Pharmacotherapeutics

Salicylates are primarily used to relieve pain and reduce fever. However, they cannot effectively relieve visceral pain or severe pain from trauma. These drugs have little or no effect on normal body temperature but cause a marked fall if body temperature is elevated.

Salicylates are used to reduce inflammation in rheumatic fever and rheumatoid arthritis. The main guideline for salicylate therapy is to use the lowest dose that provides relief.

Drug interactions

Because salicylates are highly protein-bound, they may interact with many other protein-bound drugs. They also may interact with other drugs. (For details, see Drug Interactions: *Nonnarcotic analgesic agents, antipyretic agents, and NSAIDs.*)

Adverse drug reactions

The most common adverse reactions to salicylates involve the gastrointestinal (GI) system: gastric distress, nausea, and vomiting. Other reactions may include respiratory alkalosis and metabolic acidosis, hearing problems, and hypersensitivity reactions.

Salicylates also may cause toxicity. Mild toxicity produces hearing loss, dizziness, drowsiness, headache, hyperventilation, confusion, nau-

DRUG INTERACTIONS

Nonnarcotic analgesic agents, antipyretic agents, and NSAIDs

Drug interactions involving salicylates and nonsteroidal anti-inflammatory drugs (NSAIDs) are common and sometimes severe. Interactions with acetaminophen are less common and tend to decrease acetaminophen absorption.

DRUG	INTERACTING DRUGS	POSSIBLE EFFECTS
Salicylates		
aspirin, choline magnesium trisalicylate, choline salicylate, diflunisal, salsalate, sodium salicylate	alcohol	Increased ulcerogenic effects, leading to gastrointestinal bleeding
	oral anticoagulants, heparin	Increased anticoagulant effects, increasing the risk of bleeding
	corticosteroids	Decreased plasma salicylate concentrations and increased ulcerogenic effects
	methotrexate	Increased methotrexate effects and toxicity, causing pancytopenia
	probenecid, sulfinpyrazone	Decreased uricosuric effects
	antacids	Urine alkalinization, leading to reduced renal tubular reabsorption
	oral hypoglycemic agents (sulfonylureas)	Increased hypoglycemic effects
	zidovudine	Inhibited zidovudine metabolism, possibly causing toxicity
	alkalinizing agents	Increased salicylate excretion, if salicylate dosage exceeds 50 mg/kg/day
	spironolactone	Reduced spironolactone effects
	acetazolamide	Acetazolamide intoxication
Para-aminophenol derivatives		
acetaminophen	alcohol (chronic use)	Increased risk of hepatotoxicity
	charcoal, cholestyramine, colestipol	Decreased acetaminophen effects
NSAIDs		
diclofenac, fenoprofen, flurbiprofen, ibuprofen, indomethacin, ketoprofen, meclofenamate, mefenamic acid, naproxen, naproxen sodium, piroxicam, tolmetin	corticosteroids	Increased ulcerogenic effects
	captopril, enalapril, lisinopril	Decreased antihypertensive effects of both drugs
	loop diuretics	Decreased antihypertensive and diuretic effects of both drugs
	oral anticoagulants	Increased anticoagulant effects
	lithium	Increased lithium concentration
	beta-adrenergic blockers	Hypertension
	methotrexate	Increased methotrexate toxicity
	zidovudine	Decreased zidovudine metabolism, possibly causing toxicity
sulindac	oral anticoagulants	Increased hypoprothrombinemia, causing bleeding

(continued)

DRUG INTERACTIONS

Nonnarcotic analgesic agents, antipyretic agents, and NSAIDs *(continued)*

DRUG	INTERACTING DRUGS	POSSIBLE EFFECTS
NSAIDs *(continued)*		
phenylbutazone	oral anticoagulants	Decreased anticoagulant metabolism
	oral hypoglycemic agents (sulfonylureas)	Increased hypoglycemic effects
	methotrexate	Methotrexate toxicity
	phenytoin	
indomethacin	nonamphetamine anorexigenic agents	Hypertension
ketorolac	salicylates	Increased plasma concentration of unbound ketorolac

sea, vomiting, reduced visual acuity, diaphoresis, thirst, tinnitus, and diarrhea. Severe toxicity causes electroencephalogram changes, hypoglycemia, skin eruptions, respiratory alkalosis leading to metabolic acidosis, central nervous system (CNS) depression, seizures, coma, and hemorrhagic tendencies.

In a child with a varicella infection or flulike symptoms, salicylates are contraindicated because they may lead to Reye's syndrome, a potentially fatal disorder that causes encephalopathy and fatty infiltration of the internal organs.

Para-aminophenol derivatives

Acetaminophen (Datril, Panadol, Tylenol), an analgesic and antipyretic agent, is the only para-aminophenol derivative available in the United States. Physicians frequently choose this OTC drug over a salicylate for a patient with a history of GI bleeding, ulcers, or salicylate hypersensitivity.

Pharmacokinetics

Acetaminophen is absorbed rapidly and completely from the GI tract and is absorbed well from the rectal mucosa. It is distributed widely in body fluids and readily crosses the placenta. After acetaminophen undergoes metabolism by hepatic enzymes, it is excreted by the kidneys and, in small amounts, in breast milk. The drug's peak concentration level occurs in 10 to 60 minutes, and its duration ranges from 3 to 5 hours.

Pharmacodynamics

Acetaminophen offers significant analgesic and antipyretic actions, but does not act on inflammation or platelet function. The drug may produce analgesia by inhibiting prostaglandin synthesis. It may reduce fever through its direct action on the heat-regulating center in the hypothalamus.

Pharmacotherapeutics

Acetaminophen offers an alternative for aspirin-intolerant patients and those who do not need an analgesic with anti-inflammatory properties. It is the drug of choice to treat fever and flulike symptoms in children. Acetaminophen reduces fever and relieves headache and general pain, but does not affect intense or visceral pain. Acetaminophen can be used to treat osteoarthritis because this form of arthritis does not have an inflammatory component.

Drug interactions

Few significant interactions occur between acetaminophen and other drugs. (For details, see Drug Interactions: *Nonnarcotic analgesic agents, antipyretic agents, and NSAIDs,* pages 133 and 134.)

Adverse drug reactions

Most patients tolerate acetaminophen well. Unlike the salicylates, acetaminophen rarely causes gastric irritation or hemorrhagic tendencies.

Similar to an overdose, chronic use of high doses of acetaminophen can cause hypoglycemia, methemoglobinemia, leukopenia, kidney damage, and renal failure. Ingestion of 10 grams or more of acetaminophen may cause a severe adverse reaction: hepatotoxicity that leads to coagulation defects, cyanosis, and vascular collapse. Although hepatotoxicity signs and symptoms appear with 24 hours, they mimic common illnesses in many cases and permit the real problem to go undetected.

Nonsteroidal anti-inflammatory drugs

NSAIDs have anti-inflammatory, analgesic, and antipyretic properties. Their anti-inflammatory action is equal to that of aspirin.

The NSAIDs are derived from many different chemical sources. Fenoprofen calcium (Nalfon), flurbiprofen (Ansaid), ibuprofen (Advil, Motrin, Nuprin), ketoprofen (Orudis), naproxen (Naprosyn), and naproxen sodium (Anaprox) are propionic acid derivatives (fenamates). Meclofenamate (Meclomen) and mefenamic acid (Ponstel) are anthranilic acid derivatives. Phenylbutazone (Butazolidin) is a pyrazolone derivative. Piroxicam (Feldene) is an oxicam derivative. Indomethacin (Indocin) and ketorolac tromethamine (Toradol) are indoleacetic acid derivatives. Tolmetin sodium (Tolectin) is a pyrrole acetic acid derivative. Sulindac (Clinoril) is an indeneacetic acid derivative. Diclofenac sodium (Voltaren) is a phenylacetic acid derivative.

Pharmacokinetics

All NSAIDs, except ketorolac, are absorbed from the GI tract, metabolized in the liver, and excreted by the kidneys. They differ widely in their onset, duration, and half-life. Their analgesic effects always precedes their antirheumatic effects, which may take up to 1 to 3 weeks to appear.

Pharmacodynamics

Unlike corticosteroids, NSAIDs do not reduce inflammation by stimulating the pituitary-adrenal system. Instead, they inhibit prostaglandin activity. They also retard polymorphonuclear leukocyte motility and affect the release and activity of lysosomal enzymes.

Pharmacotherapeutics

NSAIDs are used primarily to reduce inflammation and secondarily to relieve pain. Although the NSAIDs share similar indications and mechanisms of action, patient response may vary greatly. The choice of an NSAID must be made empirically. If one drug does not produce a therapeutic effect in 2 to 4 weeks, it is discontinued and another NSAID is tried. This procedure is repeated until relief is obtained.

Indications for NSAIDs include ankylosing spondylitis; moderate to severe rheumatoid arthritis; osteoarthritis in the large joints; osteoarthritis with inflammation; and acute gouty arthritis. Because of their toxicity, indomethacin and phenylbutazone usually are used after other drugs have proven ineffective.

Drug interactions

A wide variety of protein-bound and other drugs can interact with NSAIDs. (For details, see Drug Interactions: *Nonnarcotic analgesic agents, antipyretic agents, and NSAIDs,* pages 133 and 134.)

Adverse drug reactions

All NSAIDs produce similar adverse reactions that rarely require discontinuation of therapy. Generally, NSAIDs are tolerated better than salicylates or corticosteroids. However, phenylbutazone has a high incidence of adverse reactions, especially in geriatric patients.

The most common adverse reactions to NSAIDs are GI tract disturbances, such as abdominal pain, bleeding, diarrhea, nausea, ulcerations, and hepatotoxicity. Adverse CNS reactions include drowsiness, headache, dizziness, confusion, tinnitus, vertigo, and depression. Adverse renal reactions may be cystitis, hematuria, and kidney necrosis. The CNS and renal reactions are more common in geriatric patients. Blurred vision, decreased visual acuity, and corneal deposits also may occur with NSAID use.

Phenylbutazone has an unusually high incidence of adverse reactions, which include gastric ulceration and hemorrhage, vertigo, insomnia, and the combination of sodium and water retention, increased plasma volume, and decreased urine volume—which may lead to peripheral edema, acute pulmonary edema, and cardiac symptoms.

NSAIDs can cause hypersensitivity reactions, evidenced by skin rashes, urticaria, angioedema, hypotension, dyspnea, and an asthmalike syndrome.

Urinary tract analgesic   Phenazopyridine hydrochloride (Pyridium), an azo dye, produces a local analgesic effect on the urinary tract. It relieves the pain, burning, urgency, and frequency associated with urinary tract infections, usually within 24 to 48 hours.

The usual adult dosage is 100 to 200 mg P.O. t.i.d. after meals for 2 days only. The drug colors the urine orange or red, which may cause a permanent stain on any fabric it touches.

Nursing implications   When caring for a patient who is receiving a nonnarcotic analgesic agent, antipyretic agent, or NSAID, the nurse should be aware of the following implications.

- Develop appropriate nursing diagnoses for the patient. (For examples, see Sample Nursing Diagnoses: *Nonnarcotic analgesic agents, antipyretic agents, and NSAIDs,* page 138.)
- Do not administer a nonnarcotic analgesic, antipyretic, or NSAID to a patient with a condition that contraindicates its use.
- Administer a nonnarcotic analgesic, antipyretic, or NSAID cautiously to a patient at risk because of a preexisting condition.
- Observe the patient for adverse reactions and notify the physician as needed.
- Teach the patient and family the name, dose, frequency, action, and adverse effects of the nonnarcotic analgesic, antipyretic, or NSAID.
- Advise the patient to seek medical advice if the fever or pain lasts more than 3 days.

Salicylates

- Do not administer aspirin to a patient in the third trimester of pregnancy.
- Do not administer diflunisal for antipyretic therapy.
- Question any prescription of sodium salicylate for a patient with hypertension or on a sodium-restricted diet. Advise such a patient not to use effervescent aspirin products, which have a high sodium content.
- Take the patient's vital signs at least every 4 hours. If respirations increase in rate and depth, notify the physician; the patient may be compensating for or developing an acid-base imbalance.
- Administer the salicylate with at least 8 ounces of liquid.
- Monitor for hypoglycemia in a patient with diabetes who takes a salicylate and a sulfonylurea.
- Expect to discontinue aspirin 1 week before major surgery to reduce the risk of bleeding.
- Observe for early signs and symptoms of salicylate toxicity.
- Observe for these signs of bleeding if the patient receives concurrent anticoagulant therapy: gingival bleeding, black or tarry stools, blood in the urine, petechiae, bruises, or prolonged bleeding from a cut. Report these signs to the physician.
- Encourage the patient to report hearing changes because bilateral hearing loss of 30 to 40 decibels can occur with prolonged use of salicylates. Reassure the patient that hearing usually returns to normal within 2 weeks after discontinuation of salicylate therapy.

SAMPLE NURSING DIAGNOSES

Nonnarcotic analgesic agents, antipyretic agents, and NSAIDs

The following nursing diagnoses address representative problems and etiologies that a nurse may encounter when caring for a patient who is receiving a nonnarcotic analgesic agent, antipyretic agent, or nonsteroidal anti-inflammatory drug (NSAID).
• Altered protection related to hemorrhagic tendencies associated with salicylate use
• Diarrhea related to the adverse gastrointestinal effects of an NSAID
• Fluid volume excess related to sodium and water retention caused by an NSAID
• High risk for fluid volume deficit related to diaphoresis and adverse GI reactions caused by a salicylate
• High risk for injury related to adverse drug reactions
• High risk for injury related to a preexisting condition that contraindicates the use of a nonnarcotic analgesic, antipyretic, or NSAID
• High risk for injury related to a preexisting condition that requires cautious use of a nonnarcotic analgesic, antipyretic, or NSAID
• Impaired tissue integrity related to gastric ulceration caused by salicylate or NSAID use
• Knowledge deficit related to the prescribed nonnarcotic analgesic, antipyretic, or NSAID
• Pain related to ineffectiveness of the prescribed nonnarcotic analgesic, antipyretic, or NSAID
• Sensory or perceptual alterations (auditory) related to salicylate-induced hearing problems

• Discourage the use of salicylates—even "children's aspirin"—in a patient under age 18.
• Advise an aspirin-sensitive patient to read labels carefully on OTC drugs because many contain aspirin or another salicylate.
• Inform the patient that buffered aspirin contains too little antacid to reduce gastric irritation. Suggest that the patient take plain aspirin with food, milk, or 1 to 2 teaspoons of antacid to prevent GI distress more effectively at less expense.
• Inform the patient that concurrent use of alcohol and a salicylate increases the risk of bleeding.

Para-aminophenol derivatives
• Obtain a baseline liver function test before beginning acetaminophen therapy and monitor liver function test results periodically during therapy, as prescribed.
• Withhold acetaminophen and notify the physician if the patient develops a rash, unexplained fever, or angioedema.
• Inform the patient that high doses or unsupervised long-term use of this drug can cause liver damage and that excessive alcohol ingestion may increase this risk.
• Teach the patient that acetaminophen is safe and effective only when used as directed on the label. Because this drug is readily available OTC and is advertised widely, many patients assume that it is nontoxic. This assumption can lead to accidental overdose when a patient attempts to relieve severe or persistent headache, fever, or pain.

Nonsteroidal anti-inflammatory drugs

- Monitor the results of the patient's liver and kidney function tests, hemoglobin counts, and ophthalmic examinations during long-term NSAID therapy.
- Administer the prescribed NSAID with food or milk to decrease GI irritation, unless directed otherwise.
- Monitor the patient for bleeding during concurrent therapy with an NSAID and an anticoagulant.
- Evaluate the degree of pain relief during NSAID therapy. Note that 2 to 4 weeks may elapse before the prescribed NSAID provides relief. Expect to administer a different NSAID if the pain is not relieved within 4 weeks.
- Monitor the patient's blood pressure frequently during concurrent therapy with an NSAID and captopril, enalapril, lisinopril, or a loop diuretic. Expect to adjust the antihypertensive dosage or substitute sulindac for the interacting NSAID.
- Question any prescription for medications that contain alcohol, aspirin, or other drugs that may cause GI irritation and bleeding during concomitant NSAID therapy.
- Teach the patient to avoid high-sodium foods, limit fluid, and report any sudden, unexplained weight gain because fluid retention can occur.
- Advise the patient with aspirin hypersensitivity to avoid ibuprofen.

STUDY ACTIVITIES **True or false**

1. Salicylates produce their anti-inflammatory effect by stimulating prostaglandin synthesis.
   ☐ True   ☐ False

2. A child with varicella infection or flulike symptoms should take half of the usual pediatric dosage of aspirin to prevent Reye's syndrome.
   ☐ True   ☐ False

3. An aspirin-intolerant patient may use high-dose acetaminophen to reduce platelet aggregation.
   ☐ True   ☐ False

4. The physician may prescribe acetaminophen to treat osteoarthritis.
   ☐ True   ☐ False

5. Acetaminophen and NSAIDs can cause hepatotoxicity.
   ☐ True   ☐ False

Multiple choice

6. Adam Brown, age 45, has been taking aspirin (Empirin) 3.6 g P.O. daily in divided doses for rheumatoid arthritis. Which statement by him suggests the need for further patient teaching?
   A. "If I notice any ringing in my ears, I'll report it right away."
   B. "I'll list prescription and OTC drugs when I'm asked about my medications."
   C. "I plan to avoid alcohol while I'm taking aspirin to decrease the risk of GI bleeding."
   D. "If I run out of aspirin, I can substitute any other pain medication until I get more aspirin."

7. Five days ago, Joyce Greenaway, age 56, began taking ibuprofen 800 mg P.O. q.i.d. for rheumatoid arthritis. Now she states that she is not getting the pain relief she expected. What should the nurse tell her?
   A. Double the ibuprofen dosage and take 1,600 mg q.i.d.
   B. Expect to achieve pain relief after 2 to 4 weeks of therapy.
   C. Avoid the generic form of this medication because it is not a strong as the brand-name form.
   D. Ask the physician to switch her to phenylbutazone, the drug of choice for rheumatoid arthritis.

8. Ms. Greenaway asks the nurse how ibuprofen relieves pain. What is the analgesic mechanism of action for NSAIDs?
   A. Adrenal stimulation
   B. Pituitary stimulation
   C. Leukocyte infiltration
   D. Prostaglandin inhibition

9. The nurse teaches Ms. Greenaway to observe for adverse reactions to ibuprofen. What is the most common adverse reaction?
   A. Dyspnea
   B. Pruritus
   C. GI disturbances
   D. Orange or red urine

10. David Thomas, age 58, is admitted with back pain. His medical history indicates that he has had a cholecystectomy, myocardial infarction, and hemorrhoidectomy. His medications include aspirin 325 mg P.O. q.i.d. For Mr. Thomas, what is the most likely purpose of aspirin therapy?
   A. Relief of mild arthritis
   B. Control of frequent headaches
   C. Prevention of recurrence of myocardial infarction
   D. Relief of aspirin intolerance with small doses of aspirin

11. The nurse teaches Mr. Thomas about adverse reactions to aspirin. Which instruction could help him minimize adverse GI reactions?
  A. Take the medication with food or milk.
  B. Take the medication 1 hour before meals.
  C. Crush the pill and dissolve it in juice.
  D. Take the medication 2 hours after meals.

12. Ellen Barstow, age 66, has osteoarthritis. Her physician has recommended acetaminophen (Tylenol) 650 mg P.O. every 4 hours p.r.n. to relieve pain. What is the maximum recommended daily dose of acetaminophen?
  A. 2 grams
  B. 4 grams
  C. 6 grams
  D. 10 grams

13. The nurse assesses Ms. Barstow's medication history to detect potential drug interactions. Which drug could increase the risk of hepatotoxicity during acetaminophen therapy?
  A. Antacid
  B. Cholestyramine
  C. Alcohol (chronic use)
  D. Narcotic (chronic use)

Short answer
14. Why is acetaminophen preferred for treating mild pain in a patient who is receiving an oral anticoagulant?

_____

15. Aspirin may cause what two types of hearing problems?

_____

16. Which analgesic is used to relieve the pain associated with urinary tract infections?

_____

   NSAIDs can produce adverse reactions in the CNS, GI system, renal system, and eyes. Which reactions occur in each of these areas? (Name at least two for each body system.)
17. CNS

_____

18. GI system

_____

19. Renal system

_____

20. Eyes

ANSWERS

True or false

1. False. Salicylates produce analgesia and reduce inflammation by inhibiting prostaglandin synthesis.

2. False. In a child with a varicella infection or flulike symptoms, salicylates are contraindicated because they may lead to Reye's syndrome.

3. False. Acetaminophen is an effective analgesic and antipyretic agent, but it has no effect on inflammation or platelet function.

4. True.

5. True.

Multiple choice

6. D. Other pain medication may not have anti-inflammatory properties. The other comments are appropriate for a patient on aspirin therapy.

7. B. NSAIDs may take up to 2 to 4 weeks of therapy to relieve symptoms.

8. D. NSAIDs inhibit prostaglandin activity, retard polymorphonuclear leukocyte motility, and affect the release and activity of lysosomal enzymes.

9. C. GI disturbances are the most common adverse reaction to NSAIDs. Other adverse reactions commonly affect the CNS, renal system, and eyes.

10. C. Salicylates can inhibit platelet clumping, which may prevent thrombus formation and recurrence of myocardial infarction.

11. A. To reduce gastric irritation, the patient should take aspirin with food, milk, or 1 to 2 teaspoons of antacid.

12. B. The recommended maximum daily dose for adults is 4 grams.

13. C. Chronic alcohol intake increases the risk of hepatotoxicity during acetaminophen therapy. Cholestyramine may reduce acetaminophen absorption. Antacids and narcotics do not interact with acetaminophen.

Short answer

14. Salicylates and NSAIDs increase the anticoagulant effect of oral anticoagulants.

15. Hearing loss, tinnitus

16. Phenazopyridine hydrochloride (Pyridium)

17. Drowsiness, headache, dizziness, confusion, tinnitus, vertigo, depression

18. Abdominal pain, bleeding, diarrhea, nausea, ulcerations, hepatotoxicity

19. Cystitis, hematuria, kidney necrosis

20. Blurred vision, decreased visual acuity, corneal deposits

CHAPTER 10

Antianxiety, sedative, and hypnotic agents

OBJECTIVES

After studying this chapter, the reader should be able to:

1. Describe the basic similarities and differences between antianxiety, sedative, and hypnotic agents.

2. Discuss the typical sleep cycle.

3. Describe the major types of anxiety disorders and sleep disorders.

4. Compare the pharmacokinetic properties of the benzodiazepines, barbiturates, nonbenzodiazepines-nonbarbiturates, and buspirone.

5. Contrast the mechanism of action of the benzodiazepines with that of barbiturates.

6. Discuss the clinical indications for the major drugs used as antianxiety, sedative, and hypnotic agents.

7. Describe significant adverse reactions to benzodiazepines, barbiturates, nonbenzodiazepines-nonbarbiturates, and buspirone.

8. Describe how alcohol and over-the-counter products function as sleep aids.

9. Describe the nursing implications of antianxiety, sedative, or hypnotic therapy.

OVERVIEW OF CONCEPTS

With dosage adjustments, many of the drugs discussed in this chapter can be used as antianxiety agents, sedatives, and hypnotics. Only a few are used solely to reduce anxiety or induce sedation or sleep.

Antianxiety agents (anxiolytics) include benzodiazepines, buspirone hydrochloride, and barbiturates. They are among the most commonly prescribed drugs in the United States and are used to treat anxiety disorders, which affect 7% to 18% of the population.

Three main classes of drugs are used as sedatives and hypnotics: benzodiazepines, barbiturates, and nonbenzodiazepines-nonbarbiturates. Sedatives reduce activity or excitement, calming a patient. Some drowsiness commonly accompanies their use. Hypnotics are sedatives given in large doses to induce a state resembling natural sleep. (For a summary of representative drugs, see Selected Major Drugs: *Antianxiety, sedative, and hypnotic agents,* pages 144 and 145.)

SELECTED MAJOR DRUGS

Antianxiety, sedative, and hypnotic agents

The following chart summarizes the major antianxiety, sedative, and hypnotic agents currently in clinical use.

DRUG	MAJOR INDICATIONS	USUAL ADULT DOSAGES
Benzodiazepines		
alprazolam	Anxiety associated with depression	0.025 to 0.5 mg P.O. t.i.d., increased as tolerated, up to a maximum of 4 mg/day in divided doses
diazepam	Anxiety	2 to 10 mg P.O. b.i.d. to q.i.d.
	Alcohol withdrawal	10 mg P.O. t.i.d. or q.i.d. for 24 hours, then decreased to 5 mg t.i.d. or q.i.d.
	Skeletal muscle relaxation	2 to 10 mg P.O. t.i.d. or q.i.d.
	Status epilepticus	5 to 10 mg slow I.V. push, repeated every 10 to 15 minutes up to a maximum of 30 mg
flurazepam	Hypnotic for insomnia	15 to 30 mg P.O. h.s.
lorazepam	Sedative before surgery	0.05 mg/kg (up to a maximum of 4 mg) I.M. 2 hours before operative procedure
	Hypnotic for insomnia from anxiety or transient situational stress, anxiety disorders	2 to 4 mg P.O. h.s.
quazepam	Hypnotic for insomnia	15 mg P.O. h.s. until the response is measured; then decreased to 7.5 mg, if possible
temazepam	Hypnotic for insomnia	15 to 30 mg P.O. h.s.
triazolam	Hypnotic for insomnia	0.125 to 0.25 mg P.O. h.s.
Barbiturates		
amobarbital	Sedative for anxiety and tension Hypnotic for insomnia	30 to 50 mg P.O. or I.M. b.i.d. or t.i.d. 65 to 200 mg P.O. or I.M. h.s.
aprobarbital	Daytime sedative	40 mg P.O. t.i.d.
	Hypnotic	40 to 160 mg P.O. h.s.
mephobarbital	Daytime sedative	32 to 100 mg P.O. t.i.d. or q.i.d.
pentobarbital	Anxiety	20 mg P.O. t.i.d. or q.i.d.
	Daytime sedative	20 to 40 mg P.O. b.i.d. to q.i.d.
	Sedative before surgery	150 to 200 mg P.O. to I.M.
	Hypnotic for insomnia	100 mg P.O., 120 to 200 mg rectal, or 100 to 200 mg I.M.
phenobarbital	Anxiety	30 to 120 mg P.O. daily in two or three divided doses
	Daytime sedative	15 to 30 mg P.O. b.i.d. to q.i.d.
	Sedative before surgery	100 to 200 mg I.M. 60 to 90 minutes before surgery
	Hypnotic for insomnia	100 to 320 mg P.O. or I.M. h.s.

SELECTED MAJOR DRUGS

Antianxiety, sedative, and hypnotic agents *(continued)*

DRUG	MAJOR INDICATIONS	USUAL ADULT DOSAGES
Barbiturates *(continued)*		
secobarbital	Daytime sedative	30 to 50 mg P.O. t.i.d. to q.i.d., or 120 to 200 mg rectally
	Sedative before surgery	200 to 300 mg P.O. 1 to 2 hours before surgery
	Hypnotic for insomnia	100 to 200 mg P.O., 120 to 200 mg rectally, or 100 to 200 mg I.M. h.s.
Buspirone		
buspirone	Anxiety	5 mg P.O. t.i.d., increased by 5 mg every 2 to 3 days, as needed, up to a maximum of 60 mg/day
Nonbenzodiazepines-nonbarbiturates		
chloral hydrate	Daytime sedative	250 mg P.O. or 325 mg rectally t.i.d. after meals
	Hypnotic for insomnia	0.5 to 1 g P.O. or rectally 15 to 30 minutes before bedtime
ethchlorvynol	Daytime sedative	200 mg P.O. b.i.d. or t.i.d.
	Hypnotic for insomnia	0.5 to 1 g P.O. h.s.
glutethimide	Hypnotic for insomnia	250 to 500 mg P.O. h.s.
methyprylon	Hypnotic for insomnia	200 to 400 mg P.O. h.s.
paraldehyde	Sedative	5 to 10 ml P.O. or rectally
	Hypnotic for insomnia	10 to 30 ml P.O. or rectally h.s.

Anxiety disorders

Two main types of anxiety disorders exist: nonphobic and phobic. Nonphobic anxieties include generalized anxiety disorders, obsessive-compulsive disorder, and panic disorders. Phobic anxieties can take many forms, such as phobias of crowds and heights.

An anxiety disorder may be a primary medical condition or may occur secondary to another medical or social problem. The goal of treatment is to relieve the symptoms, which include nervousness, tension, tremors, tachycardia, diaphoresis, palpitations, and gastrointestinal (GI) and urinary complaints.

Sleep and sleep disorders

Sleep is an active state of unconsciousness from which a person can be awakened with appropriate stimulus. When sleeping, a person passes through several cycles. Each cycle consists of four stages of non-rapid eye movement (NREM) sleep and one stage of rapid eye movement (REM) sleep. Although the REM stage accounts for only 20% to 25% of sleep, this physiologically active period is essential for physical and mental restoration and integration of learning. A full sleep cycle of 5 stages averages 90 minutes; each time a person passes through the REM stage of sleep, a new cycle begins.

The four major types of sleep disorders are insomnia (disorders of initiating and maintaining sleep), hypersomnia (disorders of excessive somnolence), parasomnia (dysfunctions associated with sleep, such as sleepwalking, nightmares, or nocturnal enuresis), and disorders of the sleep-awake cycle (commonly experienced by shift workers and travelers who cross several time zones).

Benzodiazepines

In the United States, eight benzodiazepines are used primarily to treat anxiety: alprazolam (Xanax), chlordiazepoxide hydrochloride (Librium), clorazepate dipotassium (Tranxene), diazepam (Valium), halazepam (Paxipam), lorazepam (Ativan), oxazepam (Serax), and prazepam (Centrax). Estazolam (ProSom), flurazepam hydrochloride (Dalmane), quazepam (Doral), temazepam (Restoril), and triazolam (Halcion) are more commonly used as sedatives and hypnotics. However, with dosage adjustment, almost any drug in this list can be used as an anxiolytic, sedative, hypnotic, or anticonvulsant agent.

Pharmacokinetics

After oral administration, benzodiazepines are absorbed completely from the GI tract. After intramuscular (I.M.) injection, benzodiazepines undergo slow, erratic absorption, except for lorazepam, which is absorbed rapidly and reaches peak concentration in 60 to 90 minutes.

Benzodiazepines are distributed widely in the body, crossing the blood-brain barrier and the placenta. Because longer-acting agents are more lipophilic (have a greater affinity for fat) than shorter-acting agents, they can accumulate in fatty tissue with continued therapy. These drugs are metabolized in the liver and excreted primarily in the urine.

Most oral benzodiazepines have an onset of action of 30 minutes. They reach peak concentration in 1 to 2 hours and begin to produce therapeutic effects with the first dose. Full therapeutic effects occur after 5 to 10 days of treatment with a long-acting agent and may last several days after drug discontinuation. Short-acting agents produce full effects in 2 to 4 days. Maintenance of these effects requires multiple doses daily.

Pharmacodynamics

Benzodiazepines may act by enhancing the effects of gamma-aminobutyric acid (GABA), a natural inhibitor of excitatory stimulation. When administered at low doses, they decrease anxiety by acting on the limbic system and related brain areas that helps control emotions. At higher doses, benzodiazepines exhibit sleep-producing properties, probably by depressing the reticular activating system in the brain. Unlike barbiturates, which can depress the central nervous system

(CNS) directly, benzodiazepines work indirectly by enhancing GABA activity, which allows them to produce fewer adverse CNS reactions.

Pharmacotherapeutics

As schedule IV drugs, benzodiazepines are used for short-term treatment of generalized anxiety and production of sedative and hypnotic effects. At low dosages, they calm or sedate the patient without causing drowsiness. At higher dosages, they increase total sleep time and produce a deep, refreshing sleep. Benzodiazepines also are used to relax and calm the patient during the day or before surgery, to treat seizure disorders and skeletal muscle tension, and to manage alcohol withdrawal symptoms.

Benzodiazepines have replaced barbiturates as the drugs of choice for treating anxiety because they produce fewer adverse reactions, less respiratory depression, fewer drug interactions, less risk of overdose or physical and psychological dependence, and milder withdrawal symptoms.

Drug interactions

CNS depressants can interact with benzodiazepines, producing additive effects that can be lethal. Few other drug interactions occur. (For details, see Drug Interactions: *Antianxiety, sedative, and hypnotic agents*, pages 148 and 149.)

Adverse drug reactions

Benzodiazepines offer a wide margin of safety between therapeutic and toxic doses. Most adverse reactions to these drugs affect the CNS. Sedation is the most common reaction and may be eliminated by reducing the dosage. Motor coordination, reaction time, and cognitive reasoning may be impaired. Dose-related dizziness, ataxia, amnesia, and rebound insomnia may occur. Daytime sedation and hangover also may occur, but are less common compared to their occurrence with barbiturate use.

Fatigue, muscle weakness, respiratory depression, dry mouth, nausea, and vomiting result occasionally from benzodiazepine use. In geriatric patients, paradoxical excitation is possible. Mild allergic reactions, such as skin rash, pruritus, and urticaria, also may occur.

Benzodiazepines have a potential for abuse, tolerance, and physical and psychological dependence, especially with high doses or long-term use. Abrupt discontinuation can produce withdrawal symptoms, such as weakness, delirium, and seizures, that may appear up to 1 week after drug discontinuation.

Barbiturates Barbiturates in Schedule II include amobarbital sodium (Amytal), pentobarbital sodium (Nembutal), and secobarbital sodium (Seconal Sodium). Those in Schedule III include aprobarbital (Alurate) and butabarbital sodium (Butisol). Schedule IV barbiturates are mephobarbital (Mebaral) and phenobarbital sodium (Luminal). Like

DRUG INTERACTIONS

Antianxiety, sedative, and hypnotic agents

The most serious drug interactions occur when benzodiazepines, barbiturates, or nonbenzodiazepines-nonbarbiturates are administered with other central nervous system (CNS) depressants. Other drug interactions also may occur.

DRUG	INTERACTING DRUGS	POSSIBLE EFFECTS
Benzodiazepines		
alprazolam, chlordiazepoxide, clorazepate, diazepam, flurazepam, halazepam, lorazepam, oxazepam, prazepam, quazepam, temazepam, triazolam	CNS depressants	Increased sedative and other CNS depressant effects, possibly causing motor skill impairment and respiratory depression; possible lethal effect, especially with high doses; changes in seizures, especially in frequency and severity, with anticonvulsants
flurazepam, quazepam, triazolam	cimetidine	Increased sedation, increased CNS depression
flurazepam	oral contraceptives	Increased flurazepam effects
lorazepam, temazepam	oral contraceptives	Decreased benzodiazepine effects
Barbiturates		
amobarbital, aprobarbital, butabarbital, mephobarbital, pentobarbital, phenobarbital, secobarbital	hydantoins	Decreased phenobarbital metabolism, resulting in increased toxic effects
	beta blockers (metoprolol, propranolol)	Decreased beta-blocker effects
	chloramphenicol	Decreased chloramphenicol effects, decreased phenobarbital metabolism
	corticosteroids	Decreased corticosteroid effects
	doxycycline	Decreased doxycycline effects
	oral anticoagulants	Decreased oral anticoagulant effects
	oral contraceptives	Decreased oral contraceptive effects
	quinidine	Decreased quinidine effects
	methoxyflurane	Increased nephrotoxicity
	tricyclic antidepressants	Decreased tricyclic antidepressant effects
	CNS depressants (anxiolytics, sedatives, hypnotics, most narcotic analgesics, and alcohol)	Increased CNS effects, resulting in increased sedative toxicity
	valproic acid	Decreased hepatic metabolism of phenobarbital
	metronidazole	Increased metronidazole metabolism
	digitoxin	Decreased digitoxin effects
	theophylline	Decreased serum theophylline level
	cyclosporine	Decreased plasma cyclosporine level

DRUG INTERACTIONS

Antianxiety, sedative, and hypnotic agents *(continued)*

DRUG	INTERACTING DRUGS	POSSIBLE EFFECTS
Buspirone		
buspirone	monoamine oxidase (MAO) inhibitors	Hypertensive reactions
Nonbenzodiazepines-nonbarbiturates		
chloral hydrate, ethchlorvynol, glutethimide, methyprylon, paraldehyde	CNS depressants	Drowsiness, respiratory depression, stupor, coma, or death
chloral hydrate	oral anticoagulants	Increased bleeding
paraldehyde	disulfiram	Increased paraldehyde blood levels, causing increased CNS depression; possibly toxic disulfiram reaction (respiratory depression, cardiac arrhythmias, seizures, and unconsciousness)
glutethimide, ethchlorvynol	oral anticoagulants	Increased risk of clotting

benzodiazepines, barbiturates are CNS depressants that produce effects ranging from anxiety relief to sedation, sleep, general anesthesia, and, possibly, coma and death.

Pharmacokinetics

Barbiturates are absorbed well after oral and I.M. administration. The I.M. route usually is avoided, however, because the alkalinity of the solution causes pain and necrosis at the injection site.

Barbiturates are distributed rapidly to all body tissues and fluids. Because they are lipophilic, these drugs exhibit high concentrations in the fatty tissues of the liver and brain. They are metabolized primarily by the liver and excreted primarily by the kidneys.

The duration may be ultrashort-acting, short-acting, intermediate-acting, or long-acting, depending on the rate of drug metabolism and redistribution throughout the body. The more slowly the system metabolizes or excretes a barbiturate, the more prolonged the drug's action.

Pharmacodynamics

Researchers have not yet identified the primary sites of drug action and the mechanisms of action for barbiturates. They believe these drugs primarily affect the neuronal fibers and synapses that integrate the brain's sleep-awake center. However, barbiturates act as nonspecific CNS depressants; their sites of action are less selective than benzodiazepine sites of action. As sedative-hypnotics, these drugs depress nerve impulse transmission to the brain's sensory cortex, decreasing motor activity, altering cerebral function, and producing drowsiness, sedation, and hypnosis. The degree of depression depends on the dose, route, patient's age, and patient's emotional state.

Pharmacotherapeutics

Barbiturates have many clinical indications, including hypnotic effects, anxiety relief, anesthesia, anticonvulsant effects, and, sometimes, daytime sedation. Because of their adverse reactions and other disadvantages, however, their use is declining. Benzodiazepines now are considered the anxiolytic, sedative, and hypnotic drugs of choice.

Drug interactions

When taken with other CNS depressants (including alcohol), barbiturates can produce significant additive CNS depression. Other drug interactions may occur because barbiturates can stimulate the enzymes that degrade other drugs, decreasing their duration of action. (For details, see Drug Interactions: *Antianxiety, sedative, and hypnotic agents,* pages 148 and 149.)

Adverse drug reactions

Serious adverse reactions involve the CNS and include sedation, lethargy, ataxia, dizziness, headache, CNS depression, hangover effects, and impaired motor coordination and reaction time. Because barbiturates also produce respiratory depression, they can be especially dangerous in a patient with pulmonary disease. Barbiturate overdose can be life-threatening.

Long-term use can lead to tolerance and physical and psychological dependence. Within 8 to 12 hours after abrupt discontinuation of a barbiturate, the patient may experience withdrawal symptoms, such as anxiety, insomnia, nausea, vomiting, hallucinations, and seizures. Therefore, long-term therapy should be tapered off over 1 to 2 weeks to prevent withdrawal reactions.

Less common reactions include blood dyscrasias, allergic reactions, GI complaints, and paradoxical excitation.

Buspirone

The first of a new class of antianxiety drugs, buspirone hydrochloride (BuSpar) currently is used to treat generalized anxiety states.

Pharmacokinetics

Although buspirone is absorbed rapidly after oral administration, its bioavailability is decreased because of the first-pass effect. Metabolized occurs in the liver, and excretion occurs in the kidneys. The plasma concentration peaks 1 hour after oral administration, but the onset of action ranges from 1 to 2 weeks.

Pharmacodynamics

Unlike the benzodiazepines, buspirone does not affect GABA receptors. Rather, it seems to act in the midbrain as a modulator.

Pharmacotherapeutics

Buspirone is used to treat generalized anxiety states. It is most effective in patients who have not previously taken benzodiazepines.

Drug interactions

Buspirone interacts with monoamine oxidase (MAO) inhibitors, producing a hypertensive reaction. Unlike other antianxiety drugs, it does not interact with CNS depressants. (For details, see Drug Interactions: *Antianxiety, sedative, and hypnotic agents,* pages 148 and 149.)

Adverse drug reactions

Buspirone appears to have no abuse potential. It causes only minor adverse reactions, such as dizziness, headache, and insomnia.

Nonbenzodiazepines-nonbarbiturates

Like the barbiturates, nonbenzodiazepine-nonbarbiturate drugs act as hypnotics for short-term treatment of insomnia, but lose their effectiveness after 2 weeks. They also provide sedation before surgery and electroencephalogram (EEG) studies. They are not used as anxiolytics. Nonbenzodiazepines-nonbarbiturates in Schedule IV include chloral hydrate (Noctec, SK-Chloral Hydrate), ethchlorvynol (Placidyl), and paraldehyde (Paral). Those in Schedule III include glutethimide (Doriden) and methyprylon (Noludar).

Pharmacokinetics

These agents are absorbed rapidly from the GI tract, distributed widely, metabolized primarily in the liver, and excreted in the urine. Most of them display a rapid onset of action (10 to 45 minutes). They usually reach a peak concentration in 1 to 2 hours, except for glutethimide, which achieves its peak 1 to 6 hours because it is absorbed erratically. The duration of action varies greatly, but ranges from 4 to 8 hours for most nonbenzodiazepines-nonbarbiturates.

Pharmacodynamics

The mechanisms of action for the nonbenzodiazepines-nonbarbiturates are not fully known; but the drugs produce depressant effects similar to the barbiturates. At high doses, they can produce CNS depression of the respiratory center, causing respiratory failure and death.

Pharmacotherapeutics

Nonbenzodiazepines-nonbarbiturates are prescribed for short-term treatment of simple insomnia and for sedation before surgery.

Drug interactions

These drugs interact with other CNS depressants, causing additive CNS depression. (For details, see Drug Interactions: *Antianxiety, sedative, and hypnotic agents,* pages 148 and 149.)

Adverse drug reactions

The most common adverse reactions to nonbenzodiazepines-nonbarbiturates are GI symptoms, such as nausea, vomiting, and gastric irritation, and some hangover effects. Compared to the hangover produced by barbiturates, the hangover caused by these agents occurs less commonly, especially in geriatric patients.

At high doses, CNS depression, respiratory failure, and death can occur. Habitual use can cause tolerance and dependence. Chronic and acute toxicity can occur, and abrupt drug discontinuation can cause dangerous withdrawal symptoms, similar to those of barbiturate withdrawal.

Other antianxiety and sedative agents

Meprobamate, beta blockers, and antihistamines may be prescribed to treat anxiety disorders. Meprobamate rarely is used today because of its low degree of effectiveness, the severity of its adverse effects, and the advent of safer, more effective agents. Beta blockers are useful in treating acute situational anxiety that causes somatic symptoms. The use of antihistamines to treat anxiety is rare.

Alcohol and many over-the-counter (OTC) products often are used as sedatives. Alcohol is the most widely used and abused drug in the United States. A CNS depressant, alcohol enters the blood stream and diffuses past the blood-brain barrier. In small amounts, alcohol has been used to promote sleep and improve appetite and digestion in geriatric patients. OTC sleep aids (such as Nytol with DPH and Sleep-Eze 3) are readily available for purchase. These drugs usually contain an antihistamine, such as pyrilamine maleate or diphenhydramine, which has some sedative properties. (For more information about antihistamines, see Chapter 27, Antihistaminic agents.)

Nursing implications

When caring for a patient who is receiving an antianxiety, sedative, or hypnotic agent, the nurse should be aware of the following implications.
• Develop appropriate nursing diagnoses for the patient. (For examples, see Sample Nursing Diagnoses: *Antianxiety, sedative, and hypnotic agents.*)
• Do not administer an antianxiety, sedative, or hypnotic agent to a patient with a condition that contraindicates its use.
• Administer an antianxiety, sedative, or hypnotic agent cautiously to a patient at risk because of a preexisting condition.
• Monitor the effectiveness of the drug therapy.
• Observe the patient for adverse reactions and signs of drug interactions.
• Take safety measures if the patient develops dizziness or related CNS manifestations. Place the bed in the low position, keep the bed rails up, and supervise patient ambulation.
• Monitor the patient's vital signs frequently.
• Notify the physician if adverse reactions or drug interactions occur.
• Teach the patient and family the name, dose, frequency, action, and adverse effects of the prescribed drug. (For more information, see *Pa-*

SAMPLE NURSING DIAGNOSES

Antianxiety, sedative, and hypnotic agents

The following nursing diagnoses address representative problems and etiologies that a nurse may encounter when caring for a patient who is receiving an antianxiety, sedative, or hypnotic agent.

- Altered health maintenance related to ineffectiveness of the prescribed antianxiety, sedative, or hypnotic agent
- Altered protection related to barbiturate-induced blood dyscrasias
- Altered role performance related to benzodiazepine, barbiturate, or nonbenzodiazepine-nonbarbiturate dependence
- Altered thought processes related to the adverse central nervous system (CNS) effects of an antianxiety, sedative, or hypnotic agent
- Anxiety related to a paradoxical reaction to the barbiturate
- Diarrhea related to the adverse gastrointestinal effects of a barbiturate
- Fatigue related to the adverse effects of a benzodiazepine
- High risk for activity intolerance related to benzodiazepine-induced muscle weakness
- High risk for fluid volume deficit related to nausea and vomiting caused by a sedative or hypnotic agent
- High risk for injury related to adverse drug reactions
- High risk for injury related to a preexisting condition that contraindicates the use of an antianxiety, sedative, or hypnotic agent
- High risk for injury related to a preexisting condition that requires cautious use of an antianxiety, sedative, or hypnotic agent
- High risk for injury related to drug interactions
- High risk for injury related to the hangover effects of a sedative or hypnotic agent
- High risk for trauma related to the adverse CNS effects of an antianxiety, sedative, or hypnotic agent
- Impaired gas exchange related to the adverse respiratory effects of a sedative or hypnotic agent
- Impaired home maintenance management related to the sedative effects of the prescribed sedative or hypnotic agent
- Impaired physical mobility related to barbiturate-induced impairment of motor coordination
- Impaired skin integrity related to dermatologic allergic reactions to the prescribed benzodiazepine or barbiturate
- Ineffective breathing pattern related to respiratory depression caused by a sedative or hypnotic agent
- Knowledge deficit related to the prescribed antianxiety, sedative, or hypnotic agent
- Noncompliance related to long-term use of an antianxiety agent
- Pain related to headache caused by buspirone or a barbiturate
- Sleep pattern disturbance related to buspirone-induced insomnia
- Sleep pattern disturbance related to rebound insomnia caused by a sedative or hypnotic agent

tient-teaching tips for benzodiazepines, barbiturates, and non-benzodiazepines-nonbarbiturates, page 154.)
- Instruct the patient with insomnia or a similar sleep disorder to try other measures, such as a warm bath or relaxation techniques, before taking any medication.

Patient-teaching tips for benzodiazepines, barbiturates, and nonbenzodiazepines-nonbarbiturates

Whenever a benzodiazepine, barbiturate, or nonbenzodiazepine-nonbarbiturate is prescribed, the following patient-teaching tips apply.

• Teach the patient to take the drug exactly as prescribed and not to change the dosage without consulting the physician.

• Advise the patient not to discontinue the drug suddenly without consulting the physician because withdrawal symptoms may occur.

• Instruct the patient not to operate a motor vehicle or heavy machinery, at least until the patient is aware of the drug's effects on mental alertness.

• Instruct the patient not to drink alcohol during drug therapy because respiratory depression can occur.

• Instruct the patient to read drug labels and avoid over-the-counter drugs that contain central nervous system depressants, such as alcohol or antihistamines.

• Advise the patient to consult the physician before taking any tranquilizers, narcotics, or other prescription pain relievers.

• Instruct the patient to notify the nurse or physician when beginning or discontinuing any other drug during therapy with a benzodiazepine, barbiturate, or nonbenzodiazepine-nonbarbiturate.

• Counsel the patient not to give any prescribed drugs to family members or friends.

• Advise the patient to keep the drug and all other medications out of the reach of children.

• Instruct the patient and family to report adverse reactions to the physician.

Benzodiazepines

• Consult with the physician if other CNS depressants also are prescribed; this drug combination may cause lethal depressant effects.

• Avoid I.M. administration, if possible, because it usually produces slow, erratic drug absorption.

• Administer I.V. preparations slowly to reduce the risk of phlebitis and cardiovascular collapse.

• Do not discontinue benzodiazepine therapy abruptly. The patient may develop withdrawal symptoms, such as weakness, delirium, and tonic-clonic seizures.

• Plan nursing care and drug administration based on the hospitalized patient's daily routines and bedtime rituals. Do not awaken a patient to administer a benzodiazepine. To prevent the hangover effect, avoid giving a second p.r.n. dose during the night. Instead, try to find out why the patient cannot sleep. If pain is causing insomnia, use comfort measures, such as back rubs.

• Perform a respiratory assessment before and after giving each benzodiazepine dose. Withhold the dose and notify the physician if respiratory depression occurs.

• Watch the patient take the benzodiazepine to prevent drug hoarding for later use.

- Keep epinephrine and corticosteroids readily available for emergency care of a patient who experiences a hypersensitivity reaction to the prescribed drug.
- Assist with gastric lavage, respiratory support, and other support measures, such as intravenous fluid or drug administration, if overdose occurs. Frequently monitor vital signs and fluid intake and output.

Barbiturates

- Discontinue the drug slowly after long-term therapy, as prescribed, to prevent rebound REM sleep.
- Monitor prothrombin time, as prescribed, for a patient who also is receiving an anticoagulant. Keep in mind that abrupt withdrawal of a barbiturate many cause serious bleeding. Adjust the anticoagulant dosage as prescribed.
- Remember that the I.M. route is a poor administration route for barbiturates. If it is used, follow these precautions: Rotate (do not shake) the amobarbital ampule and mix the solution with sterile water only; discard amobarbital solutions that do not clear within 5 minutes; do not use a cloudy pentobarbital, phenobarbital, or secobarbital solution or mix the solution with other medications; use the barbiturate solution within 30 minutes after opening to minimize deterioration; and inject the solution slowly and deeply into a large muscle mass.
- Perform a respiratory assessment before and after administering each barbiturate dose. Withhold the dose and notify the physician if respiratory depression occurs.
- Position the patient to maximize respiratory function; for example, place the patient in the semi-Fowler or high Fowler position.

Buspirone

- Expect to change a patient from long-term benzodiazepine therapy to buspirone by tapering off the benzodiazepine dosage as prescribed to avoid a benzodiazepine withdrawal reaction.
- Prevent insomnia by administering the last daily dose of buspirone several hours before bedtime, if permissible.

Nonbenzodiazepines-nonbarbiturates

- Administer chloral hydrate after meals or with food to minimize gastric irritation. Dilute liquid chloral hydrate with a fluid that minimizes its unpleasant taste, such as juice or soda.
- Use paraldehyde from containers that have been opened for less than 24 hours because the drug decomposes upon exposure to light; do not give the drug if it is brown or has an acetic acid odor. Dilute the oral liquid form in iced milk, syrup, or fruit juice to disguise the taste and odor and to reduce gastric distress.
- Use glass syringes and metal needles with paraldehyde because the drug reacts with some plastics. When administering intramuscularly, inject deeply into a large muscle mass and massage the site. For rectal administration, minimize irritation by diluting the drug with vege-

table oil (one part drug to two parts diluent); then administer as a retention enema.
- Perform a respiratory assessment before and after giving each dose. Withhold the dose and notify the physician if respiratory depression occurs.
- Do not discontinue large doses abruptly.

STUDY ACTIVITIES

Fill in the blank

1. OTC sleep aids usually produce sleep because they contain

_____.

2. A full sleep cycle consists of _____ stages and averages

_____ minutes.

3. Although _____ sleep accounts for only 20% to 25% of sleep, this sleep stage is essential for physical restoration.

4. Anxiety disorders are divided into two main types: _____ and

_____.

5. Barbiturates depress nerve impulse transmission to the _____ of the brain.

True or false

6. Benzodiazepines have a wide margin of safety between therapeutic and toxic doses.
   ☐ True   ☐ False

7. After I.M. injection of most benzodiazepines, absorption is slow and erratic.
   ☐ True   ☐ False

8. Barbiturates are more selective in their sites of action than benzodiazepines.
   ☐ True   ☐ False

9. The I.M. route is the route of choice for administering barbiturates.
   ☐ True   ☐ False

10. Buspirone hydrochloride (BuSpar) has less potential for abuse than diazepam (Valium).
    ☐ True   ☐ False

11. Nonbenzodiazepine-nonbarbiturate drugs are useful for long-term treatment of insomnia.
    ☐ True   ☐ False

Multiple choice

12. Jane Ellis, age 78, is admitted to the hospital and scheduled for an exploratory laparotomy. Her physician prescribes diazepam (Valium) 2 mg P.O. b.i.d. to relieve her anxiety. Before administering this drug, the nurse reviews Ms. Ellis's medication history. Which type of drug could interact with diazepam?

    A. Antibiotic
    B. Anticoagulant
    C. CNS depressant
    D. Estrogen replacement

13. While receiving diazepam, Ms. Ellis is most likely to experience which adverse reaction?

    A. Sedation
    B. Urticaria
    C. Blood dyscrasias
    D. Nausea and vomiting

14. In which location is the highest concentration of benzodiazepines usually found?

    A. Thymus
    B. Pancreas
    C. Long bones
    D. Fatty tissue

15. Joshua Reynolds, age 49, is a painter who recently fractured his tibia. Because he cannot work and worries about his finances, he becomes anxious. His physician prescribes buspirone (BuSpar) 5 mg P.O. t.i.d. for generalized anxiety. During buspirone therapy, Mr. Reynolds should not take which of the following drugs?

    A. Beta-adrenergic blockers
    B. Antineoplastic drugs
    C. Antiparkinson drugs
    D. MAO inhibitors

16. Mr. Reynolds states that he does not like taking medication and asks if he can take buspirone only when he feels anxious. How should the nurse reply?

    A. "No. That would increase the risk of abuse and overdose."
    B. "No. That would not provide a therapeutic effect."
    C. "Yes. That would help minimize any adverse effects."
    D. "Yes. That would help minimize drug interactions."

17. How does buspirone produce its effects?

    A. It enhances the effects of GABA.
    B. It directly affects the cerebral cortex.
    C. It seems to act in the midbrain as a modulator.
    D. It produces CNS effects similar to barbiturates.

18. Mr. Reynolds is most likely to display which adverse reaction to buspirone?
   A. Insomnia
   B. Sedation
   C. Hypotension
   D. Tachycardia

19. Paul Harrell, age 59, is scheduled for cardiac catheterization the next morning. His physician prescribed secobarbital sodium (Seconal Sodium) 100 mg P.O. h.s. for sedation. What is the difference between sedatives and hypnotics?
   A. Sedatives cause predictable responses; hypnotics cause unpredictable ones.
   B. Sedatives interact with few drugs; hypnotics interact with many.
   C. Sedatives do not depress respirations; hypnotics do.
   D. Sedatives reduce excitement; hypnotics induce sleep.

20. Randolph Tuggle, age 81, is receiving chloral hydrate 250 mg P.O. t.i.d. The drug is ordered in liquid form because he cannot swallow correctly. How should the nurse administer this drug?
   A. Diluted in fruit juice
   B. With a CNS depressant
   C. Between meals
   D. With milk

ANSWERS

Fill in the blank
   1. An antihistamine
   2. 5, 90
   3. REM
   4. Nonphobic, phobic
   5. Sensory cortex

True or false
   6. True.
   7. True.
   8. False. Barbiturates act as nonspecific CNS depressants. Their sites of action are less selective than benzodiazepine sites of action.
   9. False. The I.M. route is a poor administration route for barbiturates because it causes pain and necrosis at the injection site.
   10. True.
   11. False. These drugs are used as hypnotics for short-term treatment of simple insomnia because they lose their effectiveness after 2 weeks.

Multiple choice
12. C. Concomitant use of a CNS depressant with benzodiazepines produces an additive effect that can be lethal.

13. A. Sedation is the most common reaction to benzodiazepines, such as diazepam, and may be eliminated by reducing the dosage.

14. D. Longer-acting benzodiazepines are more lipophilic (have a greater affinity for fat) than shorter-acting agents. Therefore, they can accumulate in fatty tissue.

15. D. Buspirone interacts only with MAO inhibitors, producing a hypertensive reaction.

16. D. Buspirone has an onset of action of 1 to 2 weeks, making it ineffective for p.r.n. use.

17. C. Unlike benzodiazepines, buspirone does not affect GABA receptors. Rather, it seems to act in the midbrain as a modulator.

18. A. The most common adverse reactions to buspirone are dizziness, headache, and insomnia.

19. D. Sedatives are drugs that act to reduce activity or excitement, calming a patient. Administered in large doses, sedatives act as hypnotics, which induce a state resembling natural sleep.

20. A. The nurse should dilute liquid chloral hydrate with a fluid that disguises its taste, such as fruit juice, and should administer the drug with meals to minimize gastric irritation.

CHAPTER 11

Antidepressant and antimanic agents

OBJECTIVES

After studying this chapter, the reader should be able to:

1. Discuss the clinical indications for antidepressant and antimanic agents.

2. Explain the mechanisms of action of the monoamine oxidase (MAO) inhibitors, tricyclic antidepressants, second-generation antidepressants, and lithium.

3. Identify drugs and foods that may interact with MAO inhibitors.

4. Identify the major drugs that interact with lithium.

5. Describe the major adverse effects of MAO inhibitors, tricyclic antidepressants, second-generation antidepressants, and lithium.

6. Describe the nursing implications of antidepressant or antimanic therapy.

OVERVIEW OF CONCEPTS

Depression and mania are the most common affective disorders. They affect twice as many women as men. Unipolar depression (depression not accompanied by mania) accounts for 90% of the cases. Mania and bipolar depression (alternating periods of mania and depression) account for the remainder.

Depression is characterized by the presence of several of the following signs and symptoms for at least 2 weeks: poor appetite, weight change, sleep disturbances, agitation, fatigue, feelings of worthlessness, loss of interest in activities, slowed thinking and movements, difficulty concentrating, and thoughts of death. Mania is characterized by euphoria, rapid speech, flight of ideas, reduced need for sleep, and hyperactivity.

Concentration levels of the neurotransmitters norepinephrine and serotonin are diminished in depression and excessive in mania. Drugs that treat depression and mania adjust the availability of these neurotransmitters in the brain over time. MAO inhibitors, tricyclic antidepressants, and second-generation antidepressants are used to treat unipolar disorders. Lithium is used to treat bipolar disorders. (For a sum-

SELECTED MAJOR DRUGS

Antidepressant and antimanic agents

This chart summarizes the major antidepressant and antimanic drugs currently in clinical use.

DRUG	MAJOR INDICATIONS	USUAL ADULT DOSAGES
Monoamine oxidase (MAO) inhibitors		
isocarboxazid	Atypical depression	30 mg P.O. daily in a single dose or in divided doses, reduced to 10 to 20 mg/day when condition improves
tranylcypromine	Atypical depression	10 mg P.O. b.i.d., increased to a maximum of 30 mg/day after 2 to 3 weeks, as needed
Tricyclic antidepressants		
amitriptyline	Depression	50 to 75 mg P.O. increased to 200 mg/day, then up to a maximum of 300 mg/day, as needed; or 20 to 30 mg I.M. q.i.d. or as a single dose h.s.
doxepin	Depression	Initially, 25 to 50 mg P.O. daily, increased to a maximum of 300 mg/day, as needed
Second-generation antidepressants		
trazodone	Depression	150 mg P.O. daily in divided doses, increased by 50 mg/day every 3 to 4 days, up to a maximum of 400 mg/day (or 600 mg/day for a severely ill patient)
Lithium		
lithium	Mania, bipolar disorder relapse	300 to 600 mg P.O. up to q.i.d., adjusted to achieve lithium blood level of 1 to 1.5 mEq/liter for acute mania, 0.6 to 1.2 mEq/liter to prevent bipolar disorder relapses, and 2 mEq/liter as a maximum dose

mary of representative drugs, see Selected Major Drugs: *Antidepressant and antimanic agents.*)

MAO inhibitors　MAO inhibitors include isocarboxazid (Marplan), phenelzine sulfate (Nardil), and tranylcypromine sulfate (Parnate).

Pharmacokinetics
MAO inhibitors are absorbed rapidly and completely from the gastrointestinal (GI) tract. They are metabolized in the liver to inactive metabolites, which are excreted mainly by the GI tract and secondarily by the kidneys. The onset of action ranges from 1 to 2 weeks, and a full clinical response may be delayed for 3 to 4 weeks. Therapeutic effects may last up to 2 weeks after discontinuation.

Pharmacodynamics
These agents appear to work by inhibiting synthesis and action of the enzyme monoamine oxidase (the enzyme that normally metabolizes norepinephrine and serotonin). This makes more of these neurotransmitters available to receptors, relieving the symptoms of depression.

Pharmacotherapeutics

MAO inhibitors treat atypical depression better than tricyclic antidepressants. They are used to treat typical depression when other therapies are contraindicated or have not been effective. Other uses include depression accompanied by anxiety, phobic anxieties, neurodermatitis, hypochondriasis, and narcoleptic states.

Drug interactions

Certain drugs and foods can interact with MAO inhibitors and may produce severe reactions. (For details, see Drug Interactions: *Antidepressant and antimanic agents,* pages 163 and 164, and *Foods that may interact with MAO inhibitors,* page 165.)

Adverse drug reactions

The most common adverse reactions to MAO inhibitors include restlessness, drowsiness, dizziness, headache, insomnia, constipation, anorexia, nausea, vomiting, weakness, arthralgia, dry mouth, blurred vision, edema, urine retention, rash, purpura, transient impotence, and orthostatic hypotension (which may lead to syncope with high doses).

The most serious adverse reaction is hypertensive crisis, which is characterized by increased blood pressure, severe headache, palpitations, nausea, vomiting, neck stiffness or soreness, fever, clammy skin, mydriasis, photophobia or other vision disturbances, bradycardia or tachycardia, chest pain, and intracranial hemorrhage.

Other adverse reactions include urinary frequency, increased appetite, weight gain, increased perspiration, flushing, numbness, paresthesia, muscle spasms, tremor, myoclonic jerks, and hyperreflexia. If adverse reactions do not diminish with time or dosage adjustments, the patient will be switched to a different MAO inhibitor.

Abrupt discontinuation of tranylcypromine may cause withdrawal reactions, such as anxiety, depression, confusion, and hallucinations.

Tricyclic antidepressants

Tricyclic antidepressants include amitriptyline hydrochloride (Elavil, Emitrip, Endep), clomipramine hydrochloride (Anafranil), desipramine hydrochloride (Norpramin, Pertofrane), doxepin hydrochloride (Adapin, Sinequan), imipramine hydrochloride (Janimine, Tofranil), nortriptyline hydrochloride (Aventyl, Pamelor), protriptyline hydrochloride (Vivactil), and trimipramine maleate (Surmontil).

Pharmacokinetics

After oral administration, tricyclic antidepressants are absorbed completely and distributed widely throughout the body. Because they are metabolized extensively in the liver, only small amounts of active drug are excreted in the urine. The half-lives of the tricyclic antidepressants vary from 8 to 120 hours and average 24 hours, except for protriptyline hydrochloride, which is 3 to 4 days. Because of protriptyline's long half-life, a noticeable response may not occur for 10 to 14 days; a full response, for up to 30 days.

DRUG INTERACTIONS

Antidepressant and antimanic agents

Monoamine oxidase (MAO) inhibitors and tricyclic antidepressants can interact with several commonly used drugs, causing potentially severe effects. Second-generation antidepressants may interact with the same drugs that the tricyclic antidepressants do. Lithium can interact with several drugs, but most interactions can be managed with dosage adjustments.

DRUG	INTERACTING DRUGS	POSSIBLE EFFECTS
MAO inhibitors		
isocarboxazid, phenelzine, tranyl-cypromine	amphetamines	Increased catecholamine release, increased hypertension
	fluoxetine, tricyclic antidepressants, cyclobenzaprine	Hyperpyrexia, excitation, seizures
	doxapram	Hypertension and arrhythmias; increased adverse effects of doxapram
	sympathomimetics, nonamphetamine anorexigenic agents	Increased catecholamine release, increased hypertension
	levodopa	Hypertension
	hypoglycemic agents	Hypoglycemia
	meperidine	Excitation, hypertension or hypotension, hyperpyrexia, coma
Tricyclic antidepressants		
amitriptyline, clomipramine, desipramine, doxepin, imipramine, nortriptyline, protriptyline, trimipramine	amphetamines	Hypertension
	barbiturates	Increased metabolism and decreased blood level of tricyclic antidepressant
	cimetidine	Decreased metabolism of tricyclic antidepressant, leading to toxicity
	MAO inhibitors	Hyperpyrexia, excitation, seizures
	sympathomimetics	Hypertension
	anticholinergic agents	Enhanced anticholinergic effects
	clonidine, guanethidine	Reduced antihypertensive effects
Second-generation antidepressants		
amoxapine, bupropion, fluoxetine, maprotiline, trazodone	same drugs as tricyclic antidepressants	Same effects as with tricyclic antidepressants
bupropion	carbamazepine, cimetidine, phenobarbital, phenytoin	Increased metabolism of interacting drugs
	levodopa	Increased adverse effects of levodopa
fluoxetine	diazepam	Increased half-life of diazepam
	MAO inhibitors	Hyperpyrexia, excitation, seizures
	other antidepressants	Increased serum levels of other antidepressants

(continued)

DRUG INTERACTIONS

Antidepressant and antimanic agents (continued)

DRUG	INTERACTING DRUGS	POSSIBLE EFFECTS
Second-generation antidepressants (continued)		
trazodone	CNS depressants	Increased sedation
	antihypertensives	Increased hypotensive effects
	phenytoin	Increased phenytoin levels
Lithium		
lithium	thiazide diuretics, loop diuretics	Increased lithium reabsorption in the kidneys
	nonsteroidal anti-inflammatory drugs (NSAIDs)	Decreased lithium excretion
	potassium iodide	Increased hypothyroid activity
	sodium bicarbonate	Increased lithium excretion
	sodium chloride	Altered lithium excretion in proportion to sodium chloride intake
	carbamazepine	Neurotoxicity
	phenothiazines	Neurotoxicity, seizures
	theophylline	Increased renal clearance of lithium

Pharmacodynamics

Tricyclic antidepressants increase the amount of norepinephrine and serotonin in the brain. This normalizes hyposensitive receptor sites and reduces the signs and symptoms of depression.

Pharmacotherapeutics

Tricyclic antidepressants are the drugs of choice for major depression and depressions of insidious onset accompanied by weight loss, anorexia, and insomnia. Physical signs and symptoms may resolve in 1 to 2 weeks; psychological ones may take 2 to 4 weeks.

A patient who fails to respond to one tricyclic antidepressant may respond to a different one or to a combination of lithium and a tricyclic antidepressant. Although a once-daily dosage is possible because of the tricyclic antidepressants' long half-life, the dosage is divided to decrease the risk of adverse effects or to allow the patient to adjust before changing to a once-daily dosage. Dosages should be reduced for geriatric patients.

Drug interactions

These agents can interact with many drugs, especially MAO inhibitors or sympathomimetics. (For details, see Drug Interactions: *Antidepressant and antimanic agents,* pages 163 and 164.)

Foods that may interact with MAO inhibitors

Foods that contain tyramine can produce a hypertensive crisis in a patient receiving a monoamine oxidase (MAO) inhibitor. Foods with high tyramine content should be avoided completely, those with moderate content may be eaten occasionally, and those with low tyramine levels are allowable in limited quantities.

Foods with a high tyramine content
- Red wines, such as chianti and burgundy
- Beer
- Aged cheeses, such as bleu, Swiss, and cheddar
- Aged or smoked meats, such as herring, sausage, and corned beef
- Liver, such as chicken or beef liver
- Yeast extracts, such as brewer's yeast

- Fava or broad beans, such as Italian green beans

Foods with a moderate tyramine content
- Sour cream
- Ripe avocados
- Yogurt
- Ripe bananas
- Meat extracts, such as bouillon

Foods with a low tyramine content
- Chocolate
- Figs
- American, mozzarella, cottage, and cream cheeses
- Distilled spirits, such as gin, vodka, and scotch
- White wines

Adverse drug reactions

Common reactions to tricyclic antidepressants include orthostatic hypotension, cardiovascular effects, sedation, and anticholinergic effects, such as blurred vision, constipation, and urine retention. Because adverse reactions can differ markedly among agents, the patient's therapy can be changed from one tricyclic antidepressant to another to eliminate adverse reactions. For example, a patient who develops orthostatic hypotension may be switched to nortriptyline because it is less likely to cause this reaction.

A conduction delay, demonstrated by a widening Q-T interval, also may occur with tricyclic antidepressant therapy. This adverse reaction can exacerbate congestive heart failure or an existing bundle branch block. A patient with congestive heart failure will need to be monitored for electrocardiogram (ECG) changes, palpitations, and tachycardia.

At high dosages, tricyclic antidepressants can cause seizures. Other adverse reactions include jaundice, a fine resting tremor, decreased libido, inhibited ejaculation, transient eosinophilia, and leukopenia. Rashes and photosensitivity also may occur.

Second-generation antidepressants

Second-generation antidepressants produce fewer adverse effects than tricyclic antidepressants and are chemically different from each other and from the other antidepressants. These agents include amoxapine (Asendin), bupropion hydrochloride (Wellbutrin), fluoxetine hydrochloride (Prozac), maprotiline hydrochloride (Ludiomil), and trazodone hydrochloride (Desyrel).

Pharmacokinetics

After oral administration, the second-generation antidepressants are absorbed completely and distributed throughout the body, except for cardiac tissue. The metabolism, excretion, onset, peak, and duration differ greatly among these drugs.

Pharmacodynamics

Like the tricyclic antidepressants, second-generation antidepressants inhibit the reuptake of norepinephrine and serotonin. This restores hyposensitive receptor sites to normal so that increased neurotransmitter concentrations can exert a therapeutic effect.

Pharmacotherapeutics

Second-generation antidepressants are used to treat the same depressive episodes as tricyclic antidepressants. They have the same degree of effectiveness.

Drug interactions

The same drugs that interact with tricyclic antidepressants also may interact with the second-generation antidepressants. (For details, see Drug Interactions: *Antidepressant and antimanic agents,* pages 163 and 164.)

Adverse drug reactions

Second-generation antidepressants produce fewer adverse reactions than tricyclic antidepressants. Seizures may occur, especially with high doses of maprotiline and bupropion. Amoxapine and maprotiline also may cause anticholinergic effects, orthostatic hypotension, and tachycardia. Bupropion may cause central nervous system (CNS) stimulation. Fluoxetine may cause headache, nervousness, anxiety, insomnia, nausea, anorexia, diarrhea, diaphoresis, and rash. Trazodone may result in sedation, dizziness, and priapism.

Lithium

Lithium is the drug of choice to prevent or treat mania. Two lithium salts currently are in use: lithium carbonate (Eskalith, Lithane, Lithobid) and lithium citrate (Cibalith-S).

Pharmacokinetics

After oral administration, lithium is absorbed rapidly and completely and is distributed to body tissues. It is not metabolized, but is excreted unchanged by the kidneys. Lithium crosses the placenta and is detectable in the fetus and in breast milk.

The serum concentration of lithium peaks 2 to 3 hours after administration. Initially, the half-life is 2 hours, but it increases to 20 hours as therapy continues. Steady-state concentration is reached in 6 days.

Pharmacodynamics

Although the exact mechanism of action is unknown, lithium reduces the excessive catecholamine response in mania.

Pharmacotherapeutics

Lithium is used primarily to treat acute episodes of mania and to prevent relapses of bipolar disorders. It can produce 70% to 80% improvement in manic patients within 1 to 2 weeks and can reduce the 2-year relapse incidence to 50%. After an acute manic episode, lithium therapy typically is continued for 3 to 6 months and then tapered off. A patient who experiences a relapse every 1 to 2 years, however, may require long-term prophylactic therapy.

Lithium carbonate and lithium citrate have identical effects and dosage schedules, but lithium citrate is more soluble. Because lithium's therapeutic dosage range is narrow, dosages require regular adjustment. Blood levels monitored 12 hours after the last daily dose serve as an adjustment guide.

Drug interactions

Serious interactions with other drugs can occur because of lithium's narrow therapeutic range. (For details, see Drug Interactions: *Antidepressant and antimanic agents,* pages 163 and 164.)

Adverse drug reactions

Adverse reactions to lithium affect various body systems and may occur in any phase of therapy; most are dose-related. GI complaints are most frequent during the initial phase of therapy and after dosage adjustments. About 50% of patients experience a fine tremor that may diminish with dosage reduction and worsen with dosage increase. Polyuria of 2 to 3 liters/day may appear, accompanied by polydipsia. When blood levels exceed 1.5 mEq/liter, toxicity may occur, producing confusion, lethargy, slurred speech, hyperreflexia, and seizures.

Long-term lithium therapy may result in distal tubule atrophy and decreased glomerular filtration rate (GFR). Diabetes insipidus syndrome may occur. Hypothyroidism and nontoxic goiters may affect about 4% of patients. Other adverse reactions include weight gain, skin eruptions, alopecia, and leukocytosis.

Nursing implications When caring for a patient who is receiving an antidepressant or antimanic agent, the nurse should be aware of the following implications.
- Develop appropriate nursing diagnoses for the patient. (For examples, see Sample Nursing Diagnoses: *Antidepressant and antimanic agents,* page 168.)
- Do not administer an antidepressant or antimanic agent to a patient with a condition that contraindicates its use.
- Administer an antidepressant or antimanic agent cautiously to a patient at risk because of a preexisting condition.
- Monitor the patient for adverse reactions and signs of drug interactions.

SAMPLE NURSING DIAGNOSES

Antidepressant and antimanic agents

The following nursing diagnoses address representative problems and etiologies that a nurse may encounter when caring for a patient who is receiving an antidepressant or antimanic agent.

- Altered health maintenance related to ineffectiveness of the prescribed antidepressant or antimanic agent
- Altered protection related to the adverse hematologic effects of an antidepressant or antimanic agent
- Constipation related to the anticholinergic effects of an antidepressant agent
- Diarrhea related to the adverse gastrointestinal (GI) effects of fluoxetine
- Fluid volume excess related to exacerbation of congestive heart failure caused by a tricyclic antidepressant
- High risk for fluid volume deficit related to possible adverse GI effects and excessive diaphoresis associated with fluoxetine
- High risk for fluid volume deficit related to possible lithium-induced diabetes insipidus syndrome
- High risk for injury related to adverse drug reactions
- High risk for injury related to a preexisting condition that contraindicates the use of an antidepressant or antimanic agent
- High risk for injury related to a preexisting condition that requires cautious use of an antidepressant or antimanic agent
- High risk for injury related to drug interactions
- High risk for injury related to hypertensive crisis induced by an MAO inhibitor
- High risk for trauma related to seizures caused by an antidepressant or antimanic agent
- High risk for trauma related to syncope caused by an MAO inhibitor
- Knowledge deficit related to the prescribed antidepressant or antimanic agent
- Noncompliance related to long-term use of an antidepressant or antimanic agent
- Pain related to headache caused by an MAO inhibitor or fluoxetine
- Sensory or perceptual alterations (tactile) related to paresthesias caused by an MAO inhibitor
- Sensory or perceptual alterations (visual) related to blurred vision or photosensitivity caused by an MAO inhibitor or tricyclic antidepressant
- Sexual dysfunction related to the adverse genitourinary effects of an antidepressant agent
- Sleep pattern disturbance related to insomnia caused by fluoxetine
- Urinary retention related to the adverse genitourinary effects of an antidepressant agent

---

- Take safety precautions if adverse CNS or other reactions place the patient at risk. For example, place the bed in the low position and keep the bed rails up.
- Notify the physician if adverse reactions or drug interactions occur.
- Teach the patient and family the name, dose, frequency, action, and adverse effects of the prescribed antidepressant or antimanic agent.
- Teach the patient to recognize and report any adverse reactions.

MAO inhibitors
- Monitor the patient closely for signs of hypertensive crisis, and notify the physician if signs are detected.

- Prepare for emergency interventions if hypertensive crisis occurs. For example, expect to discontinue the MAO inhibitor immediately and administer 5 to 10 mg of phentolamine by intravenous injection to reduce the blood pressure, as prescribed.
- Expect to change the administration time to early evening if drowsiness occurs or to the morning if insomnia occurs.
- Do not discontinue tranylcypromine therapy abruptly. Taper off the dosage over 2 weeks to prevent withdrawal reactions.
- Withhold the prescribed MAO inhibitor and notify the physician if the patient develops signs or symptoms of an intentional overdose, such as palpitations, frequent headaches, or severe hypertension, which typically result from a suicide attempt.
- Have the patient sit up for 1 minute before getting out of bed to reduce orthostatic hypotension; supervise ambulation.
- Monitor the patient for 7 to 10 days after discontinuing an MAO inhibitor because of its long-lasting effects.
- Record the patient's fluid intake and output to detect urine retention. Palpate and percuss the bladder after the patient voids. Notify the physician if urine retention occurs and catheterize the patient, as directed.
- Reassure the patient that drug-induced impotence should resolve when the MAO inhibitor is discontinued.
- Teach the patient which drugs and foods to avoid during MAO inhibitor therapy.
- Teach the patient and family to recognize the signs of hypertensive crisis.
- Instruct the patient to inform other physicians about MAO inhibitor therapy to prevent drug interactions or complications during surgery.

Tricyclic antidepressants
- Expect to change the patient to a different tricyclic antidepressant if intolerable adverse reactions occur.
- Ask the physician about dividing a once-daily dosage if adverse reactions occur.
- Expect to administer a lower dosage to a geriatric patient.
- Monitor the patient's blood pressure and heart rate frequently and assess for palpitations, tachycardia, and ECG changes. A geriatric patient should have an ECG before beginning therapy.
- Notify the physician if the Q-T interval widens on the ECG.
- Have the patient sit up for 1 minute before getting out of bed to reduce orthostatic hypotension; supervise ambulation.
- Take seizure precautions during high-dose therapy.
- Monitor a suicidal patient closely until the drug takes full effect.
- Reassure the patient that anticholinergic reactions should diminish.
- Record the patient's fluid intake and output to detect urine retention. Palpate and percuss the bladder after the patient voids. Notify the

physician if urine retention occurs and catheterize the patient, as directed.
- Provide a high-fiber diet and plenty of fluids to help prevent constipation. Request a stool softener, if needed.
- Reassure patient that drug-induced decreased libido and inhibited ejaculation should resolve when the drug discontinued.

Second-generation antidepressants
- Take seizure precautions. Also, expect to administer less-than-maximum dosages of maprotiline and bupropion to prevent seizures.
- Give the drug before bedtime or with food to minimize anticholinergic effects.
- Have the patient sit up for 1 minute before getting out of bed to reduce the effects of orthostatic hypotension.
- Expect to administer a fluoxetine dosage that exceeds 20 mg/day in two divided doses—in the morning and at noon.
- Expect to begin bupropion therapy with small doses and increase them slowly in a patient who is also receiving levodopa.

Lithium
- Obtain baseline tests of the patient's thyroid and renal functions, as prescribed.
- Monitor the lithium concentration regularly during therapy and after dosage adjustments. Evaluate the lithium concentration 12 hours after the last daily dose. Note a concentration that exceeds 1.5 mEq/liter, which may cause toxicity.
- Monitor the patient's white blood cell count.
- Administer lithium with food to reduce GI distress.
- Record the patient's fluid intake and output. Monitor the patient with polyuria for signs of dehydration, such as dry mucous membranes, polydipsia, and poor skin turgor. Note urine specific gravity and color.
- Notify the physician if the urine output significantly exceeds fluid intake.
- Administer fluids to replace fluid loss, as directed.

STUDY ACTIVITIES

Multiple choice
1. Ellen Farber, age 36, was brought to a psychiatric facility by her husband who stated that she had been extremely hyperactive and talking continuously, and had slept for only 3 or 4 hours each night for the last 2 weeks. Which medication is the physician most likely to prescribe for Ms. Farber?

    A. An MAO inhibitor
    B. A tricyclic antidepressant
    C. A second-generation antidepressant
    D. Lithium

2. The nurse assesses Ms. Farber's medication history before administering the prescribed drug. Which medications could cause serious drug interactions?

    A. CNS depressants and sympathomimetic agents

    B. Caffeine and hypoglycemic agents

    C. Diuretics and potassium iodide

    D. Amphetamines and levodopa

3. Which nursing intervention is routinely associated with the drug that has been prescribed for Ms. Farber?

    A. Frequent monitoring of drug concentration during therapy.

    B. Reassurance that anticholinergic effects should diminish.

    C. Instruction regarding drug-induced decreased libido.

    D. Instruction on managing orthostatic hypotension.

4. Kevin Brown, age 54, has just received a diagnosis of atypical depression. Which medication is his physician most likely to prescribe?

    A. An MAO inhibitor

    B. A tricyclic antidepressant

    C. A second-generation antidepressant

    D. Lithium

5. Allen Blake, age 41, is going to take phenelzine sulfate (Nardil) for depression accompanied by phobic anxieties. The nurse teaches him about dietary restrictions to prevent which serious adverse reaction?

    A. Diabetes insipidus syndrome

    B. Hypertensive crisis

    C. Seizures

    D. Priapism

6. Which menu is most appropriate for Mr. Blake during phenelzine sulfate therapy?

    A. Beef liver, new potatoes, fruit salad, and tea

    B. Baked turkey, rice, asparagus, cranberry sauce, and tea

    C. Corned beef, cabbage, green salad with oil and vinegar, and beer

    D. Lasagna, green salad with bleu cheese salad dressing, and red wine

7. Cecilia Curtis, age 29, seeks care for fatigue, weight loss, poor appetite, difficulty concentrating, and thoughts of death, which have persisted for 3 weeks. Her physician prescribes amitriptyline hydrochloride (Elavil). When can Ms. Curtis expect to notice relief from her physical and psychological symptoms?

    A. After 1 week

    B. After 10 to 12 days

    C. Within 2 weeks

    D. After 2 to 4 weeks

8. After 6 weeks, Ms. Curtis has not obtained relief from her symptoms. So her physician switches her to desipramine hydrochloride (Norpramin). This drug may produce which adverse reaction?
   A. Orthostatic hypotension
   B. Intracranial hemorrhage
   C. Peripheral edema
   D. Polyuria

9. Bill Griffin, age 63, is admitted to the psychiatric unit with a major depressive disorder. His physician orders fluoxetine hydrochloride (Prozac) 40 mg P.O. daily. What is the best way to administer this dosage?
   A. 40 mg P.O. at 8:00 a.m.
   B. 40 mg P.O. at 8:00 p.m.
   C. 20 mg P.O. at 8:00 a.m. and 20 mg P.O. at 8:00 p.m.
   D. 20 mg P.O. at 8:00 a.m. and 20 mg P.O. at 12:00 noon

Matching related elements
Match the antidepressant or antimanic agent on the left with its description on the right.

10. ___ Isocarboxazid   **A.** A drug of choice for treating mania

11. ___ Lithium citrate   **B.** Second-generation antidepressant that may cause insomnia

12. ___ Maprotiline   **C.** A drug of choice for treating depression of insidious onset

13. ___ Fluoxetine   **D.** A drug of choice for treating atypical depression

14. ___ Amitriptyline   **E.** Second-generation antidepressant that may have anticholinergic effects

True or false
15. MAO inhibitors are absorbed rapidly and completely from the GI tract.
   ☐ True   ☐ False

16. MAO inhibitors are the drugs of choice in typical depression.
   ☐ True   ☐ False

17. Depressions accompanied by phobias and anxiety respond best to tricyclic antidepressants.
   ☐ True   ☐ False

18. Foods that may interact with MAO inhibitors include yogurt, bananas, and figs.
   ☐ True   ☐ False

19. Tricyclic antidepressants are the drugs of choice for episodes of major depression.
   ☐ True   ☐ False

20. A patient can be safely switched from one tricyclic antidepressant to another.
☐ True ☐ False

ANSWERS

Multiple choice

1. D. Lithium is the drug of choice to treat mania.

2. C. When administered with lithium, thiazide and loop diuretics increase lithium reabsorption in the kidneys; potassium iodide increases hypothyroid activity.

3. A. Because lithium has a narrow therapeutic range and because toxicity may occur at blood levels that exceed 1.5 mEq/liter, the lithium concentration should be monitored frequently.

4. A. MAO inhibitors are the drugs of choice in atypical depression.

5. B. Hypertensive crisis can result from consumption of tyramine-rich foods during MAO inhibitor therapy.

6. B. To prevent hypertensive crisis, the patient should avoid tyramine-rich foods, such as red wine, beer, aged cheese, and liver.

7. D. Physical signs and symptoms may respond after 1 to 2 weeks of therapy; psychological symptoms may respond after 2 to 4 weeks.

8. A. Like the other tricyclic antidepressants, desipramine commonly produces orthostatic hypotension, cardiovascular effects, anticholinergic effects, and sedation.

9. D. To prevent insomnia, fluoxetine dosages above 20 mg/day should be administered in two divided doses—in the morning and at noon.

Matching related elements

10. D

11. A

12. E

13. B

14. C

True or false

15. True.

16. False. MAO inhibitors are the drugs of choice in atypical depression. They are used to treat typical depression only when it is resistant to other therapies or when other therapies are contraindicated.

17. False. MAO inhibitors also are used to treat depression accompanied by anxiety, phobic anxieties, neurodermatitis, hypochondriasis, and narcoleptic states.

18. True.

19. True.

20. True.

CHAPTER 12

Antipsychotic agents

OBJECTIVES

After studying this chapter, the reader should be able to:

1. Identify medications that are used as antipsychotic agents.

2. Discuss the clinical indications for the antipsychotic agents.

3. Describe the mechanisms of action of the antipsychotic agents.

4. Identify common adverse reactions to the antipsychotic agents.

5. Explain the importance of early detection of symptoms of dystonia and tardive dyskinesia.

6. Describe the nursing implications of antipsychotic therapy.

OVERVIEW OF CONCEPTS

Antipsychotic agents also are called major tranquilizers or neuroleptics: *antipsychotic* because they can eliminate signs and symptoms of psychoses; *major tranquilizer* because they can calm an agitated patient; *neuroleptic* because they have a neurobiological adverse effect that causes abnormal body movements.

No matter what they are called, all of these agents belong to one of two major groups: phenothiazines and nonphenothiazines. They are used to treat psychiatric disorders, primarily schizophrenia. In such disorders, antipsychotics can reduce anxiety and symptoms of sensory, thought, and affective overload, such as troublesome voices, delusional beliefs, agitation, hostility, and paranoia. Although these agents cannot cure schizophrenia or other psychoses, they can help control psychotic episodes and restore order to disordered, illogical thinking.

Nonpsychiatric uses of antipsychotics include control of nausea, vomiting, and intractable hiccups; treatment of pruritus; potentiation of narcotics for pain relief; and treatment of movement disorders of Tourette syndrome and Huntington's disease.

Researchers believe schizophrenia and other psychoses result from excess dopamine in the brain. Antipsychotics may work by blocking receptors for this neurotransmitter in the limbic system, which controls emotional behavior and drive. However, these agents also block dopamine receptors in the pyramidal and extrapyramidal tracts, which control voluntary and involuntary muscle movement, as well as other receptors. This accounts for many of their adverse effects and drug interactions.

No one antipsychotic agent is best for eliminating delusions, hallucinations, or thought disorders associated with psychoses. A specific antipsychotic agent may be selected based on its adverse effects profile and potential drug interactions. (For a summary of representative drugs, see Selected Major Drugs: *Antipsychotic agents,* page 176.)

Phenothiazines

The three groups of phenothiazines are aliphatics (which primarily cause sedation and anticholinergic effects), piperazines (which primarily cause extrapyramidal reactions), and piperidines (which primarily cause sedation). The aliphatics include chlorpromazine hydrochloride (Thorazine) and promazine hydrochloride (Sparine). The piperazines are acetophenazine maleate (Tindal), fluphenazine decanoate (Prolixin Decanoate), fluphenazine enanthate (Prolixin Enanthate), fluphenazine hydrochloride (Permitil Hydrochloride), perphenazine (Trilafon), and trifluoperazine hydrochloride (Stelazine). The piperidines include mesoridazine besylate (Serentil) and thioridazine hydrochloride (Mellaril).

Pharmacokinetics

Although the phenothiazines are absorbed erratically, they are distributed to most body tissues and are highly concentrated in the central nervous system (CNS). They are 91% to 99% bound to plasma proteins and have a high affinity for fatty tissue. Active metabolites accumulate in fatty tissues and can prolong drug activity up to 3 months after discontinuation. Phenothiazines are metabolized in the liver and excreted in urine and bile.

The onset of action varies with the type of preparation. A liquid preparation will produce effects in 2 to 4 hours. The onset with tablets is unpredictable. An intramuscular injection usually produces effects in 15 to 30 minutes. However, the antipsychotic effects may take several weeks to appear. The duration of action for a single dose is up to 24 hours.

Pharmacodynamics

The exact mechanism of action of phenothiazines is unclear, but they may act by depressing the reticular activating system, hypothalamus, chemoreceptor trigger zone, and vomiting center. They also stimulate the extrapyramidal system.

Pharmacotherapeutics

Phenothiazines are used primarily to treat schizophrenia, calm anxious or agitated patients, improve thought processes, and alleviate hallucinations and delusions.

Shortly after phenothiazine administration, a quieting and calming effect occurs, but this sedation differs from that produced by CNS depressants. With phenothiazines, the patient is aroused easily, alert, responsive, and has good motor coordination. After several days of thera-

SELECTED MAJOR DRUGS

Antipsychotic agents

This chart summarizes the major antipsychotic agents currently in clinical use.

DRUG	MAJOR INDICATIONS	USUAL ADULT DOSAGE
Phenothiazines		
chlorpromazine	Symptomatic relief of psychoses	Initially, 200 to 600 mg P.O. daily in divided doses, increased to 500 to 1,000 mg daily in divided doses for maintenance
fluphenazine decanoate	Symptomatic relief of psychoses when compliance is a problem	Initially, 12.5 to 25 mg I.M. or S.C. every 1 to 6 weeks, then 25 to 100 mg, as needed, for maintenance
Nonphenothiazines		
haloperidol, haloperidol decanoate	Symptomatic relief of psychoses, relief of dyskinesia in Tourette syndrome	0.5 to 5 mg P.O. b.i.d. or t.i.d., increased as needed, up to 100 mg/day

py, affective changes occur. After several weeks, the patient becomes more coherent, and hallucinations and delusions commonly disappear.

Initial dosing with phenothiazines can be rapid or slow, depending on the severity of symptoms and the patient's age and physical condition. In acute psychosis, the patient receives a loading dose while hospitalized so that the drug's effects and adverse reactions can be monitored.

A geriatric or debilitated patient should receive a small initial dosage that is increased gradually until a favorable response is achieved. When the symptoms are under control, the dosage is reduced gradually to the lowest effective maintenance level.

Drug interactions

When given with CNS depressants, phenothiazines may enhance depressant effects. They also may enhance the effects of antihypertensives and may increase the number or severity of adverse reactions to anticholinergic agents. (For details, see Drug Interactions: *Antipsychotic agents.*)

Adverse drug reactions

Phenothiazines produce adverse reactions that range from mild to severe. Neurologic reactions, such as extrapyramidal effects and tardive dyskinesia, are the most common and most severe. Phenothiazines also may lower the seizure threshold. (For more information, see *Common neurologic effects of antipsychotic agents,* page 178.)

Other adverse reactions may include sedation, hypotension, orthostatic hypotension, anticholinergic effects (including dry mouth, constipation, urine retention, and blurred vision), hypersensitivity reactions,

DRUG INTERACTIONS

Antipsychotic agents

Phenothiazines can interact with a wide range of drugs, most commonly with alcohol or other central nervous system (CNS) depressants. Nonphenothiazines interact with fewer drugs.

DRUG	INTERACTING DRUGS	POSSIBLE EFFECTS
Phenothiazines		
chlorpromazine, fluphenazine, mesoridazine, promazine, thioridazine, trifluoperazine	guanethidine	Decreased uptake of guanethidine
	amphetamines, nonamphetamine anorexigenic agents	Decreased effects of both drugs
	anticholinergic agents	Increased anticholinergic effects; decreased antipsychotic effects
	CNS depressants (barbiturates, narcotic analgesics, general anesthetics, alcohol)	Increased CNS depressant effects; increased phenothiazine metabolism
	levodopa	Reduced antiparkinsonian effects of levodopa
	lithium	Increased risk of neurotoxicity, seizures, delirium, and encephalopathy in manic patients; respiratory depression and hypotension
	droperidol	Increased risk of extrapyramidal effects
	anticonvulsants	Lowered seizure threshold
	tricyclic antidepressants, beta blockers	Increased serum level of either agent
Nonphenothiazines		
haloperidol, clozapine, loxapine, molindone, pimozide, chlorprothixene, thiothixene	levodopa	Decreased levodopa effects; disorientation
haloperidol	lithium	Encephalopathy
clozapine	anticholinergic agents	Increased anticholinergic effects
	antihypertensives	Increased hypotensive effects
	CNS depressants	Increased CNS depression
	bone marrow suppressants	Granulocytopenia
	highly protein-bound drugs (warfarin, phenytoin)	Increased levels of unbound drug, causing toxicity

photosensitivity, blood dyscrasias, jaundice, and neuroleptic malignant syndrome. Phenothiazines are not associated with psychological dependence, tolerance, or addiction. However, sudden discontinuation may produce withdrawal symptoms that resemble those of physical dependence, such as nausea, tremors, and sweating.

Nonphenothiazines Based on their chemical structures, nonphenothiazine antipsychotics are divided into several drug classes: butyrophenones, such as haloperi-

Common neurologic effects of antipsychotic agents

Phenothiazines and other antipsychotic drugs commonly produce adverse neurologic reactions ranging from extrapyramidal effects, such as dystonia, akathisia, and pseudoparkinsonism, to tardive dyskinesia.

Dystonia

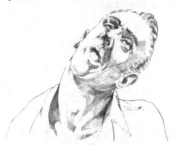

In the first week of antipsychotic therapy, the patient may exhibit an acute dystonic reaction, an extrapyramidal effect manifested by spasms in the tongue, face, neck, back, and sometimes legs that may resemble a seizure. Spasms sometimes affect certain groups of muscles only. Contracted cervical muscles can result in torticollis, an unnatural or twisted position of the neck. Opisthotonos, grimacing, perioral spasms, or pharyngeal or laryngeal spasms with dysphagia or dyspnea also can occur. Eye muscle spasms can cause oculogyrations—abnormal eye movements. Frequently accompanied by excessive salivation, these dystonic spasms typically occur when a patient receives large doses of an antipsychotic agent that is likely to produce extrapyramidal symptoms. They usually disappear with a dosage reduction or administration of 25 to 50 mg of intramuscular (I.M.) diphenhydramine (Benadryl) or 1 to 2 mg of I.M. or intravenous benztropine (Cogentin).

Akathisia

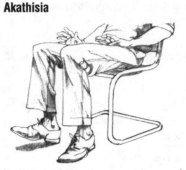

Another extrapyramidal effect, akathisia (a continuous restlessness or inability to sit or stand still) may occur in the first 90 days of therapy. The patient attempts to relieve the discomfort of remaining quiet by tapping a foot, moving about in a chair, or pacing constantly. This symptom easily can be mistaken for agitation, which requires treatment with a higher dose of an antipsychotic agent. However, akathisia should be managed by decreasing the antipsychotic dose or by giving an antiparkinsonian agent, such as benztropine.

Pseudoparkinsonism

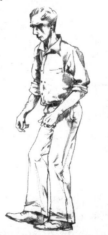

Later in the course of treatment, pseudoparkinsonism may occur. This extrapyramidal effect produces muscle tremors, cogwheel rigidity (muscle rigidity that gives way in little jerks when the muscle is stretched passively), shuffling gait, drooling, and a decrease in arm swing and associative movements when walking. Bradykinesia (slow movement) and akinesia (immobility) also may occur. Pseudoparkinsonism results from a direct blockade of dopamine receptors by antipsychotic agents. This reaction may be controlled with the use of antiparkinsonian agents, such as amantadine.

Tardive dyskinesia

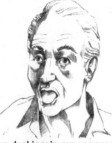

Tardive dyskinesia may appear after several months or years of treatment with antipsychotic drugs. It is characterized by abnormal muscle movement, primarily around the mouth, such as lip smacking, rhythmic darting of tongue, and constant chewing movements. Slow, aimless involuntary movements of the arms or legs also may occur. Although the exact mechanism of tardive dyskinesia is not clear, researchers believe that it may differ from that of the other extrapyramidal symptoms. Tardive dyskinesia usually affects elderly women, but can occur in younger patients as well, even after short-term antipsychotic therapy. If the medication is discontinued when the first signs, such as fine wormlike tongue movements, are detected, tardive dyskinesia sometimes can be prevented.

Prevention of this adverse reaction is vital because no effective treatment is available and the reaction usually is irreversible.

dol (Haldol) and haloperidol decanoate (Haldol Decanoate); dibenzodiazepines, such as clozapine (Clozaril); dibenzoxazepines, such as loxapine succinate (Loxitane); dihydroindolones, such as molindone hydrochloride (Moban); diphenylbutylpiperidines, such as pimozide (Orap); and thioxanthenes, such as chlorprothixene (Taractan) and thiothixene (Navane). Although chemically different from phenothiazines, the nonphenothiazines are used to treat psychotic symptoms with equal effectiveness and produce similar actions and adverse reactions.

Pharmacokinetics

Nonphenothiazines are absorbed, distributed, metabolized, and excreted in the same manner as the phenothiazines. Their onset of action, peak concentration, and duration are similar to those of the phenothiazines.

Pharmacodynamics

Except for clozapine, the mechanism of action of the nonphenothiazines resembles that of the phenothiazines—dopamine receptor blockade. Unlike other nonphenothiazines, clozapine is a weak blocker of dopamine receptors but a potent blocker of serotonin activity.

Pharmacotherapeutics

As a group, nonphenothiazines are used to treat psychotic disorders. Specific drugs may have other functions. For example, thiothixene also is used to control acute agitation. Because of its adverse effects, clozapine is reserved for patients who have not responded to therapy with other antipsychotic agents or who have developed tardive dyskinesia.

Drug interactions

Nonphenothiazines interact with fewer drugs than the phenothiazines. (For details, see Drug Interactions: *Antipsychotic agents,* page 177.)

Adverse drug reactions

Most nonphenothiazines produce the same adverse reactions as the phenothiazines: sedation, extrapyramidal symptoms, hypotension, and anticholinergic effects. Although clozapine produces comparatively fewer extrapyramidal reactions and no tardive dyskinesia, it may cause seizures and life-threatening neutropenia or granulocytopenia. (For more information, see *Common neurologic effects of antipsychotic agents.*)

Nursing implications

When caring for a patient who is receiving an antipsychotic agent, the nurse should be aware of the following implications.

- Develop appropriate nursing diagnoses for the patient. (For examples, see Sample Nursing Diagnoses: *Antipsychotic agents,* page 180.)
- Do not administer an antipsychotic agent to a patient with a condition that contraindicates its use.

Antipsychotic agents

The following nursing diagnoses address representative problems and etiologies that a nurse may encounter when caring for a patient who is receiving an antipsychotic agent.
- Altered cerebral tissue perfusion related to the hypotensive effects of an antipsychotic agent
- Altered health maintenance related to ineffectiveness of the prescribed antipsychotic agent
- Altered protection related to antipsychotic-induced blood dyscrasias
- Altered thought processes related to the sedative effects of an antipsychotic agent
- Constipation related to the anticholinergic effects of an antipsychotic agent
- High risk for injury related to adverse drug reactions
- High risk for injury related to a preexisting condition that contraindicates the use of an antipsychotic agent
- High risk for injury related to a preexisting condition that requires cautious use of an antipsychotic agent
- High risk for injury related to drug interactions
- Hyperthermia related to neuroleptic malignant syndrome caused by an antipsychotic agent
- Impaired physical mobility related to the extrapyramidal effects of an antipsychotic agent
- Knowledge deficit related to the prescribed antipsychotic agent
- Noncompliance related to long-term use of the prescribed antipsychotic agent
- Sensory or perceptual alterations (tactile) related to antipsychotic-induced photosensitivity reaction
- Urinary retention related to the anticholinergic effects of an antipsychotic agent

---

- Administer an antipsychotic agent cautiously to a patient at risk because of a preexisting condition.
- Monitor the patient for neurologic and other common adverse reactions regularly throughout antipsychotic therapy. Also observe for signs of less common, more serious adverse reactions, including blood dyscrasias, jaundice, and neuroleptic malignant syndrome. Notify the physician if the patient develops signs and symptoms of these reactions; expect to discontinue the antipsychotic or, if the patient is psychiatrically unstable, to decrease the dosage.
- Observe for extrapyramidal symptoms. Notify the physician immediately if the patient exhibits acute dystonic reactions, particularly if face or neck spasms interfere with swallowing or breathing.
- Assess the patient for early signs of tardive dyskinesia and notify the physician, as needed.
- Review the results of laboratory and diagnostic tests, including complete blood counts, liver studies, or (for a patient receiving clozapine) weekly white blood cell (WBC) counts to detect adverse hematologic and hepatic reactions.
- Observe for fever, chills, sore throat, and other signs of infection.
- Take safety precautions, such as close patient supervision and removal of harmful objects from the patient's environment, during the first

several weeks of neuroleptic therapy. Antipsychotic effects may take several weeks to appear.

- Expect to administer a small initial dosage of the prescribed antipsychotic agent and gradually increase it until a favorable response is achieved in a geriatric or debilitated patient.
- Monitor the patient's blood pressure regularly to detect hypotension.
- Have the patient sit up for 1 to 2 minutes before standing to minimize the effects of orthostatic hypotension.
- Monitor the patient closely for signs of altered cerebral perfusion, such as decreased blood pressure or a change in level of consciousness or behavior. If these signs occur, take safety precautions and notify the physician.
- Monitor the patient closely for signs of urine retention, such as urinary frequency, complaints of fullness in the lower abdomen, dullness upon percussion over the bladder, and palpation of a distended bladder. If such signs are detected, notify the physician and prepare to catheterize the patient. Expect to decrease the antipsychotic dosage or change the patient to a different drug.
- Relieve other anticholinergic effects—for example, by offering the patient sugarless gum or chipped ice to relieve dry mouth and increasing the patient's fluid and fiber intake to prevent constipation (unless otherwise contraindicated).
- Document the effects of therapy so that the patient may receive the lowest effective dosage. Note, in particular, any sedation, stimulation, agitation, or hyperactivity, and describe any changes in thought patterns and speech that might indicate hallucinations or delusions.
- Avoid abrupt discontinuation of the prescribed antipsychotic agent unless adverse reactions make this necessary.
- Monitor for signs of drug interactions, such as respiratory depression in a patient receiving a phenothiazine and a CNS depressant, and blood pressure changes in one receiving clozapine (or a phenothiazine) and an antihypertensive agent.
- Notify the physician if adverse reactions or drug interactions occur.
- Teach the patient and family the name, dose, frequency, action, and adverse effects of the prescribed antipsychotic agent.
- Stress the importance of taking the medication exactly as prescribed and not discontinuing it without physician approval because psychotic symptoms may return. Ask the family to report patient noncompliance.
- Instruct the patient to return regularly for follow-up care that includes periodic dosage adjustments and laboratory tests.
- Inform the family that they can expect to see normalization of thoughts, moods, and actions in the patient after several weeks or months of antipsychotic therapy.
- Advise the patient to obtain physician approval before ingesting other drugs.

• Teach the patient how to manage orthostatic hypotension and troublesome anticholinergic effects.
• Instruct the family to notify the physician at the first signs of tardive dyskinesia.
• Advise the patient to use a sunscreen and wear protective clothing outdoors to prevent a photosensitivity reaction.
• Teach the patient to recognize and report signs of urine retention.
• Instruct the family to use safety precautions, such as supervising the patient's ambulation, if mild sedation occurs and to alert the physician if sedation worsens or if seizures occur.
• Instruct the patient and family to notify the physician if adverse reactions or changes in psychotic symptoms occur.

Phenothiazines
• Observe for signs of an underlying disease because phenothiazines may mask nausea and suppress vomiting.
• Do not administer more than 800 mg of thioridazine daily because retinal pigmentation may occur.

Nonphenothiazines
• Expect to switch the patient to clozapine if tardive dyskinesia occurs or if the patient does not respond to standard drug therapy.
• Administer clozapine in titrated, divided doses as prescribed to minimize the risk of hypotension, sedation, and seizures.
• Monitor the patient taking chlorprothixene for an allergic reaction because it contains tartrazine.

STUDY ACTIVITIES

Fill in the blank

1. Antipsychotic agents also are called _____ or _____.

2. Although used primarily to treat psychotic disorders, nonpsychotic uses of antipsychotic drugs include _____; _____; _____; and _____.

3. Schizophrenia and other psychoses may result from excess _____ in the brain.

True or false

4. No one antipsychotic agent is superior to another for elimination of delusions, hallucinations, or thought disorders associated with psychoses.
☐ True   ☐ False

5. When administered concomitantly with levodopa, phenothiazines increase levodopa's antiparkinsonian effects.
☐ True   ☐ False

6. Phenothiazines are associated with psychological dependence.
☐ True   ☐ False

7. Patients with a history of seizures should be monitored closely because phenothiazines increase the seizure threshold.
☐ True   ☐ False

8. The four major adverse reactions to nonphenothiazines are sedation, extrapyramidal symptoms, hypotension, and antipsychotic effects.
☐ True   ☐ False

Multiple choice

9. Wallace Wheeler, age 26, is admitted to the psychiatric unit with acute onset of schizophrenia. His physician prescribes the phenothiazine chlorpromazine (Thorazine) 100 mg P.O. q.i.d. Before administering the drug, the nurse reviews Mr. Wheeler's medication history. Concomitant use of which drug is likely to increase the risk of extrapyramidal effects?

A. Guanethidine
B. Droperidol
C. Lithium
D. Alcohol

10. How soon after chlorpromazine administration should the nurse expect to see elimination of delusional thoughts and hallucinations?

A. Several minutes
B. Several hours
C. Several days
D. Several weeks

11. The physician ordered chlorpromazine to be given in liquid form rather than in tablet form. Why?

A. The liquid has a more predictable onset of action.
B. The liquid produces fewer anticholinergic effects.
C. The liquid produces fewer drug interactions.
D. The liquid has a longer duration of action.

12. After 4 months of chlorpromazine therapy, Mr. Wheeler exhibits lip smacking and constant chewing movements. What do these effects signal?

A. Akathisia
B. Dystonia
C. Pseudoparkinsonism
D. Tardive dyskinesia

13. Janet Clark, age 42, is admitted to the psychiatric unit with a tentative diagnosis of psychosis. Her physician prescribes the phenothiazine thioridazine (Mellaril) 50 mg. P.O. t.i.d. How do phenothiazines differ from CNS depressants in their sedative effects?
   A. Phenothiazines produce deeper sleep than CNS depressants.
   B. Phenothiazines produce greater sedation than CNS depressants.
   C. Phenothiazines produce a calming effect from which the patient is easily aroused.
   D. Phenothiazines produce more prolonged sedative effects, making the patient difficult to arouse.

14. The nurse tells Ms. Clark to drink fluids to help prevent dry mouth and constipation. These reactions result from which drug effects?
   A. Anticholinergic
   B. Antihistaminic
   C. Extrapyramidal
   D. Adrenergic

15. The thioridazine dosage should not exceed 800 mg/day to prevent which adverse reactions?
   A. Hypertension
   B. Respiratory arrest
   C. Tourette syndrome
   D. Retinal pigmentation

16. Holly Hamilton, age 33, begins clozapine (Clozaril) therapy after several other antipsychotic agents fail to relieve her psychotic symptoms. The nurse instructs her to return for weekly WBC counts to assess for which adverse reaction?
   A. Hepatitis
   B. Infection
   C. Granulocytopenia
   D. Systemic dermatitis

17. Clozapine may be used for patients who have developed which adverse reaction to other antipsychotic agents?
   A. Akathisia
   B. Hypertension
   C. Pseudoparkinsonism
   D. Tardive dyskinesia

18. Anne Murphy, age 43, has chronic undifferentiated schizophrenia. Because she has a history of noncompliance with antipsychotic therapy, she will receive fluphenazine decanoate (Prolixin) injections every 4 weeks. Before discharge, what should the nurse teach Ms. Murphy?
    A. Ask the physician for droperidol to control any extrapyramidal symptoms that occur.
    B. Sit up for a few minutes before standing to minimize orthostatic hypotension.
    C. Notify the physician if her thoughts do not normalize within 1 week.
    D. Expect symptoms of tardive dyskinesia to occur and be transient.

19. The nurse instructs Ms. Murphy and her family to report the first sign of tardive dyskinesia to the physician immediately. Which of the following is an early sign of tardive dyskinesia?
    A. Wormlike tongue movements
    B. Excessive salivation
    C. Cogwheel rigidity
    D. Urine retention

20. Later in fluphenazine therapy, Ms. Murphy develops pseudoparkinsonism. The physician is likely to prescribe which drug to control this extrapyramidal effect?
    A. Phenytoin
    B. Amantadine
    C. Benztropine
    D. Diphenhydramine

ANSWERS   **Fill in the blanks**
    1. Major tranquilizers, neuroleptics
    2. Control of nausea, vomiting, and intractable hiccups; treatment of pruritus; potentiation of narcotics for pain relief; and treatment of movement disorders of Tourette syndrome and Huntington's disease
    3. Dopamine

True or false
    4. True.
    5. False. Phenothiazines block the dopamine receptors in the CNS, thereby reducing the antiparkinsonian effects of levodopa.
    6. False. Phenothiazines are not associated with psychological dependence, tolerance, or addiction. However, sudden discontinuation may produce withdrawal symptoms that resemble those of physical dependence.
    7. False. Phenothiazines may lower the seizure threshold.
    8. False. The four major adverse reactions to phenothiazines and non-phenothiazines are sedation, extrapyramidal symptoms, hypotension, and anticholinergic effects.

Multiple choice

9. B. When administered with any phenothiazine, droperidol may increase the risk of extrapyramidal effects.

10. D. Although most phenothiazines produce some effects within minutes to hours, their antipsychotic effects may take several weeks to appear.

11. A. A liquid phenothiazine preparation will produce effects in 2 to 4 hours. The onset with tablets is unpredictable.

12. D. Tardive dyskinesia is characterized by abnormal muscle movement, primarily around the mouth, such as lip smacking, rhythmic darting of the tongue, and constant chewing movements.

13. C. Shortly after phenothiazine administration, a quieting and calming effect occurs, but the patient is easily aroused, alert, responsive, and has good motor coordination.

14. A. Anticholinergic effects include dry mouth, constipation, urine retention, and blurred vision.

15. D. Retinal pigmentation may occur if the thioridazine dosage exceeds 800 mg/day.

16. C. Clozapine can cause life-threatening neutropenia or granulocytopenia. To detect this adverse reaction, a WBC count should be performed weekly.

17. D. Because of its adverse effects, clozapine is reserved for patients who have not responded to therapy with other antipsychotic agents or who have developed tardive dyskinesia.

18. B. The nurse should teach the patient how to manage common adverse reactions, such as orthostatic hypotension and anticholinergic effects.

19. A. The first signs of tardive dyskinesia include wormlike tongue movements. Later signs include rhythmic darting of the tongue, lip smacking, and constant chewing movements.

20. B. An antiparkinsonian agent, such as amantadine, may be used to control pseudoparkinsonism; diphenhydramine or benztropine may be used to control other extrapyramidal effects.

CHAPTER 13

Cardiac glycoside agents and bipyridines

OBJECTIVES

After studying this chapter, the reader will be able to:

1. Describe the clinical indications of the cardiac glycosides digoxin and digitoxin and the bipyridine amrinone lactate.

2. Differentiate between the pharmacokinetic properties of digoxin and digitoxin.

3. Describe the actions of cardiac glycosides and bipyridines in treating congestive heart failure.

4. Explain why digitalis toxicity commonly occurs, and describe its signs and symptoms.

5. Describe the nursing implications of cardiac glycoside or bipyridine therapy.

OVERVIEW OF CONCEPTS

Cardiac glycosides (digitalis preparations) and bipyridines increase the force of cardiac contraction (positive inotropic effect). They also slow the heart rate (negative chronotropic effect) and slow electrical impulse conduction through the atrioventricular (AV) node (negative dromotropic effect). These actions make cardiac glycosides and bipyridines useful in treating congestive heart failure (CHF) and make cardiac glycosides useful in treating certain supraventricular arrhythmias. (For a summary of representative drugs, see Selected Major Drugs: *Cardiac glycoside agents and bipyridines,* page 188.)

Cardiac physiology

To understand how these agents improve CHF, the nurse must comprehend cardiac physiology. Cardiac output represents the amount of blood pumped from the heart in 1 minute. It equals the heart rate multiplied by the stroke volume (the amount of blood ejected by the left ventricle with each contraction). Heart rate is affected by the autonomic nervous system, the conduction system, and various drugs. Stroke volume is influenced by myocardial contractility, preload (stretch of the myofibrils, or muscle fibers, as contraction begins), and afterload (arterial resistance met by blood leaving the left ventricle).

Cardiac glycoside agents and bipyridines

This table summarizes the major cardiac glycosides and bipyridines currently in clinical use.

DRUG	MAJOR INDICATIONS	USUAL ADULT DOSAGES
Cardiac glycosides		
digoxin	Congestive heart failure, atrial and supraventricular arrhythmias	As loading dose, 10 to 15 mcg/kg I.V. or P.O.; for maintenance, 0.125 to 0.5 mg I.V. or P.O. daily
digitoxin	Congestive heart failure, atrial and supraventricular arrhythmias	As loading dose for slow digitalization, 0.2 mg P.O. b.i.d. for 4 days; as loading dose for rapid digitalization, initially, 0.6 mg P.O., followed by 0.4 mg and then 0.2 mg at 4- to 6-hour intervals; for maintenance, 0.05 to 0.3 mg P. O. daily
Bipyridines		
amrinone	Congestive heart failure	As loading dose, 0.75 mg/kg I.V. infused over 2 to 3 minutes; for maintenance, 5 to 10 mcg/kg/minute by continuous I.V. infusion

Starling's law states that although the volume of blood flowing into the heart varies, the myofibrils alter to keep the blood volume in the heart constant. This means that within limits, the heart pumps all the blood that comes to it, without allowing excessive backing up of blood in the veins. To improve cardiac output, alterations in heart rate, contractility, preload, and afterload must occur.

Cardiac glycosides

Cardiac glycosides are a group of drugs derived from digitalis. Digoxin (Lanoxicaps, Lanoxin) and digitoxin (Crystodigin) are the most frequently used agents. Both drugs have a narrow therapeutic index.

Pharmacokinetics

Intestinal absorption of digoxin varies from 60% to 100%, depending on the dosage form (liquid, capsule, or tablet) and the manufacturer. Absorption of digitoxin from the gastrointestinal (GI) tract is almost complete (90% to 100%) because the drug is more lipid-soluble than digoxin. Food in the GI tract can retard the rate, but not the extent, of absorption. Malabsorption syndromes, high-fiber foods, and certain drugs can decrease the extent of GI absorption.

Once absorbed or given by intravenous (I.V.) injection, digoxin takes about 8 hours to reach equilibrium at tissue-binding sites. It is distributed widely, bound more to skeletal muscles than to body fat, and concentrated in the cardiac tissues. Only a small percentage of digoxin is metabolized by the liver and GI flora. The remaining drug is excreted by the kidneys as unchanged drug.

The onset of action and peak concentration for digoxin and digitoxin vary with oral and I.V. administration. The duration of action varies with the patient's ability to eliminate the drug. For oral and I.V.

digoxin, it ranges from 2 to 6 days; for oral and I.V. digitoxin, 2 to 3 weeks.

Because the half-lives of digoxin (36 hours) and digitoxin (7 days) are relatively long, the patient may receive a loading, or digitalizing, dose to reach the therapeutic steady state concentration rapidly. The loading dose is followed by a regular maintenance dosage; both dosages are tailored to the individual patient.

Pharmacodynamics

Cardiac glycosides produce positive inotropic effects and negative chronotropic and dromotropic effects. They may produce these effects via three mechanisms. First, they may inhibit the sodium-potassium-adenosine triphosphatase (ATPase) pump, which normally maintains the sodium and potassium concentration differences across the cell membrane. Pump inhibition may increase intracellular sodium, which then is exchanged for calcium. This makes increased intracellular calcium available to the contractile elements of the myocardium, leading to enhanced force of contraction. Second, cardiac glycosides may enhance calcium movement into the myocardial cell. Third, these drugs may stimulate the release, or block the uptake, of norepinephrine at the adrenergic nerve terminal.

Cardiac glycosides also have electrophysiologic properties that make them useful in managing specific supraventricular arrhythmias. They stimulate the parasympathetic division of the autonomic nervous system, thereby increasing vagal tone. This vagal effect slows the heart rate, increases the refractory period, and slows conduction through the AV node and junctional tissue.

Pharmacotherapeutics

Cardiac glycosides are prescribed primarily to treat CHF and atrial arrhythmias. They may improve cardiac hemodynamics when they are used with diuretics or vasodilators in managing mild to moderate heart failure. In patients with acute myocardial infarction, cardiac glycosides must be used with caution because of their unpredictable effects on myocardial oxygen consumption.

Usually, cardiac glycosides are administered orally or intravenously. They rarely are given by intramuscular (I.M.) injection because they can cause severe pain and necrosis at the injection site. Geriatric patients require smaller doses because of their diminished lean body mass and decreased renal and hepatic blood flow.

Drug interactions

Cardiac glycosides interact with several drugs and some foods. Some drugs reduce their absorption, which can reduce their therapeutic effects; others enhance their absorption or pharmacologic effect, which can lead to digitalis toxicity. Decreased dietary potassium increases the chance of toxicity, especially if the patient also is taking a potassium-

DRUG INTERACTIONS

Cardiac glycoside agents and bipyridines

Digoxin and digitoxin interact with several drugs, which may decrease absorption, decrease therapeutic effects, increase toxic effects, and cause arrhythmias. Bipyridines interact with fewer drugs.

DRUG	INTERACTING DRUGS	POSSIBLE EFFECTS
digoxin, digitoxin	rifampin, barbiturates, phenytoin (digitoxin only), cholestyramine resin, antacids, kaolin and pectin, sulfasalazine	Decreased digoxin or digitoxin effect
	calcium preparations, quinidine, verapamil, anticholinergic agents, amiodarone, spironolactone, hydroxychloroquine	Digitalis toxicity
	amphotericin B, potassium-wasting diuretics, steroids, broad-spectrum penicillins	Hypokalemia, digitalis toxicity
	beta-adrenergic blockers	Excessive bradycardia, arrhythmias
	succinylcholine, thyroid preparations	Arrhythmias
Bipyridines		
amrinone	disopyramide	Hypotension
	digoxin, digitoxin	Enhanced atrioventricular conduction, increased ventricular response rate

wasting diuretic. (For details, see Drug Interactions: *Cardiac glycoside agents and bipyridines,* page 190.)

Adverse drug reactions

Because cardiac glycosides have a narrow therapeutic index, they produce digitalis toxicity in 8% to 35% of all hospitalized patients. The therapeutic serum concentration of digoxin typically ranges from 0.5 to 2 ng/ml; of digitoxin, from 14 to 26 ng/ml. However, patients vary greatly in their responses to cardiac glycosides. One patient may exhibit toxicity when the serum concentration falls within the therapeutic range; another may require serum concentrations above the therapeutic range to achieve the desired effect. (For more information, see *Signs and symptoms of digitalis toxicity.*) The cardiac glycoside's half-life affects the duration of adverse reactions. Because digoxin has a shorter half-life, many physicians prefer using it over digitoxin.

The following conditions may predispose a patient to digitalis toxicity: hypokalemia, hypomagnesemia, hypothyroidism, hypoxemia, advanced myocardial disease, active myocardial ischemia, and increased vagal tone.

Signs and symptoms of digitalis toxicity

Digitalis toxicity affects several body systems, most commonly the gastrointestinal tract. The most common early symptoms are anorexia, nausea, vomiting, and diarrhea.

Gastrointestinal
- anorexia
- nausea
- vomiting
- diarrhea
- abdominal pain

Neurologic
- headache
- restlessness
- irritability
- depression

- personality change
- lassitude
- confusion
- disorientation
- insomnia
- psychoses
- seizures
- coma
- blurred vision or blue-yellow color blindness
- flickering lights

- white borders on dark objects
- colored dots

Cardiac
- atrial arrhythmias
- ventricular arrhythmias
- sinoatrial arrest or block
- accelerated junctional rhythms
- atrial tachycardia with atrioventricular (AV) block
- second-degree AV block (Wenckebach)
- third-degree AV block (complete)

Bipyridines

The bipyridines, a new class of positive inotropic agents, are nonglycoside, noncatecholamine agents used to manage heart failure. Currently, amrinone lactate (Inocor) is the only approved bipyridine.

Pharmacokinetics
After I.V. administration, amrinone is distributed rapidly, metabolized by the liver, and excreted by the kidneys. The drug is rapid-acting, but has a short duration of action. After a single I.V. bolus dose of 0.5 to 1.5 mg/kg, cardiac output increases within 5 minutes. The peak effect occurs in about 10 minutes, decreasing by about half in 30 to 40 minutes. Amrinone's half-life is 3.6 hours in stable patients and 6 hours in patients with CHF. The normal therapeutic plasma level of amrinone ranges from 0.5 to 7.0 mcg/ml.

Pharmacodynamics
Amrinone improves cardiac output by increasing contractility and decreasing afterload and preload. With increased cardiac output, renal blood flow improves and urine output increases. Amrinone's only effect on the conduction system is to facilitate AV node conduction. It does not increase myocardial oxygen consumption.

Pharmacotherapeutics
Amrinone is used for short-term management of CHF in patients who have not responded to a cardiac glycoside, diuretic, or vasodilator. In a patient with atrial flutter or fibrillation with rapid ventricular response, amrinone may be given with a cardiac glycoside; this combination may increase ventricular response rates by enhancing AV node conduction.

Drug interactions
Amrinone interacts with disopyramide and cardiac glycosides. (For details, see Drug Interactions: *Cardiac glycoside agents and bipyridines.*)

Adverse drug reactions
Adverse reactions are uncommon and usually occur only during prolonged therapy. However, they may include reversible thrombocytopenia; arrhythmias and hypotension; nausea, vomiting, cramps, dyspepsia, and diarrhea; liver enzyme elevation and hepatotoxicity; burning at the injection site; and hypersensitivity. Thrombocytopenia can be reversed by reducing the amrinone dosage or discontinuing the drug.

Nursing implications
When caring for a patient who is receiving a cardiac glycoside or bipyridine, the nurse should be aware of the following implications.
• Develop appropriate nursing diagnoses for the patient. (For examples, see Sample Nursing Diagnoses: *Cardiac glycoside agents and bipyridines.*)
• Do not administer a cardiac glycoside or bipyridine to a patient with a condition that contraindicates its use.
• Administer a cardiac glycoside or bipyridine cautiously to a patient at risk because of a preexisting condition.
• Monitor the patient regularly for therapeutic and adverse effects.
• Review the patient's medication history and monitor for signs of drug interactions.
• Notify the physician if adverse reactions or drug interactions occur or if the patient responds inadequately to drug therapy.
• Teach the patient and family the name, dose, frequency, action, and adverse effects of the prescribed cardiac glycoside or bipyridine.
• Teach the patient and family to report adverse reactions.

Cardiac glycosides
• Assess the patient's apical pulse before starting therapy and before administering each dose. Withhold the drug and notify the physician if the pulse rate is below 60 beats/minute or if a significant rhythm change occurs.
• Expect to use a reduced dosage for a geriatric or pediatric patient or to one with renal dysfunction, hypoalbuminemia, or heart failure.
• Monitor the patient's serum drug levels, as prescribed.
• Monitor for electrolyte imbalances and increased creatinine levels, especially for a patient receiving digoxin. Monitor liver function studies for a patient receiving digitoxin.
• Question any order that specifies I.M. administration because this is not a preferred route.
• Expect to administer a reduced dosage of capsules or elixir because they have a higher bioavailability than tablets.

SAMPLE NURSING DIAGNOSES

Cardiac glycoside agents and bipyridines

The following nursing diagnoses address representative problems and etiologies that a nurse may encounter when caring for a patient who is receiving a cardiac glycoside or bipyridine.

- Altered health maintenance related to ineffectiveness of the prescribed cardiac glycoside or bipyridine
- Altered protection related to amrinone-induced thrombocytopenia
- Altered thought processes related to confusion caused by a cardiac glycoside
- Decreased cardiac output related to the adverse effects of a cardiac glycoside
- Diarrhea related to the adverse gastrointestinal (GI) effects of a cardiac glycoside
- High risk for fluid volume deficit related to the adverse GI effects of a cardiac glycoside or bipyridine
- High risk for injury related to adverse drug reactions
- High risk for injury related to a preexisting condition that contraindicates the use of a cardiac glycoside or bipyridine
- High risk for injury related to a preexisting condition that requires cautious use of a cardiac glycoside or bipyridine
- High risk for injury related to drug interactions
- Knowledge deficit related to the prescribed cardiac glycoside or bipyridine
- Noncompliance related to adverse drug reactions
- Pain related to abdominal or chest pain caused by a cardiac glycoside or bipyridine
- Sensory or perceptual alterations (visual) related to the central nervous system effects of a cardiac glycoside
- Sleep pattern disturbance related to insomnia caused by a cardiac glycoside

---

- Administer digoxin in two divided doses, as prescribed, for maintenance therapy in a pediatric patient to avoid a high peak serum concentration.
- Do not administer digoxin with drugs that decrease its absorption, such as antacids, kaolin, or pectin.
- Do not administer digoxin with meals or with high-bran snacks because drug absorption will be affected.
- Monitor for signs of digitalis toxicity. Withhold the drug and notify the physician immediately if such signs occur.
- Emphasize the importance of taking the drug exactly as prescribed.
- Demonstrate how to take a pulse.
- Encourage the patient to eat high-potassium foods, such as orange juice, bananas, spinach, raisins, and cantaloupes.
- Instruct the patient to store the drug in a tightly covered, light-resistant container and to consult the physician before taking any other drugs, including over-the-counter ones.

Bipyridines

- Obtain baseline platelet counts and liver enzyme, electrolyte, blood urea nitrogen, and creatinine levels before starting amrinone therapy. Monitor these values throughout therapy.

- Take bleeding precautions for a patient who develops thrombocytopenia, which can be reversed by reducing the amrinone dosage or discontinuing the drug.
- Dilute amrinone in 0.9% sodium chloride—not dextrose—solution before administration. Use the diluted solution within 24 hours.
- Administer I.V. infusions with an infusion pump, using a central or peripheral line.

STUDY ACTIVITIES

Fill in the blank

1. _____ is the amount of blood pumped from the heart in 1 minute.

2. Cardiac output = _____ × _____.

3. _____ refers to the stretch of the myofibrils as contraction begins in the heart.

4. _____ refers to the arterial resistance met by the blood leaving the left ventricle.

5. Amrinone is a _____-acting drug with a _____ duration of action.

6. Cardiac glycosides produce positive _____ effects and negative _____ and _____ effects.

7. Cardiac glycosides may produce their therapeutic effects by inhibiting _____ enhancing _____ and stimulating _____ .

Multiple choice

8. Bob Green, age 68, is admitted to the hospital with CHF. His physician orders digoxin 12 mcg/kg I.V. followed by 0.125 mg P.O. daily. Digoxin 12 mcg/kg I.V. is which type of usual adult dosage?
  A. Typical loading
  B. High loading
  C. Low loading
  D. Maintenance

9. What accounts for the need to give a loading dose of digoxin?
  A. Adverse effects profile
  B. Fast onset of action
  C. Extensive metabolism
  D. Long half-life

10. Five days after beginning digoxin therapy, Mr. Green develops headaches, nausea, and insomnia. What action should the nurse take?

    A. Notify the physician immediately.

    B. Reduce the digoxin dosage by half.

    C. Administer digoxin in two divided doses.

    D. Seek an order for an analgesic, antiemetic, and a sedative.

11. Molly Johnson, age 72, is admitted to the hospital for evaluation of digitalis toxicity. For the past 4 years, she has been taking digoxin for atrial arrhythmia. When assessing Ms. Johnson, the nurse is likely to uncover which finding?

    A. Constipation

    B. Heart rate of 72

    C. Blurred vision and flickering lights

    D. Hyperactivity, especially in the morning

12. The nurse also reviews Ms. Johnson's medication history. During digoxin therapy, use of which drug is likely to cause digitalis toxicity?

    A. Propranolol

    B. Verapamil

    C. Warfarin

    D. Aspirin

13. Ms. Johnson tells the nurse that she eats bran flakes every morning before taking digoxin. Is this likely to affect digitalis toxicity?

    A. Yes, because delayed stomach emptying increases the amount of drug in the blood.

    B. Yes, because bran flakes increase digoxin absorption.

    C. Maybe, but it depends on the digoxin dosage ordered.

    D. No, because bran flakes decrease digoxin absorption.

True or false

14. Digoxin commonly is used to treat ventricular arrhythmias.

    ☐ True   ☐ False

15. If a patient takes penicillin during digoxin therapy, no drug interaction should result.

    ☐ True   ☐ False

16. Digoxin usually is administered orally, intravenously, or intramuscularly.

    ☐ True   ☐ False

17. Decreased heart rate is a therapeutic response to digoxin.

    ☐ True   ☐ False

18. Digoxin is preferred over digitoxin because digoxin has a shorter half-life.

    ☐ True   ☐ False

19. Amrinone should be diluted in 0.9% sodium chloride solution before administration.
☐ True   ☐ False

20. Amrinone-induced thrombocytopenia can be reversed by reducing the amrinone dosage or discontinuing the drug.
☐ True   ☐ False

ANSWERS   **Fill in the blank**

1. Cardiac output
2. Heart rate, stroke volume
3. Preload
4. Afterload
5. Rapid, short
6. Inotropic, chronotropic, dromotropic
7. The sodium-potassium-adenosine triphosphatase (ATPase) pump, calcium movement into myocardial cells, norepinephrine release

Multiple choice

8. A. Usually, the loading dose for digoxin is 10 to 15 mcg/kg I.V. or P.O. It is used to promote rapid digitalization.
9. D. Because the half-life of digoxin is long (36 hours), the patient needs a loading, or digitalizing, dose to reach the therapeutic steady state concentration rapidly.
10. A. Nausea, headache, and insomnia may be signs of digitalis toxicity, which require physician notification.
11. C. Digoxin toxicity commonly produces such effects as blurred vision, flickering lights, diarrhea, lassitude, and tachycardia.
12. A. Such drugs as verapamil, calcium preparations, and quinidine may cause digitalis toxicity when combined with digoxin.
13. D. Malabsorption syndromes, high-fiber foods, and certain drugs can decrease the extent of GI absorption, which tends to decrease the risk of digitalis toxicity.

True or false

14. False. Digoxin is used to treat CHF and certain atrial and supraventricular arrhythmias.
15. False. Broad-spectrum penicillins and certain other antibiotics may interact with digoxin, causing hypokalemia or digitalis toxicity.
16. False. Usually, cardiac glycosides are administered orally or intravenously. They rarely are given by I.M. injection because they can cause severe pain and necrosis at the injection site.
17. True.
18. True.
19. True.
20. True.

CHAPTER 14

Antiarrhythmic agents

OBJECTIVES

After studying this chapter, the reader should be able to:

1. Describe the course of a normally conducted impulse from the sinus node to the ventricular myocardium.

2. Describe the mechanism of action for each class of antiarrhythmics.

3. Identify important pharmacokinetic differences among the agents in each class of antiarrhythmics.

4. Identify the clinical indications for each class of antiarrhythmics.

5. Identify adverse effects of the agents in each class of antiarrhythmics.

6. Describe the nursing implications of antiarrhythmic therapy.

OVERVIEW OF CONCEPTS

Antiarrhythmic drugs are used to treat abnormal electrical activity of the heart. They act by limiting cardiac electrical conduction to the normal pathways and decreasing abnormally fast heart rates. The drugs discussed in this chapter are grouped into seven classes, according to their effects on the action potential of cardiac cells: I, IA, IB, IC, II, III, and IV. (For a summary of representative drugs, see Selected Major Drugs: *Antiarrhythmic agents,* page 198.)

Electrophysiology and cardiac conduction

An overview of the normal electrophysiology and conduction system in the heart will help the nurse understand the action of antiarrhythmic drugs. Abnormalities of cardiac electrical activity can be diagnosed by an electrocardiogram (ECG).

Four characteristics distinguish myocardial cells from other cells: automaticity, the ability to initiate an action potential (change in intracellular charge); excitability, the ability to respond to an electrical impulse; conductivity, the ability to transmit electrical impulses to the next cell; and contractility, the ability to contract when stimulated.

Although all myocardial cells share the same characteristics, certain specialized cells generate electrical impulses. These pacemaker cells initiate electrical stimulation of the heart, which begins in the sinoatrial (SA) nodes and travels throughout the heart. (For more information, see *Pacemaker cells and pathways,* page 199.)

SELECTED MAJOR DRUGS

Antiarrhythmic agents

The following chart summarizes the major antiarrhythmic agents currently in clinical use.

DRUG	MAJOR INDICATIONS	USUAL ADULT DOSAGES
Class IA antiarrhythmics		
quinidine	Conversion of atrial fibrillation to normal sinus rhythm	300 to 400 mg quinidine sulfate P.O. every 6 hours, then 200 to 400 mg P.O. every 6 hours to maintain regular rhythm
	Suppression of atrial or ventricular ectopic beats	200 to 300 mg quinidine sulfate P.O. every 6 to 8 hours
Class IB antiarrhythmics		
lidocaine	Suppression of ventricular ectopic beats, conversion of ventricular tachycardia, prevention of ventricular arrhythmias	Initially, 50 to 100 mg I.V. bolus, followed by a second I.V. bolus of 50 to 100 mg 5 minutes later, then 1 to 4 mg/minute by continuous I.V. infusion; or 300 mg I.M., repeated in 60 to 90 minutes, as needed
Class IC antiarrhythmics		
flecainide	Prevention of sustained ventricular tachycardia	100 to 200 mg P.O. every 12 hours
Class II antiarrhythmics		
propranolol	Atrial or ventricular ectopy, sudden onset of self-limiting atrial or ventricular tachycardia	10 to 30 mg P.O. every 6 to 8 hours; for life-threatening arrhythmias, 0.5 to 3 mg I.V.
Class III antiarrhythmics		
amiodarone	Ventricular tachycardia unresponsive to other antiarrhythmics	800 to 1,600 mg P.O. daily for 1 to 3 weeks as loading dose, then reduced gradually to 200 to 400 mg P.O. daily for maintenance
Class IV antiarrhythmics		
verapamil	Paroxysmal supraventricular tachycardia	5 to 10 mg I.V. push infused over 2 minutes, followed by a second dose of 10 mg I.V. push after 15 to 30 minutes if the patient tolerates but does not respond to the first dose
	Ventricular rate control in atrial fibrillation or flutter	240 to 480 mg P.O. daily in three or four divided doses

The myocardial intracellular charge changes when sodium ions (Na^+) and calcium ions (CA^{++}) flow into the cell and potassium ions (K^+) flow out. Called the action potential, this change leads to depolarization, causing the cell to contract. Depolarization (contraction) occurs as the usual negative resting state of the cell changes to zero in the pacemaker cell or to slightly positive in the muscle cell. Repolarization (relaxation) occurs when the cell returns to its usual negative charge.

Pacemaker and muscle cells have different action potentials. The pacemaker cell undergoes more gradual excitation, whereas the muscle cell has a steeper slope of depolarization and rapid excitation (phase 0). The pacemaker cell also does not have an early rapid

Pacemaker cells and pathways

In the heart, pacemaker cells initiate electrical stimulation, which begins in the sinoatrial (SA) nodes and travels throughout the heart. Impulses spread to both atria and collect in the atrio-ventricular (AV) node, where they are delayed to allow the ventricles to fill with blood from the atria. From the AV node, impulses travel along the bundle of His, the right and left bundle branches, and the Purkinje fibers to stimulate the ventricles to contract, ejecting blood into the pulmonary artery and aorta.

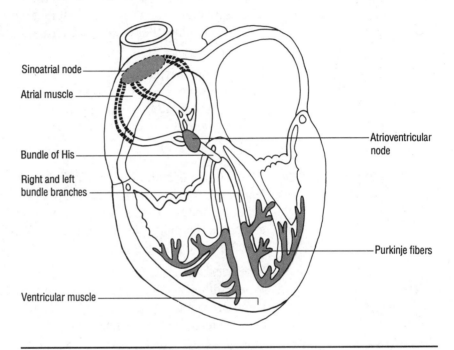

repolarization (phase 1) or a plateau (phase 2) and exhibits final rapid repolarization (phase 3) and spontaneous depolarization at rest (phase 4).

Once a muscle cell has been depolarized, it is not susceptible to a second depolarization until a certain time period has elapsed. This time period is the effective refractory period (ERP), roughly equal to the action potential duration (APD).

Class I antiarrhythmics   Moricizine hydrochloride (Ethmozine) is a new class I antiarrhythmic agent with potent anesthetic activity and myocardial membrane stabilizing effects.

Pharmacokinetics

After oral administration, about 38% of moricizine is absorbed and reaches peak concentration within 2 hours. It is highly bound to plasma proteins, extensively metabolized, and excreted in the urine.

Pharmacodynamics

Moricizine has local anesthetic and myocardial membrane stabilizing effects. It depresses the depolarization rate and decreases action potential duration and the effective refractory period.

Pharmacotherapeutics

Moricizine is used to manage life-threatening ventricular arrhythmias, such as sustained ventricular tachycardia.

Drug interactions

This class I antiarrhythmic may interact with cimetidine, propranolol, and theophylline. (For details, see Drug Interactions: *Antiarrhythmic agents.*)

Adverse drug reactions

The most serious adverse reaction is the appearance of new arrhythmias or exacerbation of existing arrhythmias. The most common reactions are dizziness, nausea, headache, fatigue, dyspnea, and palpitations.

Class IA antiarrhythmics

Class IA antiarrhythmics include disopyramide phosphate (Norpace, Norpace CR), procainamide hydrochloride (Procan SR, Pronestyl), and quinidine sulfate (Cin-Quin, Quinidex Extentabs, Quinora), quinidine gluconate (Duraquin, Quinaglute Dura-Tabs), or quinidine polygalacturonate (Cardioquin).

Pharmacokinetics

When administered orally, class IA antiarrhythmics undergo rapid absorption from the gastrointestinal (GI) tract and metabolized in the liver. For this reason, researchers have developed sustained-release forms to help maintain therapeutic levels. These drugs are excreted in the urine.

Food and extremes of gastric pH hasten or delay absorption. Quinidine's absorption rate also depends on the salt with which it is combined; quinidine polygalacturonase and quinidine gluconate are absorbed more slowly than quinidine sulfate.

The onset of action after oral administration is 30 minutes to 3 hours; sustained-release forms may have a later onset. The peak concentration occurs in 1 to 5 hours. The nurse should monitor the serum drug concentration closely to prevent toxicity.

Pharmacodynamics

Class IA antiarrhythmics alter the myocardial cell membrane by blocking the cells' fast channel. This decreases Na^+ influx, thereby depressing the rate of depolarization and prolonging repolarization. These changes reduce the rate of automaticity in ectopic foci, increase the refractory period, and decrease the conduction speed.

These drugs also interfere with autonomic nervous system control of pacemaker cells by blocking parasympathetic nervous system dis-

DRUG INTERACTIONS

Antiarrhythmic agents

Many antiarrhythmic agents interact with commonly administered drugs, causing potentially serious consequences for the patient. The nurse must be aware of these interactions to provide appropriate care.

DRUG	INTERACTING DRUGS	POSSIBLE EFFECTS
Class I antiarrhythmics		
moricizine	cimetidine	Increased plasma moricizine level
	propranolol	Increased P-R interval on electrocardiogram
	theophylline	Increased clearance and decreased half-life of theophylline
Class IA antiarrhythmics		
disopyramide	anticholinergic agents	Increased anticholinergic effects
	verapamil	Myocardial depression
procainamide	cimetidine, amiodarone	Increased serum procainamide level
quinidine	neuromuscular blockers	Increased skeletal muscle relaxation
	oral anticoagulants	Hypoprothrombinemia
	digoxin	Increased serum digoxin level
	urinary alkalinizers, cimetidine, amiodarone	Increased serum quinidine level
quinidine, disopyramide	rifampin, phenytoin, phenobarbital	Increased quinidine and disopyramide metabolism
Class IB antiarrhythmics		
lidocaine	cimetidine, propranolol	Lidocaine toxicity
mexiletine	phenytoin	Decreased mexiletine level
mexiletine, tocainide	rifampin	Decreased mexiletine or tocainide level
Class IC antiarrhythmics		
encainide	cimetidine	Decreased hepatic metabolism of encainide
	other antiarrhythmics, beta-adrenergic blockers, verapamil, diltiazem	Increased effects on conduction system
flecainide, propafenone	digoxin	Increased serum digoxin level
flecainide	alkalinizing agents, cimetidine, propranolol	Increased serum flecainide level
	disopyramide, verapamil, diltiazem, beta-adrenergic blockers	Increased negative inotropic effects
indecainide	other antiarrhythmic agents	Increased serum concentration and effects of indecainide
propafenone	warfarin	Increased prothrombin time
	metoprolol, propranolol	Increased serum concentrations and effects of metoprolol and propranolol

(continued)

Antiarrhythmic agents *(continued)*

DRUG	INTERACTING DRUGS	POSSIBLE EFFECTS
Class IC antiarrhythmics *(continued)*		
propafenone	quinidine	Inhibited propafenone metabolism
Class II antiarrhythmics		
acebutolol, esmolol, propranolol	phenothiazines	Increased hypotension
	sympathomimetics (beta agonists)	Decreased effects of sympathomimetics
	anticholinergic agents	Increased pressor effects, causing hypertension; decreased effects of the class II antiarrhythmic
	antihypertensives	Increased hypotension
	neuromuscular blockers	Increased skeletal muscle relaxation
	verapamil	Increased cardiac depression
esmolol	digoxin	Increased serum digoxin level
	morphine	Increased blood esmolol level
propranolol	cimetidine	Decreased propranolol metabolism
Class III antiarrhythmics		
bretylium, amiodarone	antihypertensives	Increased hypotension
amiodarone	warfarin	Increased hypoprothrombinemia
	digoxin	Increased serum digoxin level
	procainamide, quinidine, phenytoin	Increased serum level of the class III antiarrhythmic
Class IV antiarrhythmics		
verapamil, diltiazem	other antiarrhythmics	Additive effects
	antihypertensives	Increased hypotension; heart failure
	digoxin	Digitalis toxicity
	cimetidine	Decreased metabolism of the class IV antiarrhythmic
	rifampin	Increased metabolism of the class IV antiarrhythmic
verapamil	highly protein-bound drugs (hydantoins, salicylates, sulfonamides, sulfonylureas)	Increased adverse reactions to verapamil or the interacting drug
Other antiarrhythmic agents		
adenosine	carbamazepine	Increased cardiovascular effects
	dipyridamole	Increased adenosine effects
	methylxanthines (caffeine, theophylline)	Decreased adenosine effects

charges to the SA and atrioventricular (AV) nodes. This increases AV node conduction and makes it difficult for this class of antiarrhythmics to convert an atrial arrhythmia to a regular rhythm in a patient with rapid atrial activity.

Disopyramide produces peripheral vasoconstriction and significantly depresses contractility. Procainamide and quinidine decrease peripheral vascular resistance (afterload) and slightly depress contractility.

Pharmacotherapeutics

Class IA antiarrhythmics are used to treat various atrial and ventricular arrhythmias. The drugs (especially quinidine) act synergistically with digoxin. Disopyramide phosphate suppresses the frequency of ectopic ventricular beats and bursts of ventricular tachycardia. Procainamide is used to prevent recurrence of atrial fibrillation and suppresses the frequency and duration of atrial tachycardia, ventricular tachycardia, and ventricular ectopy. Quinidine converts atrial fibrillation to regular rhythm and prevents atrial fibrillation from recurring. It also suppresses atrial and ventricular ectopic beats and the frequency and duration of atrial and ventricular tachycardia.

Drug interactions

These antiarrhythmics may produce additive or antagonistic effects with other antiarrhythmic and anticholinergic agents. (For details, see Drug Interactions: *Antiarrhythmic agents,* pages 201 and 202.)

Adverse drug reactions

Adverse reactions to class IA antiarrhythmics include anticholinergic effects, GI changes, and a unique reaction to quinidine known as cinchonism. Also, antiarrhythmic drugs themselves can cause arrhythmias. These drugs can precipitate congestive heart failure (CHF) and produce confusion in geriatric patients.

Anticholinergic effects of disopyramide commonly include dry mouth, blurred vision, constipation, and urine retention. All class IA antiarrhythmics (especially quinidine) may produce diarrhea, cramping, nausea, vomiting, anorexia, and bitter taste.

Because its source is cinchona, quinidine may produce signs and symptoms of cinchonism, including tinnitus, headache, vertigo, fever, light-headedness, and vision disturbances. Procainamide may produce hypotension and an adverse reaction that mimics systemic lupus erythematosus.

Class IB antiarrhythmics Class IB antiarrhythmics include lidocaine hydrochloride (Xylocaine), mexiletine hydrochloride (Mexitil), and tocainide hydrochloride (Tonocard). Although they have fewer clinical indications than class IA antiarrhythmics, the class IB antiarrhythmics (especially lidocaine) are more effective for treating acute ventricular arrhythmias and cause fewer adverse reactions. Phenytoin, which resembles the class IB antiarrhythmics, also may be used to treat acute arrhythmias resulting from digitalis toxicity.

Pharmacokinetics

After oral administration, class IB antiarrhythmics are absorbed well from the GI tract, except for lidocaine, which is not available in oral form because it undergoes extensive first-pass metabolism in the liver. Their distribution and metabolism vary greatly, but all are excreted in the urine.

The onset of action depends on the administration route. After intravenous (I.V.) bolus administration, lidocaine exerts its antiarrhythmic effect in 1 to 2 minutes. Mexiletine produces its effects in 30 minutes to 2 hours; tocainide, in less than 30 minutes.

Pharmacodynamics

Class IB antiarrhythmics are used only to treat ventricular arrhythmias. These drugs depress myocardial cell depolarization and act as cell membrane stabilizers. Their major action is to decrease the action potential and the refractory period, which helps prevent reentry arrhythmias and decrease ventricular ectopy by blocking the slow influx of Na^+.

Pharmacotherapeutics

Class IB antiarrhythmics are the drugs of choice in acute care because they usually do not cause serious adverse reactions. Lidocaine is used to suppress ventricular ectopic beats in acute ischemia, to treat ventricular arrhythmias related to digitalis toxicity and other acute conditions, and to reduce the frequency and duration of sudden ventricular tachycardia. It also is used to maintain sinus rhythm after ventricular fibrillation has been defibrillated electrically. Mexiletine is used to suppress ventricular ectopy and to reduce frequency and duration of sudden ventricular tachycardia. Tocainide is considered the oral equivalent to lidocaine; it suppresses ventricular ectopy and reduces the frequency and duration of ventricular tachycardia.

Drug interactions

All class IB antiarrhythmics may interact with other antiarrhythmics. Certain ones may interact with propranolol, cimetidine, phenytoin, and rifampin. (For details, see Drug Interactions: *Antiarrhythmic agents,* pages 201 and 202.)

Adverse drug reactions

All class IB antiarrhythmics have a relatively high incidence of central nervous system (CNS) disturbances, such as confusion and drowsiness, that disappear with dosage reduction or drug discontinuation. Hypotension and bradycardia sometimes occur.

Mexiletine and tocainide may cause GI distress, which may be relieved by taking the drug with food or antacids. They also may produce allergic skin reactions. Rarely, tocainide leads to serious reactions, such as reversible blood dyscrasias and pulmonary fibrosis. It also may cause drug fever and hepatitis.

Class IC antiarrhythmics

The Food and Drug Administration (FDA) has approved four Class IC antiarrhythmics: encainide hydrochloride (Enkaid), flecainide acetate (Tambocor), indecainide hydrochloride (Decabid), and propafenone hydrochloride (Rythmol).

Pharmacokinetics

After oral administration, class IC antiarrhythmics are absorbed well, distributed in varying degrees, metabolized by the liver, and excreted in the urine, except for propafenone, which is eliminated in the feces.

Data are incomplete about the onset, peak, and duration of these agents. Encainide begins to act in 1 to 2 hours. The other drugs in this group demonstrate a peak concentration in 2 to 4 hours.

Pharmacodynamics

Most of these drugs block the influx of sodium in the cells' fast channel, decreasing depolarization. All of them prolong cardiac conduction and have minor effects on resting potential. ECG changes reflect increases in the P-R interval, QRS complex, and Q-T interval. Encainide may depress normal SA and AV node function. Flecainide and propafenone have little effect on SA and AV nodes, but depress function in dysfunctional or diseased cells. Encainide, flecainide, and propafenone all increase endocardial pacing thresholds and exert some negative inotropic effect.

Pharmacotherapeutics

Class IC antiarrhythmics are used to treat life-threatening ventricular arrhythmias, such as ventricular tachycardia. Some arrhythmias respond better to class IC agents than to class IB drugs. Class IC drugs also are being investigated for use in treating paroxysmal atrial fibrillation and supraventricular tachycardia.

Drug interactions

Class IC antiarrhythmics may exhibit additive effects with other antiarrhythmics. (For details, see Drug Interactions: *Antiarrhythmic agents,* pages 201 and 202.)

Adverse drug reactions

Class IC antiarrhythmics can produce serious adverse reactions, including new arrhythmias in the presence of existing arrhythmias, which limit the use of these drugs.

All class IC agents cause CNS disturbances, such as dizziness, paresthesia, fatigue, and blurred vision, and GI disturbances, such as nausea and vomiting. Adverse cardiovascular reactions include conduction abnormalities, exacerbation of CHF (especially with flecainide therapy), hypotension, and aggravation of existing arrhythmias. Because propafenone has beta-blocking properties, it may cause bronchospasm.

Flecainide may produce fever, rash, and allergic reactions. Flecainide, indecainide, and propafenone have been associated with hematologic disturbances.

Class II antiarrhythmics

This group of drugs includes the beta-adrenergic blockers acebutolol hydrochloride (Sectral), esmolol hydrochloride (Brevibloc), and propranolol hydrochloride (Inderal, Inderal LA). Propranolol and acebutolol also are used for their antianginal and antihypertensive effects. (For more information, see Chapter 15, Antianginal agents, and Chapter 16, Antihypertensive agents.)

Pharmacokinetics

After oral administration, acebutolol and propranolol are absorbed from the GI tract and metabolized by the liver. Propranolol is distributed more widely than acebutolol, which is less lipid soluble. Propanolol is excreted primarily in the urine; acebutolol, in the feces. Esmolol, which is administered intravenously, is immediately available systemically, hydrolyzed rapidly by blood esterases, and excreted in the urine.

Acebutolol begins to produce antiarrhythmic effects after 90 minutes and reaches a peak concentration in 3 to 8 hours. Propranolol's onset of action occurs in 30 minutes and its peak concentration occurs in 60 to 90 minutes. After I.V. administration, esmolol has a rapid onset and achieves a steady-state concentration in 10 to 30 minutes. The orally administered drugs have a longer duration of action (24 to 30 hours) than esmolol (20 to 30 minutes).

Pharmacodynamics

The class II antiarrhythmics suppress arrhythmias by blocking receptor sites in the conduction system, which slows SA and AV node function. They also exert a negative inotropic effect. By decreasing myocardial oxygen demand, this action also may decrease myocardial ischemia, which causes myocardial cells to lose their automaticity.

Pharmacotherapeutics

The class II agents are not the drugs of choice to treat arrhythmias because of their adverse effects and the possibility of breakthrough ectopy. The use of these agents with other antiarrhythmics has not been evaluated.

Drug interactions

Class II antiarrhythmics interact with phenothiazines, antihypertensive drugs, anticholinergic agents, and cimetidine. (For details, see Drug Interactions: *Antiarrhythmic agents,* pages 201 and 202.)

Adverse drug reactions

The most common adverse reactions to class II antiarrhythmics involve the cardiovascular system. Because these agents inhibit sinus node stimulation, they may produce bradycardia and hypotension. Occasionally, fluid retention and peripheral edema may occur. These agents may exacerbate or precipitate CHF and arrhythmias.

Class II antiarrhythmics may cause CNS reactions, such as dizziness, confusion, fatigue, and decreased libido, and GI disturbances, such as nausea, vomiting, and mild diarrhea or constipation. Bronchoconstriction can occur when acebutolol and propranolol block beta receptors which normally dilate bronchioles. Esmolol causes inflammation and induration at the injection site in most patients.

Class III antiarrhythmics

Antiarrhythmics in this class include amiodarone hydrochloride (Cordarone) and bretylium tosylate (Bretylol). They are used to treat ventricular arrhythmias.

Pharmacokinetics

After oral administration, amiodarone is absorbed slowly, distributed widely, metabolized in the liver, and eliminated in the feces. Bretylium's erratic GI absorption mandates parenteral administration. It is excreted unchanged in the urine.

If a loading dose of amiodarone is not given, a steady-state concentration is not attained for at least 1 month and usually not for 5 months or longer. Amiodarone's onset of action usually occurs 1 to 3 weeks after oral administration and its effects may persist for weeks or months after discontinuation. Individuals show great variation between plasma concentration and therapeutic effect. Serum concentrations greater than 2.5 mcg/ml are linked to an increased incidence of adverse reactions.

Bretylium's onset and peak concentration occur immediately after I.V. administration. Its duration of action is 6 to 24 hours, and its therapeutic serum level is 0.5 to 1.5 mcg/ml.

Pharmacodynamics

Class III antiarrhythmics lengthen the myocardial cell action potential and refractory period, which decreases the rate of automaticity of ventricular ectopic beats. They inhibit sympathetic nervous system innervation of the heart and produce some peripheral and coronary vasodilation. Amiodarone may decrease intracardiac conduction. Bretylium exerts a positive inotropic effect.

Pharmacotherapeutics

Because of their adverse effects, these drugs are not the drugs of choice for antiarrhythmic therapy. However, they are used to treat life-threatening ventricular ectopy unresponsive to other antiarrhythmics.

Drug interactions

Significant interactions may occur between these agents, particularly amiodarone, and other cardiovascular drugs. (For details, see Drug Interactions: *Antiarrhythmic agents,* pages 201 and 202.)

Adverse drug reactions

Adverse reactions to amiodarone vary widely and commonly lead to its discontinuation. They include hypotension, nausea, anorexia, CNS disturbances, pulmonary toxicity, corneal microdeposits, skin photosensitivity, and hypothyroidism or hyperthyroidism. Bretylium may cause orthostatic and supine hypotension and, with rapid injection, nausea and vomiting. Both drugs may aggravate arrhythmias, especially bradycardia, and increase ventricular ectopic beats.

Class IV antiarrhythmics

Among the class IV antiarrhythmics, or calcium channel blockers, only verapamil hydrochloride (Calan, Isoptin) has been approved by the FDA. Diltiazem hydrochloride (Cardizem) is still awaiting FDA approval. It produces similar effects and is used to treat the same arrhythmias as verapamil.

Pharmacokinetics

After oral administration, both drugs are absorbed well, extensively metabolized in the liver, and excreted mainly in the urine. Verapamil's antiarrhythmic effects begin in 3 to 5 minutes after I.V. administration and peak within 10 minutes. These effects begin 30 minutes after oral administration and peak within 1 to 2 hours. Verapamil's duration of action is usually less than 6 hours. Diltiazem tablets produce a peak concentration in 2 to 3 hours; extended-release capsules, in 6 to 11 hours.

Pharmacodynamics

Verapamil and diltiazem block the influx of calcium across the slow channel of myocardial electrical cells during the plateau (phase 2) and depolarization (phase 4) of the action potential. This increases the refractory period of the AV node and slows conduction between the atria and the ventricles.

Pharmacotherapeutics

Class IV antiarrhythmics are used to treat supraventricular arrhythmias with rapid ventricular response rates. I.V. verapamil is used to correct a rapid heart rate caused by reentry into the atria or AV nodes (paroxysmal supraventricular tachycardia [PSVT]) or after unsuccessful vagal stimulation. It also is used to decrease ventricular response in atrial flutter or fibrillation by blocking AV conduction. Oral verapamil and diltiazem are used to prevent recurrent PSVT. Diltiazem also is used to decrease ventricular response in chronic atrial flutter or fibrillation.

Drug interactions

Class IV antiarrhythmics may interact with other antiarrhythmics, antihypertensives, and other drugs. Verapamil may interact with other highly protein-bound drugs. (For details, see Drug Interactions: *Antiarrhythmic agents,* pages 201 and 202.)

Adverse drug reactions

Verapamil—especially I.V. verapamil—and diltiazem may cause hypotension (primarily orthostatic). Their effect on the SA and AV nodes may produce bradycardia, sinus block, and AV block. They may precipitate or exacerbate CHF and may cause vasodilation, which can lead to dizziness, headache, flushing, weakness, and peripheral edema.

Other reactions to class IV antiarrhythmics include GI disturbances, leg fatigue, and muscle cramps. Hypersensitivity reactions may include worsening of angina, skin eruptions, photosensitivity, pruritus, nasal congestion, and mood changes.

Other antiarrhythmic agents

Adenosine (Adenocard), an injectable antiarrhythmic agent, is used for the treatment of acute PSVT.

Pharmacokinetics

After I.V. administration, adenosine is taken up from the serum into red blood cells and vascular endothelial cells, where it is metabolized to uric acid. Its onset is almost immediate and it terminates most tachycardias within 30 seconds. The drug's duration of action is less than 2 minutes.

Pharmacodynamics

Adenosine depresses SA node function and AV node conduction, which makes it especially effective against reentry tachycardias, such as PSVT. It also produces coronary and peripheral vasodilation.

Pharmacotherapeutics

Available only as an I.V. preparation, adenosine is used to convert PSVT (including PSVT associated with accessory bypass tracts, such as Wolff-Parkinson-White syndrome) to sinus rhythm.

Drug interactions

Adenosine may interact with carbamazepine, dipyridamole, and methylxanthines. (For details, see Drug Interactions: *Antiarrhythmic agents,* pages 201 and 202.)

Adverse drug reactions

Adverse reactions may include facial flushing, shortness of breath, dyspnea, and chest pressure.

Nursing implications

When caring for a patient who is receiving an antiarrhythmic agent, the nurse should be aware of the following implications.

- Develop appropriate nursing diagnoses for the patient. (For examples, see Sample Nursing Diagnoses: *Antiarrhythmic agents,* page 210.)
- Do not administer an antiarrhythmic agent to a patient with a condition that contraindicates its use.
- Administer an antiarrhythmic agent cautiously to a patient at risk because of a preexisting condition.

SAMPLE NURSING DIAGNOSES

Antiarrhythmic agents

The following nursing diagnoses address representative problems and etiologies that a nurse may encounter when caring for a patient who is receiving an antiarrhythmic agent.

- Altered health maintenance related to ineffectiveness of the prescribed antiarrhythmic or amiodarone-induced thyroid dysfunction
- Altered peripheral tissue perfusion related to the adverse cardiac effects of an antiarrhythmic
- Altered protection related to quinidine-induced cinchonism
- Altered protection related to the adverse hematologic effects or the risk of arrhythmias caused by an antiarrhythmic
- Altered sexuality patterns related to decreased libido caused by a class II antiarrhythmic
- Altered thought processes related to confusion caused by an antiarrhythmic
- Constipation related to the anticholinergic effects of an antiarrhythmic
- Decreased cardiac output related to moricizine-induced development of new arrhythmias or exacerbation of existing arrhythmias
- Diarrhea related to the adverse gastrointestinal effects of an antiarrhythmic
- Fatigue related to the adverse central nervous system (CNS) effects of a class IV antiarrhythmic
- Fluid volume excess related to antiarrhythmic-induced congestive heart failure or the adverse myocardial effects of a class IV antiarrhythmic
- High risk for injury related to adverse drug reactions
- High risk for injury related to a preexisting condition that contraindicates the use of an antiarrhythmic
- High risk for injury related to a preexisting condition that requires cautious use of an antiarrhythmic
- High risk for injury related to drug interactions
- High risk for trauma related to the adverse CNS effects of an antiarrhythmic
- Hyperthermia related to flecainide-induced fever
- Impaired gas exchange related to the adverse pulmonary effects of an antiarrhythmic
- Ineffective breathing pattern related to amiodarone-induced pulmonary toxicity
- Knowledge deficit related to the prescribed antiarrhythmic
- Noncompliance related to long-term use of an antiarrhythmic
- Pain related to headache caused by an antiarrhythmic
- Sensory or perceptual alterations (visual) related to corneal microdeposits caused by amiodarone
- Urinary retention related to the anticholinergic effects of an antiarrhythmic

- Monitor the patient closely for adverse reactions during therapy and notify the physician if any occur.
- Keep standard emergency equipment nearby when antiarrhythmic therapy begins.
- Monitor the patient's ECG for new arrhythmias or exacerbation of existing ones.
- Monitor the patient for signs and symptoms of CHF, such as jugular vein distention, crackles, sudden weight gain, and dyspnea.
- Record the patient's fluid intake and output and weight daily.
- Monitor the patient for CNS disturbances.

- Monitor for signs of digitalis toxicity in a patient who receives a cardiac glycoside during antiarrhythmic therapy. (For more information, see Chapter 13, Cardiac glycoside agents and bipyridines.)
- Monitor the patient's vital signs regularly, particularly noting an irregular or slow pulse or hypotension.
- Monitor the serum potassium level because hypokalemia can exacerbate arrhythmias.
- Monitor the patient's serum drug concentration closely to detect early toxicity. Notify the physician if it is not within the therapeutic range.
- Teach the patient and family the name, dose, frequency, action, and adverse effects of the prescribed antiarrhythmic agent.
- Instruct the patient to recognize—and report—the signs and symptoms of CHF.
- Teach the patient to minimize fluid retention by limiting fluid and salt intake and reporting signs of fluid retention, such as shortness of breath or ankle swelling.
- Teach the patient how to take a pulse. Advise the patient to withhold the antiarrhythmic dose and notify the physician if the pulse is irregular or slow (below 60 beats/minute or the rate selected by the physician).

Class I antiarrhythmics
- Inform the patient that moricizine may cause headache or abdominal, cardiac, chest, or musculoskeletal pain. Advise the patient to report such pain, especially cardiac pain, immediately because prompt treatment is necessary.

Class IA antiarrhythmics
- Do not administer a class IA antiarrhythmic with food, unless prescribed, because food may affect drug absorption.
- Observe for signs of drug-induced systemic lupus erythematosus during procainamide therapy.
- Advise the family that a class IA antiarrhythmic may cause confusion in a geriatric patient. Instruct them to take safety measures and notify the physician if confusion occurs.

Class IB antiarrhythmics
- Do not use lidocaine solutions that contain epinephrine when lidocaine is prescribed to treat arrhythmias; such solutions are for local anesthetic use only.
- Observe for lidocaine toxicity (confusion and restlessness), especially when administering propranolol or cimetidine concomitantly.
- Use the 100-mg prefilled syringe of lidocaine for an I.V. push bolus. Use the 1- or 2-gram prefilled syringe for mixing in 250 or 500 ml dextrose 5% in water.
- Administer mexiletine or tocainide with food or antacids to reduce GI distress.

Class IC antiarrhythmics
- Monitor for additive effects in a patient who concurrently receives another antiarrhythmic.

Class II antiarrhythmics
- Inspect the esmolol solution carefully before administration. Discard the solution if it contains particles or is discolored.

Class III antiarrhythmics
- Monitor the patient receiving amiodarone for signs of pulmonary toxicity, such as dyspnea, cough, and changes in X-ray findings that show interstitial pneumonia; of hypothyroidism, such as lethargy, weight gain, cool and dry skin, bradycardia, and hypotension; and of hyperthyroidism, such as nervousness, weight loss, warm and moist skin, tachycardia, and palpitations.
- Teach the patient receiving amiodarone to use protective clothing and sunscreen products or to avoid sunlight to protect against photosensitivity.

STUDY ACTIVITIES

Fill in the blank

1. Antiarrhythmic agents treat abnormal electrical activity in the heart by limiting cardiac electrical conduction to normal pathways and

by _____ abnormally rapid heart rates.

2. Class _____ antiarrhythmics are the drugs of choice for treating ventricular arrhythmias in acute care.

3. In myocardial cells, class IA antiarrhythmics _____ the influx

of Na^+, and depress the depolarization rate; this, in turn, _____

the conduction speed.

4. The most common adverse reactions to the class IB antiarrhyth-

mics are _____.

5. _____ or _____ are the most commonly used drugs to treat arrhythmias caused by digitalis toxicity.

Multiple choice

6. Juanita Ramirez, age 62, is admitted to the critical care unit with acute myocardial infarction. Two days after admission, she develops sustained ventricular tachycardia. Her physician orders a lidocaine bolus followed by an I.V. infusion. Which dose falls within the usual adult dosage range for a lidocaine bolus?
- **A.** 50 mg, repeated in 5 minutes
- **B.** 0.5 mg/kg
- **C.** 1 mg/kg
- **D.** 150 mg

7. When should lidocaine's antiarrhythmic effect begin?
  A. 1 to 2 minutes after I.V. bolus administration
  B. 1 to 2 minutes after continuous I.V. infusion
  C. 10 to 15 minutes after I.V. bolus administration
  D. 10 to 15 minutes after continuous I.V.infusion

8. Which adverse reaction to lidocaine is the nurse most likely to detect?
  A. Necrosis at I.V. site
  B. Confusion
  C. Headache
  D. Fever

9. Charles Harding, age 72, takes digoxin and the class IA antiarrhythmic quinidine, as prescribed, to prevent recurrence of atrial fibrillation. The nurse teaches Mr. Harding and his family to watch for signs of cinchonism during quinidine therapy. What is cinchonism?
  A. Quinidine-induced arrhythmia
  B. Quinidine-induced asthma attack
  C. Quinidine-induced conversion of atrial fibrillation
  D. Quinidine-related reactions, such as tinnitus and fever

10. While receiving quinidine and digoxin, Mr. Harding develops acute arrhythmias caused by digitalis toxicity. The physician is likely to prescribe which drug to treat this type of arrhythmia?
  A. Moricizine
  B. Bretylium
  C. Phenytoin
  D. Verapamil

11. Randolph Otis, age 58, is receiving the class II antiarrhythmic esmolol to treat PSVT. Because esmolol is a beta-adrenergic blocker, the nurse should be sure to assess which parameter for Mr. Otis?
  A. Body temperature
  B. Mean arterial pressure
  C. Cerebral perfusion pressure
  D. Heart rate and blood pressure

Matching related elements
Match the drug on the left with its adverse effects on the right.

12. ___ Adenosine   **A.** Cinchonism

13. ___ Amiodarone   **B.** Exacerbation of arrhythmias

14. ___ Moricizine   **C.** Bradycardia and bronchoconstriction

15. ___ Procainamide   **D.** Hypotension and systemic lupus erythematosus-like reaction

16. ___ Propranolol   **E.** Pulmonary toxicity and photosensitivity

17. ___ Quinidine   **F.** Facial flushing and chest pressure

True or false

18. The nurse should instruct a patient to take quinidine with meals to reduce adverse GI effects.
☐ True   ☐ False

19. Lidocaine is not available in oral form because most of an absorbed dose undergoes metabolism in the liver.
☐ True   ☐ False

20. Digitalis toxicity may occur if verapamil is administered concomitantly with digoxin.
☐ True   ☐ False

21. Flecainide blocks the influx of calcium across the slow channel of myocardial cells.
☐ True   ☐ False

22. Amiodarone therapy usually begins with a loading dose of up to 1,600 mg P.O. daily.
☐ True   ☐ False

ANSWERS

Fill in the blank

1. Decreasing
2. IB
3. Reduce, decreases
4. CNS disturbances
5. Phenytoin, lidocaine

Multiple choice

6. A. The I.V. bolus dosage for lidocaine usually is 50 to 100 mg, followed by a second I.V. bolus of 50 to 100 mg 5 minutes later.

7. A. After I.V. bolus administration, lidocaine exerts its antiarrhythmic effect in 1 to 2 minutes.

8. B. All class IB antiarrhythmics have a relatively high incidence of CNS disturbances, such as drowsiness and confusion.

9. D. Quinidine may cause cinchonism, which produces such effects as tinnitus, headache, vertigo, fever, light-headedness, and vision disturbances.

10. C. Phenytoin or lidocaine may be used to correct acute arrhythmias caused by digitalis toxicity.

11. D. Because class II antiarrhythmics inhibit sinus node stimulation, they may produce bradycardia and hypotension.

Matching related elements

12. F
13. E
14. B
15. D
16. C
17. A

True or false

18. False. Class IA antiarrhythmics, such as quinidine, should not be taken with food because food may affect drug absorption.

19. True.

20. True.

21. False. Flecainide primarily blocks the influx of sodium in the cells' fast channel. Verapamil blocks the influx of calcium across the slow channel.

22. True.

CHAPTER 15

Antianginal agents

OBJECTIVES

After studying this chapter, the reader should be able to:

1. Discuss the physical causes of myocardial ischemia and its relationship to angina.

2. Compare and contrast the three forms of angina.

3. Identify the three classes of antianginal drugs and discuss the benefits of combination therapy.

4. Describe the clinical indications, administration routes, and usual adult dosages of the major antianginal agents.

5. Identify the most significant drug interactions and adverse effects associated with antianginal agents.

6. Describe the nursing implications of antianginal therapy.

OVERVIEW OF CONCEPTS

Antianginal agents are used to relieve angina pain. They fall into three classes: nitrates, beta-adrenergic blockers, and calcium channel blockers. Combining drugs from different classes provides antianginal effects from different mechanisms of action and reduces the risk of adverse reactions from high doses of any one drug. Combination drug therapy also lets the patient receive the lowest amount of drug possible to achieve the desired therapeutic effect of pain relief. (For a summary of representative drugs, see Selected Major Drugs: *Antianginal agents.*)

Cardiac blood supply

To pump effectively, the heart requires its own blood supply. The coronary arteries, which arise from the aorta and penetrate throughout the heart muscle, provide oxygenated blood and nutrients to the myocardium. During diastole (relaxation), blood flows through the coronary arteries. With physical exercise or exertion, the heart rate increases and the diastolic period shortens. This increases the oxygen demand while decreasing the time available for the arteries to supply it.

Angina

When the myocardial oxygen demand exceeds the supply, areas become ischemic, causing chest pain. Symptomatic myocardial ischemia is known as angina pectoris or angina. Angina's painful symptoms may result from decreased coronary artery blood flow, as in atheroscle-

SELECTED MAJOR DRUGS

Antianginal agents

This chart summarizes the major antianginal agents currently in clinical use.

DRUG	MAJOR INDICATIONS	USUAL ADULT DOSAGES
Nitrates		
nitroglycerin	Relief of acute angina attack	0.15 to 0.6 mg sublingually repeated up to three times, or 5 mcg/minute I.V., increased by 5 to 20 mcg every 3 to 5 minutes, up to a maximum of 400 mcg/minute, until pain is relieved
	Prevention of expected attack	0.15 to 0.6 mg sublingually repeated up to three times
	Long-term prevention of angina	1 to 3 mg of a sustained-release tablet between the upper gum and lip t.i.d. or q.i.d., or a sustained-release transdermal patch that releases 2.5 to 15 mg over 24 hours
Beta-adrenergic blockers		
propranolol	Long-term prevention of angina	10 to 20 mg P.O. b.i.d. to q.i.d., increased up to 320 mg P.O. in two to four divided doses, as needed; or 80 to 160 mg of the long-acting form P.O. daily
Calcium channel blockers		
nifedipine	Long-term prevention of angina, especially Prinzmetal's angina	10 mg P.O. t.i.d., gradually increased to 40 mg P.O. q.i.d.; or 30 to 120 mg of the sustained-release form P.O. daily

rosis; from decreased oxygen-carrying capacity of the blood, as in anemia; or from increased work load of the heart, as from exertion.

Angina may cause crushing chest pain or a feeling of pressure under the sternum, sometimes radiating into the neck, jaw, shoulders, and arms. At first, symptoms may be mild; the patient may mistake the angina for indigestion or heartburn.

Angina usually takes one of three main forms:
• Stable (predictable or chronic) angina, which occurs at a predictable level of physical or emotional stress, builds gradually, and reaches maximum intensity quickly.
• Unstable angina (preinfarction or crescendo angina, acute coronary insufficiency, or impending myocardial infarction), which is unpredictable and more severe than stable angina.
• Prinzmetal's (variant) angina, which usually produces pain at rest that resembles the pain of unstable angina. A patient may have both stable and Prinzmetal's angina.

Although all three forms of angina cause chest pain, the antianginal drugs are not analgesics. They relieve this pain by reducing myocardial oxygen demand, increasing myocardial oxygen supply, or both. (For a summary of their function, see *How antianginal agents relieve angina*, page 218.)

How antianginal agents relieve angina

Angina occurs when the coronary arteries, the heart's primary source of oxygen, supply insufficient oxygen to the myocardium. This increases the heart's work load, thereby increasing the heart rate, preload (blood volume in the ventricle at the end of diastole), afterload (arterial pressure that must be overcome for ejection to occur), and force of myocardial contractility. The antianginal agents (nitrates, beta-adrenergic blockers, and calcium channel blockers) relieve angina by decreasing one or more of these four factors, as shown in the diagram below.

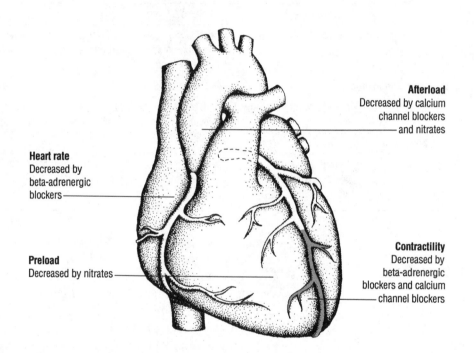

Heart rate
Decreased by
beta-adrenergic
blockers

Preload
Decreased by nitrates

Afterload
Decreased by calcium
channel blockers
and nitrates

Contractility
Decreased by
beta-adrenergic
blockers and calcium
channel blockers

Nitrates   This group of drugs includes erythrityl tetranitrate (Cardilate), isosorbide dinitrate (Isordil, Sorbitrate), isosorbide mononitrate (Ismo), nitroglycerin (Nitro-Bid, Nitrostat), and pentaerythritol tetranitrate (Duotrate, Peritrate).

Pharmacokinetics
Sublingual, buccal, and chewable tablets and lingual aerosols are absorbed almost completely by the oral mucosa. Nitrate tablets or capsules that are swallowed are absorbed through the gastric and intestinal mucosa; their absorption reaches only 50% to 60%. Transdermal nitrates are absorbed slowly in varying percentages, depending on the amount of drug administered, location of administration, and cuta-

neous circulation. Nitrates are distributed widely in the body, metabolized primarily in the liver, and excreted by the kidneys.

The nitrate's onset of action begins within 1 to 3 minutes of intravenous (I.V.), sublingual, buccal, or lingual administration; 20 to 30 minutes of other oral administration; and 30 to 60 minutes of transdermal administration. Their peak concentration occurs almost simultaneously with their onset. Their duration of action varies greatly, from 20 minutes for sublingual nitroglycerin to nearly 24 hours for some transdermal nitrates.

Pharmacodynamics

Nitrates act primarily as vasodilators, working directly on vascular smooth muscle to reduce vasoconstriction. They decrease preload by dilating veins and decrease afterload by dilating arteries. Nitrates also promote coronary artery autoregulation, improving blood flow to the ischemic areas and decreasing blood flow to unaffected areas.

Pharmacotherapeutics

Nitrates are indicated for immediate relief of angina, prevention of angina when an attack can be expected, and long-term prevention of chronic angina. Rapidly absorbed nitrates, such as nitroglycerin, are the drugs of choice to relieve acute angina. Daily application of a nitroglycerin transdermal patch effectively prevents chronic angina, especially for patients who have difficulty complying with a regimen of frequent oral doses.

Drug interactions

Nitrates can interact with alcohol and anticholinergic agents. They are synergistic with other antianginal agents, such as beta blockers and calcium channel blockers. (For details, see Drug Interactions: *Antianginal agents,* page 220.)

Adverse drug reactions

Adverse reactions to nitrates, such as hypotension, orthostatic hypotension, tachycardia, and cardiovascular collapse, result from changes in the cardiovascular system. Headache, the most common adverse reaction, usually disappears after several days and can be treated with acetaminophen. Transdermal nitrates sometimes cause local skin irritation. Other reactions to nitrates include blurred vision, dry mouth, increased peripheral edema, and methemoglobinemia.

Nitrate tolerance may develop over time, especially with high-dose, long-term therapy. To minimize tolerance, nitrate therapy should be individualized, using the lowest effective dose and an intermittent dosage schedule. Long-term, high-dose I.V. nitroglycerin can produce alcohol intoxication.

DRUG INTERACTIONS

Antianginal agents

Drug interactions with the antianginal agents commonly affect the cardiovascular system and may affect other body systems.

DRUG	INTERACTING DRUGS	POSSIBLE EFFECTS
Nitrates		
erythrityl, isosor-bide, nitroglycerin, pentaerythritol	alcohol	Severe hypotension
	anticholinergic agents	Delayed sublingual nitrate absorption caused by dry mouth (an anticholinergic effect)
Beta-adrenergic blockers		
atenolol, metoprolol, nadolol, propranolol	antacids	Delayed beta blocker absorption from gastrointestinal tract
	lidocaine	Increased plasma levels of lidocaine (possibly causing toxicity); increased cardiac depressant effects
	insulin, oral hypoglycemic agents	Hypoglycemia or hyperglycemia; masking of tachycardia as a sign of hypoglycemia (diaphoresis and agitation still present)
	anti-inflammatory drugs (indomethacin, salicylates)	Decreased hypotensive effects of beta blocker
	barbiturates	Increased metabolism of beta-adrenergic blocker that is metabolized extensively
	cardiac glycosides	Increased bradycardia, depressed atrioventricular conduction
	calcium channel blockers	Increased pharmacologic and toxic effects of both drugs
	epinephrine, dobutamine, dopamine, isoproterenol, terbutaline, metaproterenol, albuterol, ritodrine	Hypertension, reflex bradycardia
	cimetidine, flecainide, propafenone	Decreased metabolism of beta blocker; enhanced ability of beta blocker to reduce pulse rate
	rifampin	Reduced therapeutic response to metoprolol and propranolol
	theophyllines	Decreased bronchodilating effects of theophyllines by nonselective beta blockers
	clonidine	Increased antihypertensive and bradycardiac effects
Calcium channel blockers		
diltiazem, nicardi-pine, nifedipine, verapamil	cimetidine	Decreased hepatic clearance of calcium channel blocker
	calcium salts, vitamin D	Reduced response to calcium channel blocker
diltiazem, verapamil	digoxin	Increased serum digoxin level
verapamil	disopyramide phosphate, beta-adrenergic blockers	Myocardial depression
	nondepolarizing blocking agents	Increased muscle relaxation
	carbamazepine	Increased carbamazepine effects
diltiazem	cyclosporine	Increased cyclosporine effects

Beta-adrenergic blockers

Beta-adrenergic blockers used to prevent angina include atenolol (Tenormin), metoprolol tartrate (Lopressor), nadolol (Corgard), and propranolol hydrochloride (Inderal, Inderal LA). Of this class, propranolol is the most commonly prescribed drug.

Pharmacokinetics

Only oral preparations of beta-adrenergic blockers are used to treat angina. Metoprolol and propranolol are absorbed almost completely from the gastrointestinal (GI) tract; less than 50% of atenolol and nadolol is absorbed. Beta-adrenergic blockers are distributed widely, but only metoprolol and propranolol cross the blood-brain barrier. Metoprolol and propranolol are metabolized in the liver and excreted in the urine. Atenolol and nadolol are excreted unchanged in the urine and feces.

Because beta-adrenergic blockers are not used for relief of acute angina, their onset of action is difficult to measure. Their peak concentration varies from 1 to 6 hours, and their duration ranges from 6 to 24 hours.

Pharmacodynamics

Beta-adrenergic blockers decrease blood pressure, heart rate, and the force of myocardial contraction by blocking beta receptor sites in the myocardium and in the electrical conduction system of the heart. This reduces the heart's oxygen demands considerably. The drugs also increase the patient's maximal exercise tolerance by preventing the angina that often accompanies exertion.

Pharmacotherapeutics

Beta-adrenergic blockers are used for long-term prevention of angina. When administered with nitrates, they help limit the reflex tachycardia that accompanies nitrate administration.

Drug interactions

Beta-adrenergic blockers may interact with insulin, oral hypoglycemic agents, digoxin, antiarrhythmics, antihypertensives, phenothiazines, theophyllines, and cimetidine. They act synergistically with other antianginal agents. (For details, see Drug Interactions: *Antianginal agents.*)

Adverse drug reactions

The most common adverse reactions to beta-blockers involve the cardiovascular system and occur when the drug is administered initially. These reactions include bradycardia, hypotension, fluid retention, peripheral edema, angina, syncope, shock, exacerbation of congestive heart failure (CHF), and arrhythmias.

Adverse central nervous system reactions may include dizziness, fatigue, lethargy, confusion, depression, and decreased libido. Nausea, vomiting, or diarrhea are transient GI reactions. Bronchoconstriction may result from bronchial beta receptor blockade.

Calcium channel blockers

This class of drugs includes bepridil hydrochloride (Vascor), diltiazem hydrochloride (Cardizem), nicardipine hydrochloride (Cardene), nifedipine (Adalat, Procardia), and verapamil hydrochloride (Calan, Isoptin).

Pharmacokinetics

Because calcium channel blockers vary in their chemical structures, their pharmacokinetic processes vary also. After sublingual administration, nifedipine is absorbed quickly and almost completely. After oral administration, at least 80% of the calcium channel blockers is absorbed in the GI tract. However, their bioavailability is lower, ranging from 20% to 70%. These agents are metabolized in the liver, but their metabolites differ in their activity. They are excreted in the urine and feces. The onset of action ranges from 10 to 60 minutes; the peak concentration, from 30 minutes to 3 hours.

Pharmacodynamics

Unlike other antianginal agents, calcium channel blockers produce antianginal effects by preventing the influx of calcium ions into the myocardial and vascular smooth muscle cells, blocking the interaction of actin and myosin, and inhibiting myocardial cell contraction. This decreases the force of myocardial contractility—and oxygen demand.

Calcium channel blockers also prevent calcium ions from entering arteriolar smooth muscle cells, which decreases afterload and further decreases myocardial oxygen demand. These drugs increase oxygen supply to the myocardium by dilating coronary arteries.

Pharmacotherapeutics

These agents are used only for long-term prevention of angina, and are the drugs of choice for preventing Prinzmetal's angina. They commonly are prescribed when nitrates or beta-blockers have been ineffective. Calcium channel blockers also are used to slow rapid heart rates by decreasing conduction velocity in the heart's conduction system.

Drug interactions

Calcium channel blockers can interact with beta-adrenergic blockers, digoxin, drugs that affect hepatic metabolism, and other antianginal agents. (For details, see Drug Interactions: *Antianginal agents,* page 220.)

Adverse drug reactions

The most common and serious adverse reactions to calcium channel blockers affect the cardiovascular system and may include hypotension, orthostatic hypotension, arrhythmias, and exacerbation or precipitation of CHF. Because these drugs are vasodilators, they may cause dizziness, headache, flushing, weakness, and peripheral edema. They also may produce GI disturbances, muscle fatigue and cramps, skin eruptions, photosensitivity, pruritus, and mood changes.

SAMPLE NURSING DIAGNOSES

Antianginal agents

The following nursing diagnoses address representative problems and etiologies that a nurse may encounter when caring for a patient who is receiving an antianginal agent.
- Altered health maintenance related to ineffectiveness of the prescribed antianginal agent
- Altered nutrition: less than body requirements, related to the adverse gastrointestinal (GI) effects of an antianginal agent
- Altered protection related to arrhythmias caused by an antianginal agent
- Altered sexuality patterns related to decreased libido caused by a beta-adrenergic blocker
- Altered thought processes related to alcohol intoxication caused by intravenous nitroglycerin
- Decreased cardiac output related to hypotension caused by an antianginal agent
- Diarrhea related to the adverse GI effects of an antianginal agent
- Fatigue related to the adverse central nervous system (CNS) effects of a beta-adrenergic blocker
- Fluid volume excess related to fluid retention caused by an antianginal agent
- High risk for injury related to adverse drug reactions
- High risk for injury related to a preexisting condition that contraindicates the use of an antianginal agent
- High risk for injury related to a preexisting condition that requires cautious use of an antianginal agent
- High risk for injury related to drug interactions
- High risk for trauma related to the adverse CNS effects of an antianginal agent
- Impaired skin integrity related to skin eruptions caused by a calcium channel blocker
- Ineffective breathing pattern related to bronchoconstricting effects of a beta-adrenergic blocker
- Knowledge deficit related to the prescribed antianginal agent
- Noncompliance related to adverse reactions caused by the prescribed antianginal agent
- Pain related to nitrate-induced headache or the adverse muscular effects of a calcium channel blocker
- Sensory or perceptual alterations (visual) related to nitrate-induced blurred vision

---

Nursing implications   When caring for a patient who is receiving an antianginal agent, the nurse should be aware of the following implications.
- Develop appropriate nursing diagnoses for the patient. (For examples, see Sample Nursing Diagnoses: *Antianginal agents.*)
- Do not administer an antianginal agent to a patient with a condition that contraindicates its use.
- Administer an antianginal agent cautiously to a patient at risk because of a preexisting condition.
- Monitor the patient for adverse reactions, especially cardiovascular ones.
- Have the patient sit up for a few minutes before standing to minimize the effects of orthostatic hypotension.
- Take safety precautions if the patient develops dizziness, syncope, or similar symptoms. For example, keep the bed in a low position and supervise the patient's ambulation.

- Monitor the effectiveness of the antianginal agent.
- Monitor the patient for signs of drug interactions.
- Notify the physician if adverse reactions or drug interactions occur or if the antianginal agent is ineffective.
- Teach the patient and family the name, dose, frequency, action, and adverse effects of the prescribed antianginal agent.
- Teach the patient to recognize and report signs and symptoms of hypotension. Also describe how to minimize the effects of orthostatic hypotension.
- Instruct the patient to notify the physician if adverse reactions occur or if the drug is ineffective.

Nitrates

- Do not administer more than 5 mg of chewable isosorbide dinitrate as an initial dose.
- Administer the first nitrate dose with the patient seated or lying down. Take the pulse and blood pressure before drug administration and again at the onset of action.
- Assess the degree of pain relief. Notify the physician if the nitrate is ineffective.
- Prepare I.V. infusions of nitroglycerin with dextrose 5% in water or 0.9% sodium chloride solution in a glass bottle. Use tubing supplied by the manufacturer because nitroglycerin readily migrates into standard polyvinyl chloride tubing.
- Begin infusing I.V. nitroglycerin at 5 mcg/minute and increase the rate, as prescribed, every 3 to 5 minutes until pain is relieved. Monitor the blood pressure and heart rate every 5 to 15 minutes while titrating the dosage and every hour thereafter.
- Instruct the patient to store sublingual nitroglycerin tablets in the original container away from heat, to carry the nitroglycerin tablets at all times, to discard the cotton filler because it can absorb some of the drug, and to replace the tablets every 3 months because they lose their potency.
- Instruct the patient to take a sublingual nitrate dose a few minutes before engaging in activities known to induce angina.
- Instruct the patient to go to the nearest emergency department and to notify the physician if angina is not relieved by three tablets taken 5 minutes apart while resting. Explain that pain may indicate an acute myocardial infarction.
- Advise the patient to take nitrate tablets 30 minutes before or 1 hour after meals for better absorption.
- Instruct the patient to change a long-acting transdermal patch, as frequently as prescribed, using a different, hairless site each time.
- Teach the patient to consult the physician before discontinuing the drug; abrupt discontinuation of a nitrate may cause vasospasm.
- Advise the patient to avoid drinking alcohol during nitrate therapy.

Beta-adrenergic blockers

- Monitor the patient's blood pressure and heart rate, noting decreased blood pressure or heart rate or irregular rhythm. Withhold the dose and notify the physician if the systolic pressure is less than 90 mm Hg or the pulse is less than 60 beats/minute.
- Do not administer metoprolol or propranolol with food because the presence of food in the GI tract delays their peak concentration levels.
- Instruct the patient not to discontinue the drug abruptly, but to notify the physician because the drug must be tapered off slowly.
- Reassure the patient that adverse GI reactions usually are transient.
- Teach the patient with diabetes to test blood glucose regularly and to expect a change in the insulin or oral hypoglycemic agent dosage.

Calcium channel blockers

- Take the patient's vital signs regularly and monitor the electrocardiogram (ECG) for arrhythmias.
- Monitor the patient for signs of CHF, such as jugular vein distention, crackles, dyspnea, or peripheral edema.
- Withhold the dose and notify the physician if the patient's systolic blood pressure is less than 90 mm Hg or the heart rate is less than 60 beats/minute.
- Monitor hydration if the patient experiences GI distress.
- Monitor the patient for muscle cramps or headache.
- Administer diltiazem before meals; administer the once-daily dose of a sustained-release tablet in the morning.
- Demonstrate how to take a pulse and tell the patient to take a pulse before each dose of calcium channel blocker. Advise the patient to delay the dose and notify the physician if the pulse is less than 60 beats/minute.

STUDY ACTIVITIES   Fill in the blank

1. Symptomatic myocardial ischemia also is known as _____.

2. Angina pain may result from decreased coronary artery blood flow, as in _____, or increased in myocardial work load, as from _____.

3. Antianginal agents relieve pain by reducing myocardial _____, increasing myocardial _____, or both.

4. Nitrates work directly on vascular smooth muscle, producing _____.

5. Beta-adrenergic blockers decrease _____, _____, and the force of myocardial contraction by blocking beta receptor sites in the myocardium and in the electrical _____ of the heart.

6. Calcium channel blockers prevent the influx of _____ into the myocardial and vascular smooth muscle cells, block the interaction of _____ and _____, and inhibit _____ contraction.

Matching related elements

Match the antianginal agent on the left with its clinical indication on the right.

7. ___ Nitroglycerin   **A.** Long-term prevention of Prinzmetal's angina

8. ___ Propranolol   **B.** Relief of acute anginal attack

9. ___ Nifedipine   **C.** Limitation of reflex tachycardia caused by a nitrate

Match the antianginal agent on the left with a sample drug interaction on the right.

10. ___ Isosorbide   **A.** May alter insulin or oral hypoglycemic agent requirements

11. ___ Nadolol   **B.** May cause severe hypotension when combined with alcohol

12. ___ Diltiazem   **C.** May exhibit decreased effects when taken with vitamin D

Multiple choice

13. Benjamin Young, age 63, is admitted to the hospital with chest pain and shortness of breath. The physician prescribes sublingual nitroglycerin tablets p.r.n. for chest pain. Before administering the first dose to relieve Mr. Young's chest pain, what should the nurse do?
   A. Ascertain the time of Mr. Young's last meal.
   B. Have Mr. Young lie down and take his pulse and blood pressure.
   C. Take a detailed health history, including a complete medication history.
   D. Calm Mr. Young and explain that he is experiencing symptoms of a heart attack.

14. After receiving three sublingual nitroglycerin tablets, Mr. Young's chest pain is not relieved. What should the nurse do next?
   A. Notify the physician immediately.
   B. Encourage Mr. Young to relax, take deep breaths, and elevate his legs.
   C. Monitor Mr. Young's ECG, heart rate, and blood pressure every 5 to 15 minutes.
   D. Have Mr. Young take a sip of water before taking the next dose of nitroglycerin in 5 minutes.

15. Later, the physician orders a nitroglycerin infusion, titrated to relieve Mr. Young's pain. How often should the nurse expect to increase the dosage?

    A. Every 1 to 2 minutes
    B. Every 3 to 5 minutes
    C. Every 10 to 15 minutes
    D. Every 15 to 30 minutes

16. The nurse should monitor Mr. Young for which adverse reaction to I.V. nitroglycerin?

    A. Hypotension
    B. Clammy skin
    C. Muscle cramps
    D. Fluid overload

True or false

17. Beta-adrenergic blockers are used widely as antianginal agents because they cause few adverse cardiovascular reactions.
    ☐ True   ☐ False

18. For a patient receiving a calcium channel blocker, the nurse should monitor for such adverse effects as GI disturbances and exacerbation of CHF.
    ☐ True   ☐ False

19. When teaching a patient about diltiazem therapy, the nurse should instruct the patient to take the drug before meals.
    ☐ True   ☐ False

20. Combination antianginal therapy reduces the risk of adverse reactions from high doses of any one drug.
    ☐ True   ☐ False

ANSWERS

Fill in the blank

    1. Angina
    2. Atherosclerosis, exertion
    3. Oxygen demand, oxygen supply
    4. Vasodilation
    5. Heart rate, blood pressure, conduction system
    6. Calcium ions, actin, myosin, myocardial cell

Matching related elements

    7. B
    8. C
    9. A
    10. B
    11. A
    12. C

Multiple choice

13. B. The nurse should administer the first nitrate dose by having the patient sit or lie down and taking the pulse and blood pressure before administration and again at the onset of action.

14. A. If angina is not relieved by three tablets taken 5 minutes apart while the patient is resting, the physician should be notified because the pain may indicate an acute myocardial infarction.

15. B. The nurse should begin infusing I.V. nitroglycerin at 5 mcg/minute and increase the infusion rate, as prescribed, every 3 to 5 minutes until pain is relieved.

16. A. The decreased afterload produced by arteriolar dilation can cause hypotension that may be compounded by the reduced cardiac output after decreased preload.

True or false

17. False. The most common adverse reactions to beta blockers involve the cardiovascular system and include bradycardia, hypotension, fluid retention, peripheral edema, angina, syncope, shock, exacerbation of CHF, and arrhythmias.

18. True.

19. True.

20. True.

CHAPTER 16

Antihypertensive agents

OBJECTIVES

After studying this chapter, the reader should be able to:

1. Describe the various types of hypertension.
2. Identify nondrug interventions that help manage hypertension.
3. List at least three examples of sympatholytics, vasodilators, and angiotensin-converting enzyme (ACE) inhibitors.
4. Compare the mechanisms of action of drugs in the three classes of antihypertensive agents.
5. Identify the major adverse reactions to each of the three major classes of antihypertensive agents.
6. Describe the nursing implications of antihypertensive therapy.

OVERVIEW OF CONCEPTS

Blood pressure is regulated by several homeostatic mechanisms. Cardiac output and peripheral resistance determine systolic and diastolic pressures, respectively. The nervous system stimulates the sympathetic pathways to increase blood pressure by releasing epinephrine and norepinephrine. The renin-angiotensin-aldosterone system, a hormonal regulator, helps control blood pressure by affecting angiotensin II and aldosterone levels. Baroceptors, located in the carotid arteries and aortic arch, also respond to pressure changes by adjusting the heart rate and peripheral resistance.

Hypertension is a disorder characterized by elevation in systolic pressure, diastolic pressure, or both. Essential (primary) hypertension, which affects about 95% of all hypertensive patients, arises spontaneously. Secondary hypertension, which affects the remaining 5%, results from such underlying disorders as aortic regurgitation, renal stenosis, pheochromocytoma, and neurologic disease.

Either form of hypertension can occur to varying degrees. (For details, see *Classification of blood pressure,* page 230.) Hypertensive crisis is a medical emergency manifested by a diastolic pressure above 140 mm Hg. Another medical emergency, malignant hypertension is characterized by a diastolic pressure above 140 mm Hg and papilledema.

Classification of blood pressure

Blood pressure is classified into three categories: normal, high normal, and hypertension. Hypertension is divided into four stages of increasing risk of cardiovascular or renal disease. A patient's blood pressure is based on the average of two of more readings taken at each of two or more visits after an initial screening. If the systolic and diastolic blood pressures fall into two different categories, the higher risk category is used to determine a patient's blood pressure category.

CATEGORY	SYSTOLIC BLOOD PRESSURE (mm Hg)	DIASTOLIC BLOOD PRESSURE (mm Hg)
Normal	less than 130	less than 85
High normal	130 to 139	85 to 89
Hypertension		
stage 1 (mild)	140 to 159	90 to 99
stage 2 (moderate)	160 to 179	100 to 109
stage 3 (severe)	180 to 209	110 to 119
stage 4 (very severe)	210 or more	120 or more

Source: U.S. Department of Health and Human Services. National Institutes of Health. National Heart, Lung, and Blood Institute. The Fifth Report of the Joint National Committee on Detection, Evaluation, and Treatment of High Blood Pressure (JNC V). Washington, D.C.: Government Printing Office, 1992.

Stepped-care approach to antihypertensive therapy

As soon as hypertension is diagnosed, the patient should begin the stepped-care approach to antihypertensive therapy. This cumulative, systematic approach begins with step 1—nondrug therapy, including sodium and alcohol restriction, weight control, aerobic exercise, and cessation of smoking.

If the patient does not respond, step 2 begins. In this step, nondrug therapy continues and drug therapy begins, usually with a beta-adrenergic blocker or diuretic. (An ACE inhibitor, calcium channel blocker, alpha-adrenergic blocker, or mixed alpha- and beta-adrenergic blocker may be used as an alternative.)

If the patient still does not respond, therapy moves to step 3, in which the physician may increase the drug dosage, substitute another drug, or add a second hypertensive agent from a different class.

If the patient's response remains inadequate, step 4 begins. In this step, the physician may add a second or third agent or a diuretic. (For a summary of representative drugs, see Selected Major Drugs: *Antihypertensive agents.*)

Sympatholytic agents

Sympatholytic agents, which reduce blood pressure by inhibiting or blocking motor and secretory action in the sympathetic nervous system, are divided into several groups. They are classified by their site or mechanism of action and include central-acting sympathetic nervous system inhibitors, ganglionic blocking agents, beta-adrenergic blocking

SELECTED MAJOR DRUGS

Antihypertensive agents

This chart summarizes the major antihypertensive agents currently in clinical use.

DRUG	MAJOR INDICATIONS	USUAL ADULT DOSAGES
Sympatholytic agents		
Calcium channel blockers		
clonidine	Mild to moderate hypertension	Initially, 0.1 mg P.O. b.i.d., increased by 0.1 or 0.2 mg daily every 2 to 4 days; for maintenance, 0.1 to 0.2 mg P.O. b.i.d. to q.i.d., up to a maximum of 2.4 mg daily
methyldopa	Mild to moderate hypertension	Initially, 250 mg P.O. b.i.d. or t.i.d., increased biweekly to a maintenance dosage of 500 mg to 2 g P.O. daily in two to four divided doses or up to a maximum of 3 g daily
	Hypertensive crisis	250 to 500 mg I.V. in 100 ml of dextrose 5% in water infused over 30 to 60 minutes, repeated every 6 hours, as needed
Beta-adrenergic blockers		
metoprolol	Hypertension	Initially, 100 mg P.O. daily in a single dose or in divided doses, increased by 50 mg daily every week, up to a maximum of 450 mg daily
propranolol	Mild to moderate hypertension	40 mg P.O. b.i.d., or 80 mg P.O. daily of extended-release capsules, increased gradually to a maximum of 640 mg daily
Alpha-adrenergic blockers		
prazosin	Hypertension	Initially, 0.5 to 1 mg P.O. b.i.d. or t.i.d., increased gradually to a maintenance dosage of 6 to 15 mg P.O. daily when given alone or 1 to 2 mg P.O. t.i.d. when given with a diuretic or another antihypertensive
Mixed alpha- and beta-adrenergic blockers		
labetalol	Mild to severe hypertension	100 mg P.O. b.i.d., increased as needed up to 400 mg P.O. b.i.d.
	Hypertensive crisis	20 to 80 mg slow I.V. bolus every 10 minutes or 2 mg/minute by continuous I.V. infusion, up to a maximum of 300 mg
Norepinephrine depletors		
guanethidine	Moderate to severe hypertension	Initially, 10 to 12.5 mg P.O. once daily, increased by 10 to 12.5 mg every 5 to 7 days, as needed, up to a maintenance dosage of 25 to 50 mg P.O. daily
Vasodilating agents		
Direct vasodilators		
hydralazine	Moderate to severe hypertension	40 mg P.O. daily for the first 2 to 4 days, then increased gradually to a maximum of 300 mg P.O. daily
	Hypertensive crisis	10 to 40 mg I.V. or I.M., repeated as needed
Calcium channel blockers		
nifedipine	Hypertension	30 to 60 mg sustained-release tablets P.O. daily, increased to a maximum of 120 mg P.O. daily

(continued)

SELECTED MAJOR DRUGS

Antihypertensive agents (continued)

DRUG	MAJOR INDICATIONS	USUAL ADULT DOSAGES
Vasodilating agents (continued)		
Calcium channel blockers (continued)		
nifedipine	Hypertensive crisis	10 mg sublingually, administered by placing the contents of a punctured capsule under the tongue or having the patient bite and swallow the capsule
Angiotensin-converting enzyme (ACE) inhibitors		
captopril	Mild to moderate hypertension	Initially, 12.5 to 25 mg P.O. t.i.d., increased to 50 mg P.O. t.i.d. after 1 to 2 weeks and up to a maximum of 450 mg P.O. daily

agents, alpha-adrenergic blocking agents, mixed alpha- and beta-blocking agents, and norepinephrine depletors.

The centrally-acting agents include clonidine hydrochloride (Catapres), guanabenz acetate (Wytensin), guanfacine hydrochloride (Tenex), and methyldopa (Aldomet). Ganglionic blockers include mecamylamine hydrochloride (Inversine) and trimethaphan camsylate (Arfonad). Beta-adrenergic blockers are numerous: acebutolol hydrochloride (Sectral), atenolol (Tenormin), betaxolol hydrochloride (Kerlone), carteolol hydrochloride (Cartrol), metoprolol tartrate (Lopressor), nadolol (Corgard), penbutolol sulfate (Levatol), pindolol (Visken), propranolol hydrochloride (Inderal), and timolol maleate (Blocadren). Alpha-adrenergic blockers are fewer: doxazosin mesylate (Cardura), phentolamine mesylate (Regitine), prazosin hydrochloride (Minipress), and terazosin (Hytrin). Labetalol hydrochloride (Normodyne, Trandate) is a mixed alpha- and beta-adrenergic blocker. Sometimes called peripheral-acting sympatholytic agents, norepinephrine depletors include guanadrel sulfate (Hylorel), guanethidine sulfate (Ismelin), and reserpine (Serpasil).

Pharmacokinetics

Most central-acting nervous system inhibitors are absorbed well from the gastrointestinal (GI) tract after oral administration. Methyldopa is the exception, because its absorption is variable and incomplete. These agents are distributed widely to body tissues, metabolized in the liver, and excreted in the urine.

After oral administration, most ganglionic blockers are absorbed well from the GI tract. However, trimethaphan must be administered intravenously because of its erratic and incomplete absorption after oral administration. Oral mecamylamine also is absorbed erratically. The ganglionic blockers are distributed widely throughout the body, metabolized by the liver and excreted in the urine. Mecamylamine crosses the blood-brain barrier.

Beta-adrenergic blockers are absorbed well from the GI tract, except for atenolol and nadolol. These drugs achieve wide distribution in the body; metoprolol and propranolol readily cross the blood-brain barrier. The beta blockers are metabolized primarily by the liver, except for atenolol. They are excreted in the urine.

Most alpha-adrenergic blocking agents are absorbed well from the GI tract, distributed widely, metabolized in the liver (except for terazosin and phentolamine), and excreted in the bile and feces. The pharmacokinetics of phentolamine and the metabolism of terazosin are unknown.

Labetalol, the mixed alpha- and beta-adrenergic blocker, is absorbed well and distributed widely in the body. It is metabolized by the liver and excreted in the bile and urine.

Among the norepinephrine depletors, guanadrel is absorbed well; guanethidine and reserpine are not. These agents are distributed widely in the body and partially metabolized in the liver. Guanadrel is excreted primarily in the urine. Guanethidine and reserpine are excreted primarily in the urine and feces.

The onset of action, peak concentration, and duration of action vary greatly among the sympatholytics and depend on the administration route and the specific drug.

Pharmacodynamics

All sympatholytic agents inhibit stimulation of the sympathetic nervous system, which decreases blood pressure (caused by peripheral vasodilation) or decreases cardiac output.

Central-acting sympathetic nervous system inhibitors act in the central nervous system (CNS) to reduce sympathetic activity. This reduces peripheral resistance, heart rate, cardiac output, and blood pressure. Ganglionic blockers interfere with the transmission of sympathetic and parasympathetic nerve impulses through the ganglia, producing vasodilation and reducing cardiac output and blood pressure.

Beta-adrenergic blockers decrease heart rate, cardiac output, blood pressure, and the effects of the renin-angiotensin-aldosterone system by inhibiting epinephrine at beta-adrenergic receptor sites. Alpha-adrenergic blockers directly relax arteriolar smooth muscle. This results in vasodilation and decreased peripheral resistance without causing reflex tachycardia or decreased cardiac output. However, nonselective alpha-adrenergic blockers, such as phentolamine, may produce reflex tachycardia. Labetalol acts by decreasing peripheral and renal vascular resistance, renin levels, and cardiac output.

Norepinephrine depletors act by depleting catecholamine stores and inhibiting norepinephrine transport. This action decreases cardiac output, peripheral resistance, vasomotor tone, and heart rate. Guanadrel is not associated with decreased cardiac output; however, it may increase fluid retention. Guanethidine can cause increased peripheral vasodilation, which may decrease blood flow to the vital organs and alter plasma renin activity.

Pharmacotherapeutics

Sympatholytics typically are used to lower blood pressure in patients with mild to severe essential hypertension. Using the stepped-care approach to antihypertensive therapy, the physician can change the type of drug used and alter the dosage to achieve effective therapeutic effects with the fewest adverse reactions.

Central-acting nervous system inhibitors generally are used in step 3 to control mild to moderate hypertension. Ganglionic blockers are used to treat moderate to severe hypertension (mecamylamine hydrochloride) and hypertensive crisis (trimethaphan camsylate).

Beta-adrenergic blockers commonly are used in step 2 of antihypertensive therapy and may be continued in step 3. Alpha-adrenergic blockers or labetalol sometimes are used as alternates to beta-adrenergic blockers in step 2. They also may be prescribed in step 3. Administered intravenously or intramuscularly, phentolamine also is used to prevent or control hypertensive crisis associated with pheochromocytoma surgery and to diagnose pheochromocytoma. Intravenous (I.V.) labetalol also is effective for treating hypertensive crisis.

Norepinephrine depletors are used in steps 3 or 4 of antihypertensive therapy.

Drug interactions

Sympatholytic agents may interact with many drugs, frequently producing blood pressure changes and other effects. (For details, see Drug Interactions: *Antihypertensive agents*.)

Adverse drug reactions

Central-acting nervous system inhibitors typically produce adverse CNS reactions, such as sedation, drowsiness, and depression. Other reactions include forgetfulness, inability to concentrate, vivid dreams, edema, hepatic dysfunction, vertigo, paresthesia, weakness, dry mouth (especially with clonidine), fever, nasal congestion, decreased libido, impotence, and lactation. Guanabenz also is associated with chest pain, arrhythmias, edema, palpitations, blurred vision, ataxia, and anxiety. Clonidine and guanabenz can produce rebound hypertension if they are discontinued suddenly.

Ganglionic blockers may cause adverse CNS reactions similar to those of the central-acting agents. They also may produce shortness of breath, respiratory depression, and tachycardia. Trimethaphan may decrease serum potassium levels. They should be used cautiously in a patient with cardiac disease, benign prostatic hypertrophy, fever, hemorrhage, glaucoma, sodium depletion, renal disorder, Addison's disease, diabetes, and respiratory, hepatic, or cerebrovascular disease.

DRUG INTERACTIONS

Antihypertensive agents

Sympatholytic agents interact with many drugs to produce blood pressure changes as well as other severe reactions. Vasodilating agents and angiotensin-converting enzyme (ACE) inhibitors may interact with several drugs, including other antihypertensives.

DRUG	INTERACTING DRUGS	POSSIBLE EFFECTS
Sympatholytic agents		
clonidine	tricyclic antidepressants	Increased blood pressure
	beta-adrenergic blockers	Paradoxical hypertensive response
trimethaphan	nondepolarizing muscle relaxants, especially spinal anesthetics	Increased hypotensive effects; prolonged apnea
labetalol	halothane anesthesia	Increased hypotensive effects of labetalol
guanadrel	sympathomimetics	Decreased antihypertensive effects of guanadrel
guanethidine	sympathomimetics, phenothiazines, tricyclic antidepressants, amphetamines	Decreased antihypertensive effects of guanethidine
reserpine	levodopa	Decreased levodopa effects
acebutolol, atenolol, betaxolol, carteolol, metoprolol, nadolol, penbutolol, pindolol, propanolol, timolol	antacids	Delayed drug absorption from gastrointestinal tract
	lidocaine	Increased plasma level of lidocaine
	insulin, oral hypoglycemic agents	Hypoglycemia; masking of tachycardia as a sign of hypoglycemia (diaphoresis and agitation still present)
	anti-inflammatory drugs	Decreased hypotensive effects of beta-adrenergic blocker
	barbiturates, rifampin	Increased metabolism of beta-adrenergic blocker that is metabolized extensively
	cardiac glycosides	Additive bradycardia, depressed atrioventricular conduction
	calcium channel blockers	Increased pharmacologic and toxic effects of both drugs
	sympathomimetics (epinephrine, dobutamine, dopamine, isoproterenol, terbutaline, metaproterenol, albuterol, ritodrine)	Hypertension, reflex bradycardia
	cimetidine	Decreased metabolism of beta-adrenergic blocker; enhanced ability of beta-adrenergic blocker to reduce pulse rate
	theophyllines	Decreased bronchodilating effects of theophyllines (with nonselective beta-adrenergic blockers)
	clonidine	Attenuation or reversal of antihypertensive effects; life-threatening increase in blood pressure
Vasodilating agents		
hydralazine, minoxidil	other antihypertensives	Increased antihypertensive effects
	nitrates	Increased effects of both drugs

(continued)

DRUG INTERACTIONS

Antihypertensive agents (continued)

DRUG	INTERACTING DRUGS	POSSIBLE EFFECTS
Vasodilating agents (continued)		
diltiazem, verapamil	digoxin	Digitalis toxicity
verapamil	digitoxin	Digitalis toxicity
diltiazem, nicardipine, verapamil	drugs that affect the hepatic microsomal system	Altered metabolism of either drug
nicardipine	cimetidine	Increased plasma nicardipine level
ACE inhibitors		
All ACE inhibitors	diuretics, other antihypertensives	Increased hypotensive effects
captopril, enalapril, lisinopril	nonsteroidal anti-inflammatory drugs	Decreased effects of ACE inhibitor

Beta-adrenergic blockers produce many of the same adverse CNS reactions as the central-acting agents. They also may cause adverse cardiovascular reactions, including bradycardia, hypotension, congestive heart failure, exacerbation of peripheral vascular disease, and increased cholesterol and triglyceride levels. Other reactions may include nausea, vomiting, diarrhea, insomnia, nightmares, depression, hallucinations, dry eyes, paresthesia, transient thrombocytopenia, granulocytopenia, sore throat, fever, and difficulty breathing.

The alpha-adrenergic blockers doxazosin and prazosin are associated with orthostatic hypotension and first-dose syncope. Terazosin commonly produces orthostatic hypotension, dizziness, and precipitation of angina. Phentolamine also can precipitate angina attacks and may cause rebound tachycardia, hypotension, palpitations, dizziness, weakness, flushing, nausea, vomiting, diarrhea, and nasal congestion.

Adverse reactions to labetalol resemble those of the beta-adrenergic blockers. Others include scalp tingling, alopecia, orthostatic hypotension, intermittent claudication, bronchospasm, drug-induced systemic lupus erythematosus, eye irritation, myalgia, and rash.

Norepinephrine depletors may produce many adverse reactions. Guanadrel and guanethidine may cause orthostatic hypotension and generalized weakness. Guanadrel also produces fainting, nocturia, and dyspnea. Guanethidine also results in explosive diarrhea; sexual dysfunction; reduced myocardial contractility; fluid retention; increased blood urea nitrogen (BUN), aspartate aminotransferase (AST, formerly SGOT), and alanine aminotransferase (ALT, formerly SGPT) levels; decreased prothrombin time; and decreased serum glucose and urine catecholamine levels. Common reactions to reserpine may include drowsiness, sleep pattern disturbances, weight gain, and nasal congestion. Other adverse reactions include abdominal cramps, diarrhea, depression, uterine contractions, and bronchoconstriction.

Vasodilating agents   Two types of vasodilating agents exist: direct vasodilators and calcium channel blockers. Direct vasodilators include diazoxide (Hyperstat), hydralazine hydrochloride (Apresoline), minoxidil (Loniten, Minodyl), and nitroprusside sodium (Nipride). Calcium channel blockers include amlodipine besylate (Norvasc), diltiazem hydrochloride (Cardizem SR), felodipine (Plendil), isradipine (DynaCirc), nicardipine hydrochloride (Cardene), nifedipine (Procardia XL), and verapamil hydrochloride (Calan, Isoptin, Verelan). Both types reduce blood pressure by relaxing arteriolar smooth muscle, which dilates arteries and decreases peripheral resistance.

Pharmacokinetics
Most vasodilators are absorbed rapidly and distributed well. They are metabolized in the liver, and are excreted in the urine, bile, or feces. Vasodilators vary greatly in their onset of action (from less than 1 minute to 1 hour), peak concentration (from less than 1 minute to 3 hours), and duration of action (from 1 minute to 72 hours).

Pharmacodynamics
The direct vasodilators relax peripheral vascular smooth muscles, lowering blood pressure by increasing blood vessel caliber and reducing total peripheral resistance. Calcium channel blockers prevent calcium transport across the cell membrane. This reduces the activity of the vascular smooth muscle, producing vasodilation and lowering the blood pressure.

Pharmacotherapeutics
Vasodilating agents are used as adjuncts to control moderate to severe hypertension. Although the calcium channel blockers may be part of step-2 antihypertensive therapy, all vasodilating agents may be used in step 3 or 4. Many of these agents also are used to treat hypertensive crisis or malignant hypertension.

Drug interactions
The vasodilating agents may interact with other antihypertensives, nitrates, cardiac glycosides, cimetidine, and drugs that affect the hepatic microsomal system. (For details, see Drug Interactions: *Antihypertensive agents,* pages 235 and 236.)

Adverse drug reactions
Direct vasodilators commonly produce palpitations, angina, tachycardia, increased myocardial work load, electrocardiogram changes, edema, breast tenderness, fatigue, headache, and rash. Severe pericardial effusions may develop. Alkaline phosphatase, BUN, and creatinine levels may increase. Unlike the other vasodilators, calcium channel blockers do not produce rebound tachycardia or significant edema.

Other adverse reactions depend on the specific drug used. Diazoxide may cause headache, anorexia, nausea, diaphoresis, rash, drug fever, urticaria, polyneuritis, GI hemorrhage, anemia, pancytopenia, excessive hypotension, hyperglycemia (in patients with diabetes). Hydralazine may cause headache, diarrhea or constipation, dizziness or light-headedness, orthostatic hypotension, facial flushing, shortness of breath, nasal congestion, urinary hesitancy, lacrimation, conjunctivitis, paresthesia, edema, tremor, and muscle cramps. Minoxidil may produce hypertrichosis (excessive hair growth), fluid retention, and reflex tachycardia. Nitroprusside may cause headache, dizziness, nausea, vomiting, and abdominal pain.

Adverse reactions to diltiazem, nifedipine, and verapamil may include hypotension, bradycardia, flushing, palpitations, somnolence or insomnia, tremor, headache, edema, nausea, rash, and elevated liver enzymes. Additional reactions to nifedipine and verapamil include peripheral edema, dizziness, light-headedness; to verapamil alone, atrioventricular heart block and constipation. Reactions to nicardipine commonly include flushing, headache, and facial edema.

Angiotensin-converting enzyme (ACE) inhibitors

ACE inhibitors include benazepril (Lotensin), captopril (Capoten), enalapril maleate (Vasotec), enalaprilat (Vasotec I.V.), fosinopril (Monopril), lisinopril (Prinivil, Zestril), quinapril (Accupril), and ramipril (Altace).

Pharmacokinetics

The ACE inhibitors are absorbed from the GI tract, distributed to most body tissues, metabolized somewhat by the liver, and excreted primarily in the urine. Ramipril also is excreted in the feces. Because enalapril is a prodrug (precursor), it has little pharmacologic activity until hydrolyzed in the liver to enalaprilat.

Captopril and enalapril reach peak concentration in 30 to 90 minutes; enalaprilat, in 3 to 4 hours; lisinopril, within 6 hours. Captopril's duration of action ranges from 6 to 12 hours. Enalapril and lisinopril have a duration of up to 24 hours. The other ACE inhibitors vary in their onset, peak, and duration.

Pharmacodynamics

ACE inhibitors lower blood pressure by interfering with the renin-angiotensin-aldosterone system. They inhibit the enzyme that converts angiotensin I to angiotensin II, a potent vasoconstrictor. This inhibition decreases aldosterone release and reduces peripheral arterial resistance, which ultimately decreases blood pressure.

Pharmacotherapeutics

These agents may be used as step 2 drugs for treating mild to moderate hypertension. They also may be used alone or with another agent in step 3 or 4. Captopril is especially effective in treating hypertension associated with high or normal renin levels. Enalaprilat, which is administered intravenously, is especially useful for patient who cannot take it orally.

Drug interactions

ACE inhibitors may interact with other antihypertensives, diuretics, and nonsteroidal anti-inflammatory drugs. (For details, see Drug Interactions: *Antihypertensive agents,* pages 235 and 236.)

Adverse drug reactions

Severe adverse reactions, such as proteinuria, blood dyscrasias, rash, and loss of taste, occur most commonly with captopril. All ACE inhibitors can cause adverse CNS reactions, such as headache, dizziness, syncope, and fatigue, and adverse GI reactions, such as nausea, vomiting, diarrhea, and abdominal pain. Other common reactions include transient elevations of BUN, serum creatinine, and serum potassium levels; scratchy throat; nonproductive cough; and angioedema.

Nursing implications   When caring for a patient who is receiving an antihypertensive agent, the nurse should be aware of the following implications.

- Develop appropriate nursing diagnoses for the patient. (For examples, see Sample Nursing Diagnoses: *Antihypertensive agents,* page 240.)
- Do not administer an antihypertensive agent to a patient with a condition that contraindicates its use.
- Administer an antihypertensive agent cautiously to a patient at risk because of a preexisting condition.
- Monitor the patient for adverse reactions.
- Review the results of laboratory studies, as prescribed.
- Measure the patient's fluid intake and output daily; also weigh the patient daily.
- Assess the patient's standing, sitting, and supine blood pressures and pulse before administering each dose and during peak concentration times.
- Take safety precautions if the patient develops such symptoms as dizziness or syncope. For example, raise the bed rails and keep the bed in the low position.
- Monitor the patient for signs of drug interactions.
- Assess the drug's effectiveness periodically.
- Notify the physician if adverse reactions or drug interactions occur or if the drug is ineffective.
- Limit the patient's dietary sodium intake.
- Have the patient sit on the edge of the bed before rising from a supine position to minimize the effects of orthostatic hypotension.
- Teach the patient and family the name, dose, frequency, action, and adverse effects of the prescribed antihypertensive agent.

SAMPLE NURSING DIAGNOSES

Antihypertensive agents

The following nursing diagnoses address representative problems and etiologies that a nurse may encounter when caring for a patient who is receiving an antihypertensive agent.

- Altered health maintenance related to ineffectiveness of the prescribed antihypertensive
- Altered nutrition: less than body requirements, related to the adverse gastrointestinal (GI) effects of an antihypertensive
- Altered nutrition: more than body requirements, related to weight gain caused by a norepinephrine depletor
- Altered peripheral tissue perfusion related to exacerbation of peripheral vascular disease caused by an antihypertensive
- Altered protection related to masking of the early signs of hypoglycemia by a beta-adrenergic agent in a patient with diabetes
- Altered protection related to the adverse hematologic effects of an antihypertensive
- Altered thought processes related to the adverse central nervous system (CNS) effects of an antihypertensive
- Altered urinary elimination related to guanadrel-induced nocturia
- Anxiety related to the adverse CNS effects of an antihypertensive
- Body image disturbance related to minoxidil-induced hypertrichosis
- Constipation related to the adverse GI effects of an antihypertensive
- Decreased cardiac output related to arrhythmias caused by an antihypertensive
- Diarrhea related to the adverse GI effects of an antihypertensive
- Fatigue related to the adverse CNS effects of a direct vasodilator
- Fluid volume excess related to antihypertensive-induced fluid retention
- High risk for injury related to adverse drug reactions
- High risk for injury related to a preexisting condition that contraindicates the use of an antihypertensive
- High risk for injury related to a preexisting condition that requires cautious use of an antihypertensive
- High risk for injury related to drug interactions
- High risk for trauma related to the adverse CNS effects of an antihypertensive
- Hyperthermia related to fever caused by an antihypertensive
- Ineffective breathing pattern related to the adverse respiratory effects of an antihypertensive
- Knowledge deficit related to the prescribed antihypertensive
- Noncompliance related to the adverse effects and duration of antihypertensive therapy
- Pain related to antihypertensive-induced anginal attacks or vasodilator-induced headache, angina, or muscle cramps
- Sensory or perceptual alterations (tactile) related to paresthesia caused by an antihypertensive
- Sensory or perceptual alterations (visual) related to blurred vision caused by an antihypertensive
- Sexual dysfunction related to the adverse genitourinary effects of an antihypertensive
- Sleep pattern disturbance related to sleep alterations caused by an antihypertensive

- Teach the patient to take the drug exactly as prescribed and never to double the dose, take other medications, or abruptly discontinue therapy without consulting the physician.
- Instruct the patient to avoid sudden position changes and physical exertion in hot weather, which can increase dizziness or fainting. Also

advise the patient to avoid driving and operating potentially dangerous machinery until the drug's effects are known.
- Teach the patient to report adverse reactions to the physician, to return for follow-up visits as directed, and to try to reduce factors that
increase blood pressure, such as smoking, obesity, lack of exercise,
and excessive sodium intake.

Sympatholytic agents
- Anticipate gradual discontinuation of beta blockers, clonidine, or
guanabenz.
- Monitor the patient regularly for signs of CHF, such as increasing
dyspnea, crackles, jugular vein distention, fatigue, and pallor.
- Discontinue trimethaphan immediately if hypotension occurs.
- Give labetalol, metoprolol, or propranolol between meals; give reser-
pine with food or milk.
- Discontinue guanethidine 72 hours before elective surgery, as pre-
scribed, to prevent drug interactions with sympathomimetics.
- Teach the patient to avoid orthostatic hypotension by remaining su-
pine for 3 hours after the first dose of an alpha-adrenergic blocker.

Vasodilating agents
- Assess the patient's blood pressure continuously or at least every 5
minutes during nitroprusside therapy.
- Administer nitroprusside via an infusion pump.
- Administer I.V. diazoxide in a peripheral vein to prevent arrhythmias.
- Administer oral hydralazine with meals to promote absorption.
- Monitor the patient closely for signs of fluid excess. For example,
weigh the patient daily and monitor fluid intake and output to detect
fluid retention. Auscultate breath sounds regularly to detect crackles.

ACE inhibitors
- Observe for signs of angioedema, such as flushing or pallor and swelling of the face, arms, legs, lips, tongue, or throat. If angioedema occurs, withhold the drug, notify the physician, and begin emergency
treatment.
- Instruct the patient to take captopril on an empty stomach, preferably
1 hour before meals, for maximum effectiveness.

STUDY ACTIVITIES   Fill in the blank

1. Peripheral resistance determines the _____ blood pressure;

cardiac output determines the _____ blood pressure.

2. The nervous system stimulates the sympathetic pathways to

increase blood pressure by releasing _____ and _____.

3. The _____ system provides hormonal regulation of blood
pressure.

4. Baroceptors respond to pressure changes in the arterial system by adjusting the _____ and _____.

Multiple choice

5. Sue Li, age 67, is receiving I.V. nitroprusside for hypertensive crisis. How frequently should the nurse assess her blood pressure?

A. At least every 5 minutes

B. Every 15 minutes and as needed

D. Every hour and when she changes position

C. Every 4 hours and as needed

6. Michael Morgan, age 44, takes the beta-adrenergic blocker propranolol for hypertension. How do beta blockers reduce blood pressure?

A. They directly relax arteriolar smooth muscle.

B. They increase renin levels in the vasculature.

C. They inhibit epinephrine at beta receptor sites.

D. They enhance aldosterone secretion in the nephron.

7. Alice Newell, age 59, is about to begin methyldopa therapy for moderate hypertension. What is the recommended initial dosage for methyldopa?

A. 12.5 mg P.O. t.i.d.

B. 50 mg P.O. q.i.d.

C. 250 mg P.O. b.i.d.

D. 4 g P.O. q.i.d.

8. Thomas Anderson, age 52, is diagnosed with moderate hypertension. The physician orders clonidine hydrochloride (Catapres) 0.1 mg P.O. b.i.d. What should the nurse do before administering this drug?

A. Ensure that the patient has an empty stomach.

B. Assess supine, sitting, and standing blood pressures.

C. Review the patient's serum potassium levels.

D. Check the patient for signs of diuresis.

9. In addition to drug therapy, which action would help reduce Mr. Anderson's blood pressure?

A. Eating high-fiber foods.

B. Eating low-sodium foods.

C. Drinking at least 68 oz (2,000 ml) fluid daily.

D. Restricting fluid intake to less than 34 oz (1000 ml) daily.

10. Sheryl Kohl, age 48, comes to the clinic for a routine checkup. She has been taking atenolol (Tenormin) 50 mg P.O. daily for moderate hypertension. Which statement by Ms. Kohl indicates the need for more teaching?
- **A.** "I'm increasing the distance I walk every day."
- **B.** "I'm trying to cut back on my salt intake."
- **C.** "I've lost 14 pounds so far, and I'm going to try to lose 10 more."
- **D.** "When I feel light-headed, I don't take my pill for a couple of days."

True or false

11. A patient should take captopril between meals.
□ True   □ False

12. Beta-adrenergic blockers, such as atenolol, can produce adverse reactions in the central nervous, cardiovascular, and GI systems.
□ True   □ False

13. Prazosin is less likely to cause orthostatic hypotension than the other sympatholytics.
□ True   □ False

14. Daily weight and fluid intake and output measurements help the nurse monitor the effectiveness of antihypertensive therapy.
□ True   □ False

15. Sexual dysfunction rarely is associated with antihypertensive therapy.
□ True   □ False

Matching related elements

Match the drug on the left with its drug class on the left.

16. ___ Trimethaphan camsylate   **A.** Norepinephrine depletor

17. ___ Nadolol   **B.** Calcium channel blocker

18. ___ Minoxidil   **C.** Centrally-acting nervous system inhibitor

19. ___ Verapamil   **D.** Alpha-adrenergic blocker

20. ___ Reserpine   **E.** Ganglionic blocker

21. ___ Guanabenz   **F.** Direct vasodilator

22. ___ Enalapril   **G.** Mixed alpha- and beta-adrenergic blocker

23. ___ Labetalol   **H.** ACE inhibitor

24. ___ Prazosin   **I.** Beta-adrenergic blocker

ANSWERS

Fill in the blank

1. Diastolic, systolic
2. Epinephrine, norepinephrine
3. Renin-angiotensin-aldosterone
4. Heart rate, peripheral resistance

Multiple choice

5. A. The nurse should assess the patient's blood pressure continuously or at least every 5 minutes during nitroprusside therapy.

6. B. Beta-blocking agents decrease heart rate, cardiac output, blood pressure, and the effects of the renin-angiotensin-aldosterone system by inhibiting epinephrine at the beta-adrenergic receptor sites. Alpha-adrenergic blockers directly relax arteriolar smooth muscle.

7. C. The usual adult dosage for methyldopa is: initially, 250 mg b.i.d. or t.i.d., increased biweekly to a maintenance dosage of 500 mg to 2 g daily in two to four divided doses or up to a maximum of 3 g daily.

8. B. The nurse should assess the patient's standing, sitting, and supine blood pressures and pulse before administering each dose and during peak concentration times.

9. B. Factors that can increase blood pressure include smoking, obesity, lack of exercise, and excessive sodium intake.

10. D. The patient should take the drug exactly as prescribed. If adverse reactions occur, she should notify the physician. Abrupt discontinuation of a beta-blocker may cause serious problems.

True or false

11. True.
12. True.
13. False. The alpha-adrenergic blockers doxazosin and prazosin are associated with orthostatic hypotension and first-dose syncope.
14. True.
15. False. Sexual dysfunction, including decreased libido and impotence, is a common adverse reaction to certain antihypertensives.

Matching related elements

16. E
17. I
18. F
19. B
20. A
21. C
22. H
23. G
24. D

CHAPTER 17

Diuretic agents

OBJECTIVES

After studying this chapter, the reader should be able to:

1. Compare the mechanisms of action of thiazide and thiazide-like, loop, potassium-sparing, and osmotic diuretics.

2. Identify the major clinical indications for the various types of diuretics.

3. Describe the major drug interactions that can occur with the various types of diuretics.

4. Describe the fluid and electrolyte imbalances that commonly result from diuretic therapy.

5. Describe the nursing implications of diuretic therapy.

OVERVIEW OF CONCEPTS

Most diuretic agents promote renal excretion of water and electrolytes by increasing the glomerular filtration rate (GFR), decreasing sodium reabsorption, or increasing the rate of sodium excretion. They are used clinically to increase urine volume by acting at different sites in the nephrons (structural and functional units of the kidneys). (For an illustration, see *Principal sites of diuretic action,* page 246. For a summary of representative drugs, see Selected Major Drugs: *Diuretic agents,* pages 247 and 248.)

Thiazide and thiazide-like diuretics

The thiazide diuretics include bendroflumethiazide (Naturetin), benzthiazide (Aquatag, Proaqua), chlorothiazide (Diuril), hydrochlorothiazide (Esidrix, HydroDIURIL), hydroflumethiazide (Diucardin, Saluron), methyclothiazide (Aquatensen, Enduron), polythiazide (Renese), and trichlormethiazide (Metahydrin, Naqua). The thiazide-like diuretics include chlorthalidone (Hygroton), indapamide (Lozol), metolazone (Diulo, Zaroxolyn), and quinethazone (Hydromox).

Pharmacokinetics

After oral administration, these diuretics are absorbed rapidly but incompletely from the gastrointestinal (GI) tract. Although they differ greatly in their distribution and metabolism, all are eliminated rapidly and primarily in the urine; metolazone is also excreted in the feces.

Principal sites of diuretic action

Diuretics increase the urinary excretion of water and sodium, primarily by decreasing sodium chloride reabsorption in the renal tubules. Different diuretics act at different sites in the nephron, as illustrated below.

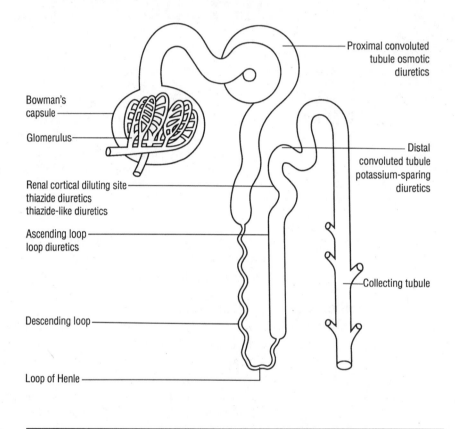

The onset of action of thiazide and thiazide-like diuretics is rapid, usually occurring within 1 hour of oral administration. Optimal antihypertensive effects typically do not appear for 3 to 4 weeks after therapy begins—but they may appear within 3 or 4 days. For most of these diuretics, the peak concentration occurs within 4 to 6 hours; the duration of action ranges from 6 to 24 hours.

Pharmacodynamics

Thiazide and thiazide-like diuretics are sulfonamide derivatives that inhibit sodium reabsorption, which increases sodium and water excretion. They also increase the excretion of chloride, potassium, and bicarbonate ions, which can lead to electrolyte imbalances. These actions are related directly to the drug's ability to interfere with sodium ion transport across the renal tubular epithelium at the distal segment of the nephrons.

SELECTED MAJOR DRUGS

Diuretic agents

This chart summarizes the major diuretics currently in clinical use.

DRUG	MAJOR INDICATIONS	USUAL ADULT DOSAGES
Thiazide and thiazide-like diuretics		
benzthiazide	Edema	50 to 200 mg P.O. daily in a single dose or in divided doses
	Hypertension	50 mg P.O. once daily or b.i.d., depending on patient's response
chlorothiazide	Edema	500 mg to 2 g P.O. or I.V. daily in a single dose or in two divided doses
	Hypertension	500 mg to 1 g P.O. or I.V. daily in a single dose or in divided doses
hydrochlorothiazide	Edema	25 to 200 mg P.O. daily or intermittently
	Hypertension	25 to 100 mg P.O. daily in a single dose or in divided doses
metolazone	Edema caused by congestive heart failure (CHF)	5 to 10 mg P.O. daily
	Edema caused by renal or hepatic disease	5 to 20 mg P.O. daily
	Hypertension	2.5 to 5 mg P.O. daily
Loop diuretics		
bumetanide	Edema and hypertension	0.5 to 2 mg P.O. in a single daily dose or repeated at 4- to 5-hour intervals up to a total of 10 mg daily; maintenance dosages usually are given intermittently with 1- to 2-day rest periods; or 0.5 to 1 mg I.M. or I.V. given over 1 to 2 minutes; I.V. doses may be repeated every 2 to 3 hours up to a total of 10 mg daily
ethacrynate sodium, ethacrynic acid	Acute pulmonary edema	50 to 100 mg ethacrynate sodium I.V., infused slowly over several minutes
	Other forms of edema	50 to 200 mg ethacrynic acid P.O. once daily after meals or on alternate days; or up to 200 mg P.O. b.i.d. to obtain a therapeutic effect
furosemide	Acute pulmonary edema	40 mg I.V. slowly, then repeated every 2 hours as needed
	Other forms of edema	20 to 80 mg P.O. once daily or b.i.d., up to a maximum of 600 mg daily, or 20 to 40 mg I.M. or I.V. with repeated doses of 20 mg I.M. or I.V. every 2 hours until therapeutic effect is reached
	Hypertensive crisis, acute renal failure	100 to 200 mg I.V. over 1 to 2 minutes
	Chronic renal failure	Initially, 80 mg P.O. daily; increased up to 120 mg daily until therapeutic effect is achieved
	Hypertension	20 to 80 mg P.O. daily

(continued)

Diuretic agents *(continued)*

DRUG	MAJOR INDICATIONS	USUAL ADULT DOSAGES
Potassium-sparing diuretics		
amiloride	Hypertension or edema associated with CHF	Initially, 5 to 10 mg P.O. daily, increased up to 20 mg daily, as needed
spironolactone	Essential hypertension	50 to 100 mg P.O. daily in a single dose or two divided doses
	Edema	Initially, 25 to 200 mg P.O. daily in a single dose or two divided doses, with the total dosage adjusted to patient response
Osmotic diuretics		
mannitol	Oliguria, prevention of acute renal failure	50 to 100 g I.V. of 5% to 25% solution
	Increased intracranial or intraocular pressure	1.5 to 2 g/kg I.V. of 15% to 20% solution infused over 30 to 60 minutes; for preoperative medication, give same dosage 1 to $1\frac{1}{2}$ hours before surgery
	Drug intoxication from secobarbital, imipramine, aspirin, or carbon tetrachloride use	Up to 200 g I.V. of 5% to 10% solution infused over 24 hours

Pharmacotherapeutics

These diuretics are used alone and with other drugs, primarily to treat hypertension and edema resulting from mild to moderate congestive heart failure (CHF). They also are used to treat edema associated with hepatic disease, renal disease, and corticosteroid and estrogen therapy. Because thiazide diuretics decrease urinary calcium levels, these drugs can be used to prevent the development and recurrence of calcium nephrolithiasis. Metolazone is the only drug in this class that is effective when the patient's GFR is less than 20 ml/minute.

Drug interactions

Thiazide and thiazide-like diuretics may interact with a variety of drugs. Most of these interactions result in altered fluid volume, blood pressure, or serum electrolyte levels. (For details, see Drug Interactions: *Diuretic agents.*)

Adverse drug reactions

The most common adverse reactions to thiazide and thiazide-like diuretics are blood volume depletion, orthostatic hypotension, hyponatremia, and hypokalemia. Other reactions include glucose intolerance, hypercalcemia, hypophosphatemia, hyperuricemia, and GI reactions, such as anorexia, nausea, and pancreatitis. Hypersensitivity reactions include purpura, photosensitivity, rash, urticaria, necrotizing vasculitis, and blood abnormalities.

DRUG INTERACTIONS

Diuretic agents

Drug interactions related to diuretics may cause severe fluid and electrolyte imbalances and other serious problems.

DRUG	INTERACTING DRUGS	POSSIBLE EFFECTS
Thiazide and thiazide-like diuretics		
all thiazide and thiazide-like diuretics	oral hypoglycemic agents, insulin	Hyponatremia, thiazide resistance, hyperglycemia
	corticosteroids, corticotropin	Hypokalemia
	lithium carbonate	Lithium toxicity
	skeletal muscle relaxants (tubocurarine, gallamine)	Increased responsiveness to the skeletal muscle relaxant
	cardiac glycosides	Increased risk of digitalis toxicity (as a result of hypokalemia)
	probenecid	Decreased renal excretion of uric acid, which may precipitate or worsen gout
	cholestyramine, colestipol	Decreased therapeutic effects of the diuretic
	indomethacin, other nonsteroidal anti-inflammatory drugs (NSAIDs)	Decreased antihypertensive effects
Loop diuretics		
bumetanide, ethacrynate sodium, ethacrynic acid, furosemide	oral hypoglycemic agents	Hyperglycemia
	aminoglycosides	Ototoxicity
	lithium carbonate	Decreased lithium excretion, resulting in lithium toxicity
	cisplatin	Increased ototoxicity
	cardiac glycosides	Electrolyte disturbances that may predispose the patient to digitalis-induced arrhythmias
	NSAIDs	Reduced antihypertensive and diuretic effects
furosemide	neuromuscular blockers	Enhanced neuromuscular blockade
	phenytoin	Decreased furosemide absorption and effects
Potassium-sparing diuretics		
amiloride, spironolactone, triamterene	potassium supplements, other potassium-sparing diuretics, angiotensin-converting enzyme (ACE) inhibitors (captopril, enalapril, lisinopril)	Hyperkalemia
spironolactone	cardiac glycosides	Decreased renal excretion of cardiac glycoside
	salicylates	Decreased spironolactone effects

Loop diuretics Loop, or high-ceiling, diuretics are highly potent agents. They include bumetanide (Bumex), ethacrynate sodium (Edecrin Sodium), ethacrynic acid (Edecrin), and furosemide (Lasix).

Pharmacokinetics

Loop diuretics are absorbed well and distributed rapidly. Extensively protein-bound, these drugs undergo partial or complete metabolism in the liver except for furosemide, which is excreted primarily unchanged. They are excreted primarily in the urine, but also in the bile and feces.

These diuretics have a more rapid onset of action and produce a much greater volume of diuresis than other types of diuretics. After oral administration, the onset ranges from 30 to 60 minutes; after intravenous (I.V.) administration, onset occurs within a few minutes. For most loop diuretics, the duration is 6 to 8 hours after oral administration and up to 2 hours after I.V. administration.

Pharmacodynamics

Loop diuretics inhibit sodium and chloride reabsorption in the renal tubules and inhibit sodium, chloride, and water reabsorption in the proximal tubule. Because of their potency, these drugs can cause profound diuresis and water and electrolyte depletion.

Pharmacotherapeutics

The most potent diuretics available, loop diuretics are used primarily to treat edema associated with CHF, hepatic or renal disease, or nephrotic syndrome. They also are used to treat mild hypertension, and some may be prescribed to treat edema resulting from various causes, cancer-related ascites, nephrogenic diabetes insipidus, and hypercalcemia. These agents are valuable in treating patients who do not respond to less potent diuretics or who have impaired renal function.

Drug interactions

Loop diuretics may interact with various drugs, including aminoglycosides, cardiac glycosides, hypoglycemic agents, and nonsteroidal anti-inflammatory drugs. (For details, see Drug Interactions: *Diuretic agents,* page 249.)

Adverse drug reactions

Because loop diuretics are potent, adverse reactions may be severe. Common adverse reactions include volume depletion, orthostatic hypotension, hypokalemia, hypochloremia, hypochloremic alkalosis, asymptomatic hyperuricemia, hyponatremia, hypocalcemia, and hypomagnesemia. Transient deafness, abdominal discomfort or pain, diarrhea, impaired glucose tolerance, dermatitis, paresthesia, hepatic dysfunction, and thrombocytopenia also can occur. Hypersensitivity reactions include purpura, photosensitivity, rash, pruritus, urticaria, and erythema multiforme.

Potassium-sparing diuretics

These diuretics include amiloride hydrochloride (Midamor), spironolactone (Aldactone), and triamterene (Dyrenium). They have weaker diuretic and antihypertensive effects than other types of diuretics.

Pharmacokinetics

After oral administration, potassium-sparing diuretics are absorbed to varying degrees from the GI tract and distributed widely in body tissues and fluids. They are metabolized in the liver (except for amiloride, which is not metabolized) and excreted in the urine and feces.

The onset of action for the potassium-sparing diuretics ranges from 2 to 4 hours. Their peak concentration occurs in 1 to 4 hours. Their duration ranges from 12 to 72 hours and increases with repeated doses.

Pharmacodynamics

These diuretics act in the distal renal tubule, increasing urinary excretion of sodium, chloride, and calcium ions and decreasing excretion of potassium and hydrogen ions.

Pharmacotherapeutics

Because the potassium-sparing diuretics conserve potassium, they usually are combined with other diuretics to potentiate their action or counteract their potassium-wasting effects. These diuretics are used chiefly to treat edema and diuretic-induced hypokalemia in patients with CHF, cirrhosis, nephrotic syndrome, or hypertension. Spironolactone also is used to treat hyperaldosteronism and hirsutism.

Drug interactions

The potassium-sparing effects of these diuretics are responsible for most of their drug interactions. (For details, see Drug Interactions: *Diuretic agents,* page 249.)

Adverse drug reactions

The potassium-sparing effects of these agents can lead to hyperkalemia, especially if the patient consumes a potassium supplement or a high-potassium diet. Other dose-related reactions include megaloblastic anemia, dizziness, orthostatic hypotension, sore throat, dry month, nausea, and vomiting. Hypersensitivity reactions include urticaria, pruritus, erythematous eruptions, rash, photosensitivity, and anaphylaxis.

Amiloride also may produce headache, anorexia, diarrhea or constipation, muscle cramps, abdominal pain, impotence, and metabolic disturbances. Spironolactone also may cause headache, abdominal cramps, diarrhea, gynecomastia in men, and breast soreness and menstrual abnormalities in women.

Osmotic diuretics

The primary drugs in this class are mannitol (Osmitrol) and urea (Ureaphil), which also is known as carbamide.

Pharmacokinetics

After I.V. administration, mannitol and urea are distributed rapidly. They are filtered primarily by the glomeruli and are excreted primarily unchanged in the urine. Diuresis occurs in 1 to 3 hours after mannitol administration and in 1 to 2 hours after urea administration. The peak concentration ranges from 30 to 60 minutes for mannitol; 1 to 2 hours for urea. Depending on the dosage used and the clinical indication, the duration of action for mannitol is 3 to 8 hours; for urea, 3 to 10 hours.

Pharmacodynamics

Osmotic diuretics act by increasing the osmolality of the plasma, glomerular filtrate, and tubular fluid. This causes increased water, chloride, and sodium excretion.

Pharmacotherapeutics

Mannitol and urea are used primarily to reduce increased intracranial and intraocular pressure and to prevent oliguria and acute renal failure. Mannitol also is useful in treating some types of drug intoxication.

Drug interactions

Osmotic diuretics produce no significant interactions.

Adverse drug reactions

Common adverse reactions to osmotic diuretics include circulatory overload, tachycardia, electrolyte imbalances, volume depletion, cellular dehydration, headache, nausea, and vomiting. Other reactions may include local irritation and thrombophlebitis (caused by extravasation) and hypersensitivity reactions. In addition, mannitol may cause rebound increased intracranial pressure, angina-like pain, blurred vision, rhinitis, thirst, and urine retention.

Nursing implications When caring for a patient who is receiving a diuretic agent, the nurse should be aware of the following implications.
- Develop appropriate nursing diagnoses for the patient. (For examples, see Sample Nursing Diagnoses: *Diuretic agents*.)
- Do not administer a diuretic to a patient with a condition that contraindicates its use.
- Administer a diuretic cautiously to a patient at risk because of a preexisting condition.
- Monitor the patient for adverse reactions and signs of drug interactions.
- Review the patient's serum electrolyte levels and other laboratory studies to detect any imbalances or abnormalities.
- Monitor the effectiveness of the diuretic. Measure and document the patient's fluid intake and output. Also weigh the patient daily under controlled conditions (at the same time each morning, after the patient voids, before the patient eats, with the patient wearing similar clothing at each weigh-in, and on the same scale).

SAMPLE NURSING DIAGNOSES

Diuretic agents

The following nursing diagnoses address representative problems and etiologies that a nurse may encounter when caring for a patient who is receiving a diuretic agent.

- Altered urinary elimination related to the urinary effects of a diuretic
- Constipation related to the adverse gastrointestinal (GI) effects of amiloride
- Diarrhea related to the adverse GI effects of a diuretic
- Fluid volume excess related to ineffectiveness of the prescribed diuretic
- High risk for fluid volume deficit related to diuretic-induced volume depletion or the adverse GI effects of a diuretic
- High risk for impaired skin integrity related to a dermatologic hypersensitivity reaction to a diuretic
- High risk for injury related to adverse drug reactions
- High risk for injury related to a preexisting condition that contraindicates the use of a diuretic
- High risk for injury related to preexisting condition that requires cautious use of a diuretic
- High risk for injury related to drug interactions
- High risk for trauma related to diuretic-induced orthostatic hypotension
- Impaired tissue integrity related to necrotizing vasculitis caused by a thiazide or thiazide-like diuretic
- Knowledge deficit related to the prescribed diuretic
- Noncompliance related to long-term use of the prescribed diuretic
- Pain related to loop diuretic-induced abdominal pain
- Sensory or perceptual alterations (auditory, tactile) related to transient deafness or paresthesias caused by a loop diuretic
- Sexual dysfunction related to amiloride-induced impotence

- Notify the physician if adverse reactions or drug interactions occur or if the drug is ineffective.
- Teach the patient and family the name, dose, frequency, action, and adverse effects of the prescribed diuretic.

Thiazide, thiazide-like, loop, and potassium-sparing diuretics

- Have patient sit up for a few minutes before standing to minimize the effects of orthostatic hypotension.
- Offer fluids regularly to combat dehydration.
- Keep a urinal or bedpan within reach of a bedridden patient; ensure that the bathroom is easily accessible for an ambulatory patient.
- Administer the diuretic in the morning, if possible, to prevent nocturia from upsetting the patient's normal sleep pattern.
- Provide high-potassium foods to a patient who also is receiving a potassium-wasting diuretic.
- Notify the physician immediately if the diuretic does not cause diuresis as expected.
- Store spironolactone in a light-resistant container away from light.
- Use the Z-track injection method when administering furosemide intramuscularly to minimize tissue irritation.

- Administer I.V. loop diuretics slowly over 1 to 2 minutes to prevent adverse reactions.
- Teach the patient to take the diuretic exactly as prescribed.
- Advise the patient to expect an increase in urinary frequency and amount voided.
- Teach the patient to recognize and report adverse reactions, such as hypokalemia (characterized by drowsiness, paresthesia, muscle cramps, and hyporeflexia) or hyperkalemia (characterized by confusion, hyperexcitability, muscle weakness, paresthesia, and arrhythmias), to the physician.
- Instruct the patient to obtain a daily weight under the same conditions every time and to notify the physician of any sudden weight gain.

Osmotic diuretics

- Measure the patient's vital signs hourly during osmotic diuretic therapy because these drugs can cause rapid changes in the patient's fluid status.
- Administer mannitol 1 to $1\frac{1}{2}$ hours before surgery when it is used as preoperative medication.
- Redissolve parenteral mannitol, which crystallizes at low temperatures, by warming it in a hot-water bath and shaking the container vigorously. Then let the solution return to room temperature before administration. Do not administer crystallized medication.
- Administer mannitol at the prescribed rate using an in-line I.V. filter.
- Do not add blood products to I.V. lines used for mannitol administration because they are incompatible.
- Store mannitol at 59° to 86° F (15° to 30° C) unless otherwise directed. Do not allow it to freeze.
- Provide mouth care and offer ice chips to relieve thirst.
- Instruct the patient to notify the nurse if angina-like chest pain occurs during mannitol therapy.
- Explain the need for frequent tests to monitor drug therapy.
- Reassure the patient that blurred vision, rhinitis, and thirst should subside when therapy is discontinued.

STUDY ACTIVITIES

Fill in the blank

1. Clinically, diuretics are used to increase _____ volume by acting at different sites in the _____.

2. The four major classes of diuretics are _____, _____, _____, and _____ diuretics.

3. Thiazide diuretics are _____ derivatives that inhibit sodium reabsorption.

4. Because thiazide diuretics decrease urinary calcium levels, they can be used to prevent _____.

5. After I.V. administration of furosemide, the onset of action occurs _____.

6. The signs and symptoms of hypokalemia include _____, _____, _____, and _____.

7. The signs and symptoms of hyperkalemia include _____, _____, _____, _____, and _____.

Multiple choice

8. Joseph Upton, age 68, is admitted with a diagnosis of hypertension. His physician orders chlorothiazide 1 g P.O. b.i.d. The nurse reviews Mr. Upton's medication history, which shows that he has been taking digoxin for 3 years. What effect is this likely to have on his diuretic therapy?

    A. It may enhance the effects of the chlorothiazide.
    B. It may increase the risk of digitalis toxicity.
    C. It may increase the risk of hyponatremia.
    D. It should cause no unusual problems.

9. The nurse weighs Mr. Upton every day. What else should the nurse do during chlorothiazide therapy?

    A. Assess for signs and symptoms of hypokalemia.
    B. Assess for signs and symptoms of hyperkalemia.
    C. Monitor the patient for signs of fluid overload.
    D. Teach the patient to take the drug upon arising and before bedtime.

10. The nurse notes that Mr. Upton's fluid output does not exceed his intake. What should the nurse do next?

    A. Contact the physician immediately.
    B. Increase Mr. Upton's fluid intake to 2,000 ml daily.
    C. Discontinue the medication immediately.
    D. Determine the patient's serum potassium level.

11. William Golden, age 31, sustained a head injury in an automobile accident. The physician orders mannitol to treat Mr. Golden's increased intracranial pressure. How frequently should the nurse assess the patient's vital signs?

    A. Once every shift
    B. Every 4 hours
    C. Every 2 hours
    D. Every hour

12. Before administering mannitol, the nurse should take which precaution?

    A. Evaluate the patient's blood type.

    B. Add a blood product to the I.V. line.

    C. Place an in-line filter in the I.V. line.

    D. Refrigerate mannitol for 2 hours before administering.

13. Two hours after the mannitol infusion, Mr. Golden reports chest pain. What should the nurse do?

    A. Assess the patient's vital signs.

    B. Inquire about pain in other areas.

    C. Obtain an order for an analgesic.

    D. Notify the physician immediately.

True or false

14. Loop diuretics commonly are prescribed for patients who do not respond to less potent diuretics.

    ☐ True   ☐ False

15. The nurse should assess fluid intake and output regularly for a patient receiving a potassium-sparing diuretic.

    ☐ True   ☐ False

16. I.V. bumetanide should be administered slowly over 10 minutes to a patient with edema and hypertension.

    ☐ True   ☐ False

17. Loop diuretics reduce potassium loss from the kidneys.

    ☐ True   ☐ False

18. Potassium-sparing diuretics are the strongest diuretics available.

    ☐ True   ☐ False

19. The nurse should use the Z-track method when administering furosemide intramuscularly.

    ☐ True   ☐ False

20. A patient taking a thiazide diuretic can reduce the effects of orthostatic hypotension by sitting up for a few minutes before standing.

    ☐ True   ☐ False

ANSWERS

Fill in the blank

1. Urine, nephrons

2. Thiazide and thiazide-like, loop, potassium-sparing, osmotic

3. Sulfonamide

4. Calcium nephrolithiasis

5. Within a few minutes

6. Drowsiness, paresthesia, muscle cramps, hyporeflexia

7. Confusion, hyperexcitability, muscle weakness, paresthesia, arrhythmias

Multiple choice

8. B. Chlorothiazide and the other thiazide diuretics increase the risk of digitalis toxicity as a result of hypokalemia.

9. A. Thiazide diuretics can produce hypokalemia and volume depletion. Because they also can cause nocturia, they should not be administered in the evening, if possible.

10. A. A therapeutic response to diuretic agents is increased urine output. If output does not increase, the diuretic is ineffective; this requires physician notification.

11. D. The nurse should measure the patient's vital signs hourly during mannitol therapy because osmotic diuretics can cause rapid changes in the patient's fluid status.

12. C. An in-line filter prevents large crystals from being infused. Mannitol crystallizes at low temperatures and is incompatible with blood products.

13. D. Chest pain may indicate an adverse reaction, which should be reported to the physician.

True or false

14. True.

15. True.

16. False. Like several other loop diuretics, I.V. bumetanide should be administered over 1 to 2 minutes.

17. False. Loop diuretics cause potassium loss; potassium-sparing diuretics counteract that loss.

18. False. Loop diuretics are the most potent diuretics available. Potassium-sparing diuretics have weaker diuretic and antihypertensive effects.

19. True.

20. True.

CHAPTER 18

Antilipemic agents

OBJECTIVES After studying this chapter, the reader should be able to:
1. Describe the blood lipid components and lipoproteins.
2. Discuss the various types of hyperlipoproteinemia and identify the antilipemic agents that usually are used to treat each type.
3. Describe the mechanism of action and major adverse reactions for each of the three major classes of antilipemic agents.
4. Explain how bile-sequestering agents and fibric acid derivatives interact with other drugs.
5. Describe how niacin acts as an antilipemic agent and identify its major adverse reactions.
6. Describe the nursing implications of antilipemic therapy.

OVERVIEW OF CONCEPTS Antilipemic agents lower abnormally high blood levels of lipids (fatty substances). Excessive lipids lead to the formation of excess cholesterol, which results in atherosclerosis and increased risk of coronary artery disease (CAD).

Lipids are composed of free fatty acids (FFAs), triglycerides, sterols, and phospholipids. They can be exogenous (derived from the diet) or endogenous (produced by the liver). Combinations of these lipids form the various lipoproteins that transport lipids throughout the body: chylomicrons, chylomicron fragments, very-low-density lipoproteins (VLDLs), low-density lipoproteins (LDLs), intermediate-density lipoproteins, and high-density lipoproteins (HDLs). HDLs may serve a protective role by excreting cholesterol from body tissues.

Hyperlipidemia (an excess of any type of lipid in the blood) can cause hyperlipoproteinemia (an excess of lipoproteins), hypercholesterolemia (an excess of cholesterol), or hypertriglyceridemia (an excess of triglycerides). These conditions contribute to hypertension and CAD, may be familial, and can vary for men and women of different ages. Therefore, the nurse must consider the patient's age and sex when interpreting blood lipid levels.

Antilipemic agents can reduce cholesterol and other lipid levels, but are not the first treatment of choice. Initial therapy should include proper diet, weight loss, and exercise to reduce blood lipid levels. If this

Antilipemic agents

This chart summarizes the major antilipemic agents currently in clinical use.

DRUG	MAJOR INDICATIONS	USUAL ADULT DOSAGES
Bile-sequestering agents		
cholestyramine	Type IIa hyperlipoproteinemia (hypercholesterolemia)	4 g resin P.O. one to six times daily mixed with 120 to 180 ml of fluid, soup, cereal, or pulpy fruit; or one chewable bar P.O. one to six times daily followed by adequate fluid consumption
Folic acid derivatives		
gemfibrozil	Type III hyperlipoproteinemia; types II, IV, and V hyperlipoproteinemia	1,200 mg P.O. daily in two divided doses
Cholesterol synthesis inhibitors		
lovastatin	Primary type IIa and IIb hyperlipoproteinemia	20 to 80 mg P.O. daily

regimen does not lower blood lipid levels sufficiently, antilipemic therapy may begin. (For a summary of representative drugs, see Selected Major Drugs: *Antilipemic agents.*)

Bile-sequestering agents Bile-sequestering agents include cholestyramine (Cholybar, Questran, Questran Light) and colestipol hydrochloride (Colestid).

Pharmacokinetics
These agents are not absorbed from the gastrointestinal (GI) tract because of their high molecular weight. Instead, they combine with bile acids in the GI tract for about 5 hours and then are excreted in the feces.

Pharmacodynamics
Cholestyramine and colestipol combine with bile acids in the GI tract, which decreases bile acid levels in the gallbladder. This triggers the liver to synthesize more bile acids from cholesterol. As cholesterol leaves the bloodstream to replace the lost bile acids, blood cholesterol levels decrease. The overall effect is a decrease in blood LDL levels.

Pharmacotherapeutics
Bile-sequestering agents are the drugs of choice for treating type IIa hyperlipoproteinemia (familial hypercholesterolemia) in patients who do not respond to dietary management. Cholestyramine is available as a powder or chewable bar; each scoop, packet, or bar contains 4 grams of resin. Colestipol is available in 5-gram packets.

DRUG INTERACTIONS

Antilipemic agents

Of the antilipemic agents, the bile-sequestering agents interact with the widest range of drugs.

DRUG	INTERACTING DRUGS	POSSIBLE EFFECTS
Bile-sequestering agents		
cholestyramine, colestipol	oral anticoagulants	Increased risk of clotting
	corticosteroids	Decreased corticosteroid effects
	acetaminophen	Reduced pain relief
	cardiac glycosides	Decreased cardiac glycoside effects
	iron preparations	Reduced serum iron level
	thiazide diuretics	Decreased diuretic effects
	thyroid hormones	Reduced triiodothyronine (T_3) and thyroxine (T_4) levels
	methotrexate	Decreased methotrexate absorption
Fibric acid derivatives		
clofibrate, gemfibrozil	oral anticoagulants	Increased anticoagulant effect
	sulfonylureas	Increased hypoglycemic effects
Cholesterol synthesis inhibitors		
probucol	clofibrate	Decreased high-density lipoprotein level
	drugs that prolong the Q-T interval, affect the atrial rate, or produce atrioventricular block	Increased cardiovascular effects
lovastatin, pravastatin, simvastatin	immunosuppressants (especially cyclosporine), gemfibrozil, niacin (in antilipemic dosages)	Increased risk of myopathy or rhabdomyolysis

Drug interactions
Bile-sequestering agents bind with acidic drugs and other drugs normally absorbed in the GI tract. They also interact with oral anticoagulants, corticosteroids, acetaminophen, and many other drugs. (For details, see Drug Interactions: *Antilipemic agents.*)

Adverse drug reactions
Adverse reactions to bile-sequestering agents usually result from long-term therapy. Common GI reactions include constipation, fecal impaction, abdominal pain, distention, flatulence, belching, nausea, vomiting, diarrhea, and hemorrhoid irritation. Less common GI reactions are peptic ulcers and bleeding, cholelithiasis, and cholecystitis. GI reactions are more likely to affect patients over age 60 or those who take more than 24 grams of cholestyramine daily. Headache, dizziness, weakness, and fatigue also may occur.

Fibric acid derivatives

These agents include clofibrate (Atromid-S) and gemfibrozil (Lopid).

Pharmacokinetics

Fibric acid derivatives are absorbed readily from the GI tract, highly protein-bound, metabolized in the liver, and excreted in the urine. They begin to reduce VLDL levels in 2 to 5 days. Clofibrate's action peaks in 4 weeks; gemfibrozil peaks in 3 weeks. The duration of action for clofibrate is unknown; for gemfibrozil, 3 weeks.

Pharmacodynamics

The exact mechanism of action of these drugs is unknown. These agents may work by reducing cholesterol formation early in its biosynthesis. Gemfibrozil has two other effects. It increases blood HDL levels and increases the serum's capacity to dissolve additional cholesterol.

Pharmacotherapeutics

Fibric acid derivatives are used primarily to reduce high triglyceride levels and secondarily to reduce high cholesterol levels. They are used chiefly in patients with types II, III, IV, and mild type V hyperlipoproteinemia. However, they should be used only in patients at severe risk for CAD who have not responded adequately to diet changes; who exhibit other risk factors, such as hypertension or obesity; or who have a family history of CAD. Fibric acid derivatives are most effective in those patients with no history of CAD or angina. In patients with types IIa, IIb, and IV hyperlipoproteinemia, niacin is used as adjunct therapy to fibric acid derivative treatment.

Drug interactions

Fibric acid derivatives can interact with anticoagulants and sulfonylureas. They also may displace other acidic drugs, such as barbiturates, phenytoin, thyroid derivatives, and cardiac glycosides, although this interaction has not been demonstrated in studies. (For details, see Drug Interactions: *Antilipemic agents.*)

Adverse drug reactions

The most common adverse reactions to fibric acid derivatives are GI effects that resemble those of the bile-sequestering agents. Because clofibrate increases the incidence of cholelithiasis and malignant tumors, the drug is not recommended for long-term use. Other adverse reactions to this drug include pancreatitis, arrhythmias, intermittent claudication, thromboembolic events, angina, flulike symptoms, and elevated creatinine phosphokinase (CPK) level. Gemfibrozil may cause cholelithiasis.

Both drugs may produce a wide range of hypersensitivity reactions, such as skin rash, urticaria, dry skin, alopecia, brittle hair, hepatomegaly, impotence, leukopenia, weight gain, muscle pain, and abnormal liver function test results.

Cholesterol synthesis inhibitors

These antilipemic agents include lovastatin (Mevacor), pravastatin sodium (Pravachol), probucol (Lorelco), and simvastatin (Zocor).

Pharmacokinetics

After oral administration, lovastatin is absorbed incompletely. Its distribution in the body is unknown. The drug is metabolized extensively in the liver and excreted in the urine and feces. It usually produces a therapeutic response in 2 weeks and maximal changes in lipoprotein and cholesterol concentrations in 4 to 6 weeks.

Pravastatin is rapidly but incompletely absorbed after oral administration and undergoes first-pass metabolism in the liver. It is excreted primarily in the feces with a small amount eliminated in the urine.

Probucol is not absorbed well from the GI tract, although its absorption improves somewhat when given with food. The drug is distributed primarily in fatty acid depots. Although probucol's metabolism has not been identified, the drug is excreted in the urine. It begins to produce effects 2 to 4 weeks after therapy begins.

Simvastatin's pharmacokinetic properties are to similar to those of pravastatin. However, it is more than 95% protein-bound, whereas only 50% of pravastatin is protein-bound.

Pharmacodynamics

Although these agents are known to lower lipid levels by interfering with cholesterol synthesis, their exact mechanisms of action have not been identified. Lovastatin may inhibit the conversion of mevalonic acid to cholesterol, thus reducing cholesterol biosynthesis. It also reduces LDL levels, possibly by increasing clearance of serum LDLs by liver receptors and inhibiting LDL production.

Pravastatin may increase the number of LDL receptors on cell surfaces, receptor-mediated catabolism, and circulating LDL clearance. It also may inhibit LDL production.

Probucol may inhibit cholesterol transport from the intestine, inhibit cholesterol synthesis, and increase cholesterol and bile acid secretion. It decreases cholesterol and LDL levels.

Simvastatin may reduce VLDL cholesterol concentration and induce the LDL receptors, leading to reduced production and increased catabolism of LDL cholesterol.

Pharmacotherapeutics

Lovastatin is used to decrease serum levels of total and LDL cholesterol in familial types IIa and IIb hyperlipoproteinemia. It may be used in combination with a bile-sequestering agent. Pravastatin is used as an adjunct for type IIa and IIb hypercholesterolemia. Probucol may be used alone or with colestipol to treat type IIa hyperlipoproteinemia. Simvastatin is prescribed as adjunct therapy for hypercholesterolemia and mixed hyperlipidemia.

Drug interactions

Cholesterol synthesis inhibitors may interact with clofibrate, immuno-suppressants, gemfibrozil, niacin, and other drugs. (For details, see Drug Interactions: *Antilipemic agents,* page 260.)

Adverse drug reactions

Cholesterol synthesis inhibitors commonly produce adverse GI reactions similar to those caused by the other antilipemic agents. Probucol's other adverse effects also resemble those of the other antilipemics. Animal studies have shown that probucol prolongs the Q-T interval of the cardiac cycle.

In addition to GI distress, lovastatin may cause headache, elevated liver enzymes, elevated CPK level, myalgia, muscle cramps, myopathy, lens opacities, blurred vision, rash, and pruritus.

Other antilipemic agents Ethinyl estradiol, norethindrone acetate, nandrolone and other anabolic agents, neomycin, and niacin sometimes are used to treat hyperlipoproteinemia. However, only niacin has received Food and Drug Administration approval for this indication. (For more information about drugs other than niacin, see Chapter 33, Other major drugs, and Chapter 29, Antibacterial agents.) Dextrothyroxine sodium has been approved to treat hypercholesterolemia. Its serious cardiovascular effects, however, limit its use.

Niacin

Also known as nicotinic acid and vitamin B_3, niacin (Nicobid, Nicolar) decreases blood levels of LDL, VLDL, and phospholipids and increases the HDL level in types II, III, IV, and V hyperlipoproteinemia. With oral administration, niacin begins to produce therapeutic effects in 1 to 2 weeks, possibly by inhibiting the release of FFAs from lipid tissues.

Niacin's adverse reactions may limit its usefulness. It commonly produces skin flushing and GI effects that disappear in 2 to 6 weeks. Other adverse reactions include abnormal liver function test results, jaundice, abnormal prothrombin time, hypoalbuminemia, hyperglycemia, and hyperuricemia. (For more information, see Chapter 33, Other major drugs.)

Nursing implications When caring for a patient who is receiving an antilipemic agent, the nurse should be aware of the following implications.
- Develop appropriate nursing diagnoses for the patient. (For examples, see Sample Nursing Diagnoses: *Antilipemic agents,* page 264.)
- Do not administer an antilipemic agent to a patient with a condition that contraindicates its use.
- Administer an antilipemic agent cautiously to a patient at risk because of a preexisting condition.

Antilipemic agents

The following nursing diagnoses address representative problems and etiologies that a nurse may encounter when caring for a patient who is receiving an antilipemic agent.

- Altered cardiopulmonary tissue perfusion related to clofibrate-induced thromboembolic events
- Altered health maintenance related to ineffectiveness of the prescribed antilipemic agent
- Altered nutrition: less than body requirements, related to the adverse gastrointestinal (GI) effects of an antilipemic agent
- Altered nutrition: more than body requirements, related to weight gain caused by a fibric acid derivative
- Altered peripheral tissue perfusion related to clofibrate-induced intermittent claudication
- Altered protection related to the adverse hematologic effects of a fibric acid derivative or the increased risk of malignant tumors caused by clofibrate therapy
- Body image disturbance related to alopecia, dry skin, brittle hair, and weight gain caused by a fibric acid derivative
- Constipation related to the adverse GI effects of an antilipemic agent
- Decreased cardiac output related to clofibrate-induced arrhythmias
- Diarrhea related to the adverse GI effects of an antilipemic agent
- Fatigue related to the adverse effects of a bile-sequestering agent
- High risk for fluid volume deficit related to the adverse GI effects of an antilipemic agent
- High risk for injury related to adverse drug reactions
- High risk for injury related to a preexisting condition that contraindicates the use of an antilipemic agent
- High risk for injury related to a preexisting condition that requires cautious use of an antilipemic agent
- High risk for injury related to drug interactions
- Impaired physical mobility related to weakness caused by a bile-sequestering agent
- Impaired tissue integrity related to peptic ulcers caused by a bile-sequestering agent
- Knowledge deficit related to the prescribed antilipemic agent
- Noncompliance related to the adverse reactions to and duration of therapy with the prescribed antilipemic agent
- Pain related to biliary colic resulting from drug-induced cholelithiasis
- Sensory or perceptual alterations (visual) related to lovastatin-induced lens opacities or blurred vision
- Sexual dysfunction related to the adverse genitourinary effects of a fibric acid derivative

---

- Monitor the patient for adverse reactions and signs of drug interactions.
- Obtain baseline blood cholesterol and lipid levels before therapy begins. Then monitor blood cholesterol and lipid levels periodically for a patient receiving long-term therapy to assess the drug's effectiveness.
- Notify the physician if adverse reactions or drug interactions occur or if the drug is ineffective.
- Teach the patient and family the name, dose, frequency, action, and adverse effects of the prescribed antilipemic agent.
- Instruct the patient to notify the physician if adverse reactions occur.

Bile-sequestering agents

- Introduce and titrate the bile-sequestering agent slowly to minimize adverse GI reactions.
- Mix the powder form with 120 to 180 ml of liquid (such as water, carbonated beverage, or soup) or a pulpy fruit with a high moisture content (such as applesauce). Never administer the dry powder because the patient may inhale it accidentally.
- Have the patient chew a cholestyramine bar and then drink at least 8 oz (240 ml) of water or other liquid.
- Monitor prothrombin times regularly for a patient who also is taking an oral anticoagulant.
- Administer drugs that bind with bile-sequestering agents 1 hour before or 6 hours after giving the agent.
- Encourage the patient to drink at least 68 to 100 oz (2 to 3 liters) of fluid daily, increase dietary fiber intake, and get plenty of exercise to prevent constipation.
- Instruct the patient to have blood cholesterol levels checked every 3 to 6 months and to inform all other physicians about bile-sequestering agent therapy. The dosages of the other drugs may need to be adjusted.

Fibric acid derivatives

- Monitor the patient for biliary colic, which may be the first sign of cholelithiasis.
- Monitor the patient's liver function studies and white blood cell count to detect adverse reactions; also monitor prothrombin time (if the patient is taking an oral anticoagulant) to detect drug interactions.
- Observe closely for warning signs of cancer, adverse GI effects (especially abdominal pain, nausea, or vomiting, which may suggest biliary colic), decreased peripheral tissue perfusion resulting from intermittent claudication, and decreased cardiopulmonary tissue perfusion caused by a pulmonary embolism.
- Explain the importance and purpose of liver function studies and triglyceride and cholesterol level tests. Advise the patient that they require a blood sample after fasting from midnight the previous night.
- Instruct the patient to notify the physician of pain, swelling, or redness in legs and to go to the emergency department if shortness of breath develops.
- Teach the patient how to manage adverse GI effects.
- Teach the patient the warning signs of cancer.
- Instruct the patient who also is taking an anticoagulant that the physician may need to reduce the anticoagulant dosage to prevent bleeding during fibric acid derivative therapy. Teach the patient to take bleeding precautions, such as avoiding cuts and bruises, using a soft toothbrush, and using an electric razor.

Cholesterol synthesis inhibitors

- Administer probucol with morning and evening meals and lovastatin with the evening meal to enhance absorption.
- Obtain an electrocardiogram (ECG) when probucol treatment begins and after 6 and 12 months of therapy to detect adverse cardiac effects, such as a prolonged Q-T interval.
- Monitor liver function tests before lovastatin therapy begins, every 4 to 6 weeks during the first 12 to 15 months of therapy, and periodically thereafter to detect liver function abnormalities.
- Instruct the patient to take lovastatin or probucol with meals to enhance absorption; pravastatin at bedtime; or simvastatin in the evening
- Inform the patient that cholesterol level, ECG, and liver function must be assessed periodically.

STUDY ACTIVITIES

Fill in the blank

1. Abnormally high blood levels of lipids can lead to _____ and increased risk of _____.

2. When interpreting blood lipid levels, the nurse should consider the patient's _____ and _____.

3. Bile-sequestering agents are the drugs of choice for treating type _____ in patients who do not respond to dietary management.

4. _____ can be used as an adjunct to fibric acid derivative therapy in patients with types IIa, IIb, and IV hyperlipoproteinemia.

5. Because of its adverse effects, the cholesterol synthesis inhibitor lovastatin should be used cautiously in a patient with a history of _____ disease.

Matching related elements

Match the drug on the left with the best definition of its mechanism of action on the right.

6. ___ Cholestyramine   **A.** May inhibit cholesterol transport from the intestine and increases cholesterol and bile acid secretion

7. ___ Clofibrate   **B.** Inhibits the release of FFAs from lipid tissues

8. ___ Probucol   **C.** Removes excess bile acids from the GI tract

9. ___ Niacin   **D.** May reduce cholesterol formation early in its biosynthesis

Multiple choice

10. Jonas Smithers, age 60, has type III hyperlipoproteinemia that has not responded to a low-fat diet and exercise program. His physician is most likely to prescribe which type of antilipemic agent?
  A. Bile-sequestering agent
  B. Fibric acid derivative
  C. Cholesterol synthesis inhibitor
  D. Other antilipemic agent

11. For Monica Mason, age 53, the physician prescribes gemfibrozil 1,200 mg P.O. daily. During a patient-teaching session, the nurse should provide which instruction?
  A. Take the medication in a single dose with food.
  B. Return for regular hemoglobin and hematocrit testing.
  C. Stop taking the drug immediately if constipation occurs.
  D. Notify the physician if abdominal pain, nausea, or vomiting occurs.

12. Where is gemfibrozil metabolized?
  A. In the liver
  B. In the plasma
  C. In the kidneys
  D. In the GI tract

13. Samuel Greenbaum, age 66, takes colestipol for hypercholesterolemia. What adverse reaction can result from long-term use and what are its nursing implications?
  A. Cancer. The nurse should teach the patient to observe for early warning signs, such as a change in bowel or bladder habits.
  B. GI reactions. The nurse should titrate the drug slowly to the maximum dosage to minimize these effects.
  C. Hypoglycemia. The nurse should expect to see adjustments in the insulin or oral hypoglycemic agent dosage.
  D. Liver disease. The nurse should monitor liver function studies every 3 months after therapy begins.

14. Lisa Wellman, age 35, begins niacin therapy to decrease her blood LDL and VLDL levels. What is the most common adverse reaction to niacin?
  A. Flushing
  B. Hemorrhage
  C. Hypouricemia
  D. Hyperalbuminemia

True or false

15. Antilipemic therapy is the first treatment of choice in reducing cholesterol and other lipid levels.
☐ True ☐ False

16. Adverse reactions to bile-sequestering agents include GI reactions, peptic ulcers, and fatigue.
☐ True ☐ False

17. For a patient who must receive an oral anticoagulant concomitantly with a fibric acid derivative, the nurse should monitor the prothrombin time closely to prevent anticoagulant overdosage.
☐ True ☐ False

18. A patient may mix cholestyramine powder with a liquid or may take it in dry form.
☐ True ☐ False

19. Niacin is used primarily to treat type I hyperlipoproteinemia.
☐ True ☐ False

20. Bile-sequestering agents may interact with cardiac glycosides, thiazide diuretics, and thyroid hormones.
☐ True ☐ False

ANSWERS

Fill in the blank

1. Atherosclerosis, coronary artery disease (CAD)
2. Age, sex
3. IIa hyperlipoproteinemia
4. Niacin
5. Liver

Matching related elements

6. C
7. D
8. A
9. B

Multiple choice

10. B. Fibric acid derivatives are used chiefly in patients with types II, III, IV, and mild type V hyperlipoproteinemia.
11. D. Abdominal pain, nausea, and vomiting may be signs of cholelithiasis and should be reported to the physician.
12. A. After absorption in the GI tract, gemfibrozil is extensively metabolized in the liver.
13. B. The nurse should introduce and titrate the bile-sequestering agent slowly to minimize adverse GI reactions, such as constipation, fecal impaction, abdominal pain, nausea, and vomiting.
14. A. Niacin commonly produces skin flushing and GI effects that disappear in 2 to 6 weeks.

True or false

15. False. Initial therapy should include a proper diet, weight loss, and exercise. If this regimen does not lower blood lipid levels sufficiently, antilipemic therapy may begin.

16. True.

17. True.

18. False. Cholestyramine powder should be mixed with a liquid or a pulpy fruit. It must not be taken in dry form because the patient may inhale the powder accidentally.

19. False. Niacin is used to treat types II, III, IV, and V hyperlipoproteinemia.

20. True.

CHAPTER 19

Bronchodilators

OBJECTIVES

After studying this chapter, the reader should be able to:
1. Describe the main functions of the respiratory system.
2. Explain the pharmacokinetics and pharmacodynamics of methylxanthine agents.
3. Describe the clinical indications for methylxanthine agents.
4. Discuss the adverse reactions to methylxanthine agents.
5. Explain how adrenergic agents are used as bronchodilators.
6. Describe the nursing implications of bronchodilator therapy.

OVERVIEW OF CONCEPTS

The respiratory system extends from the nose to the pulmonary capillaries. It provides oxygen to tissues, removes carbon dioxide, regulates acid-base balance, and defends against airborne infection.

Air flows into the lungs through the conducting airways (nose to bronchioles) and reaches the alveoli, where gas exchange occurs. There, oxygen diffuses into the pulmonary capillaries and enters the red blood cells. At the same time, carbon dioxide diffuses from the blood into the alveoli, for exhalation from the lungs.

The rate and depth of respirations influence the acid-base balance of the blood, which normally ranges from a pH of 7.35 to 7.45. Hypoventilation causes carbon dioxide retention, which lowers the blood pH to more acidic levels; hyperventilation causes excess carbon dioxide removal, which raises the blood pH to more alkaline levels.

To defend the body against infection, the upper airways filter, humidify, and warm air during inhalation. Also, the mucosa and cilia trap infectious particles and remove them from the airway. Coughing rapidly expels air and particles from the airways; sneezing clears the nasal passages. (For an illustration, see *Normal respiratory anatomy and physiology*.)

When the body's defense mechanisms fail, the patient may develop a disorder, such as asthma, chronic bronchitis, or emphysema. These disorders commonly are treated with methylxanthine agents and other bronchodilators. (For a summary of representative drugs, see Selected Major Drugs: *Bronchodilators*, page 272.)

Normal respiratory anatomy and physiology

The respiratory system's major structures are illustrated below. The insert below right shows the partial pressures of the carbon dioxide and oxygen exchanged. The insert below left, which is an enlargement of the alveolus and surrounding vessels, shows intrapulmonary blood circulation around the alveolus.

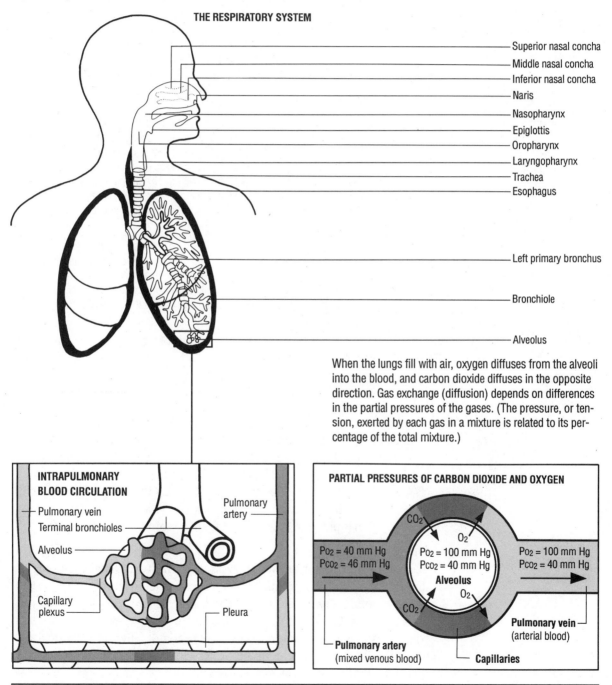

THE RESPIRATORY SYSTEM

- Superior nasal concha
- Middle nasal concha
- Inferior nasal concha
- Naris
- Nasopharynx
- Epiglottis
- Oropharynx
- Laryngopharynx
- Trachea
- Esophagus

- Left primary bronchus
- Bronchiole
- Alveolus

When the lungs fill with air, oxygen diffuses from the alveoli into the blood, and carbon dioxide diffuses in the opposite direction. Gas exchange (diffusion) depends on differences in the partial pressures of the gases. (The pressure, or tension, exerted by each gas in a mixture is related to its percentage of the total mixture.)

INTRAPULMONARY BLOOD CIRCULATION

- Pulmonary vein
- Terminal bronchioles
- Alveolus
- Capillary plexus
- Pulmonary artery
- Pleura

PARTIAL PRESSURES OF CARBON DIOXIDE AND OXYGEN

CO_2
O_2

P_{O_2} = 40 mm Hg
P_{CO_2} = 46 mm Hg

P_{O_2} = 100 mm Hg
P_{CO_2} = 40 mm Hg
Alveolus

P_{O_2} = 100 mm Hg
P_{CO_2} = 40 mm Hg

O_2
CO_2

Pulmonary artery
(mixed venous blood)

Capillaries

Pulmonary vein
(arterial blood)

Bronchodilators

This chart summarizes the major methylxanthine agents currently in clinical use.

DRUG	MAJOR INDICATIONS	USUAL ADULT DOSAGES
Methylxanthine agents		
anhydrous theophylline	Asthma, bronchitis, and emphysema; neonatal apnea (rapid-release oral liquids)	Specific dosage based on serum theophylline concentration, patient response, and occurrence of adverse reactions; the daily dosage is divided into 6- or 8-hour doses for rapid-release products and 8-, 12-, or 24-hour doses for slow-release products; initial maximum dosage is 13 mg/kg/day or a total of 800 mg/day, whichever is less
aminophylline	Asthma, chronic bronchitis, emphysema	Dosage based on theophylline content and specific dosage based on serum theophylline concentration, patient response, and occurrence of adverse reactions; the daily dosage is divided into 6- or 8-hour doses for rapid-release products and 8- or 12-hour doses for slow-release products; after an I.V. loading dose of 5 to 6 mg/kg is given over 20 to 30 minutes, the patient may receive a maintenance dosage of 0.4 to 0.7 mg I.V./kg/hour; initial maximum dosage in adults is 13 mg/kg/day of theophylline or a total of 800 mg/day, whichever is less
oxtriphylline	Asthma, chronic bronchitis, emphysema, similar chronic obstructive pulmonary diseases	200 mg P.O. every 6 to 8 hours; the daily dosage should be divided into 6- or 8-hour doses for rapid-release products and 8- to 12-hour doses for slow-release products; the specific dosage is based on serum theophylline concentration, patient response, and occurrence of adverse reactions; the initial maximum dosage in adults is 13 mg/kg/day of theophylline or a total of 800 mg/day, whichever is less
dyphylline	Asthma, chronic bronchitis, emphysema	Up to 15 mg/kg P.O. every 6 hours, or 250 to 500 mg I.M. up to a maximum of 15 mg/kg, every 6 hours

Methylxanthine agents
Also called xanthines, methylxanthine agents are used primarily to treat asthma, chronic bronchitis, emphysema, and neonatal apnea. Commonly used methylxanthines include anhydrous theophylline (Slo-bid Gyrocaps, Theo-24, Theo-Dur), theophylline salts, dyphylline (Dylline, Lufyllin), and caffeine. Theophylline salts include aminophylline (Aminophyllin, Somophyllin-DF), oxtriphylline (Brondecon, Choledyl), theophylline sodium glycinate (Asbron G, Synophylate).

Pharmacokinetics
The pharmacokinetics of methylxanthines vary with the agent used, its dosage form, and its administration route. These differences are particularly significant with the theophylline salts, which were developed to increase the solubility of theophylline because it is only slightly water-soluble. When administered orally or parenterally, the salts dissociate and appear as theophylline in the blood. However, they vary greatly in their theophylline content.

Theophylline generally is absorbed rapidly and completely. However, gastric pH and the presence of food in the stomach can alter the absorption rate. Therefore, oral theophylline products should be administered with a small amount of food or when the patient's stomach is empty. The volume of distribution of theophylline averages 0.5 liter/kg; the drug is not distributed well into adipose tissue. Theophylline is metabolized primarily in the liver and excreted in the urine.

Theophylline's absorption, metabolism, and excretion rates vary and can be affected by circulatory or metabolic dysfunction, fever, smoking, or drug interactions. Therefore, the drug dosage must be individualized based on the patient's body weight and condition, and serum theophylline levels must be monitored closely.

The onset and duration of action of theophylline depend on the serum theophylline level. To achieve a therapeutic level rapidly, a loading dose usually is administered; this is followed by a maintenance dosage to keep the serum drug level within the therapeutic range. To treat respiratory disease, the therapeutic serum level is 10 and 20 mcg/ml; to treat neonatal apnea, 5 to 10 mcg/ml. The maximum benefit from theophylline therapy occurs when the amount of drug excreted equals the amount of drug absorbed (steady-state concentration or level).

The half-life of theophylline varies from preparation to preparation and from patient to patient. Age and smoking directly affect the half-life of theophylline. In general, the half-life for children averages 3 to 4 hours; for smoking adults, 4 to 5 hours; and for nonsmoking adults, 7 to 8 hours.

Dyphylline, which is freely water-soluble, is not dissociated to theophylline in blood. It is absorbed incompletely after oral or intramuscular (I.M.) administration and is not metabolized by the liver. Most of a dyphylline dose is excreted unchanged in the urine. Its half-life is about 2.5 hours.

Caffeine, which is more water-soluble than theophylline, is absorbed well and distributed widely after oral administration. It is metabolized by the liver and excreted in the urine. Its half-life decreases with age, averaging 3 to 6 hours in adults.

Pharmacodynamics

Methylxanthines display similar pharmacologic activity, but may differ in the intensity of their effects on the target organs. In the respiratory system, they are powerful bronchodilators. They decrease nonspecific airway reactivity and, in the presence of bronchospasm, relax bronchial smooth muscle. Their specific mechanism of action in reversible obstructive airway disease is unknown. In nonreversible obstructive airway disease, methylxanthines seem to increase the central respiratory center's sensitivity to carbon dioxide and to stimulate the respiratory drive. In chronic bronchitis and emphysema, they decrease diaphragmatic fatigue and improve ventricular function.

Most methylxanthines also are powerful central nervous system (CNS) stimulants. They stimulate the respiratory center in the medulla and increase reflex excitability in the spinal cord. Slight depression usually follows this CNS excitation.

In the cardiovascular system, these agents increase myocardial contractility and dilate coronary, pulmonary, and systemic blood vessels. They strengthen skeletal muscle contractions, reduce muscle fatigability, cause diuresis, increase sodium and chloride excretion, and stimulate gastric acid secretion.

Pharmacotherapeutics

Theophylline, its salts, and dyphylline are used to treat asthma, bronchitis, and emphysema because they are effective bronchodilators. In neonates with apnea, theophylline and caffeine are equally effective. Theophylline also is a powerful cardiac stimulant, CNS stimulant, smooth muscle relaxant, diuretic, and gastric acid stimulant. Caffeine is used primarily as a CNS stimulant.

Drug interactions

Other drugs and food can interact with theophylline and its salts. Smoking cigarettes or marijuana can increase its elimination. Dyphylline and caffeine also may interact with various drugs. (For details, see Drug Interactions: *Bronchodilators.*)

Adverse drug reactions

Adverse reactions to theophylline can be transient (especially at the beginning of therapy) or can be symptomatic of toxicity. These reactions most commonly affect the CNS, gastrointestinal (GI) tract, and cardiovascular system. Adverse CNS reactions can include irritability, insomnia, headache, anxiety, and restlessness. Seizures may occur with very high serum drug levels. Adverse GI reactions can include nausea, vomiting, abdominal cramps, epigastric pain, anorexia, and diarrhea. Adverse cardiovascular symptoms, which result from myocardial irritation, are tachycardia, palpitations, extrasystoles, arrhythmias, peripheral vasodilation, and hypotension.

Other bronchodilators Some adrenergic agents are used as bronchodilators, including catecholamine and noncatecholamine agents. Catecholamine bronchodilators include epinephrine (Adrenalin, Medihaler-Epi, Primatene Mist) and isoproterenol (Isuprel, Medihaler-Iso). Noncatecholamine bronchodilators include albuterol (Proventil), metaproterenol sulfate (Alupent, Metaprel), and terbutaline sulfate (Brethaire, Brethine, Bricanyl). Although these drugs are available in many forms, they commonly are used as inhalants for fast relief of bronchospasm.

Pharmacologically, adrenergic agents cause biological responses similar to those produced by activation of the sympathetic nervous system. Agents with beta$_2$ adrenergic activity dilate the bronchial passages, which makes them useful in treating acute and chronic bronchial

DRUG INTERACTIONS

Bronchodilators

In many cases, interactions between theophylline and other drugs increase the risk of toxicity or subtherapeutic levels.

DRUG	INTERACTING DRUGS	POSSIBLE EFFECTS
Methylxanthine agents		
anhydrous theophylline, aminophylline, oxtriphylline, theophylline sodium glycinate	cimetidine, ciprofloxacin, norfloxacin	Increased theophylline concentration, resulting in a potentially toxic concentration
	erythromycin, troleandomycin	Increased theophylline concentration
	allopurinol (high doses), disulfiram, thiabendazole	Increased theophylline concentration
	oral contraceptives	Increased serum theophylline concentration
	beta-adrenergic blockers	Increased theophylline concentration; decreased bronchodilating effects of theophylline
	phenobarbital, phenytoin, rifampin, carbamazepine	Decreased serum theophylline concentration
	halothane, enflurane, isoflurane, methoxyflurane	Increased risk of cardiac toxicity
	lithium	Increased lithium clearance
	thyroid hormones, antithyroid agents	Increased or decreased theophylline metabolism
dyphylline	probenecid	Decreased dyphylline excretion, resulting in prolonged effects
caffeine	adrenergic agents, beverages containing caffeine	Additive adverse reactions; methylxanthine toxicity

asthma, bronchitis, emphysema, and acute hypersensitivity reactions. (For detailed information, see Chapter 5, Autonomic agents.)

When caring for a patient receiving an adrenergic bronchodilator, the nurse should monitor for adverse reactions, such as headache, flushing, restlessness, nausea, vomiting, arrhythmias, and vital sign changes. During isoproterenol therapy, the nurse should also assess the patient's respiratory rate to detect rebound bronchospasm. The nurse should avoid administering isoproterenol and inhaled epinephrine concomitantly, and should space their administration 4 hours apart to help prevent cardiac stimulation.

In patient-teaching sessions, the nurse should demonstrate how to use the inhalant device properly, emphasize using the lowest number of inhalations possible, and encourage rinsing the mouth after inhalation to minimize dryness and irritation. Other teaching points include instructing the patient to avoid contact between the drug and the eyes, teaching the patient to take the drug only as prescribed and to main-

SAMPLE NURSING DIAGNOSES

Bronchodilators

The following nursing diagnoses address representative problems and etiologies that a nurse may encounter when caring for a patient who is receiving a methylxanthine agent.

- Altered cerebral tissue perfusion related to methylxanthine-induced hypotension
- Altered health maintenance related to the ineffectiveness of the prescribed methylxanthine
- Altered protection related to methylxanthine-induced arrhythmias
- Altered renal tissue perfusion related to methylxanthine-induced hypotension
- Anxiety related to the adverse central nervous system effects of a methylxanthine
- Diarrhea related to the adverse gastrointestinal (GI) effects of a methylxanthine
- Fluid volume deficit related to the adverse GI effects of a methylxanthine
- High risk for fluid volume deficit related to the adverse GI effects of a methylxanthine
- High risk for injury related to adverse drug reactions
- High risk for injury related to a preexisting condition that contraindicates the use of a methylxanthine
- High risk for injury related to a preexisting condition that requires cautious use of a methylxanthine
- High risk for injury related to drug interactions
- High risk for trauma related to seizures caused by a high serum concentration of the prescribed methylxanthine
- Knowledge deficit related to the prescribed methylxanthine
- Pain related to methylxanthine-induced headache
- Sleep pattern disturbance related to methylxanthine-induced insomnia

---

tain the prescribed interval between inhalations, and advising the patient not to use another other aerosol bronchodilator during terbutaline inhalation therapy. Finally, the nurse should instruct the patient to perform inhalation therapy before meals to improve lung ventilation and reduce fatigue caused by eating.

Nursing implications When caring for a patient who is receiving a methylxanthine agent, the nurse should be aware of the following implications.

- Develop appropriate nursing diagnoses for the patient. (For examples, see Sample Nursing Diagnoses: *Bronchodilators.*)
- Do not administer a methylxanthine to a patient with a condition that contraindicates its use.
- Administer a methylxanthine cautiously to a patient at risk because of a preexisting condition.
- Monitor the patient closely for symptoms of adverse CNS, GI, or cardiovascular reactions, particularly when therapy begins or when the serum drug concentration exceeds 20 mcg/ml. If adverse reactions occur, withhold the drug and notify the physician. If vomiting occurs shortly after oral administration, consult the physician before repeating the dose.

- Obtain a prescription for an analgesic if the patient experiences a methylxanthine-induced headache. Also obtain one for an antiemetic or antidiarrheal agent if needed.
- Monitor the patient's blood pressure for hypotension, the pulse for changes in the rate or pattern, and electrocardiogram for arrhythmias.
- Monitor the patient's serum drug levels closely throughout therapy. Notify the physician if elevations occur. Take seizure precautions if the drug level becomes very high.
- Observe for toxic drug interactions with such drugs as cimetidine or erythromycin. Monitor for signs of theophylline toxicity, such as palpitations and restlessness.
- Use the peak serum concentration to monitor oral methylxanthine therapy. The peak concentration of rapid-release products occurs 1 to 2 hours after administration; of slow-release products, about 4 hours. If no adverse reactions occur, measure the peak serum concentration when the steady-state level has been reached. Reaching the steady-state level requires that the patient receive the drug at regular intervals for 48 to 72 hours.
- Mix the loading dose for intravenous (I.V.) aminophylline in dextrose 5% in water (D_5W)or 0.9% sodium chloride solution. Administer this dose over 20 to 30 minutes.
- Administer the I.V. maintenance dosage in a standard concentration, using an infusion pump.
- Change a patient from I.V. to oral theophylline by stopping the infusion when starting the oral drug, as prescribed.
- Encourage the patient receiving a theophylline enema or rectal solution to retain it as long as possible. Do not use the rectal route if rectal irritation or infection is present.
- Administer an oral methylxanthine with a full glass of water and on an empty stomach or with only a small amount of food. Slow-release products should not be crushed or chewed.
- Encourage relaxation techniques, such as warm baths, reading, and soft music, if the patient develops insomnia. Notify the physician if insomnia persists because a change in dosage or administration time may be needed.
- Notify the physician if adverse reactions or drug interactions occur.
- Teach the patient and family the name, dose, frequency, action, and adverse effects of the prescribed methylxanthine.
- Stress the importance of returning regularly for drug level testing (except with dyphylline therapy).
- Advise the patient to withhold the drug and notify the physician if adverse reactions occur.
- Instruct the patient to take an oral preparation with 8 oz (240 ml) of water and preferably on an empty stomach or with a small amount of food. Advise the patient taking a slow-release product not to crush or chew it.

- Advise the patient not to adjust the dosage without consulting the physician.
- Instruct the patient to avoid using products that contain methylxanthines during methylxanthine therapy. The additional agents may not contribute to the therapy's effectiveness and may cause adverse reactions.
- Advise the patient to inform all personal physicians about methylxanthine therapy to prevent drug interactions.

STUDY ACTIVITIES

Fill in the blank

1. The rate and depth of respirations influence the_____ balance of the blood, which normally remains between a pH of

_____ and _____.

2. Hyperventilation _____ the blood pH; hypoventilation

_____ the blood pH.

3. The absorption rate of theophylline can be affected by the presence of _____ in the stomach and by gastric _____.

4. A serum theophylline level of _____ to _____ mcg/ml usually produces a therapeutic effect in a patient with respiratory disease.

5. Adverse reactions to theophylline generally affect the _____,

_____, and _____ systems.

6. The nurse should measure the serum theophylline level at its

_____, which usually occurs _____ to _____ hours

after administering a rapid-acting oral agent or _____ hours after administering a slow-acting oral agent.

7. The nurse should mix an I.V. loading dose of aminophylline in

_____ or _____ and should administer it over _____

to _____ minutes.

8. The nurse should not administer a theophylline rectally if rectal

_____ or _____ is present.

True of false

9. Adrenergic agents cause responses similar to those produced by the parasympathetic nervous system.
   ☐ True   ☐ False

10. Adverse reactions to adrenergic bronchodilators include headache, vomiting, arrhythmias, and vital sign changes.
☐ True　　　　　　　☐ False

11. The patient should perform adrenergic bronchodilator inhalation after meals to prevent drug-food interactions.
☐ True　　　　　　　☐ False

Multiple choice

12. Joyce Reynolds, age 40, is admitted to the hospital for treatment of acute asthma. She receives a loading dose of aminophylline, 5 mg/kg I.V. Which statement accurately characterizes aminophylline administration?
    A. The nurse should administer the loading dose over 50 to 60 minutes.
    B. The nurse should mix aminophylline with D_5W or 0.9% sodium chloride solution.
    C. The nurse should administer the loading dose after the patient's last meal of the day.
    D. The nurse should follow up by administering a maintenance dosage of aminophylline via I.V. bolus.

13. Thomas Keller, age 57, must receive an injectable form of dyphylline, 10 mg/kg every 6 hours, for emphysema. Which route is appropriate for this medication?
    A. I.V.
    B. S.C.
    C. I.M.
    D. I.V.P.B.

14. Later, the physician changes Mr. Keller to oral dyphylline. While Mr. Keller is receiving oral dyphylline, which parameter should the nurse monitor closely?
    A. Cardiovascular status
    B. Prothrombin time
    C. Fluid intake and output
    D. Serum theophylline level

15. Calvin Grove, age 63, is receiving oral theophylline (Theo-Dur) for chronic bronchitis. When the nurse brings him the afternoon dose of Theo-Dur, Mr. Grove says that he is nauseous and that he vomited after taking his last pill. What should the nurse do?
    A. Withhold the afternoon dose and notify the physician.
    B. Omit this dose, but double the dose after the nausea has subsided.
    C. Explain that vomiting is a common, but transient, adverse reaction.
    D. Insist that he take this dose because the medication schedule must not be interrupted.

16. Mr. Grove's serum theophylline level is far above the therapeutic level. After notifying the physician, what should the nurse do?

   A. Have the laboratory repeat the test.
   B. Administer a diuretic immediately.
   C. Transfer Mr. Grove to the intensive care unit.
   D. Take seizure precautions.

ANSWERS

Fill in the blanks

1. Acid-base, 7.35, 7.45
2. Raises, lowers
3. Food, pH
4. 10, 20
5. Central nervous, gastrointestinal, cardiovascular
6. Peak, 1, 2, 4
7. Dextrose 5% in water (D_5W), 0.9% sodium chloride solution, 20, 30
8. Irritation, infection

True or false

9. False. Adrenergic agents cause responses similar to those produced by the sympathetic nervous system.
10. True.
11. False. The patient should perform inhalation therapy before meals to improve lung ventilation and to reduce fatigue caused by eating.

Multiple choice

12. B. After mixing the loading dose of aminophylline with D_5W or 0.9% sodium chloride solution, the nurse should administer it over 20 to 30 minutes. The maintenance dosage should be given by I.V. infusion, using an infusion pump.
13. C. Dyphylline should be administered by the I.M. or oral route.
14. A. Like the other methylxanthines, dyphylline may cause adverse reactions in the central nervous, GI, and cardiovascular systems. Because the drug does not dissociate to theophylline in the blood, dyphylline therapy does not require monitoring of the serum theophylline level.
15. A. If vomiting occurs shortly after oral administration, the nurse should consult the physician before repeating the dose.
16. D. The nurse should monitor the patient's serum theophylline level closely throughout therapy. If very high elevations occur, the nurse should notify the physician and take seizure precautions.

CHAPTER 20

Expectorant, antitussive, mucolytic, and decongestant agents

After studying this chapter, the reader should be able to:

1. Explain the actions of expectorants, antitussives, mucolytics, and decongestants.

2. Describe the pharmacologic differences among these agents and explain the appropriate use of each.

3. Differentiate between systemic and topical decongestants.

4. Discuss rebound nasal congestion.

5. Describe the nursing implications of expectorant, antitussive, mucolytic, or decongestant therapy.

OVERVIEW OF CONCEPTS

The respiratory system is the first line of defense against microbial invasion of the body. The mucociliary clearance mechanism and the cough mechanism play important roles in this function. In the mucociliary clearance mechanism, ciliated epithelial cells and mucus secretions trap debris and bacteria and facilitate their removal. In addition to acting as a clearance agent, mucus acts as a barrier to prevent water loss from the epithelium.

The cough mechanism facilitates mucus removal from the respiratory tract. Triggered by nerve receptor stimulation, the cough helps cilia remove materials from the respiratory tract. It can be productive or nonproductive. Although coughing is useful and protective, it may be exhausting and irritating. Treatment of a cough depends on its cause, effectiveness, and interference with the patient's sleep and activities of daily living.

When invading organisms elude these defense mechanisms, they trigger the release of histamines and other substances, causing edema and swelling of the nasal passages.

This chapter discusses expectorants and mucolytics, which enhance mucus removal; antitussives, which suppress coughing; and de-

SELECTED MAJOR DRUGS

Expectorant, antitussive, mucolytic, and decongestant agents

The following chart summarizes the major expectorant, antitussive, mucolytic, and decongestant agents currently in clinical use.

DRUG	MAJOR INDICATIONS	USUAL ADULT DOSAGES
Expectorants		
guaifenesin	Cough associated with common cold and upper respiratory infection	200 to 400 mg P.O. every 4 hours, not to exceed 2.4 g daily
Antitussives		
codeine	Nonproductive cough	10 to 20 mg P.O. every 4 to 6 hours, not to exceed 120 mg daily
dextromethorphan	Nonproductive cough	10 to 20 mg P.O. every 4 hours or 30 mg P.O. every 6 to 8 hours, not to exceed 120 mg daily; long-acting preparations, 60 mg P.O. every 12 hours
Mucolytics		
acetylcysteine	Bronchopulmonary diseases (chronic bronchitis, emphysema, bronchiectasis, pneumonia, atelectasis, cystic fibrosis)	Nebulization: 3 to 5 ml (20% solution) t.i.d. or q.i.d. or 6 to 10 ml (10% solution) t.i.d. or q.i.d.; direct instillation: 1 to 2 ml of a 10% to 20% solution every hour
Systemic decongestants		
phenylpropanolamine	Nasal congestion associated with acute or chronic rhinitis, sinusitis, the common cold, hay fever, or other allergies	25 mg P.O. every 4 hours or 75 mg P.O. of the sustained-release preparation every 12 hours, not to exceed 150 mg P.O. daily
pseudoephedrine	Nasal congestion associated with acute or chronic rhinitis, sinusitis, the common cold, hay fever, or other allergies	60 mg P.O. every 4 to 6 hours or 120 mg P.O. of the sustained-release preparation every 12 hours
Topical decongestants		
naphazoline	Nasal congestion associated with acute or chronic rhinitis, sinusitis, the common cold, hay fever, or other allergies	2 drops or sprays of 0.05% solution in each nostril, repeated every 3 to 6 hours
phenylephrine	Nasal congestion associated with acute or chronic rhinitis, sinusitis, the common cold, hay fever, or other allergies	1 or 2 sprays or small amount of jelly in each nostril, repeated every 4 hours
oxymetazoline	Nasal congestion associated with acute or chronic rhinitis, sinusitis, the common cold, hay fever, or other allergies	2 or 3 drops or 1 or 2 sprays of 0.05% solution in each nostril b.i.d.
tetrahydrozoline	Nasal congestion associated with acute or chronic rhinitis, sinusitis, the common cold, hay fever, or other allergies	2 to 4 drops or sprays of 0.1% solution in each nostril, repeated every 3 hours, as needed
xylometazoline	Nasal congestion associated with acute or chronic rhinitis, sinusitis, the common cold, hay fever, or other allergies	2 or 3 drops or sprays of 0.1% solution in each nostril every 8 to 10 hours, not to exceed three times in 24 hours

congestants, which relieve upper respiratory tract signs and symptoms associated with the common cold. (For a summary of representative drugs, see Selected Major Drugs: *Expectorant, antitussive, mucolytic, and decongestant agents.*)

Expectorants

Expectorants include guaifenesin (Breonesin, Robitussin), iodinated glycerol (Organidin), potassium iodide (Pima, SSKI), and terpin hydrate.

Pharmacokinetics

Expectorants are absorbed from the gastrointestinal (GI) tract and distributed to the bronchial glands. The iodides also are distributed to the salivary, lacrimal, and thyroid glands, as well as across the placenta. Guaifenesin is metabolized by the liver. Potassium iodide is not metabolized and is excreted basically unchanged. Excretion of expectorants is primarily renal, although the iodides also are excreted in breast milk. The onset of action for expectorants is immediate to 30 minutes.

Pharmacodynamics

Expectorants may promote mucus removal from the respiratory tract by acting on the bronchial glands or by reducing the adhesiveness and surface tension of the mucus.

Pharmacotherapeutics

Expectorants are used for symptomatic relief of coughs caused by colds, minor bronchial irritations, and other respiratory disorders. Guaifenesin, the most commonly used expectorant, is safe when taken as directed. The iodides are prescribed less frequently because of their potential for toxic effects. Because it has a high alcohol content, terpin hydrate may be abused. It is contraindicated in a pregnant patient or one with peptic ulcer disease or severe diabetes.

Drug interactions

Expectorants are involved in few interactions with other drugs or food. (For details, see Drug Interactions: *Expectorant, antitussive, mucolytic, and decongestant agents,* page 284.)

Adverse drug reactions

Although adverse reactions to guaifenesin are uncommon, vomiting, nausea, diarrhea, drowsiness, and abdominal pain may occur. The iodides possess the greatest potential for adverse reactions, which include thyroid gland hyperplasia, urticaria, fever, goiter, and iodism (burning of the mouth and throat, soreness of gums and teeth, and minor cold symptoms). Potassium toxicity also may occur in a patient receiving potassium iodide. Terpin hydrate often causes drowsiness and may cause nausea and vomiting.

Antitussives

The major antitussives include benzonatate (Tessalon), codeine, dextromethorphan hydrobromide (Robitussin-DM), and hydrocodone bi-

DRUG INTERACTIONS

Expectorant, antitussive, mucolytic, and decongestant agents

Various drugs may interact with expectorants, antitussives, mucolytics, and decongestants. Because many of these respiratory drugs are available over-the-counter, patient teaching about possible drug interactions is especially important.

DRUG	INTERACTING DRUGS	POSSIBLE EFFECTS
Expectorants		
guaifenesin	anticoagulants	Increased risk of bleeding
iodinated glycerol, potassium iodide	lithium, antithyroid agents	Increased hypothyroid and goitrogenic effects
potassium iodide	potassium-sparing diuretics, potassium-containing drugs	Increased serum potassium level, possibly leading to arrhythmias and cardiac arrest
terpin hydrate	disulfiram	Alcohol-disulfiram reaction
Antitussives		
codeine, hydrocodone bitartrate	monoamine oxidase (MAO) inhibitors (isocarboxazid, phenelzine, tranylcypromine)	Excitation, hypertension or hypotension, coma
codeine	central nervous system (CNS) depressants (alcohol, barbiturates, sedative-hypnotics, phenothiazines)	Increased CNS depressant effects (drowsiness, lethargy, stupor, respiratory depression, coma, death)
dextromethorphan	MAO inhibitors	Excitation, hyperpyrexia, hypotension, coma
Mucolytics		
acetylcysteine	amphotericin B, chlortetracycline hydrochloride, erythromycin lactobionate, oxytetracycline hydrochloride, ampicillin sodium, tetracycline hydrochloride, iodized oil, hydrogen peroxide, chymotrypsin, trypsin	Drug incompatibility
	activated charcoal	Decreased acetylcysteine effects
Systemic decongestants		
ephedrine, phenylpropanolamine, pseudoephedrine	other sympathomimetic amines, including epinephrine, norepinephrine, dopamine, dobutamine, isoproterenol, metaproterenol, terbutaline, phenylephrine, tyramine	Increased CNS stimulation
	MAO inhibitors	Severe hypertension or hypertensive crisis
pseudoephedrine	alkalinizing agents	Decreased urinary excretion of pseudoephedrine
Topical decongestants		
ephedrine, epinephrine, naphazoline, oxymetazoline, phenylephrine, propylhexedrine, tetrahydrozoline, xylometazoline	MAO inhibitors	Increase CNS stimulation, increased hypertension or hypertensive crisis
	beta-adrenergic blockers, methyldopa, reserpine, guanethidine	Decreased hypotensive effects

tartrate (Hycodan). Diphenhydramine hydrochloride (Benadryl, Benylin) and lidocaine hydrochloride (Xylocaine) also provide antitussive effects, but are used infrequently for this purpose.

Pharmacokinetics
The antitussives are absorbed well through the GI tract, metabolized in the liver, and excreted in the urine. The narcotic antitussives codeine and hydrocodone are distributed across the placenta and also are excreted in breast milk. The distribution of benzonatate and dextromethorphan is unknown. All antitussives begin to act within 30 minutes. Their duration of action varies from 3 to 8 hours.

Pharmacodynamics
Antitussives inhibit irritating, nonproductive coughs. The centrally-acting antitussives codeine, hydrocodone bitartrate, and dextromethorphan suppress the coughing reflex directly by depressing the cough center in the medulla. The peripherally-acting agent benzonatate acts by anesthetizing the cough receptors throughout the bronchi, alveoli, and pleura.

Pharmacotherapeutics
Antitussives are used to treat a serious, nonproductive cough that interferes with a patient's ability to rest or carry out activities of daily living. Benzonatate also is administered before bronchial diagnostic tests to suppress cough during the procedure. Dextromethorphan is the most widely used antitussive because it produces few adverse reactions and is nonaddictive. Codeine and hydrocodone have a potential for abuse, but the risk of addiction is low in short-term antitussive therapy.

Drug interactions
With the exception of benzonatate, the antitussives may interact with other central nervous system (CNS) depressants and monoamine oxidase (MAO) inhibitors. (For details, see Drug Interactions: *Expectorant, antitussive, mucolytic, and decongestant agents.*)

Adverse drug reactions
Benzonatate can cause dizziness, sedation, GI upset, constipation, and rash. Dextromethorphan rarely causes adverse reactions. However, an overdose can cause CNS depression. Antitussive dosages of codeine and hydrocodone may cause drowsiness or impaired coordination. Repeated doses increase the chance for GI upset, constipation, and CNS depression. Long-term use may result in physical dependence.

Mucolytics
The only mucolytic used clinically in the United States is acetylcysteine (Mucomyst).

Pharmacokinetics
Acetylcysteine is absorbed from the pulmonary epithelium and metabolized in the liver. Its onset of action occurs 1 minute after inhalation

and immediately after direct application or instillation. Its maximal effect occurs 5 to 10 minutes after inhalation.

Pharmacodynamics
Acetylcysteine decreases the viscosity of respiratory tract secretions by altering the molecular composition of mucus. The drug's free sulfhydryl group disrupts glycoprotein strands and decreases mucus viscosity.

Pharmacotherapeutics
Acetylcysteine is used in lung disorders in which mucus overproduction and accumulation interfere with gas exchange and provide a medium for infection. It also may be used to treat acetaminophen overdose. The drug usually is administered via a nebulizer.

Drug interactions
Acetylcysteine is incompatible with many drugs. (For details, see Drug Interactions: *Expectorant, antitussive, mucolytic, and decongestant agents,* page 284.)

Adverse drug reactions
Acetylcysteine has a wide margin of safety. However, its "rotten egg" odor can cause nausea, and prolonged use may produce stomatitis, vomiting, drowsiness, and severe rhinorrhea. Bronchospasm can occur.

Decongestants
Most decongestants are primarily synthetic versions of epinephrine. They are classified as systemic or topical agents. The major systemic decongestants are ephedrine sulfate, phenylpropanolamine hydrochloride (Propagest, Rhindecon), and pseudoephedrine hydrochloride (Novafed, Sudafed), and pseudoephedrine sulfate (Afrinol Repetabs). Common topical agents include ephedrine sulfate (Efedron Nasal Jelly), epinephrine hydrochloride (Adrenalin Chloride), naphazoline hydrochloride (Privine), oxymetazoline hydrochloride (Afrin, Dristan), phenylephrine (Neo-Synephrine, Sinex), propylhexedrine (Benzedrex Inhaler), tetrahydrozoline hydrochloride (Tyzine Drops), and xylometazoline hydrochloride (Otrivin).

Pharmacokinetics
After oral administration, the systemic decongestants are absorbed readily from the GI tract, distributed widely throughout the body, slowly and incompletely metabolized by the liver, and excreted primarily unchanged in the urine. The onset of nasal decongestion is 15 to 30 minutes, peaking within 60 to 90 minutes. The duration of action is 3 to 6 hours for tablets and syrups, and 8 to 12 hours for sustained-release capsules and tablets.

After direct application to the mucous membranes, topical decongestants undergo minimal absorption. Onset of action immediately follows application, and drug action peaks quickly. The duration of symptom relief, however, usually is short.

Pharmacodynamics

As sympathomimetic amines, the systemic decongestants stimulate alpha-adrenergic receptors in vascular smooth muscle, constricting arterioles of the nasal mucosa, which reduces blood flow and edema. These actions open the nasal passages, increase air flow, and promote sinus drainage. Systemic agents also indirectly stimulate beta-adrenergic receptors, which increases the heart rate, force of myocardial contractions, and cardiac output.

Topical decongestants work by a similar mechanism of action. However, they display more alpha-receptor specificity and provide a faster onset of action, shorter duration, and fewer systemic effects.

Pharmacotherapeutics

All decongestants help relieve the swelling of the nasal passages associated with the common cold and other upper respiratory disorders. Systemic decongestants offer prolonged symptom relief and OTC availability. However, their systemic adverse effects contraindicate their use in certain patients.

Generally inhaled as drops or sprays, topical decongestants rapidly relieve symptoms with minimal adverse reactions. However, rebound nasal congestion occurs with frequent or long-term use.

Drug interactions

Systemic decongestants may interact with other sympathomimetic amines and other drugs. Topical decongestants seldom interact with other drugs. (For details, see Drug Interactions: *Expectorant, antitussive, mucolytic, and decongestant agents,* page 284.)

Adverse drug reactions

Adverse reactions to systemic decongestants primarily are dose-related and may include CNS stimulation (nervousness, restlessness, insomnia), nausea, palpitations, urinary difficulty, and blood pressure elevation. Hypersensitivity reactions and teratogenic effects also may occur.

The most common adverse reaction to topical decongestants is rebound nasal congestion, which usually resolves a few days after drug discontinuation. Other common adverse reactions are burning and stinging of the oral mucosa upon application, sneezing, and mucosal dryness or ulceration. Overuse or inadvertent swallowing of a topical decongestant may produce adverse reactions similar to those of a systemic decongestant.

Nursing implications When caring for a patient who is receiving an expectorant, antitussive, mucolytic, or decongestant, the nurse should be aware of the following implications.
- Develop appropriate nursing diagnoses for the patient. (For examples, see Sample Nursing Diagnoses: *Expectorant, antitussive, mucolytic, and decongestant agents,* page 289.)

- Do not administer an expectorant, antitussive, mucolytic, or decongestant to a patient with a condition that contraindicates its use.
- Administer an expectorant, antitussive, mucolytic, or decongestant cautiously to a patient at risk because of a preexisting condition.
- Monitor the patient for adverse reactions and signs of drug interactions.
- Take safety measures if drowsiness or dizziness occurs.
- Assess the effectiveness of the prescribed agent periodically.
- Notify the physician if adverse reactions or drug interactions occur or if drug therapy is ineffective.
- Teach the patient and family the name, dose, frequency, action, and adverse effects of the prescribed drug.
- Instruct the patient to avoid activities that require alertness or coordination if excessive drowsiness or dizziness occurs.

Expectorants
- Monitor the patient's hydration status. Encourage the patient to drink 2 to 3 liters (68 to 100 oz) of fluid daily, unless contraindicated, to help thin and mobilize secretions.
- Monitor for signs of iodism in a patient receiving an iodide expectorant.
- Dilute potassium iodide solution in a glass of water or juice and give the patient a glass drinking straw to prevent discoloration of teeth.
- Discard any potassium iodide solution that has turned brown; such discoloration indicates decomposition.
- Monitor the patient's serum potassium level if potassium iodide is administered with a potassium-sparing diuretic or potassium-containing drug.
- Teach the patient and family to recognize the signs and symptoms of iodism.

Antitussives
- Do not administer an antitussive to a patient with a productive cough or one who can benefit from coughing.
- Monitor for signs of respiratory depression.
- Monitor for constipation. To prevent or relieve constipation, encourage the patient to drink 2 to 3 liters (68 to 100 oz) of fluid daily, unless contraindicated.
- Instruct the patient to report a cough that lasts longer than 7 days or a cough that changes from nonproductive to productive.
- Instruct the patient not to take the antitussive with a CNS depressant—including alcohol—or an MAO inhibitor.

Mucolytics
- Prepare the patient for the drug's "rotten egg" smell. Have the patient gargle after administration to relieve mouth odor and dryness.
- Avoid contamination of the solution and refrigerate an opened vial. Discard opened vials after 96 hours.

SAMPLE NURSING DIAGNOSES

Expectorant, antitussive, mucolytic, and decongestant agents

The following nursing diagnoses address representative problems and etiologies that a nurse may encounter when caring for a patient who is receiving an expectorant, antitussive, mucolytic, or decongestant.

- Altered health maintenance related to ineffectiveness of the prescribed expectorant, antitussive, mucolytic, or decongestant
- Altered oral mucous membrane related to acetylcysteine-induced stomatitis
- Altered protection related to iodide-induced thyroid disorder
- Altered role performance related to physical dependence on codeine
- Altered thought processes related to central nervous system (CNS) depression caused by extremely high dosages of an antitussive
- Constipation related to the adverse gastrointestinal (GI) effects of an antitussive
- Diarrhea related to the adverse GI effects of guaifenesin
- High risk for impaired skin integrity related to benzonatate-induced skin eruptions
- High risk for injury related to adverse drug reactions
- High risk for injury related to a preexisting condition that requires cautious use of an expectorant, antitussive, mucolytic, or decongestant
- High risk for injury related to a preexisting condition that requires cautious use of an expectorant, antitussive, mucolytic, or decongestant
- High risk for injury related to drug interactions
- High risk for injury related to the teratogenic effects of a decongestant
- High risk for trauma related to decongestant-induced hypertension
- High risk for trauma related to the adverse CNS effects of an expectorant, antitussive, or decongestant
- Impaired gas exchange related to the adverse respiratory effects of a mucolytic
- Impaired tissue integrity related to mucosal dryness and ulcerations caused by a topical decongestant
- Knowledge deficit related to the prescribed expectorant, antitussive, mucolytic, or decongestant
- Pain related to burning and stinging of the nasal mucosa caused by application of a topical decongestant
- Pain related to guaifenesin-induced abdominal pain
- Sleep pattern disturbance related to decongestant-induced insomnia
- Urinary retention related to the adverse genitourinary effects of a decongestant

---

- Know that acetylcysteine may discolor to a light purple, but that it may be used safely.
- Assess respiratory status before and after each administration.
- Encourage coughing and deep breathing after administration.
- Rinse the patient's mouth with a warm water solution—not an antiseptic mouthwash—if stomatitis occurs; also notify the physician of this adverse effect.
- Use a 10% or 20% acetylcysteine solution undiluted, as prescribed. For further dilution, use 0.9% sodium chloride solution or sterile water.

Decongestants

- Monitor the patient's vital signs, observing closely for hypertension or changes in cardiac rate or rhythm.
- Do not administer a systemic decongestant with other sympathomimetic amines because increased CNS stimulation can occur.
- Observe the patient for urinary changes. Be aware that alkaline urine decreases the excretion rate of a decongestant.
- Observe for signs of CNS stimulation and notify the physician if they occur. Take safety precautions, as needed.
- Inform the patient that the systemic decongestant may interfere with sleep, and suggest taking the drug a few hours before bedtime to minimize insomnia.
- Teach the patient not to take other OTC medications because they might interact with the systemic decongestant.
- Inspect the patient's oral and nasal mucosa for signs of dryness or ulceration. Encourage the patient to use a humidifier if dryness occurs.
- Teach the patient not to exceed the recommended dosage or to continue topical decongestant therapy for more than 4 days.
- Inspect the patient for signs of rebound nasal congestion, such as red, boggy, swollen nasal mucosa. If such signs occur, withhold the drug and notify the physician.
- Teach the patient using a topical agent to recognize the signs of rebound nasal congestion and to discontinue the drug if they occur.

STUDY ACTIVITIES

Fill in the blank

1. _____ agents suppress coughing.

2. _____ agents alter the molecular composition of mucus.

3. _____ agents relieve nasal swelling and edema.

4. A potassium iodide solution should be mixed in a glass of _____ or _____ and should be administered through a _____.

5. Most antitussives should not be used concomitantly with _____ or _____.

6. Adverse GI reactions to codeine include GI upset and _____.

7. A patient receiving an antitussive should report a cough that changes from _____ to _____.

8. The nurse should _____ an opened vial of acetylcysteine after _____ hours.

9. The most common adverse reaction to topical decongestants is

_____.

Multiple choice

10. The physician orders potassium iodide 300 mg P.O. t.i.d. for Anna Reynolds, age 31. Which statement by Ms. Reynolds should make the nurse question this order?
    A. "I have a headache."
    B. "I have false teeth."
    C. "I think I'm pregnant."
    D. "My mother died of breast cancer."

11. Lynette Kimball, age 46, is taking codeine for a severe cough. A drug from which class could interact with codeine?
    A. Anticoagulant
    B. MAO inhibitor
    C. Topical decongestant
    D. Potassium-sparing diuretic

12. Gregory Towner, age 62, has a discharge order for acetylcysteine 3 ml via nebulizer t.i.d. When teaching Mr. Towner about acetylcysteine therapy, the nurse is most likely to make which statement?
    A. "Dilute the medication with dextrose 5% in water."
    B. "Use an antiseptic gargle if your mouth becomes sore."
    C. "Discard the medication if it discolors to light purple."
    D. "You may notice an unpleasant odor when you use this drug."

13. Bill Upton, age 24, is taking an OTC systemic decongestant to relieve his hay fever symptoms. How do topical and systemic decongestants differ?
    A. Topical decongestants have a faster onset of action.
    B. Topical decongestants produce greater CNS depression.
    C. Topical decongestants have a longer duration of action.
    D. Topical decongestants are more likely to produce adverse reactions.

Matching related elements
Match the drug on the left with its class on the right.

14. ___ Dextromethorphan   **A.** Expectorant

15. ___ Pseudoephedrine   **B.** Antitussive

16. ___ Phenylephrine   **C.** Mucolytic

17. ___ Acetylcysteine   **D.** Topical decongestant

18. ___ Potassium iodide   **E.** Systemic decongestant

ANSWERS

Fill in the blank

1. Antitussive
2. Mucolytic
3. Decongestant
4. Water, juice, glass straw
5. MAO inhibitors, CNS depressants
6. Constipation
7. Nonproductive, productive
8. Discarded, 96
9. Rebound nasal congestion

Multiple choice

10. C. The iodides should not be used in a pregnant or breast-feeding patient or one with iodide sensitivity, thyroid disease, tuberculosis, or acute bronchitis.

11. B. MAO inhibitors and CNS depressants (including alcohol, barbiturates, sedative-hypnotics, and phenothiazines) may interact with codeine.

12. D. The nurse should prepare the patient for acetylcysteine's "rotten egg" odor. The drug may be used even if it discolors to light purple. If stomatitis occurs, the patient should rinse the mouth with a warm-water solution. If the drug must be diluted, the patient should use 0.9% sodium chloride solution or sterile water.

13. A. Topical decongestants offer faster relief of symptoms and fewer adverse reactions than systemic decongestants. However, topical decongestants have a shorter duration of action.

Matching related elements

14. B
15. E
16. D
17. C
18. A

CHAPTER 21

Peptic ulcer agents

OBJECTIVES   After studying this chapter, the reader should be able to:

1. Explain peptic ulcer formation, concentrating on the role played by acetylcholine, prostaglandin, gastrin, and histamine.

2. Describe the mechanisms of action for antacids, histamine$_2$ (H$_2$)-receptor antagonists, and other agents used in peptic ulcer healing.

3. Discuss why H$_2$-receptor antagonists are the drugs of choice for duodenal and gastric ulcers.

4. Identify the major indications for oral and parenteral H$_2$-receptor antagonists.

5. Describe the nursing implications of peptic ulcer therapy.

OVERVIEW OF   A peptic ulcer is an open lesion of the epithelial, mucosal lining of the
CONCEPTS   lower esophagus, stomach, or duodenum. Some peptic ulcers develop when increased acid secretions overcome the protective mechanism of the gastrointestinal (GI) tract; others develop from impaired protective mechanisms. Factors that contribute to peptic ulcer disease include smoking and the use of aspirin, nonsteroidal anti-inflammatory drugs (NSAIDs), or corticosteroids.

Many patients with duodenal ulcers display hypersecretion of acid and pepsin. Factors that can lead to such hypersecretion include increased mass of parietal (acid-secreting) cells and chief (pepsin-secreting) cells in the stomach; cholinergic stimulation via the vagus nerve; and gastrin release in the postprandial state. Gastrin, histamine, and acetylcholine stimulate acid and pepsin secretion.

The parietal cells of the stomach contain an acid pump (proton pump) that helps maintain gastric acidity. Blockage of this pump inhibits acid secretion and helps prevent peptic ulcer formation. The timing of acid hypersecretion also is important in preventing peptic ulcer formation. Nocturnal acid secretion, which is unopposed by the presence of food in the stomach, is higher in some patients; it can inhibit peptic ulcer therapy.

Not all ulcers result from hypersecretion of acid and pepsin. Some duodenal and gastric ulcers are caused by a breakdown in mucosal resistance to the effects of acids, pepsin, and other stomach contents. The gastric mucosal barrier is a complex defense system that allows hydrochloric acid to diffuse into the lumen of the stomach but prevents the return of such acid, thereby protecting the gastric mucosa from digesting itself. This protective response is referred to as cytoprotection. Cytoprotective drugs, such as sucralfate, help prevent mucosal damage and enhance the protective effects of the gastric mucosal barrier.

Mucus and bicarbonate secretion by the epithelial cells of the stomach and duodenum also provide a protective layer along the walls of the stomach and duodenum. This mucus barrier helps protect against pepsin and other injurious agents. Mucosal perfusion and cellular repair also help protect the mucosal barrier.

Endogenous prostaglandins also help maintain normal mucosal defenses. Prostaglandins increase mucus and bicarbonate secretion, increase mucosal perfusion, and enhance cellular repair after injury. Thus, they are cytoprotective. Aspirin and NSAIDs can damage the gastric mucosa because they inhibit prostaglandin synthesis. Once the mucosal defense system is impaired, peptic ulcer disease may occur.

Drug therapy for peptic ulcers includes antacids, H_2-receptor antagonists, and other peptic ulcer agents. These agents act by neutralizing acid in the GI tract, reducing acid secretion, protecting the mucosal barrier, or blocking the proton pump. (For a summary of representative drugs, see Selected Major Drugs: *Peptic ulcer agents.*)

Antacids

Over-the-counter medications, antacids may be used alone or in combination with other drugs to treat peptic ulcer disease. Drug forms include suspensions, tablets, and chewable tablets. Common antacids include calcium carbonate (Alka-Mints, Calcilac, Dicarbosil, Tums), magaldrate or aluminum-magnesium complex (Riopan), and magnesium hydroxide and aluminum hydroxide with simethicone (Gelusil-II, Maalox TC, Mylanta).

Pharmacokinetics

Acid neutralization, the primary action of antacids, takes place in the stomach. Absorption of acid is neither necessary nor desired. Depending on the patient's physical condition, problems may develop if absorption takes place. For example, a patient with renal failure may develop hypermagnesemia if the kidneys do not excrete the magnesium absorbed from the antacid.

The speed at which antacids neutralize acids depends on the rate of solubilization. Sodium bicarbonate is the most rapidly solubilized antacid, but it is no longer recommended because of its high sodium content and its ability to cause acid rebound (production of more acid in the stomach in response to the rapid neutralization). Antacids are eliminated primarily in the feces.

Antacids have a relatively short duration of action. When taken on an empty stomach, they act for about 1 hour; when taken with food, for about 3 hours.

SELECTED MAJOR DRUGS

Peptic ulcer agents

The following chart summarizes the major peptic ulcer agents currently in clinical use.

DRUG	MAJOR INDICATIONS	USUAL ADULT DOSAGES
Antacids		
magaldrate or aluminum-magnesium complex	Symptomatic and therapeutic treatment of peptic ulcer disease	540 to 1,080 mg (5 to 10 ml) of suspension P.O. with water between meals and h.s., or 480 to 960 mg (1 to 2 tablets) P.O. with water between meals and h.s.
magnesium hydroxide and aluminum hydroxide with simethicone	Symptomatic and therapeutic treatment of peptic ulcer disease	10 to 30 ml P.O. 1 and 3 hours after each meal and h.s.
Histamine$_2$-receptor antagonists		
cimetidine	Treatment or prevention of peptic ulcer disease	800 mg P.O. h.s. daily, or 300 mg I.V. every 6 to 8 hours up to a maximum of 24 g in 24 hours
famotidine	Treatment or prevention of peptic ulcer disease	20 mg P.O. b.i.d. with the second dose at h.s., 40 mg P.O. h.s., or 20 mg I.V. every 12 hours
nizatidine	Treatment or prevention of peptic ulcer disease	300 mg P.O. h.s. or 150 mg P.O. b.i.d.
ranitidine	Treatment or prevention of peptic ulcer disease	150 mg P.O. b.i.d. with the second dose at h.s., 300 mg P.O. h.s., or 50 mg I.V. or I.M. every 6 to 8 hours
Other peptic ulcer agents		
misoprostol	Prevention of nonsteroidal anti-inflammatory drug-induced gastric ulcers	200 mcg P.O. q.i.d. with food or, if the patient cannot tolerate this dosage, 100 mcg P.O. q.i.d.
omeprazole	Severe, erosive or symptomatic esophagitis	20 mg P.O. daily for 4 to 8 weeks
	Pathologic hypersecretory conditions	Initially, 60 mg P.O. daily, then individualized based on the severity of the condition
sucralfate	Short-term treatment of duodenal ulcers	1 g P.O. q.i.d. for 4 to 8 weeks

Pharmacodynamics

Antacids generally do not neutralize all of the stomach acid, nor do they increase the pH above 4.0 or 5.0. By increasing gastric pH from the normal 1.3 to 2.3, an antacid neutralizes about 90% of the gastric acid; by increasing the pH to 3.3, it further neutralizes about 99% of the acid. Increasing the pH also decreases the proteolytic activity of pepsin.

Pharmacotherapeutics

Antacids are administered orally to relieve esophageal reflux, acid indigestion, heartburn, and dyspepsia. During periods of severe physical stress in critically ill patients, antacids may be administered by nasogastric tube to prevent stress ulcers and GI bleeding. Antacids also may be used with H_2-receptor antagonists to help control or prevent pain. Because of the need for frequent, regular (rather than p.r.n.) doses and the use of the liquid form of the antacid, patient acceptance and compliance may be lower than with other peptic ulcer medications.

Many antacids are available over-the-counter, and most of them contain aluminum hydroxide and magnesium hydroxide. Because aluminum has a constipating effect and magnesium has a laxative effect, this combination helps offset these effects.

Drug interactions

All antacids can interfere with the absorption of concomitantly administered oral drugs. They also can increase the excretion of weakly acidic drugs. (For details, see Drug Interactions: *Peptic ulcer agents.*)

Adverse drug reactions

Most adverse reactions affect the GI tract and commonly include diarrhea or constipation. Other reactions include hyperaluminemia (in patients with renal failure who take aluminum-containing antacids), hypermagnesemia (in patients taking magnesium-containing antacids), and hypophosphatemia. All adverse reactions are dose-related; no hypersensitivity reactions have been reported.

H₂-receptor antagonists

The most commonly prescribed antiulcer drugs in the United States, H_2-receptor antagonists include cimetidine (Tagamet), famotidine (Pepcid), nizatidine (Axid), and ranitidine hydrochloride (Zantac).

Pharmacokinetics

Cimetidine, nizatidine, and ranitidine are absorbed rapidly and completely from the GI tract; famotidine is absorbed incompletely. Food and antacids may impair absorption of these drugs. All H_2-receptor antagonists are distributed widely, metabolized in the liver, and excreted primarily in the urine.

Pharmacodynamics

H_2-receptor antagonists promote healing of gastric and duodenal ulcers by blocking histamine receptor sites, thereby inhibiting histamine-stimulated acid secretion by the parietal cells, as well as basal-, postprandial-, and gastrin-stimulated acid secretion.

Pharmacotherapeutics

The drugs of choice in treating peptic ulcers, H_2-receptor antagonists also are used in long-term treatment of pathologic GI hypersecretory conditions, such as Zollinger-Ellison syndrome and hyperhistaminemia. Physicians also prescribe these drugs to reduce gastric acid output and to prevent stress ulcers in severely ill patients and in those with reflux esophagitis or upper GI bleeding.

DRUG INTERACTIONS

Peptic ulcer agents

The nurse should be aware of the following drug interactions with peptic ulcer agents and their possible effects.

DRUG	INTERACTING DRUGS	POSSIBLE EFFECTS
Antacids		
calcium carbonate, magaldrate or aluminum-magnesium complex, magnesium hydroxide and aluminum hydroxide with simethicone	digoxin, digitoxin, iron salts, isoniazid, quinolones, tetracyclines	Decreased rate or extent of absorption of digoxin or other drugs
	amphetamines, quinidine	Increased urine pH; decreased excretion of weakly basic drugs, such as amphetamines and quinidine
	salicylates	Increased urine pH; increased excretion of weakly acidic drugs, such as salicylates
	methenamine compounds	Decreased activity of methenamine compounds
H$_2$-receptor antagonists		
cimetidine, famotidine, nizatidine, ranitidine	antacids	Decreased H$_2$-receptor antagonist absorption
cimetidine	oral anticoagulants, propranolol, possibly other beta blockers, benzodiazepines, tricyclic antidepressants, theophylline, procainamide, quinidine, lidocaine, phenytoin, calcium channel blockers, cyclosporine, carbamazepine, narcotic analgesics	Decreased hepatic enzyme metabolism of these drugs, thereby increasing their levels and effects
	carmustine (BCNU)	Increased bone marrow toxicity
	ethyl alcohol	Increased absorption and decreased metabolism of alcohol
Other peptic ulcer agents		
misoprostol	antacids	Decreased misoprostol absorption
omeprazole	diazepam, phenytoin, warfarin	Increased half-life and plasma concentration of these agents
	ketoconazole, ampicillin esters, iron salts, other drugs that depend on gastric pH for absorption	Interfered absorption of these agents
sucralfate	antacids	Decreased antacid activity
	cimetidine	Decreased bioavailability of cimetidine

Drug interactions

H$_2$-receptor antagonists may interact with antacids. Cimetidine may interact with many other drugs. (For details, see Drug Interactions: *Peptic ulcer agents.*)

Adverse drug reactions H$_2$-receptor antagonists may produce adverse central nervous system (CNS) reactions, including headache, dizziness, malaise, and somno-

Monitoring for adverse reactions to H₂-receptor antagonists

The following chart should help the nurse assess a patient receiving an H₂-receptor antagonist and help implement appropriate interventions.

ADVERSE REACTIONS	SIGNS AND SYMPTOMS	INTERVENTIONS
Headache	General, sometimes severe, headache	Administer mild analgesics, as prescribed.
Blood dyscrasias	Easy bruising, more frequent infections, granulocytopenia, leukopenia, thrombocytopenia	Consult with the physician about discontinuing the drug.
Mental status changes	Confusion, agitation, depression, hallucinations, especially in severely ill or geriatric patients or patients with renal failure	Consult with the physician about substituting another H₂-receptor antagonist or to discontinue drug use for a patient receiving cimetidine; discontinue drug use as prescribed for a patient receiving famotidine, nizatidine, or ranitidine.
Anti-androgenic effects	Gynecomastia, impotence	Consult with the physician about discontinuing the drug or altering the dosing schedule.
Changes in blood chemistry	Small increases in serum creatinine level without corresponding increase in blood urea nitrogen level	Continue to monitor the patient's renal function.
	Increased hepatic enzymes	Monitor the patient for hepatotoxicity, especially in one receiving high-dose I.V. therapy.

lence. They also may cause reversible confusion, agitation, depression, and hallucinations, especially in a severely ill or geriatric patient receiving cimetidine or a patient who has decreased renal function or has had an overdose. Adverse GI reactions are nausea and diarrhea or constipation. Other reactions include gynecomastia, rash, and pruritus. Rapid intravenous (I.V.) injection may cause profound bradycardia and other cardiotoxic effects. (For more information, see *Monitoring for adverse reactions to H₂-receptor antagonists.*)

Other peptic ulcer agents The following agents also may be used to treat peptic ulcers: misoprostol (Cytotec), omeprazole (Prilosec), and sucralfate (Carafate).

Pharmacokinetics

After oral administration, misoprostol is absorbed rapidly and extensively. It is metabolized to misoprostol acid, which is responsible for its clinical activity, is 90% protein-bound, and is excreted primarily in the urine.

Omeprazole also is absorbed rapidly after oral administration. Because the drug is affected by stomach acid, the capsules are formulated with delayed-release, enteric-coated granules that are absorbed in the small intestine. Omeprazole is 95% protein-bound, extensively metabolized, and excreted in the urine.

Sucralfate is absorbed minimally from the GI tract, which is appropriate because sucralfate exerts its effects locally. It rapidly reacts with hydrochloric acid in the GI tract to form a highly condensed, viscous, adhesive, pastelike substance that adheres to the gastric mucosa and especially to ulcer sites. The drug is distributed minimally and is excreted in the feces.

Pharmacodynamics

Misoprostol is a synthetic prostaglandin E_1 analogue with antisecretory and mucosal protective properties. NSAIDs inhibit prostaglandin synthesis, which may diminish bicarbonate and mucus secretion and promote mucosal damage and ulcer formation in the GI tract. Misoprostol counteracts these effects by replacing the endogenous prostaglandins.

Omeprazole suppresses gastric acid formation by inhibiting the hydrogen/potassium adenosine triphosphatase (H^+/K^+ ATPase) enzyme in gastric parietal cells. This enzyme is part of the proton pump. Because omeprazole blocks this step in acid production, it is considered a proton pump inhibitor.

In an acid environment, sucralfate becomes a negatively charged pastelike material that binds with positively charged proteins, such as albumin, fibrinogen, damaged mucosal cells, and dead leukocytes, found at the base of the ulcer. By forming a barrier at the ulcer site, sucralfate protects the ulcer against the erosive effects of gastric acid, pepsin, and bile; this allows the ulcer to heal.

Pharmacotherapeutics

Misoprostol is used to prevent NSAID-induced gastric ulcers in patients at high risk for complications from gastric ulcer. Omeprazole is used for short-term treatment of GI reflux disease (severe, erosive esophagitis) or symptomatic esophagitis that responds poorly to other treatments. It also is used for long-term treatment of pathologic hypersecretory conditions, such as Zollinger-Ellison syndrome.

Sucralfate is used for short-term treatment of duodenal, gastric, recurrent, NSAID-induced, and stress ulcers. Although sucralfate effectively treats these ulcers, it requires a cumbersome dosage schedule and produces minor adverse reactions that can lead to patient noncompliance.

Drug interactions

Misoprostol may interact with antacids. Omeprazole may interfere with diazepam, phenytoin, warfarin, and drugs that depend on an acid medium for absorption. Sucralfate may interact with antacids and cimetidine. (For details, see Drug Interactions: *Peptic ulcer agents,* page 297.)

Adverse drug reactions

Misoprostol commonly produces adverse GI reactions, such as diarrhea, abdominal pain, flatulence, nausea, and vomiting. It also can affect the uterus, causing spotting, cramps, hypermenorrhea, other menstrual disorders, and miscarriage.

Omeprazole generally is tolerated well for short-term therapy. However, it may cause headache, dizziness, weakness, back pain, diarrhea, abdominal pain, nausea, vomiting, constipation, upper respiratory tract infection, cough, and rash.

Usually, sucralfate also is tolerated well. However, its adverse reactions include constipation, diarrhea, indigestion, dry mouth, metallic taste, back pain, dizziness, sleepiness, vertigo, rash, and pruritus.

Nursing implications

When caring for a patient who is receiving a peptic ulcer agent, the nurse should be aware of the following implications.
- Develop appropriate nursing diagnoses for the patient. (For examples, see Sample Nursing Diagnoses: *Peptic ulcer agents.*)
- Do not administer a peptic ulcer agent to a patient with a condition that contraindicates its use.
- Administer a peptic ulcer agent cautiously to a patient at risk because of a preexisting condition.
- Monitor the patient closely for adverse reactions and signs of drug interactions.
- Notify the physician if adverse reactions or drug interactions occur.
- Teach the patient and family the name, dose, frequency, action, and adverse effects of the prescribed drug.
- Advise the patient and family that ulcer healing may take 4 to 6 weeks.
- Monitor for compliance with the prescribed drug regimen. Notify the physician if noncompliance is suspected.

Antacids
- Avoid administering calcium carbonate for long-term therapy because gastric hypersecretion and acid rebound may occur.
- Have the patient thoroughly chew any chewable antacid tablet before swallowing and then drink 6 to 8 oz (180 to 240 ml) of water. If a tablet is used, have the patient drink 6 to 8 ounces of water with it. If a suspension is used, have the patient take a few sips of water after taking the antacid.
- Avoid giving other oral medications within 1 to 2 hours of antacid administration because antacids impair the absorption of many other drugs.
- Monitor the patient for constipation, which may become severe, especially with use of an aluminum-containing antacid.

Histamine$_2$-receptor antagonists
- Monitor the patient for profound bradycardia and other cardiotoxic effects when giving an H$_2$-receptor antagonist by rapid I.V. injection.
- Stress the importance of having laboratory studies done.

SAMPLE NURSING DIAGNOSES

Peptic ulcer agents

The following nursing diagnoses address representative problems and etiologies that a nurse may encounter when caring for a patient who is receiving a peptic ulcer agent.

- Altered cardiopulmonary tissue perfusion related to the cardiotoxic effects of a histamine$_2$ (H_2)-receptor antagonist
- Altered protection related to the adverse hematologic effects of an H_2-receptor antagonist
- Altered thought processes related to the adverse central nervous system effects of an H_2-receptor antagonist
- Constipation related to the adverse gastrointestinal effects of a peptic ulcer agent
- Decreased cardiac output related to profound bradycardia caused by an H_2-receptor antagonist
- Diarrhea related to the laxative effects of a peptic ulcer agent
- Fluid volume excess related to sodium and fluid retention caused by a high-sodium antacid
- High risk for injury related to adverse drug reactions
- High risk for injury related to a preexisting condition that contraindicates the use of a peptic ulcer agent
- High risk for injury related to a preexisting condition that requires cautious use of a peptic ulcer agent
- High risk for injury related to an electrolyte or mineral disturbance caused by an antacid
- High risk for injury related to drug interactions
- High risk for trauma related to hemorrhoids, rectal fissures, or fecal impaction secondary to antacid-induced constipation
- Knowledge deficit related to the prescribed peptic ulcer agent
- Noncompliance related to long-term antacid therapy
- Pain related to headache caused by a peptic ulcer agent
- Sexual dysfunction related to the adverse genitourinary effects of an H_2-receptor antagonist

---

- Dilute cimetidine, famotidine, and ranitidine before I.V. administration in a compatible I.V. solution, such as 0.9% sodium chloride solution, dextrose 5% or 10% in water, lactated Ringer's solution, or 5% sodium bicarbonate. Do not use sterile water as a diluent.

Other peptic ulcer agents

- Administer sucralfate at least 1 hour before meals and at bedtime for best results. If the patient also is receiving cimetidine, administer the drugs at least 2 hours apart.
- Administer misoprostol with food to help prevent adverse GI reactions.
- Provide verbal and written warnings to a woman of childbearing age that misoprostol may induce miscarriage. To prevent miscarriage, advise such a patient to obtain a serum pregnancy test within 2 weeks of beginning therapy, to use an effective contraceptive during therapy, and to notify her physician if she is pregnant or plans to become pregnant.

STUDY ACTIVITIES

Fill in the blank

1. An open lesion of the epithelial, mucosal lining of the lower esophagus, stomach, or duodenum is called a _____.

2. In the stomach, _____ cells secrete acid and _____ cells secrete pepsin.

3. The _____ cells of the stomach contain an acid pump known as the _____.

Matching related elements
Match the drug on the left with its mechanism of action on the right.

4. ___ Aluminum hydroxide

5. ___ Cimetidine

6. ___ Misoprostol

7. ___ Omeprazole

8. ___ Sucralfate

A. Suppresses gastric acid formation by inhibiting the proton pump

B. Replaces endogenous prostaglandins

C. Forms a protective coating at the ulcer site

D. Neutralizes stomach acid

E. Inhibits histamine-stimulated acid secretion by the parietal cells

Multiple choice

9. Sam Jones, age 46, is admitted to the hospital for active duodenal ulcer disease. The physician prescribes magnesium hydroxide and aluminum hydroxide 30 ml P.O. every 2 hours when awake. Where is this drug's site of action?
  A. Esophagus
  B. Stomach
  C. Small intestine
  D. Large intestine

10. Frequent doses of a liquid antacid preparation may lead to which problem?
  A. Acid rebound
  B. Metabolic alkalosis
  C. Fluid imbalance
  D. Noncompliance

11. The physician adds ranitidine 150 mg. P.O. b.i.d. and h.s. to Mr. Jones's regimen. When should the nurse administer the antacid in relation to ranitidine?
  A. Simultaneously with ranitidine
  B. 30 minutes after ranitidine
  C. 3 hours after ranitidine
  D. Within 1 to 2 hours of ranitidine

12. The bedtime dose of ranitidine helps control duodenal ulcer disease by affecting which nocturnal occurrence?
   A. Increased acid secretion
   B. Increased bicarbonate secretion
   C. Increased prostaglandin secretion
   D. Increased activity of the protective barrier

13. Jim Franklin, age 26, is admitted to the burn unit with first-, second-, and third-degree burns on his left arm, trunk, and upper thigh. The physician prescribes ranitidine 50 mg I.V. every 8 hours. How does ranitidine help prevent peptic ulcer formation?
   A. By neutralizing gastric acid
   B. By creating a barrier at the ulcer site
   C. By blocking the action of histamine on gastric parietal cells
   D. By blocking the action of histamine on gastric chief cells

14. The nurse prepares the ranitidine for I.V. administration. Which solution is incompatible for diluting ranitidine?
   A. 0.9% sodium chloride
   B. Sterile water
   C. Dextrose 5% in water
   D. 5% sodium bicarbonate

15. By monitoring and adjusting the I.V. flow rate of ranitidine, the nurse can prevent which adverse reaction?
   A. Profound bradycardia
   B. Nausea and vomiting
   C. Fluid overload
   D. Confusion

16. During a skiing accident, Rita Frost, age 22, dislocates her right knee. The physician prescribes misoprostol 200 mcg P.O. q.i.d. in conjunction with an NSAID to prevent gastric irritation. Before Ms. Frost begins misoprostol therapy, the nurse should expect the physician to order which laboratory test?
   A. Bleeding and clotting time
   B. Complete blood count
   C. Blood urea nitrogen
   D. Serum pregnancy test

17. The nurse should teach Ms. Frost to take misoprostol:
   A. On an empty stomach
   B. With food
   C. 1 hour after meals
   D. As needed for pain

Short answer

18. Frank Hamilton, age 66, has chronic renal failure and a peptic ulcer. His physician prescribes aluminum hydroxide antacid therapy. Edna Hamilton asks the nurse if she can buy Maalox tablets (magnesium and aluminum hydroxide) for her husband at the grocery store. How should the nurse reply?

_____

19. Although sodium bicarbonate is an effective antacid, it is not advocated for use as an antacid. Why?

_____

ANSWERS

Fill in the blank
  1. Peptic ulcer
  2. Parietal, chief
  3. Parietal, proton

Matching related elements
  4. D
  5. E
  6. B
  7. A
  8. C

Multiple choice
  9. B. Antacids act locally on the lining of the stomach, neutralizing acid.

10. D. Because of the need for frequent, regular (rather than p.r.n.) doses and the use of the liquid form of the antacid, patient acceptance and compliance with an antacid regimen may be lower than with another peptic ulcer medication.

11. C. The nurse should avoid giving other oral medications within 1 to 2 hours of antacid administration because antacids impair the absorption of many other drugs.

12. A. The timing of acid hypersecretion is important in preventing peptic ulcer formation. Nocturnal acid secretion, which is unopposed by presence of food in the stomach, is higher in some patients.

13. C. H_2-receptor antagonists inhibit histamine-stimulated acid secretion by the parietal cells as well as basal-, postprandial-, and gastrin-stimulated acid secretion.

14. B. Before I.V. administration, ranitidine should be diluted in a compatible I.V. solution, such as 0.9% sodium chloride, dextrose 5% or 10% in water, lactated Ringer's solution, or 5% sodium bicarbonate. Sterile water should not be used for dilution.

15. A. Rapid I.V. injection of an H_2-receptor antagonist can cause profound bradycardia and other cardiotoxic effects.

16. D. A female patient should obtain a serum pregnancy test 2 weeks before beginning misoprostol therapy because the drug may induce miscarriage.

17. B. Taking misoprostol with food may prevent adverse GI reactions.

Short answer

18. "No, because a patient with renal failure may develop hyper-magnesemia if the kidneys do not excrete the magnesium absorbed from the antacid."

19. Sodium bicarbonate is the most rapidly solubilized antacid, but it is no longer recommended because of its high sodium content and its ability to cause acid rebound.

CHAPTER 22

Adsorbent, antiflatulent, digestive, antiemetic, and emetic agents

OBJECTIVES

After studying this chapter, the reader should be able to:

1. Explain the physiology of nausea and vomiting.

2. Explain how an adsorbent works to treat an acute poisoning.

3. Describe the mechanism of action by which antiflatulent agents work in the gastrointestinal tract.

4. Identify the action of each of the three major groups of digestive agents.

5. Identify the adverse reactions to digestive agents.

6. Describe the therapeutic uses of and adverse reactions to the antiemetic and emetic agents.

7. Describe the proper technique for administering transdermal scopolamine.

8. Describe the nursing implications of therapy with an adsorbent, antiflatulent, digestive, antiemetic, or emetic agent.

OVERVIEW OF CONCEPTS

The drugs in this chapter are used to treat acute poisonings by acting in the gastrointestinal (GI) tract or to manage GI disturbances. An adsorbent attracts molecules of a liquid, gas, or dissolved substance to its surface. Adsorbents are used to prevent drug or toxin absorption in the GI tract in acute poisoning. Emetics are prescribed primarily to induce vomiting in the emergency treatment of acute poisonings. The induced vomiting empties the stomach and prevents absorption of the ingested toxin. Adsorbents also are used as adjuncts to emetic therapy; they are administered after emesis has occurred and bind with the remaining drug or toxin in the GI tract. (For detailed information, see *Emetic agents.*)

Antiflatulents are used to treat gastric bloating with or without flatulence; digestive agents (digestants), to treat inadequate or incomplete digestion. Antiemetics, which act in opposition to emetics, are pre-

Emetic agents

When a patient ingests a toxin, an emetic is used to induce vomiting and prevent toxin absorption. Although mechanical stimulation and such substances as detergents and salt solutions were used in the past to induce vomiting, ipecac syrup is the only emetic currently in clinical use. Ipecac syrup is administered orally, is highly effective, and causes fewer severe adverse reactions. For these reasons, it is considered the drug of choice to treat toxin ingestion.

Ipecac syrup is available over-the-counter (OTC) in 1 oz (30 ml) containers. It induces vomiting by producing a local effect on the gastric mucosa and a central effect on the chemoreceptor trigger zone. The usual adult dose is 15 to 30 ml followed by 200 to 300 ml of water. After oral administration, about 50% of patients begin vomiting in less than 15 to 20 minutes; about 90% vomit within 30 minutes.

If vomiting does not occur within 30 minutes, the dose is repeated. If the second dose does not produce emesis, the nurse should expect to use other measures, such as gastric lavage and administration of activated charcoal. These measures minimize absorption and prevent toxicity from ipecac syrup and the poison.

Ipecac syrup rarely produces adverse reactions when used in recommended dosages. However, high doses or long-term use (which may occur in patients with bulimia or anorexia nervosa) can produce cardiac arrhythmias or fatal myocarditis. Long-term use also may cause skin eruptions as well as esophageal tears. Other adverse reactions may include prolonged vomiting, lethargy, and diarrhea.

Before administering ipecac syrup, the nurse should assess for preexisting conditions that contraindicate or require cautious use of the drug. After administering the drug, the nurse should monitor closely for adverse reactions. If the patient develops a fluid volume deficit, the nurse should replace lost fluids and electrolytes, as prescribed, and continue to monitor hydration status. If lethargy occurs, the nurse should take safety precautions, such as placing the bed in low position, keeping the side rails up, and supervising ambulation.

Because ipecac syrup is an OTC drug and many families keep a bottle at home for childhood emergencies, the nurse should teach family members how to use it. Here are some important points to include in the teaching session:
• Keep ipecac syrup and all other medications out of children's reach.
• Contact the physician, poison control center, or emergency department before using ipecac syrup to induce vomiting after a poisoning.
• Do not give ipecac syrup to an unconscious or very drowsy child because vomited material may enter the lungs.
• Give the poisoned child or adult a glass of water immediately after taking ipecac syrup to help induce vomiting. Do not give milk, unless otherwise instructed, because it can bind with ipecac and prevent its emetic effect.
• Induce early emesis after drug administration by gently bouncing a child or moving an adult.
• If vomiting does not occur within 30 minutes, repeat the dose and take the child or adult to the emergency department.

scribed to decrease nausea and, hence, the urge to vomit. (For a summary of representative drugs, see Selected Major Drugs: *Adsorbent, antiflatulent, digestive, antiemetic, and emetic agents,* page 308.)

Physiology of nausea and vomiting

The vomiting center, located in the reticular formation of the medulla of the brain, integrates the nausea response and coordinates the resulting vomiting reflex. The nausea response can be initiated when the upper GI tract sends nerve impulses to the vomiting center. These nerve impulses can be stimulated by radiation therapy, injury to the GI mucosa, malignant disease of the GI tract, or an emetic drug.

Nausea and vomiting also can be induced by activation of the chemoreceptor trigger zone (CTZ), located in the medulla near the vomiting center. The CTZ contains dopamine receptors that can be activated by narcotics, chemotherapeutic drugs, vestibular motion or inflammation, ketoacidosis, or uremia.

SELECTED MAJOR DRUGS

Adsorbent, antiflatulent, digestive, antiemetic, and emetic agents

The following chart summarizes the major adsorbent, antiflatulent, digestive, antiemetic, and emetic agents currently in clinical use.

DRUG	MAJOR INDICATIONS	USUAL ADULT DOSAGES
Adsorbents		
activated charcoal	Acute toxic poisoning	5 to 10 times the estimated weight of the drug or chemical ingested, or a minimum dose of 30 grams P.O. mixed in 250 ml of water
Antiflatulents		
simethicone	Excess gas in the gastrointestinal tract	160 to 500 mg P.O. daily in divided doses, given after each meal and h.s.
Digestants		
dehydrocholic acid	Insufficient bile production	244 to 500 mg P.O. t.i.d. after meals for 4 to 6 weeks
glutamic acid hydrochloride	Hypochlorhydria, achlorhydria	1 to 3 capsules (340 mg to 1 g) P.O. t.i.d. before meals
hydrochloric acid (dilute)	Hypochlorhydria, achlorhydria	5 to 10 ml in 125 to 250 ml of water P.O. in several divided doses at 15-minute intervals
pancreatin	Insufficient pancreatic enzymes	1 to 3 tablets P.O. after meals
pancrelipase	Insufficient pancreatic enzymes, steatorrhea	1 to 3 capsules or tablets P.O. before or with meals and 1 capsule or tablet P.O. with snacks; or 0.7 g of powder P.O. before meals and snacks
Antiemetics		
dimenhydrinate	Prevention of motion sickness	50 to 100 mg P.O. every 4 to 6 hours up to a maximum of 400 mg daily
meclizine	Prevention of motion sickness	25 to 50 mg P.O. daily at least 1 hour before travel
trimethobenzamide	Prevention or treatment of mild to moderate nausea and vomiting	250 mg P.O. t.i.d. or q.i.d. or 200 mg I.M. or rectally t.i.d. or q.i.d.
prochlorperazine	Prevention or treatment of severe nausea and vomiting from various causes	5 to 10 mg P.O. or I.M. t.i.d. or q.i.d. or 25 mg rectally b.i.d.
promethazine	Prevention or treatment of severe nausea and vomiting from various causes	12.5 to 25 mg P.O., I.M., or rectally every 4 to 6 hours
Emetics		
ipecac syrup	Emesis of ingested poisons	15 to 30 ml P.O. followed by 200 to 300 ml of water; dose may be repeated in 30 minutes if vomiting is not induced

If not controlled, nausea and vomiting may lead to many other problems, such as esophageal injury or suture disruption. Prolonged vomiting may lead to dehydration and loss of gastric secretions, which can cause electrolyte, acid-base, nutritional, and fluid abnormalities.

Adsorbents The major adsorbent in clinical use is activated charcoal (Charcocaps), a black powder residue obtained from the distillation of various organic materials.

Pharmacokinetics

Adsorbents, which are not absorbed or metabolized by the body, are excreted unchanged in the feces. Activated charcoal must be administered soon after poison ingestion because it only can bind drugs or toxins that have not yet been absorbed from the GI tract. Its duration of action depends on transit time through the bowel and the resultant contact time for adsorption to occur.

Pharmacodynamics

Chemically inert powders, adsorbents attract dissolved or suspended substances, such as gases, toxins, and bacteria, and bind with them in the intestinal lumen. This inhibits their absorption from the GI tract.

Pharmacotherapeutics

Activated charcoal is a general-purpose antidote used for acute oral poisoning with amphetamines, antimony, aspirin, atropine, barbiturates, camphor, carbon tetrachloride, cardiac glycosides, cocaine, phenothiazines, potassium permanganate, propoxyphene, quinine, sulfonamides, or tricyclic antidepressants. However, it is not effective in acute poisoning with cyanide, ethanol, methanol, iron, sodium chloride alkalies, inorganic acids, or organic solvents.

Drug interactions

Activated charcoal interacts with food or drug in the GI tract by binding to them. However, the nurse or physician must be careful when administering this drug in combination with ipecac syrup or acetylcysteine. (For details, see Drug Interactions: *Adsorbent, antiflatulent, digestive, antiemetic, and emetic agents,* page 310.)

Adverse drug reactions

Adverse reactions to activated charcoal include black stools and constipation. Activated charcoal commonly is administered in a sorbitol-based formulation; the sorbitol acts a laxative.

Antiflatulents Antiflatulents are preparations that disperse gas pockets in the GI tract. They are available alone or in combination with antacids. The major antiflatulent is simethicone (Mylicon).

Pharmacokinetics

Antiflatulents are physiologically inactive and are not absorbed in the GI tract. Because they are not absorbed, they do not interfere with gas-

DRUG INTERACTIONS

Adsorbent, antiflatulent, digestive, antiemetic, and emetic agents

The antiflatulents produce no significant drug interactions. However, the following chart presents drug interactions for the major adsorbent, digestive, antiemetic, and emetic agents.

DRUG	INTERACTING DRUGS	POSSIBLE EFFECTS
Adsorbents		
activated charcoal	ipecac syrup	Vomiting of activated charcoal or inactivation of ipecac
	acetylcysteine	Decreased effectiveness in treating acetaminophen overdose, possibly leading to acetaminophen-induced hepatotoxicity
Digestants		
pancreatin, pancrelipase	antacids	Negation of digestant's effects
Antiemetics		
antihistamine antiemetics, including buclizine, cyclizine, dimenhydrinate, diphenhydramine, hydroxyzine, meclizine, trimethobenzamide	central nervous system (CNS) depressants, including barbiturates, tranquilizers, alcohol, and opiates	Additive CNS depression
	anticholinergic drugs, including tricyclic antidepressants, phenothiazines, and antiparkinsonian drugs	Additive anticholinergic effects
	ototoxic medications	Masked signs and symptoms of ototoxicity
phenothiazine antiemetics, including chlorpromazine, perphenazine, prochlorperazine, promethazine, thiethylperazine	guanethidine	Inhibited uptake of guanethidine
	amphetamines, nonamphetamine anorexigenic agents	Inhibited effects of both drugs
	anticholinergic drugs	Increased anticholinergic effects; decreased antiemetic effects
	barbiturates	Increased CNS depressant effects; increased phenothiazine metabolism
	levodopa	Reduced antiparkinsonian effects of levodopa
	lithium	Increased chance of neurotoxicity, seizures, delirium, and encephalopathy in manic patients; respiratory depression and hypotension
	droperidol	Increased risk of extrapyramidal effects
Emetics		
ipecac syrup	phenothiazines	Decreased emetic effect of ipecac
	activated charcoal	Vomiting of activated charcoal or inactivation of ipecac syrup

tric secretion or nutrient absorption. Antiflatulents are distributed only in the intestinal lumen and are eliminated intact in the feces. They provide an immediate onset of action, with a duration of action of approximately 3 hours.

Pharmacodynamics

Antiflatulents provide defoaming action in the GI tract. By producing a film in the intestines that collapses gas bubbles, simethicone disperses and helps prevent the formation of mucus-enclosed gas pockets.

Pharmacotherapeutics

Physicians prescribe antiflatulents to treat conditions in which excess gas is a problem, such as functional gastric bloating, postoperative gaseous bloating, diverticulitis, spastic or irritable colon, air swallowing, and peptic ulcer disease. Simethicone is available in these forms: drops, oral suspensions, chewable tablets, regular tablets, and capsules.

Drug interactions

Simethicone produces no significant drug interactions.

Adverse drug reactions

Simethicone does not cause adverse reactions.

Digestants   Digestants aid digestion in patients who lack one or more of the substances that naturally digest food. Dehydrocholic acid (Cholan, Decholin) stimulates bile output. Glutamic acid hydrochloride and hydrochloric acid (dilute, 10% solution) convert pepsinogen in the stomach into pepsin. Pancreatin (Dizymes) and pancrelipase (Cotazym, Ilozyme, Pancrease, Viokase) replace normal pancreatic enzymes.

Pharmacokinetics

Because the digestants are natural body substances (bile acids, hydrochloric acid, and pancreatic secretions), they are absorbed, distributed, metabolized, and excreted as they would be if they were produced by the patient rather than taken therapeutically. Their onset of action, peak concentration level, and duration of action also resemble those of the body substances they replace. Onset and duration depend on the type and amount of food ingested.

Pharmacodynamics

The action of digestants resembles the action of the body substances they replace.

Pharmacotherapeutics

Digestants are prescribed to treat conditions in which the patient produces little or none of the substances that naturally digest food. The bile acid dehydrocholic acid corrects insufficient bile production by stimulating bile flow from the liver. Glutamic acid hydrochloride and hydrochloric acid are used to treat hypochlorhydria, achlorhydria, and gastric achylia. Pancreatin and pancrelipase replace endogenous pancreatic enzymes and aid in digestion. Pancrelipase also is useful in treating steatorrhea.

Drug interactions
No significant drug interactions occur with dehydrocholic acid, glutamic acid hydrochloride, or hydrochloric acid. However, antacids may interact with pancreatin and pancrelipase. (For details, see Drug Interactions: *Adsorbent, antiflatulent, digestive, antiemetic, and emetic agents,* page 310.)

Adverse drug reactions
Dehydrocholic acid can produce abdominal cramping and diarrhea. If a dislodged gallstone is obstructing a biliary duct, this choleretic drug can produce biliary colic. Hydrochloric acid can damage tooth enamel. A massive overdose of hydrochloric acid can cause acid-base abnormalities (specifically metabolic acidosis). Pancreatic enzymes typically cause nausea and diarrhea.

Antiemetics

Antiemetic agents fall into three general categories: antihistamine, phenothiazine, and other antiemetics. The antihistamine antiemetics block histamine$_1$ (H$_1$) receptors and decrease nausea, vomiting, and vertigo. Antihistamines with the greatest antiemetic activity are the ethanolamine derivatives dimenhydrinate (Dramamine) and diphenhydramine hydrochloride (Benadryl); the piperazine derivatives buclizine hydrochloride (Bucladin-S), cyclizine hydrochloride (Marezine), cyclizine lactate (Marezine), hydroxyzine hydrochloride (Atarax), hydroxyzine pamoate (Vistaril), and meclizine hydrochloride (Antivert, Bonine); and trimethobenzamide hydrochloride (Tigan), which is related structurally to the ethanolamine antihistamines.

Although phenothiazines are used primarily to treat psychotic disorders, some of these drugs are used to prevent or treat severe nausea and vomiting (but not nausea resulting from motion sickness or vestibular dysfunction). The phenothiazines most commonly used for their antiemetic effects include chlorpromazine hydrochloride (Thorazine), perphenazine (Trilafon), prochlorperazine maleate (Compazine), promethazine hydrochloride (Phenergan), and thiethylperazine (Torecan). (For more information, see Chapter 12, Antipsychotic agents.)

Other drugs also effectively prevent or treat nausea and vomiting. These drugs include benzquinamide hydrochloride (Emete-Con), diphenidol (Vontrol), dronabinol (Marinol), metoclopramide hydrochloride (Reglan), and scopolamine (Transderm-Scop). Scopolamine may be the most effective drug for motion sickness; however, its use may be limited by its adverse sedative and anticholinergic effects. (For more information, see *Other emetic agents.*)

Pharmacokinetics
Antihistamine antiemetics are absorbed well from the GI tract, may be distributed to the central nervous system (CNS) and breast milk, and

Other antiemetic agents

Other drugs unrelated to the antihistamines or phenothiazines also act effectively to prevent or treat nausea and vomiting.

Benzquinamide hydrochloride (Emete-Con), a benzoquinolizine derivative, is used to treat nausea and vomiting associated with anesthesia and surgery. Its antiemetic effect may result from direct suppression of the chemoreceptor trigger zone (CTZ). After intramuscular injection, benzquinamide is absorbed rapidly. Its adverse effects include central nervous system (CNS) reactions—especially drowsiness—and anticholinergic reactions.

Diphenidol (Vontrol) prevents vertigo and prevents or treats generalized nausea and vomiting. Its dual antiemetic effects may stem from inhibition of impulse conduction from the ear's vestibular area to the vomiting center and direct suppression of the CTZ. The drug produces typical anticholinergic adverse reactions. Its use is limited because it may cause auditory and visual hallucinations, confusion, and disorientation.

Dronabinol (Marinol) is a Schedule II drug that is prescribed for nausea and vomiting resulting from cancer chemotherapy in patients who do not adequately respond to conventional antiemetics. The most prominent adverse reactions occur in the CNS and include mood changes (euphoria, panic, and paranoia), memory loss, sleep pattern disturbances, hallucinations, alterations of time perception, and poor impulse control. A responsible adult should monitor the patient taking this drug.

Metoclopramide hydrochloride (Reglan) is used to manage gastrointestinal (GI) motility disorders and prevent cancer chemotherapy-induced nausea and vomiting. It antagonizes dopamine receptors in the CNS and CTZ, thereby suppressing the impulse to vomit. It also may decrease direct impulses from the GI tract to the vomiting center.

Scopolamine (Transderm-Scop) may be the most effective drug for motion sickness. However, its use may be limited by its sedative and anticholinergic effects. One transdermal scopolamine preparation (Transderm-Scop) provides highly effective action without producing the drug's usual adverse effects. It acts by reducing the activity of nerve fibers in the vestibular apparatus of the inner ear. It produces minimal adverse reactions by releasing minute amounts of scopolamine that permeate the skin at a programmed rate.

The patch is a flexible adhesive disk of four layers, as shown below. The drug passes by diffusion through the membrane from the higher concentration inside the reservoir in the patch to the lower concentration outside the reservoir. For optimal effect, the patient should apply the patch behind the ear at least 4 hours before the need for its antiemetic action. The patient should remove the patch after it is no longer needed or after 72 hours.

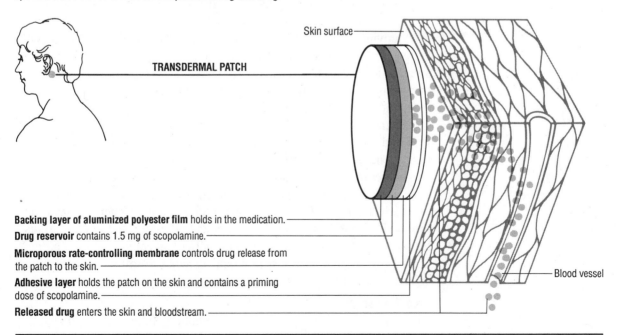

Skin surface

TRANSDERMAL PATCH

Blood vessel

Backing layer of aluminized polyester film holds in the medication.

Drug reservoir contains 1.5 mg of scopolamine.

Microporous rate-controlling membrane controls drug release from the patch to the skin.

Adhesive layer holds the patch on the skin and contains a priming dose of scopolamine.

Released drug enters the skin and bloodstream.

are metabolized primarily by the liver. Their inactive metabolites are excreted in the urine. Most of these drugs produce an onset of action 30 minutes after oral administration, a peak concentration in 1 to 2 hours, and a duration of up to 6 hours. Hydroxyzine and meclizine may provide a duration of up to 24 hours. After intramuscular (I.M.) injection of trimethobenzamide, the onset of antiemetic action occurs in 15 to 35 minutes, and the duration is from 2 to 3 hours.

Phenothiazine antiemetics are absorbed well after oral, rectal, or I.M. administration. They are metabolized extensively by the liver and excreted in the urine and feces. Phenothiazines are distributed to most body tissues and fluids, including breast milk, and cross into the CNS.

Pharmacodynamics

Antihistamine antiemetics prevent nausea and vomiting by inhibiting impulses from the inner ear to the vestibular nuclei and by inhibiting cholinergic stimulation of the CTZ and vomiting center from the vestibular nuclei. The vestibular pathway produces the nausea and vomiting of motion sickness and other labyrinthine disorders. Trimethobenzamide directly inhibits dopaminergic stimulation of the CTZ, thus providing a general antiemetic effect.

Phenothiazines produce their antiemetic effect by blocking the dopamine receptors in the CTZ. These drugs also may depress the vomiting center directly.

Pharmacotherapeutics

With the exception of trimethobenzamide, the antihistamines are antiemetics specifically used for nausea and vomiting caused by inner ear stimulation. As a consequence, these drugs prevent or treat motion sickness. They prove most effective when given prophylactically before activities that produce motion sickness; the drugs are much less effective when nausea or vomiting has already begun. The antihistamine antiemetics are used extensively to relieve the symptoms of diseases that produce vertigo by affecting the vestibular system, such as labyrinthitis and Ménière's disease.

Phenothiazines are the drugs of choice when vomiting becomes severe and potentially hazardous. These drugs are equally effective in treating nausea and vomiting caused by viral illness, uremia, cancer chemotherapy, radiotherapy, anesthesia, or drug toxicity. However, their use is limited to short-term therapy because of the potential for serious adverse reactions. Parenteral administration of phenothiazines is reserved for patients under direct medical observation. Rectal administration is used more commonly in an outpatient setting, where parenteral administration proves less practical, or when vomiting reduces the effectiveness of the oral preparations.

Drug interactions

Antihistamine and phenothiazine antiemetics can interact with drugs that have anticholinergic or sedative effects. (For details, see Drug Interactions: *Adsorbent, antiflatulent, digestive, antiemetic, and emetic agents,* page 310.)

Adverse drug reactions

Most adverse reactions to antihistamine antiemetics are predictable, mild, and easy to control. All antihistamines produce some dose-related drowsiness. Other CNS effects include dizziness, headache, lassitude, and paradoxical CNS stimulation. They also may cause mild nausea, epigastric distress, anorexia, rashes, photosensitivity reactions, and blood dyscrasias. Their anticholinergic effects may produce constipation, dry mouth, blurred vision, tinnitus, dysuria, urine retention, and impotence. Trimethobenzamide may produce extrapyramidal symptoms, such as dystonia and dyskinesia, that require drug discontinuation.

Used in larger dosages as antipsychotics, phenothiazines can produce numerous adverse reactions. When used as antiemetics, however, the drugs primarily produce sedation, hypotension, and extrapyramidal effects. They also may lower the seizure threshold and cause headache, blood dyscrasias, dermatologic reactions, and photosensitivity reactions.

Nursing implications   When caring for a patient who is receiving an adsorbent, antiflatulent, digestant, antiemetic, or emetic, the nurse should be aware of the following implications.
- Develop appropriate nursing diagnoses for the patient. (For examples, see Sample Nursing Diagnoses: *Adsorbent, antiflatulent, digestive, antiemetic, and emetic agents,* page 316.)
- Do not administer an adsorbent, antiflatulent, digestant, antiemetic, or emetic to a patient with a condition that contraindicates its use.
- Administer an adsorbent, antiflatulent, digestant, antiemetic, or emetic cautiously to a patient at risk because of a preexisting condition.
- Monitor the patient for adverse reactions and signs of drug interactions.
- Assess the patient regularly to determine the effectiveness of drug therapy.
- Notify the physician if adverse reactions or drug interactions occur or if the drug is ineffective.
- Teach the patient and family the name, dose frequency, action, and adverse effects of the prescribed adsorbent, antiflatulent, digestant, antiemetic, or emetic.

Adsorbents
- Do not administer activated charcoal to a patient who has ingested a poison for which activated charcoal is ineffective.
- Administer activated charcoal within 30 minutes of the poisoning for maximum effect.
- Expect to administer large doses of activated charcoal to treat the poisoning if food is present in the patient's stomach.

SAMPLE NURSING DIAGNOSES

Adsorbent, antiflatulent, digestive, antiemetic, and emetic agents

The following nursing diagnoses address representative problems and etiologies that a nurse may encounter when caring for a patient who is receiving an adsorbent, antiflatulent, digestant, antiemetic, or emetic.

- Altered health maintenance related to drug interactions with pancreatin or pancrelipase
- Altered health maintenance related to ineffectiveness of the prescribed digestant
- Altered nutrition: less than body requirements, related to anorexia caused by long-term use of an antihistamine antiemetic
- Altered protection related to the adverse hematologic effects of an antiemetic
- Altered thought processes related to central nervous system depression caused by an antiemetic
- Constipation related to the adverse gastrointestinal (GI) effects of activated charcoal or the anticholinergic effects of an antiemetic
- Diarrhea related to the adverse GI effects of a digestant or ipecac syrup
- Health-seeking behaviors related to GI discomfort caused by ineffectiveness of simethicone
- High risk for fluid volume deficit related to ineffectiveness of the prescribed antiemetic
- High risk for fluid volume deficit related to prolonged vomiting induced by an emetic
- High risk for injury related to adverse drug reactions
- High risk for injury related to a preexisting condition that contraindicates the use of an adsorbent, antiflatulent, digestant, antiemetic, or emetic
- High risk for injury related to a preexisting condition requires cautious use of an adsorbent, antiflatulent, digestant, antiemetic, or emetic
- High risk for injury related to drug interactions
- High risk for injury related to ipecac-induced generalized myopathy or cardiomyopathy
- High risk for poisoning related to ineffectiveness of activated charcoal
- High risk for trauma related to esophageal tears caused by ipecac syrup abuse
- High risk for trauma to tooth enamel related to hydrochloric acid administration
- Impaired physical mobility related to the extrapyramidal effects of trimethobenzamide or a phenothiazine antiemetic
- Knowledge deficit related to the prescribed adsorbent, antiflatulent, digestant, antiemetic, or emetic
- Noncompliance related to long-term use of a digestant
- Pain related to antiemetic-induced headache
- Sensory or perceptual alterations (visual, auditory) related to the anticholinergic effects of an antiemetic
- Sexual dysfunction related to impotence caused by an antihistamine antiemetic
- Urinary retention related to the anticholinergic effects of an antiemetic

---

- Add fruit juice to the charcoal and water mixture to make it more palatable.
- Do not administer activated charcoal simultaneously with ipecac syrup. Give ipecac syrup first and allow emesis to occur before administering activated charcoal because emesis enhances the effectiveness of the activated charcoal by decreasing the amount of toxin in the GI tract.
- Advise the patient to anticipate black stools from the activated charcoal.

Antiflatulents

- Administer simethicone after each meal and at bedtime for maximum effectiveness.
- Teach the patient to shake a simethicone suspension before taking each dose or to chew thoroughly chewable tablets before swallowing.
- Encourage the patient with functional gastric bloating to increase activity and exercise, unless contraindicated.

Digestants

- Instruct the patient to take the digestant before, with, or after meals, as prescribed, to enhance effectiveness.
- Teach the patient to take dilute hydrochloric acid at 15-minute intervals in divided doses, as prescribed, and to use a glass straw to prevent damage to tooth enamel.
- Instruct the patient taking a pancreatic enzyme to balance fat, protein, and carbohydrate intake to avoid indigestion.
- Advise the patient not to take a pancreatic enzyme with an antacid.
- Inform the patient that the number of bowel movements will decrease during digestant therapy and that the stool consistency will improve when replacement therapy reaches a therapeutic level. Advise the patient, however, to report diarrhea to the physician.

Antiemetics

- Take safety precautions if drowsiness or dizziness occurs. Expect to reduce the dosage, as prescribed, if the patient experiences drowsiness.
- Monitor the patient closely for signs of other adverse CNS reactions.
- Take seizure precautions when administering a phenothiazine antiemetic to a patient who is predisposed to seizures because these drugs lower the seizure threshold.
- Obtain a prescription for a mild analgesic if the patient experiences a headache.
- Monitor closely for signs of urine retention. If urine retention is present, notify the physician. Catheterize the patient and discontinue the antiemetic, as prescribed.
- Evaluate hematologic studies to detect signs of blood dyscrasias. Alert the physician to any abnormalities.
- Avoid skin contact with oral solutions and injections when preparing or administering a phenothiazine antiemetic.
- Teach the patient how to relieve the antiemetic's anticholinergic effects, such as dry mouth (by drinking sips of water or sucking on sugarless candy) and constipation (by increasing fluid and fiber intake).
- Advise the patient not to drive or participate in other activities that require mental alertness if sedation occurs. Advise the patient not drink alcohol or take other CNS depressants in order to prevent additive sedative effects.

• Advise the patient to avoid prolonged exposure to sunlight or to wear protective clothing and sunscreen when outside because antiemetics may cause photosensitivity reactions.
• Instruct the patient to take an antihistamine antiemetic with food or milk to decrease the nausea caused by the drug.
• Advise the patient to ingest an antihistamine antiemetic 30 to 60 minutes before engaging in an activity that causes motion sickness.
• Instruct the patient to remain recumbent for 30 to 60 minutes after taking a phenothiazine antiemetic to prevent hypotension.

STUDY ACTIVITIES

Fill in the blank

1. The vomiting center is located in the reticular formation of the

_____ of the brain.

2. Nausea and vomiting can be induced by activation of the

_____.

3. An _____ or _____ is used to prevent _____ of an ingested toxin.

True or false

4. Ipecac syrup is available as an over-the-counter drug.
☐ True   ☐ False

5. Antihistamine antiemetics produce additive effects when administered with a CNS depressant.
☐ True   ☐ False

6. Most adverse reactions to antihistamine antiemetics are predictable and easy to control.
☐ True   ☐ False

Matching related elements
Match the drug on the left with its description on the right.

7. ___ Activated charcoal

A. Digestant used to treat hypochlorhydria or achlorhydria

8. ___ Simethicone

B. Digestant used to treat steatorrhea

9. ___ Dehydrocholic acid

C. Adsorbent used for acute poisoning

10. ___ Pancrelipase

D. Digestant used to stimulate bile flow

11. ___ Hydrochloric acid

E. Antiflatulent agent used to treat excessive GI gas

Multiple choice

12. Brad Campbell, age 25, is admitted to the emergency department with a barbiturate overdose. The physician orders immediate administration of activated charcoal. How does activated charcoal exert its therapeutic effect?

A. It binds with toxins and prevents their absorption in the GI tract.

B. It absorbs the metabolic end products of toxins in the GI tract.

C. It produces emesis, which removes toxins from the GI tract.

D. It neutralizes toxins in the GI tract.

13. Mr. Campbell is likely to receive which type of drug in addition to activated charcoal?

A. Emetic

B. Antacid

C. Laxative

D. Antiflatulent

14. When teaching Mr. Campbell about activated charcoal, the nurse should advise him to anticipate which adverse reaction?

A. Vomiting

B. Flatulence

C. Black stools

D. Tooth discoloration

15. Chris Thomson, age 46, seeks care for abdominal fullness and bloating after meals. The physician prescribes simethicone 160 mg P.O. daily in divided doses. For optimum effect, when should Mr. Thomson take simethicone?

A. With food

B. After meals

C. With an antacid

D. On an empty stomach

16. How does simethicone produce its antiflatulent effects?

A. By increasing peristalsis to prevent flatulence

B. By increasing bile flow to aid in fat digestion

C. By inhibiting the absorption of gas-producing foods

D. By producing a film in the intestines that collapses gas bubbles

17. What should the nurse teach Ms. Thomson about simethicone therapy?

A. Store simethicone in the refrigerator.

B. Chew the chewable tablets well before swallowing.

C. Thoroughly dissolve simethicone in 250 ml of water.

D. Avoid taking simethicone with over-the-counter drugs.

18. Olivia Anders, age 76, is about to begin hydrochloric acid (dilute) therapy for achylia. Which instruction should the nurse give Ms. Anders?

    A. Take hydrochloric acid at 30-minute intervals before meals.
    B. Sip the hydrochloric acid solution through a glass straw.
    C. Store hydrochloric acid in the refrigerator.
    D. Increase food consumption at mealtimes.

19. Lawrence Steele, age 52, has developed pancreatic enzyme deficiency secondary to pancreatitis. His physician has prescribed pancrelipase (Cotazym) 1 capsule P.O. before meals and snacks. The nurse should instruct Mr. Steele to avoid which type of drug during pancrelipase therapy?

    A. Antacid
    B. Antiflatulent
    C. Anticoagulant
    D. Anti-inflammatory drug

20. The nurse also should teach Mr. Steele to observe for which adverse reaction to pancrelipase?

    A. Tarry stools
    B. Constipation
    C. Steatorrhea
    D. Nausea

21. Polly Nolan, age 46, is planning to go on a 7-day cruise. She asks her physician for a prescription for an antiemetic because she suffers from motion sickness. The physician prescribes a transdermal scopolamine patch (Transderm-Scop) to be applied behind the ear. How long before she departs for the cruise should she apply the patch?

    A. 30 minutes
    B. 1 hour
    C. 2 hours
    D. 4 hours

22. When should Ms. Nolan remove the first patch?

    A. In 12 hours
    B. In 24 hours
    C. In 48 hours
    D. In 72 hours

23. After abdominal surgery, Bernie Hayes, age 36, experiences severe nausea and vomiting. His physician prescribes the phenothiazine antiemetic promethazine (Phenergan) 25 mg I.M. every 6 hours. Which adverse reaction is Mr. Hayes likely to experience?

    A. Sedation
    B. Hypothermia
    C. Hypertension
    D. Increased salivation

24. Andrea Clark calls the poison control center because her daughter Amy, age 2, has ingested half a bottle of children's acetaminophen. She is instructed to give Amy 15 ml of ipecac syrup followed by 200 ml of water. When should Amy begin to vomit?
   A. Immediately
   B. Within 30 minutes
   C. Within 1 hour
   D. Within 2 hours

ANSWERS

Fill in the blank
   1. Medulla
   2. Chemoreceptor trigger zone (CTZ)
   3. Adsorbent, emetic, absorption

True or false
   4. True.
   5. True.
   6. True.

Matching related elements
   7. C
   8. E
   9. D
   10. B
   11. A

Multiple choice
12. A. Activated charcoal attracts dissolved or suspended substances, such as gases, toxins, and bacteria, and binds with them in the intestinal lumen. This inhibits their absorption from the GI tract.
13. C. A laxative, such as sorbitol, commonly is given with activated charcoal to prevent constipation.
14. C. Adverse reactions to activated charcoal include black stools and constipation.
15. B. Simethicone should be administered after each meal and at bedtime for maximum effectiveness.
16. D. By producing a film in the intestines that can collapse gas bubbles, simethicone disperses and helps prevent the formation of mucus-enclosed gas pockets.
17. B. The nurse should teach the patient to chew thoroughly chewable tablets before swallowing or to shake a simethicone suspension before taking each dose.
18. B. The nurse should teach the patient to take dilute hydrochloric acid at 15-minute intervals in divided doses, as prescribed, and to use a glass straw to prevent damage to tooth enamel.
19. A. Antacids negate the effects of pancrelipase and pancreatin.
20. D. Pancreatic enzymes, such as pancrelipase, typically cause nausea and diarrhea.

21. D. A transdermal scopolamine patch should be applied at least 4 hours before its antiemetic effect is needed.

22. D. A transdermal scopolamine patch should be removed after 72 hours or when it is no longer needed.

23. A. When used as antiemetics, phenothiazines primarily produce sedation, hypotension, and extrapyramidal effects.

24. B. Approximately 90% of patients vomit within 30 minutes of receiving ipecac syrup.

CHAPTER 23

Antidiarrheal and laxative agents

OBJECTIVES

After studying this chapter, the reader should be able to:

1. Identify the antidiarrheal agents indicated for acute, nonspecific, and chronic diarrhea.

2. Explain the mechanisms of action of the various antidiarrheal agents.

3. Identify adverse reactions to the antidiarrheal agents.

4. Describe the general mechanism of action of laxatives.

5. Compare the clinical indications for various laxatives.

6. Identify adverse reactions to laxatives.

7. Describe the nursing implications of antidiarrheal or laxative therapy.

OVERVIEW OF CONCEPTS

Diarrhea and constipation are the two major symptoms of disturbances of the large intestine. These symptoms may lead to physiologic problems that interfere with the patient's ability to perform activities of daily living. Diarrhea may precipitate abdominal discomfort, malaise, and lethargy resulting from dehydration. Constipation may be harmful to a patient who should not strain during defecation, such as one who has recently had a myocardial infarction. Fortunately, drug therapy can control most diarrhea and constipation. (For a summary of representative drugs, see Selected Major Drugs: *Antidiarrheal and laxative agents,* page 324.)

Diarrhea

Diarrhea refers to the increased frequency or weight and liquidity of stools produced by the rapid movement of fecal matter through the large intestine. Acute diarrhea may be caused by a viral or bacterial infection of the large intestine; chronic diarrhea, by a disorder such as ulcerative colitis (a nonspecific inflammatory disease marked by acute exacerbations and remissions). Brief episodes of self-limiting diarrhea may be psychogenic.

Antidiarrheals reduce the fluidity of the stool and the frequency of defecation. They act systemically or locally. Opium tincture, paregoric, loperamide, difenoxin, and diphenoxylate are systemic agents. The

SELECTED MAJOR DRUGS

Antidiarrheal and laxative agents

The following chart summarizes the major antidiarrheal and laxative agents currently in clinical use.

DRUG	MAJOR INDICATIONS	USUAL ADULT DOSAGES
Antidiarrheals		
difenoxin (with atropine)	Acute, nonspecific diarrhea	Initially, 2 mg P.O., followed by 1 mg P.O. every 3 to 4 hours, as needed, up to a maximum of 8 mg daily
diphenoxylate (with atropine)	Acute, nonspecific diarrhea	Initially, 5 mg P.O. q.i.d., with dosage adjusted to patient response
kaolin and pectin mixture	Mild to moderate nonspecific diarrhea	60 to 120 ml regular-strength suspension or 45 to 90 ml concentrated-strength suspension P.O. after each loose bowel movement, usually up to eight doses per day
loperamide	Acute, nonspecific diarrhea; chronic diarrhea	Initially, 4 mg P.O., then 2 mg after each unformed stool; up to a maximum of 16 mg daily
opium tincture	Acute, nonspecific diarrhea	0.6 ml (range 0.3 to 1 ml) P.O. q.i.d., up to a maximum of 6 ml daily
paregoric (camphorated opium tincture)	Acute, nonspecific diarrhea	5 to 10 ml P.O. once daily to q.i.d., until acute diarrhea subsides
Laxatives		
bisacodyl	Chronic constipation	10 to 15 mg P.O. in the evening or before breakfast, or 10 mg as a rectal suppository or 1.25 oz enema
	Bowel evacuation before delivery, surgery, or rectal or bowel examination	Up to 30 mg P.O.
docusate sodium	Stool softening for patients who should not strain during defecation	50 to 500 mg P.O. daily until bowel movements are normal
glycerin	Reestablishment of proper bowel patterns in laxative-dependent adults	3 g by suppository or 5 to 15 ml as an enema
lactulose	Chronic constipation	10 to 20 g (15 to 30 ml) P.O. daily
	Reduction of ammonia level in patients with systemic portal encephalopathy	20 to 30 g (30 to 45 ml) P.O. t.i.d. or q.i.d. until two to three soft stools are produced daily; or 200 g (300 ml) diluted in 700 ml of water or 0.9% sodium chloride solution, given via rectal balloon catheter and retained 30 to 60 minutes, every 4 to 6 hours
methylcellulose	Constipation	5 to 20 ml liquid P.O. t.i.d. with 8 oz (240 ml) of water
mineral oil	Constipation or maintenance of soft stools for patients who should not strain during defecation	15 to 30 ml P.O., usually h.s., or 4 oz enema

SELECTED MAJOR DRUGS

Antidiarrheal and laxative agents *(continued)*

DRUG	MAJOR INDICATIONS	USUAL ADULT DOSAGES
Laxatives *(continued)*		
psyllium hydrophilic mucilloid	Constipation	1 to 2 teaspoonfuls or 1 packet P.O. dissolved in 8 oz of water b.i.d. or t.i.d., followed by another 8 oz of water
saline compounds (magnesium salts, sodium biphosphate, sodium phosphate)	Prompt and complete bowel evacuation	10 to 15 g magnesium sulfate P.O. in a glass of water; 240 ml magnesium citrate h.s.; 20 to 30 ml oral sodium phosphate or sodium biphosphate solution mixed with 8 oz water; or 120 ml (4 oz) sodium phosphate or sodium biphosphate as an enema

combination of kaolin and pectin is a local agent. Diarrhea caused by a specific pathogen also may be treated with an antimicrobial agent.

Constipation

Constipation refers to the decreased movement of fecal matter through the large intestine. Common causes of constipation include poor bowel habits established in childhood, long-term laxative abuse, poor dietary habits, and the use of certain drugs.

Laxatives and cathartics include various drugs that stimulate defecation. Laxatives exert their effects by increasing the water content of the feces and increasing the movement of intestinal materials from the colon and rectum. The term *cathartic* implies a fluid evacuation; the term *laxative,* the elimination of the soft, formed stool.

Excessive use of laxatives may result in habitual dependence, fluid and electrolyte imbalances, acid-base abnormalities, dehydration, and cardiac arrhythmias. For a patient who habitually uses laxatives, the nurse should institute a bowel retraining program and teach how to prevent chronic constipation.

Antidiarrheals Clinicians recognize three groups of antidiarrheals: opium preparations; difenoxin, diphenoxylate, and loperamide; and kaolin and pectin. Antidiarrheal opium preparations include opium tincture (a Schedule II drug) and paregoric or camphorated opium tincture (a Schedule III drug). Difenoxin hydrochloride (Motofen), diphenoxylate hydrochloride (Lomotil), and loperamide (Imodium) are synthetic drugs related to meperidine. Kaolin, which is hydrated aluminum silicate, and pectin, which is a purified carbohydrate product obtained from fruit, are combined as kaolin and pectin mixtures (Kaopectate, Kapectolin) that are available over-the-counter.

Pharmacokinetics

After oral administration, opium preparations are absorbed quickly from the gastrointestinal (GI) tract and distributed to the kidneys, lungs, liver, and spleen. They are metabolized by the liver and excreted primarily by the kidneys. Their onset of action occurs within 1 hour of administration. Concentration levels peak within 2 to 3 hours. Their duration of action is about 4 hours.

After oral administration, difenoxin and diphenoxylate are absorbed readily in the GI tract; loperamide is not absorbed well. These agents are distributed in the serum, metabolized in the liver, and excreted primarily in the feces. Difenoxin and diphenoxylate have a faster onset of action and a shorter duration of action than loperamide.

Kaolin and pectin mixtures are not absorbed and, therefore, not distributed throughout the body. They are metabolized in the GI tract and excreted in the feces. Their onset of action is 30 minutes after oral administration; duration of action, 4 to 6 hours.

Pharmacodynamics

The morphine in opium tincture and paregoric causes antidiarrheal effects by decreasing GI motility and peristalsis. It does this through a direct central action on the brain and a local action in nerve plexuses and exocrine glands of the stomach and intestines.

Difenoxin, diphenoxylate, and loperamide decrease GI motility by depressing intestinal muscle action, which decreases peristalsis. Difenoxin (a Schedule IV drug) and diphenoxylate (a Schedule V drug) can penetrate the central nervous system (CNS), especially the brain. Loperamide does not enter the CNS readily. Atropine is combined with difenoxin and diphenoxylate to discourage the abuse of these drugs; this is effective because the toxic effects of atropine occur before the narcotic effects of difenoxin and diphenoxylate.

Kaolin and pectin mixtures act locally on the intestinal mucosa as adsorbents and protectants. They bind with bacteria, toxins, and other irritants on the intestinal mucosa. Pectin decreases intestinal pH and provides a soothing, demulcent effect on irritated mucosa.

Pharmacotherapeutics

Opium preparations are used to treat acute, nonspecific diarrhea. They commonly are used with kaolin, pectin, and bismuth salts because these three drugs offer adsorbent and protective effects. Opium preparations are contraindicated for treatment of diarrhea caused by toxic chemicals or pathogens.

Difenoxin, diphenoxylate, and loperamide are used to treat acute, nonspecific diarrhea. Loperamide also is used to treat chronic diarrhea because of its minimal effects on the CNS.

Kaolin and pectin mixtures are used to relieve mild to moderate acute diarrhea. They also may be used temporarily to relieve chronic

DRUG INTERACTIONS

Antidiarrheal and laxative agents

Although hyperosmolar and dietary fiber and bulk-forming laxatives cause no significant drug interactions, drugs from other laxative classes and antidiarrheal drugs may be associated with various interactions.

DRUG	INTERACTING DRUGS	POSSIBLE EFFECTS
Antidiarrheals		
difenoxin, diphenoxylate, loperamide	central nervous system (CNS) depressants	Increased CNS depression
kaolin and pectin mixture	lincomycin	Decreased lincomycin absorption
	digoxin and drugs that undergo similar type of absorption	Decreased absorption from intestinal mucosa
opium tincture, paregoric	CNS depressants, including alcohol, barbiturates, and tranquilizers	Increased CNS depression
	anticholinergic agents	Increased constipation
Laxatives		
bisacodyl, cascara sagrada, castor oil, phenolphthalein, senna	other oral drugs, especially sustained-release formulations	Decreased absorption of other oral drugs
mineral oil	oral fat-soluble vitamins (A, D, E, and K), oral contraceptives, oral anticoagulants	Decreased absorption of the vitamin, contraceptive, or anticoagulant
	sulfonamides	Decreased antibacterial activity of sulfonamide
oral docusate salts, poloxamer 188	oral mineral oil	Increased systemic absorption and tissue deposition of mineral oil
	other oral drugs	Increased absorption of other oral drugs

diarrhea until the cause has been determined and definitive treatment instituted. They generally are effective within 48 hours.

Drug interactions

Antidiarrheals can interact with various drugs. (For more information, see Drug Interactions: *Antidiarrheal and laxative agents*.)

Adverse drug reactions

Adverse reactions to opium tincture and paregoric commonly are mild and dose-related. They include nausea, vomiting, dizziness, malaise, constipation, and increased biliary tract pressure. Patients over age 60 are more likely to experience allergic reactions, such as urticaria and contact dermatitis. Anaphylactic reactions are rare.

Adverse reactions to difenoxin, diphenoxylate, and loperamide include nausea, vomiting, abdominal discomfort or distention, drowsiness, fatigue, CNS depression, tachycardia, hypoperistalsis, and paralytic ileus. Allergic responses, such as rash and urticaria, may occur. Adverse reactions to the atropine in difenoxin and diphenoxylate include flushing, diminished salivary and bronchial secretions, hyperthermia, tachycardia, urine retention, miosis, nystagmus, and blurred vision.

Kaolin and pectin mixtures cause few adverse reactions. Constipation may occur, especially in a geriatric or debilitated patient or with overdose and prolonged use; it is generally mild and transient.

Laxatives

A high-fiber diet is the most natural way of preventing or treating constipation. However, the following types of laxatives also may be used: hyperosmolar, bulk-forming, emollient, stimulant, and lubricant agents. Hyperosmolar laxatives include glycerin, lactulose (Cephulac, Chronulac), and saline compounds, such as magnesium salts (Milk of Magnesia), sodium biphosphate (Fleet Enema, Phospho-Soda), or sodium phosphate. Bulk-forming laxatives resemble dietary fiber and include methylcellulose (Citrucel), polycarbophil (Fibercon, Mitrolan), and psyllium hydrophilic mucilloid (Metamucil).

Emollients, or stool softeners, include docusate calcium (Surfak), docusate potassium (Dialose, Kasof), and docusate sodium (Colace, Regutol). Stimulant laxatives, or irritant cathartics, include bisacodyl (Dulcolax), cascara sagrada (Cas-Evac), castor oil (Neoloid), phenolphthalein (Alophen Pills, Ex-Lax), and senna (Senokot, X-Prep). The most commonly used lubricant laxative is mineral oil (Agoral Plain, Fleet Mineral Oil).

Pharmacokinetics

Hyperosmolar laxatives are absorbed poorly. Glycerin and lactulose are distributed in the intestines, where they exert their laxative action. Lactulose is metabolized by intestinal microflora and excreted in the feces. When saline compounds are introduced to the GI tract, some absorption of component ions (magnesium and sodium) occurs. Glycerin generally causes bowel evacuation in 15 to 30 minutes; lactulose, in 1 to 2 days; and saline compounds, in 1 to 3 hours.

Like dietary fiber, bulk-forming laxatives are not absorbed systemically. They act primarily in the small intestine and colon, and are excreted in the feces. Fecal softening occurs 1 to 3 days after administration and reaches maximum effect after 3 to 4 days of continued use.

Administered orally, emollients are absorbed somewhat through the duodenum and jejunum. They concentrate in the liver and are excreted in the feces. Stool softening occurs within several days after administration.

Most stimulant laxatives are absorbed slightly and metabolized in the liver. The metabolites are excreted in the urine or feces. Bisacodyl and phenolphthalein are distributed to breast milk. Cascara sagrada and senna are distributed to body tissues and breast milk. Castor oil is hydrolyzed to its active ingredient, ricinoleic acid, in the small intestine. Bisacodyl and phenolphthalein act within 6 to 8 hours after oral administration and 15 to 60 minutes after rectal administration. Cascara sagrada and senna act within 6 to 12 hours after oral administration and 30 minutes to 2 hours after rectal administration. Castor oil acts within 2 to 3 hours after oral administration.

Nonemulsified mineral oil is absorbed minimally; about half of emulsified mineral oil is absorbed. Absorbed mineral oil is distributed to the mesenteric lymph nodes, intestinal mucosa, liver, and spleen. It is metabolized by the liver and excreted in the feces. Defecation occurs 6 to 8 hours after oral administration and about 2 hours after rectal administration.

Pharmacodynamics

Hyperosmolar laxatives produce bowel evacuation by drawing water into the intestinal lumen. Distention of the bowel from fluid accumulation promotes peristalsis and bowel movement.

Bulk-forming laxatives act like dietary fiber, increasing fecal bulk and water content, which promotes peristalsis and elimination.

Emollients are surface-acting agents that soften the stool and ease defecation by emulsifying fat and water in feces. This detergent action allows water and lipids to penetrate the feces, producing a net fluid accumulation.

All stimulant laxatives stimulate peristalsis and induce evacuation by irritating the intestinal mucosa and stimulating nerve endings of the intestinal smooth muscle. They also alter fluid and electrolyte absorption.

Mineral oil lubricates the feces and intestinal mucosa by preventing water reabsorption from the bowel. The increased fluid content of the feces increases peristalsis. Rectally administered mineral oil produces laxation by physical distention.

Pharmacotherapeutics

Among the hyperosmolar laxatives, glycerin suppositories are helpful in bowel retraining. Lactulose sometimes is used to treat chronic constipation and primarily is used to reduce liver ammonia levels in a patient with systemic portal encephalopathy. Saline compounds are natural substances used primarily for prompt bowel evacuation.

Bulk-forming agents are used to treat simple constipation. They also may be used to manage patients with irritable bowel syndrome and diverticulosis.

Usually safe, emollients are the drugs of choice for softening the stools of patients who should avoid straining during defecation, such as those who have recently experienced a myocardial infarction (to avoid Valsalva's maneuver) or increased intracranial pressure.

Stimulant laxatives are preferred for emptying the bowel before general surgery and GI tests or procedures. They also are used to treat constipation caused by prolonged bed rest, neurologic dysfunction of the colon, and such constipating drugs as narcotics. Because these laxatives may stimulate uterine contractions, milder laxatives usually are preferred to treat constipation associated with pregnancy or delivery. Stimulant laxatives are never administered to women who breast-feed their infants.

The lubricant agent mineral oil is used to treat constipation in patients who must avoid straining. Administered orally or by enema, it also may be used to treat patients with fecal impaction. Bulk-forming and emollient laxatives provide milder action than mineral oil.

Drug interactions

Dietary fiber and hyperosmolar and bulk-forming laxatives do not interact significantly with other drugs. However, emollient, stimulant, and lubricant laxatives may interact with a variety of drugs. (For details, see Drug Interactions: *Antidiarrheal and laxative agents,* page 327.)

Adverse drug reactions

Adverse reactions to hyperosmolar laxatives involve fluid and electrolyte imbalances. Glycerin is quite safe, but may cause weakness and fatigue. Lactulose may cause adverse GI reactions, such as abdominal distention, flatulence, and abdominal cramps. It also may produce hypokalemia, hypovolemia, increased blood glucose level, and increased systemic portal encephalopathy. Saline compounds may result in hypernatremia, hypermagnesemia, hyperphosphatemia, hypocalcemia, and hypovolemic shock.

Because they resemble dietary fiber, bulk-forming laxatives pose little risk of toxicity when used in recommended amounts. Flatulence, abdominal fullness, fecal impaction, and diarrhea may occur.

Emollients rarely cause adverse reactions. However, bitter taste, diarrhea, throat irritation, and mild, transient abdominal cramping may occur.

Adverse reactions to stimulant laxatives include weakness, nausea, abdominal cramps, and mild proctitis. Long-term use or overdose can lead to fluid and electrolyte imbalances, malabsorption, and weight loss. Habitual use may lead to cathartic colon accompanied by atony and dilation. Phenolphthalein allergy may result in renal, cardiac, and respiratory dysfunction.

Mineral oil's adverse reactions include nausea, vomiting, diarrhea, and abdominal cramping. Seepage from the rectum may result in anal irritation, pruritus ani, infection, and impaired healing in the area. Lipid pneumonitis may result from aspiration of mineral oil.

Nursing implications

When caring for a patient who is receiving an antidiarrheal or laxative, the nurse should be aware of the following implications.
• Develop appropriate nursing diagnoses for the patient. (For examples, see Sample Nursing Diagnoses: *Antidiarrheal and laxative agents.*)
• Do not administer an antidiarrheal or laxative to a patient with a condition that contraindicates its use.

SAMPLE NURSING DIAGNOSES

Antidiarrheal and laxative agents

The following nursing diagnoses address representative problems and etiologies that a nurse may encounter when caring for a patient who is receiving an antidiarrheal or laxative.
- Activity intolerance related to hyperosmolar laxative-induced weakness and lethargy
- Altered health maintenance related to ineffectiveness of the prescribed antidiarrheal or laxative
- Altered nutrition: less than body requirements, related to impaired absorption of nutrients and fat-soluble vitamins caused by long-term use of mineral oil or a stimulant laxative
- Altered protection related to electrolyte imbalance caused by a hyperosmolar or stimulant laxative
- Constipation related to the adverse gastrointestinal (GI) effects of an antidiarrheal or laxative
- Diarrhea related to the adverse GI effects of an antidiarrheal or laxative
- Fluid volume deficit related to hypovolemia caused by lactulose or a saline compound
- High risk for fluid volume deficit related to decreased intake caused by the adverse GI effects of an antidiarrheal
- High risk for injury related to adverse drug reactions
- High risk for injury related to a preexisting condition that contraindicates the use of an antidiarrheal or laxative
- High risk for injury related to a preexisting condition that requires cautious use of an antidiarrheal or laxative
- High risk for injury related to drug interactions
- High risk for trauma related to central nervous system (CNS) depression, hypoperistalsis, or intestinal or esophageal obstruction caused by an antidiarrheal
- Hyperthermia related to the adverse CNS effects of atropine
- Impaired skin integrity related to seepage of mineral oil after rectal administration
- Knowledge deficit related to the prescribed antidiarrheal or laxative
- Pain related to rectal administration of bisacodyl
- Sensory or perceptual alterations (visual) related to the adverse CNS effects of atropine
- Urinary retention related to the adverse genitourinary effects of atropine

---

- Administer an antidiarrheal or laxative cautiously to a patient at risk because of a preexisting condition.
- Monitor the patient for adverse reactions, such as GI disturbances and fluid and electrolyte imbalances, and signs of drug interactions.
- Evaluate the effectiveness of the prescribed agent by assessing the patient's bowel pattern.
- Notify the physician if adverse reactions or drug interactions occur or if the prescribed agent is ineffective.
- Monitor hydration in a patient with diarrhea.
- Teach the patient and family the name, dose, frequency, action, and adverse effects of the prescribed antidiarrheal or laxative.
- Instruct the patient to notify the physician of any adverse reactions.
- Advise the patient to take the drug exactly as prescribed.
- Encourage the patient to maintain a fluid intake of 68 to 100 oz (2 to 3 liters) daily to replace the fluid lost through diarrhea.

Preventing constipation

The nurse should review the following measures when teaching a patient how to avoid constipation and minimize laxative use.

- Eat a regular diet with adequate amounts of dietary fiber (6 to 10 g daily) and fluids (at least eight 8-oz [240 ml] glasses daily).
- Consume meals at about the same time each day.
- Allow time each day to use the toilet; do not ignore the urge to defecate.
- Maintain a regular exercise regimen.
- Avoid habitual use of laxatives or cathartics.

- Describe the proper use of laxatives to a patient with constipation. Caution the patient about laxative dependence.
- Teach the patient how to avoid constipation. (For details, see *Preventing constipation.*)

Antidiarrheals: Opium preparations

- Be alert for allergic reactions and decreased sensitivity to pain in a patient over age 60. Notify the physician if such reactions occur.
- Expect a milky fluid to form when paregoric is added to water.
- Take safety precautions if the patient experiences dizziness. For example, place the bed in a low position, keep the side rails up, and supervise ambulation.
- Monitor for enhanced CNS depression in a patient who also is receiving another CNS depressant.
- Consult the physician if the patient's diarrhea lasts longer than 48 hours or if fever and abdominal pain develop during therapy. If an opium preparation is ineffective, the patient may require a different drug.
- Monitor for constipation, especially if the patient also is receiving an anticholinergic agent.

Antidiarrheals: Difenoxin, diphenoxylate, and loperamide

- Monitor for signs of atropine-induced hypoperistalsis. If it occurs, withhold the next dose and notify the physician.
- Perform neurologic checks to assess for CNS depression, especially during concomitant therapy with another CNS depressant.
- Take safety precautions if drowsiness occurs.
- Withhold the drug and consult the physician if the patient shows signs of abdominal distention (which may indicate toxic megacolon, especially with ulcerative colitis); if the patient with acute, nonspecific diarrhea shows no improvement in 48 hours; or if patient with chronic diarrhea shows no improvement after 10 days.

- Monitor for urine retention in a patient receiving difenoxin or diphenoxylate made with atropine, especially if the patient has benign prostatic hypertrophy.

Antidiarrheals: Kaolin and pectin

- Monitor closely for constipation during kaolin and pectin therapy. Fecal impaction can result from severe constipation, especially in an infant or debilitated patient. Withhold the drug and notify the physician if constipation occurs.
- Advise the patient to avoid self-medication for longer than 48 hours and to consult the physician if diarrhea persists or if fever is present.
- Instruct the patient who experiences more than eight bowel movements a day—even when following the prescribed regimen—to consult the physician.

Hyperosmolar laxatives

- Assess for signs of fluid or electrolyte imbalance. If the patient develops signs of hypovolemic shock, such as hypotension, tachycardia, or oliguria, notify the physician and prepare to take supportive measures.
- Take safety precautions if the patient develops weakness or fatigue.
- Monitor the patient's blood glucose levels once every shift or as prescribed for a patient with impaired glucose tolerance who is receiving lactulose. Observe for signs of hyperglycemia, such as polyuria, polydipsia, polyphagia, and weakness.
- Teach the patient to recognize and report signs of fluid and electrolyte imbalance and, if they occur, to discontinue the drug.
- Instruct the patient with impaired glucose tolerance to observe for signs of hyperglycemia and to monitor blood glucose level regularly during lactulose therapy.
- Instruct the patient who experiences diarrhea to withhold the drug, notify the physician, and increase fluid intake (unless contraindicated).

Bulk-forming laxatives

- Be especially alert for adverse GI reactions and notify the physician if they occur.
- Administer a bulk-forming laxative with 8 oz (240 ml) of water to prevent esophageal obstruction. Ensure that the patient follows each dose of psyllium hydrophilic mucilloid with a second 8-oz glass of water to prevent intestinal obstruction.
- Advise the patient to avoid bulk-forming laxatives if sugar and salt intake is restricted. Recommend sugar-free products for the patient with diabetes.

Emollient laxatives

- Monitor hydration and notify the physician if the patient develops di-

arrhea. Replace fluids and electrolytes, as prescribed.
• Store the emollient laxative at 59° to 86° F (15° to 30° C). Protect liquid preparations from light.
• Avoid administering an emollient laxative with mineral oil or an oral drug to prevent alterations in drug absorption.
• Caution the patient to swallow—not to chew or open—emollient capsules.

Stimulant laxatives
• Be especially alert for fluid and electrolyte imbalances, rash, and pruritus. Also monitor for renal, cardiac, or respiratory dysfunction in a patient receiving phenolphthalein.
• Store castor oil below 40° F (4.5° C), but do not freeze.
• Administer castor oil on an empty stomach.
• Alert the patient that phenolphthalein may color urine red; cascara sagrada and senna, red-pink or brown.
• Instruct the patient not to chew enteric-coated bisacodyl tablets (to prevent GI irritation) and not to take them with antacids.

Lubricant laxatives
• Inspect the anal area regularly for irritation, pruritus ani, infection, and impaired lesion healing in a patient who receives the drug rectally.
• Administer mineral oil cautiously to prevent aspiration and lipid pneumonitis.
• Avoid administering mineral oil with other oral medications.
• Monitor the patient on long-term mineral oil therapy for early signs of fat-soluble vitamin deficiency.
• Do not administer the drug with or shortly after meals or with fat-soluble vitamins.
• Instruct the patient that mineral oil interferes the absorption of fat-soluble vitamins and oral medications.

STUDY ACTIVITIES   **Fill in the blank**

1. Diarrhea refers to increased _____ or _____ and _____ of stools.

2. Acute diarrhea may be caused by a _____ or _____ infection of the large intestine. Chronic diarrhea may result from _____ .

3. Constipation refers to _____ movement of fecal matter through the _____ .

Matching related elements
Match the drug on the left with its description on the right.

4. ___ Paregoric   **A.** Stimulant laxative

5. ___ Glycerin   **B.** Adsorbent-protectant antidiarrheal

6. ___ Kaolin and pectin   **C.** Emollient laxative (stool softener)

7. ___ Docusate sodium   **D.** Antidiarrheal opium preparation

8. ___ Bisacodyl   **E.** Hyperosmolar laxative

True or false
9. Excessive use of laxatives may result in habitual dependence.
   ☐ True   ☐ False

10. Constipation may be caused by poor bowel habits established in childhood.
    ☐ True   ☐ False

11. Opium preparations are used to treat diarrhea caused by toxic chemicals or pathogens.
    ☐ True   ☐ False

12. The nurse should notify the physician if diarrhea persists for more than 18 hours in a patient receiving an opium preparation.
    ☐ True   ☐ False

13. The patient should take a bulk-forming laxative with 4 to 6 ounces of fluid.
    ☐ True   ☐ False

14. Stimulant laxatives, such as bisacodyl, are used to prepare the bowel before general surgery or GI tests.
    ☐ True   ☐ False

Multiple choice
15. Brenda Adams, age 28, comes to the emergency department with severe, chronic diarrhea. While awaiting the results of a stool culture, Ms. Adams is most likely to receive which antidiarrheal agent?
    A. Paregoric
    B. Diphenoxylate
    C. Opium tincture
    D. Kaolin and pectin

16. Don Bowden, age 44, has acute viral enteritis. His physician orders loperamide (Imodium). The nurse should monitor Mr. Bowden for which adverse reaction?
    A. Polyuria
    B. Mydriasis
    C. Bradycardia
    D. Hypoperistalsis

17. Andrew Howe, age 58, is recovering from a myocardial infarction. To prevent Mr. Howe from straining during defecation, the physician prescribes docusate sodium. During docusate sodium therapy, Mr. Howe should avoid which drug?
  A. Subcutaneous insulin
  B. Intramuscular furosemide
  C. Oral mineral oil
  D. Intravenous penicillin G

18. A nursing home resident, Martha Jansen, age 86, has developed constipation. The physician prescribes psyllium hydrophilic mucilloid (Metamucil) 1 packet P.O. in a glass of water. Which statement accurately characterizes this bulk-forming laxative?
  A. It only interacts with fat-soluble vitamins.
  B. It promotes peristalsis and elimination.
  C. It will be effective within 8 to 12 hours of administration.
  D. It is likely to cause hypercalcemia.

19. The nurse teaches Ms. Jansen to prevent constipation by increasing fiber and fluid intake and exercising moderately. How much dietary fiber should Ms. Jansen consume daily?
  A. 1 to 2 grams
  B. 3 to 6 grams
  C. 6 to 10 grams
  D. 12 to 14 grams

20. Maureen Bender gives her son Tod, age 5, a kaolin and pectin mixture for mild nonspecific diarrhea. How does this preparation produce its antidiarrheal effects?
  A. It acts as an intestinal adsorbent.
  B. It prevents ammonia buildup in the GI tract.
  C. It encourages the growth of intestinal flora.
  D. It produces an osmotic effect in the intestine.

ANSWERS

Fill in the blank
  1. Frequency, weight, liquidity
  2. Viral, bacterial, ulcerative colitis
  3. Decreased, large intestine

Matching related elements
  4. D
  5. E
  6. B
  7. C
  8. A

True or false
  9. True.
  10. True.

11. False. Opium preparations are contraindicated for treatment of diarrhea caused by toxic chemicals or pathogens.

12. False. The nurse should consult the physician if the patient's diarrhea lasts longer than 48 hours or if fever and abdominal pain develop during therapy.

13. False. The nurse should administer a bulk-forming laxative with 8 oz (240 ml) of water to prevent esophageal obstruction.

14. True.

Multiple choice

15. D. Kaolin and pectin may be used temporarily to relieve chronic diarrhea until the cause has been determined and definitive treatment instituted.

16. D. Adverse reactions to loperamide include GI disturbances, CNS depression, tachycardia, hypoperistalsis, and paralytic ileus.

17. C. Oral docusate salts and other emollients enhance the systemic absorption of mineral oil and many oral drugs.

18. B. Bulk-forming laxatives increase fecal bulk and water content, which promotes peristalsis and elimination. They do not cause drug interactions and primarily cause adverse GI reactions.

19. C. The patient should consume 6 to 10 grams of fiber per day to prevent constipation.

20. A. Kaolin and pectin act as adsorbents, binding with bacteria, toxins, and other irritants on the intestinal mucosa.

CHAPTER 24

Hypoglycemic agents and glucagon

OBJECTIVES

After studying this chapter, the reader should be able to:

1. Differentiate between Type I and Type II diabetes mellitus and describe the patient's needs in each.

2. Identify the different sources of insulins and describe how they are classified.

3. Describe the mechanism of action by which insulin decreases the blood glucose level.

4. Explain what the nurse should teach a patient with diabetes about taking insulin.

5. Explain why different insulin regimens exist.

6. Discuss the pharmacokinetics and clinical uses of oral hypoglycemic agents.

7. Explain how glucagon increases the blood glucose level.

8. Describe the nursing implications of hypoglycemic agent or glucagon therapy.

OVERVIEW OF CONCEPTS

Scattered throughout the pancreas are cell clusters known as islets of Langerhans. Beta cells in the islets of Langerhans produce insulin and alpha cells produce glucagon. Insulin decreases the blood glucose level; glucagon increases it.

During normal carbohydrate metabolism, insulin facilitates glucose uptake, storage (in the form of glycogen and fat), and metabolism. Insulin also plays an important role in protein and fat metabolism. Without insulin, the body cannot metabolize glucose, and must break down protein and fat for fuel.

Glucagon opposes the actions of insulin. It stimulates glycogenolysis (conversion of glycogen to glucose) and gluconeogenesis (glucose production from plasma amino acids resulting from protein breakdown or from lipid breakdown). Glucagon also increases lipolysis (fat breakdown) and inhibits triglyceride storage.

Diabetes mellitus that results from an *absolute* insulin deficiency is known as Type I or insulin-dependent diabetes mellitus (IDDM). Dia-

SELECTED MAJOR DRUGS

Hypoglycemic agents and glucagon

The following chart summarizes the major hypoglycemic agents currently in clinical use. It also lists glucagon.

DRUG	MAJOR INDICATIONS	USUAL ADULT DOSAGES
Insulin		
insulin	Hyperglycemia	Individualized according to the patient's blood glucose level
Oral hypoglycemic agents		
chlorpropamide	Hyperglycemia	100 to 750 mg P.O. daily
glipizide	Hyperglycemia	2.5 to 40 mg P.O. daily
glyburide	Hyperglycemia	1.25 to 20 mg P.O. daily
tolbutamide	Hyperglycemia	250 to 3,000 mg P.O. daily
Glucagon		
glucagon	Emergency treatment of severe hypoglycemia	0.5 to 1 mg S.C., I.M., or I.V., repeated once or twice if patient does not awaken after the first injection

betes mellitus caused by a *relative* insulin deficiency is known as Type II or noninsulin-dependent diabetes mellitus (NIDDM). A patient with Type I diabetes mellitus must depend on exogenous sources of insulin for normal carbohydrate metabolism; one with Type II diabetes simply may need to modify diet and exercise patterns to maintain normal blood glucose levels.

Other types of diabetes usually are temporary. These types of diabetes may result from drug therapy, another disorder, or the stress of pregnancy. Patients with blood glucose levels that are above normal but not indicative of diabetes mellitus are considered to have impaired glucose tolerance.

Insulin and oral hypoglycemic agents are classified as antidiabetic or hypoglycemic agents. Glucagon is classified as a hyperglycemic agent. (For a summary of representative drugs, see Selected Major Drugs: *Hypoglycemic agents and glucagon.*)

Insulin   Insulin is used to control the blood glucose level in all patients with Type I diabetes and in some patients with Type II and other types of diabetes mellitus. In the United States, many different insulin preparations are available and may vary in concentration and source. Insulin comes in two concentrations: U-100 (100 units of insulin/ml) and U-500 (500 units of insulin/ml). The source of these insulins may be beef (derived from the bovine pancreas), pork (derived from the porcine pancreas), or "human" sources (derived from genetically altered *Escherichia coli* bacteria or enzymatically altered pork insulin).

Pharmacokinetics of insulins

An insulin's onset of action, peak concentration level, and duration of action can vary from patient to patient and from injection to injection in the same patient. However, these pharmacokinetic properties can be estimated for the three categories of insulins shown in the chart below.

TYPE	ONSET OF ACTION	PEAK CONCENTRATION	DURATION OF ACTION
rapid-acting	$\frac{1}{2}$ to 1 hour	2 to 10 hours	5 to 16 hours
intermediate-acting	1 to 2 hours	4 to 15 hours	22 to 28 hours
long-acting	4 to 8 hours	10 to 30 hours	36 hours or more

Pharmacokinetics

The absorption, distribution, metabolism, and excretion of different insulins are similar. They are *not* effective when taken orally because they are broken down in the gastrointestinal (GI) tract breakdown. Therefore, all insulins are given by subcutaneous (S.C.) injection. Regular (unmodified) insulin also may be given by the intravenous (I.V.) or intramuscular (I.M.) routes or by peritoneal dialysis (in dialysate fluid).

Insulin absorption varies with the injection site and the site's vascular supply and degree of tissue hypertrophy. For example, after S.C. administration, insulin is absorbed most rapidly from abdominal sites, more slowly from arm sites, and slowest from anterior thigh sites. Insulin is distributed throughout the body. Insulin-responsive tissues are located in the liver, adipose tissue, and muscle. Insulin is metabolized primarily in the liver and secondarily in the kidneys, adipose tissue, and muscle. It is excreted in the feces and the urine.

Insulin preparations, which are categorized as regular-acting, intermediate-acting, and long-acting, differ in their onset of action, peak concentration, and duration of action. (For more information, see *Pharmacokinetics of insulins*.)

Pharmacodynamics

Insulin is an anabolic (building) hormone. It decreases blood glucose levels by promoting glucose uptake and storage of insulin-dependent cells, increasing protein and fat synthesis, and inhibiting the breakdown of glycogen, protein, and fat. By decreasing the serum osmotic effect of elevated glucose levels, insulin corrects the polyuria and polydipsia associated with hyperglycemia. Insulin also facilitates the movement of potassium from extracellular fluid into the cell.

Pharmacotherapeutics

Insulin is indicated for Type I diabetes mellitus. It also is administered to patients with gestational, Type II, and other types of diabetes mellitus when other methods of glucose control are ineffective or contraindicated. Insulin also is used for two types of complications that are related to diabetes: diabetic ketoacidosis (DKA), more common with Type I, and hyperosmolar nonketotic syndrome (HNKS), more common with Type II.

Because insulin stimulates cellular uptake of potassium, it sometimes is given with hypertonic glucose to nondiabetic patients with severe hyperkalemia. This insulin and glucose mixture causes a shift of potassium into cells, lowering the serum potassium level.

The physician selects an insulin preparation that will provide a normal or near-normal blood glucose level throughout the day with minimal risk and disruption to the patient's life-style. To achieve this goal, the physician chooses a particular insulin category (rapid-, intermediate-, or long-acting) or a combination of categories. Insulin doses usually are administered 30 minutes before breakfast, dinner, or both.

Although U-100 insulin is the most commonly used concentration, the U-500 concentration may be prescribed for patients who need very large amounts of insulin in one injection.

Adult doses of insulin vary widely and represent the amount needed to keep the blood glucose at a normal or near-normal level. The dose varies not only from person to person, but also in the same person at different times. Insulin requirements are increased by growth, pregnancy, increased food intake, stress, surgery, infection, illness, increased insulin antibodies, and some medications. Insulin requirements are decreased by hypothyroidism, decreased food intake, exercise, and some medications.

Drug interactions

Insulin may interact with a variety of drugs. (For details, see Drug Interactions: *Hypoglycemic agents and glucagon,* page 342.)

Adverse drug reactions

The patient may experience dose-related or idiosyncratic reactions to contaminants in the insulin. However, hypoglycemia (below-normal blood glucose levels) is a relatively frequent adverse reaction to insulin. Specific signs include nervousness or shakiness, diaphoresis, weakness, light-headedness, confusion, paresthesia, irritability, headache, hunger, tachycardia, and changes in speech, hearing, or vision. If untreated, symptoms may progress to unconsciousness, seizures, coma, and death.

Insulin may produce local hypersensitivity reactions, such as redness, itching, or burning at the injection site, but these reactions usually disappear after 1 to 2 months of therapy. However, the patient may be switched to a purified insulin and given an antihistamine, if needed. A small percentage of patients may develop an allergy to animal insulins, with beef insulin considered more antigenic than pork insulin. Human insulin is the least antigenic. Although rare, insulin may cause systemic hypersensitivity reactions, including hives, angioedema, dyspnea, tachy-

Hypoglycemic agents and glucagon

Numerous drugs can interact with insulin and oral hypoglycemic agents, altering blood glucose levels substantially. As a normal body protein, glucagon only interacts with one class of drugs.

DRUG	INTERACTING DRUGS	POSSIBLE EFFECTS
Insulin		
insulin	alcohol	Hypoglycemia
	anabolic steroids, salicylates, monoamine oxidase (MAO) inhibitors	Hypoglycemia
	corticosteroids, sympathomimetic agents, thiazide diuretics, dextrothyroxine	Hyperglycemia
	beta blockers	Masked signs of hypoglycemia (except diaphoresis); delayed recovery from hypoglycemia
Oral hypoglycemic agents		
acetohexamide, chlorprop-amide, tolazamide, tolbutamide, glipizide, glyburide	alcohol	Hypoglycemia or hyperglycemia
	dicumarol	Hypoglycemia, increased anticoagulant effects of dicumarol
	anabolic steroids, chloramphenicol, clofibrate, gemfibrozil, MAO inhibitors, phenylbutazone, salicylates, sulfonamides	Hypoglycemia
	corticosteroids, dextrothyroxine, rifampin, sympathomimetic agents, thiazide diuretics	Hyperglycemia
	beta blockers, clonidine	Masked signs of hypoglycemia (except diaphoresis)
Glucagon		
glucagon	oral anticoagulants	Increased anticoagulant effects

cardia, and anaphylactic shock. In such situations, the offending insulin is discontinued and an insulin from a different source is substituted.

Two kinds of lipodystrophy may result from insulin use: lipohypertrophy (thickening of subcutaneous fat tissue) and lipoatrophy (loss of fat tissue at injection site). These adverse reactions can be avoided by rotating the insulin injection sites.

Insulin resistance may occur in patients with Type II diabetes mellitus. It usually results from a decreased number of insulin receptors, a postreceptor defect in insulin action, or an excess of hormones antagonistic to insulin.

Two phenomena also may occur with insulin therapy. The Somogyi phenomenon occurs during the late night or early morning. As the patient sleeps, insulin is absorbed from the S.C. injection site, producing a rapid drop in blood glucose level (hypoglycemia). In response, the body secretes glucagon, norepinephrine, and corticosteroids, producing an overshoot phenomenon (hyperglycemia). Although the patient awakens with symptoms of hyperglycemia, hypoglycemia is the condition that must be corrected. The dawn phenomenon (an early morning rise in blood glucose level) may result from nocturnal secretion of growth hormone, which causes insulin resistance. Unlike the Somogyi phenomenon, the dawn phenomenon is not preceded by hypoglycemia.

Oral hypoglycemic agents

All oral hypoglycemic agents approved for use in the United States are sulfonylureas. First-generation sulfonylureas include acetohexamide (Dymelor), chlorpropamide (Diabinese, Glucamide), tolazamide (Tolinase), and tolbutamide (Orinase). The second-generation sulfonylureas include glipizide (Glucotrol) and glyburide (DiaBeta, Micronase).

Pharmacokinetics
After oral administration, sulfonylureas are absorbed from the GI tract and distributed via the bloodstream throughout the body. They bind rapidly to plasma proteins; only a small portion of a sulfonylurea dose is left free to produce an effect. The sulfonylureas are metabolized primarily in the liver and excreted primarily in the urine. Patients with renal dysfunction taking these drugs require careful monitoring for signs of hypoglycemia and metabolite accumulation.

Their onset of action varies greatly, from 30 minutes (for tolbutamide) to 6 hours (for tolazamide). The oral hypoglycemic agents reach peak concentration levels 2 to 6 hours after administration. Their half-life and duration of action vary considerably.

Pharmacodynamics
First- and second-generation sulfonylureas probably work by stimulating the pancreas to release endogenous insulin; therefore, the pancreas already must be functioning at a minimal level. Within a few weeks to months of the initial response to sulfonylureas, pancreatic insulin secretion drops to pretreatment levels. However, the drugs' extrapancreatic actions maintain blood glucose at normal or near-normal levels. These actions may include a decrease in glucose production by the liver and an increase in the number of cellular insulin receptors.

Pharmacotherapeutics
Oral hypoglycemic agents are given to patients with Type II diabetes mellitus when they cannot maintain normal or near-normal blood glucose levels with exercise and diet. Patients with Type I diabetes mellitus (IDDM) cannot benefit from these drugs because they have insufficient pancreatic beta-cell activity. These agents should be taken on a regular schedule to minimize wide fluctuations in the blood glucose level.

Sulfonylureas have one major advantage over insulin: oral administration. However, they have several disadvantages. These agents only can be used in patients with functioning beta cells. They cannot be used by patients who have been instructed to take nothing by mouth and may not control blood glucose sufficiently during periods of acute injury, stress, or infection. Also, these agents are contraindicated during pregnancy and lactation because their effects on the fetus and nursing infant are unknown.

Drug interactions

Oral hypoglycemic agents can interact with various drugs. (For details, see Drug Interactions: *Hypoglycemic agents and glucagon,* page 342.)

Adverse drug reactions

Hypoglycemia, the major adverse reaction to oral hypoglycemic agents, usually results from eating too little food or taking too much medication. It also can be caused by drug or metabolite accumulation in the body. Patients with decreased hepatic or renal function and those also taking chlorpropamide must be monitored carefully.

Another common adverse reaction, primary drug failure (that is, no initial response to sulfonylurea therapy) occurs in about 20% of patients by an unknown mechanism. Secondary drug failure occurs when the sulfonylurea maintains a normal or near-normal blood glucose level for a time, but then, for unknown reasons, no longer does so. Secondary failure occurs in 5% to 10% of patients taking oral hypoglycemic agents. However, 25% to 60% of affected patients will respond to another agent. Therefore, trial with a different sulfonylurea may be warranted.

Relatively uncommon reactions to oral hypoglycemic agents include GI effects (nausea, vomiting), skin reactions (rash, photosensitivity), hematologic reactions (leukopenia, thrombocytopenia), hepatic effects (abnormal liver function tests), and renal effects (severe diuretic or antidiuretic effect). Allergic reactions also may occur.

Glucagon

Glucagon is a hormone normally produced by the alpha cells of the islets of Langerhans in the pancreas. The hyperglycemic agent glucagon increases the blood glucose level.

Pharmacokinetics

After S.C, I.M., or I.V. injection, glucagon is absorbed rapidly and distributed throughout the body. It is degraded extensively in the liver and removed from the body by the liver and kidneys. The blood glucose level begins to rise 5 to 20 minutes after glucagon administration; the half-life of glucagon in plasma is about 3 to 6 minutes.

Pharmacodynamics

Glucagon acts primarily in the liver, where it increases glycogenolysis and gluconeogenesis. It also inhibits fat storage and increases fat breakdown. A glucagon deficiency results in hypoglycemia. Although glucagon stimulates insulin secretion, insulin antagonizes glucagon's actions through a negative feedback system.

Pharmacotherapeutics
Glucagon is used for emergency treatment of severe hypoglycemia. It also is used as a diagnostic aid during radiologic examination of the GI tract to decrease motility. For glucagon to be effective, the patient must have glycogen stores in the liver. Therefore, a patient who is poorly nourished or starving would not benefit from glucagon treatment.

Drug interactions
Glucagon can interact with oral anticoagulants. (For details, see Drug Interactions: *Hypoglycemic agents and glucagon,* page 342.)

Adverse drug reactions
Nausea and vomiting occasionally result from glucagon administration, probably from the drug's inhibitory effect on GI motility or from hypoglycemia. With large doses or prolonged treatment, hypokalemia can result. Other adverse reactions are rare, but may include allergy to glucagon (because it is a protein) and the development of antibodies against it.

Nursing implications
When caring for a patient who is receiving a hypoglycemic agent or glucagon, the nurse should be aware of the following implications.
- Develop appropriate nursing diagnoses for the patient. (For examples, see Sample Nursing Diagnoses: *Hypoglycemic agents and glucagon,* page 346.)
- Do not administer a hypoglycemic agent or glucagon to a patient with a condition that contraindicates its use.
- Administer a hypoglycemic agent or glucagon cautiously to a patient at risk because of a preexisting condition.
- Monitor the patient closely for adverse reactions and signs of drug interactions.
- Notify the physician if adverse reactions or drug interactions occur.
- Monitor the patient for signs and symptoms of hypoglycemia and hyperglycemia.
- Assess the effectiveness of the prescribed agent regularly. Notify the physician if the drug or dosage is ineffective.
- Monitor the patient's compliance with the prescribed regimen.
- Notify the physician if the patient is not complying with the regimen and try to determine the patient's reasons for doing so.
- Teach the patient and family the name, dose, frequency, action, and adverse effects of the prescribed drug.
- Review factors that may affect the hypoglycemic agent dosage requirement, such as diet, exercise, stress, and illness.
- Teach the patient to recognize the signs of hypoglycemia and hyperglycemia. Instruct the patient to take some form of glucose if signs of

SELECTED NURSING DIAGNOSES

Hypoglycemic agents and glucagon

The following nursing diagnoses address representative problems and etiologies that a nurse may encounter when caring for a patient who is receiving a hypoglycemic agent or glucagon.

- Altered health maintenance related to ineffectiveness of the prescribed hypoglycemic agent
- Altered health maintenance related to the development of insulin resistance
- Altered protection related to hypoglycemia caused by a hypoglycemic agent
- Altered protection related to insulin-induced Somogyi or dawn phenomenon
- Altered protection related to the adverse hematologic or hepatic effects of an oral hypoglycemic agent
- Altered urinary elimination related to the adverse renal effects of an oral hypoglycemic agent
- High risk for fluid volume deficit related to the adverse gastrointestinal effects of an oral hypoglycemic agent
- High risk for injury related to adverse drug reactions
- High risk for injury related to a preexisting condition that contraindicates the use of a hypoglycemic agent or glucagon
- High risk for injury related to a preexisting condition that requires cautious use of a hypoglycemic agent or glucagon
- High risk for injury related to a systemic hypersensitivity reaction to insulin
- High risk for injury related to drug interactions
- Impaired tissue integrity related to a local reaction to insulin
- Knowledge deficit related to the prescribed hypoglycemic agent or glucagon
- Noncompliance related to long-term use of a hypoglycemic agent

---

hypoglycemia occur. If hyperglycemia persists, instruct the patient to notify the physician; the insulin regiment may need to be changed.
- Teach the patient how to monitor the blood glucose level.
- Teach the patient to recognize the signs and symptoms of drug failure, such as polyuria, polydipsia, polyphagia, weight loss, and fatigue. Instruct the patient to check the blood glucose level and notify the physician immediately if these effects occur.
- Emphasize the importance of eating meals at regular times to prevent glucose alterations.
- Instruct the patient to wear medical identification and to keep a source of glucose, such as hard candy, readily available.

Insulin
- Avoid dosage errors by measuring U-100 insulin in U-100 insulin syringes.
- Do not shake insulin because the resulting froth prevents withdrawal of an accurate dose and may damage protein molecules.
- Expect to administer insulin subcutaneously. If prescribed, however, administer regular insulin intravenously or intramuscularly, or mix it with dialysate fluid and infuse it into the peritoneal cavity.

- Mix insulins in the same order every time, withdrawing the long-acting insulin last. Administer mixed insulins within 5 minutes after mixing.
- Do not administer regular insulin that appears cloudy or any insulin solution that contains particles.
- Store insulin at a temperature of 36° F to 80° F (2° C to 27° C). Do not freeze insulin or leave it in direct sunlight.
- Administer a once-daily morning dosage of insulin 30 minutes before breakfast or a split morning and evening dosage 30 minutes before breakfast and 30 minutes before dinner, unless otherwise prescribed.
- Rotate and document insulin injection sites.
- Observe the S.C. or I.M. injection site for signs of a local hypersensitivity reaction, such as redness, itching, or burning.
- Observe the patient closely during initial or episodic insulin therapy, particularly noting systemic hypersensitivity reactions, such as generalized urticaria, angioedema, dyspnea, tachycardia, and, possibly, anaphylactic shock. Have standard emergency equipment readily available.
- Monitor the patient with hyperglycemia for signs of DKA or HNKS, such as Kussmaul's respirations or electrolyte imbalances, and test the patient's urine for ketones.
- Monitor the patient for signs of insulin resistance, such as hyperglycemia that persists despite adherence to the insulin regimen, and a progressive increase in the amount of insulin needed to achieve blood glucose control.
- Administer only human insulin, as prescribed, for episodic insulin therapy.
- Instruct the patient not to change the manufacturer, type, purity, species, or dosage of insulin unless told to do so by the physician.
- Advise the patient to obtain guidelines for alcohol use from the physician.
- Instruct the patient who must mix insulins always to follow the same order when drawing the insulins into the syringe. Typically, the rapid-acting insulin is drawn first.

Oral hypoglycemic agents
- Monitor the patient's laboratory tests for results that suggest leukopenia, thrombocytopenia, hemolytic anemia, or liver dysfunction.
- Give an oral hypoglycemic agent 30 minutes before breakfast; if the daily drug dosage is divided, give the second dose 30 minutes before dinner. A patient who also is taking tolbutamide three times a day should take a dose of insulin before each meal.
- Inform the patient that the oral hypoglycemic agent may cause photosensitivity, and advise the patient to avoid exposure to the sun. When this is not possible, the patient should use protective measures, such as sunglasses, sunscreen, and a hat.

• Advise the patient to obtain guidelines for alcohol use from the physician.

Glucagon

• Monitor hydration if the patient experiences nausea or vomiting after glucagon administration.
• Observe the patient receiving high-dose or long-term therapy for signs of hypokalemia, such as arrhythmias, mental status changes, or irritability.
• Monitor the patient receiving concomitant therapy with oral anticoagulants for signs of bleeding, such as epistaxis, bleeding gums, hematuria, and bruising. Notify the physician if these occur.
• Give the patient with Type I diabetes mellitus who requires glucagon a complex carbohydrate snack as soon as possible to restore liver glycogen and prevent secondary hypoglycemia.
• Contact the physician immediately to obtain a prescription for I.V. glucose if the patient does not respond to glucagon because of the potential harmful effects of cerebral hypoglycemia.
• Mix glucagon powder only with the diluent provided.
• Do not administer I.V. glucagon in a solution that contains calcium, potassium, or sodium chloride because precipitation may occur.
• Teach the patient and family to recognize the signs and symptoms of hypoglycemia. Also show them how to prepare and administer glucagon in an emergency.
• Instruct the family to provide a complex carbohydrate snack after the patient awakens from hypoglycemic coma.
• Advise the family to seek emergency help immediately if the patient does not respond to glucagon therapy.

STUDY ACTIVITIES   **Fill in the blank**

1. Type _____ diabetes mellitus is characterized by an absolute lack of insulin.

2. Oral hypoglycemic agents may stimulate the _____ to produce more endogenous insulin.

3. Insulin increases the uptake and storage of _____ and increases _____ and _____ synthesis.

4. Glucagon acts primarily in the liver, where it increases _____ and _____.

Multiple choice

5. Ted Overstreet, age 33, has Type I diabetes mellitus and has been self-administering 6 units of intermediate-acting insulin every morning. To achieve better control of Mr. Overstreet's blood glucose level, the physician adds 3 units of regular (rapid-acting) insulin to the regimen. Which insulin should the nurse draw into the syringe first?

A. Intermediate-acting insulin
B. Regular insulin
C. Either insulin (order is not important)
D. Neither insulin (they should not be mixed)

6. The nurse administers the first dose of the new insulin regimen to Mr. Overstreet at 7:30 a.m. When should the onset of action occur?

A. Between 8:00 a.m. and 8:30 a.m.
B. Between 9:00 a.m. and 9:30 a.m.
C. Between 10:00 a.m. and 10:30 a.m.
D. Between 11:00 a.m. and 11:30 a.m.

7. Mr. Overstreet develops sinusitis and otitis media accompanied by a fever of 100.8° F. What effect may this have on his need for insulin?

A. It will have no effect.
B. It will decrease the need for insulin.
C. It will increase the need for insulin.
D. It will cause wide fluctuations in the need for insulin.

8. During a patient-teaching session with Mr. Overstreet, the nurse should instruct him to administer the morning insulin dose at what time?

A. Immediately upon arising
B. 30 minutes before breakfast
C. 1 hour before breakfast
D. 1 hour after breakfast

9. The nurse teaches Mr. Overstreet to recognize the signs and symptoms of hypoglycemia. What should he do if they occur?

A. Count his pulse and take his temperature.
B. Drink a caffeine-containing beverage.
C. Immediately lie down and rest.
D. Eat some hard candy.

10. Carrie Burns, age 36, has just received a diagnosis of Type II diabetes mellitus (NIDDM). Her physician prescribes chlorpropamide (Diabinese) 100 mg P.O. daily. The nurse takes a careful medication history. Which agent could interact with chlorpropamide?

A. Potassium supplement
B. Oral contraceptives
C. Acetaminophen
D. Dicumarol

11. Ms. Burns asks the nurse if she needs to take any special precautions during chlorpropamide therapy. The nurse should advise her to avoid which substance?
   A. Codeine
   B. Alcohol
   C. Diazepam
   D. Iron supplement

Matching related elements
Match the term on the left with the phrase on the right.

12. ___ Lipodystrophy   **A.** Is caused by hypoglycemia and produces an overshoot of glucagon production

13. ___ Somogyi phenomenon   **B.** Is more common in Type II diabetes mellitus

14. ___ Thrombocytopenia   **C.** May be avoided by rotating insulin injection sites

15. ___ Hyperosmolar nonketotic syndrome (HNKS)   **D.** Is an adverse reaction to oral hypoglycemic agents

True or false
16. Insulin produces local reactions, but does not cause systemic reactions.
   ☐ True   ☐ False

17. Glucagon may be given by S.C., I.M., or I.V. injection.
   ☐ True   ☐ False

18. U-100 insulin is the most concentrated form of insulin available.
   ☐ True   ☐ False

19. Concomitant use of anabolic steroids may cause hypoglycemia in a patient taking insulin.
   ☐ True   ☐ False

20. Hypoglycemia and drug failure are the most common adverse reactions to sulfonylureas.
   ☐ True   ☐ False

ANSWERS

Fill in the blank
1. I or insulin-dependent
2. Pancreas
3. Glucose, protein, fat
4. Glycogenolysis, gluconeogenesis

Multiple choice
5. B. When drawing insulins into a syringe, the nurse always should follow the same order. Typically, the rapid-acting insulin is drawn first.

6. A. The onset of action of rapid-acting insulin occurs $\frac{1}{2}$ to 1 hour after administration.

7. C. Insulin requirements are increased by growth, pregnancy, increased food intake, stress, surgery, infection, illness, increased insulin antibodies, and some medications.

8. B. The patient should administer a once-daily morning dosage of insulin 30 minutes before breakfast or a split morning and evening dosage 30 minutes before breakfast and 30 minutes before dinner, unless otherwise prescribed.

9. D. If hypoglycemia occurs, the patient should ingest some form of glucose, such as hard candy.

10. D. Concomitant use of dicumarol and chlorpropamide may cause hypoglycemia and increase the anticoagulant effects of dicumarol.

11. B. Alcohol and chlorpropamide may interact, causing hypoglycemia or hyperglycemia.

Matching related elements
12. C
13. A
14. D
15. B

True or false
16. False. Although rare, insulin may cause systemic reactions, including hives, angioedema, dyspnea, tachycardia, and anaphylactic shock.
17. True.
18. False. U-500 insulin is the most concentrated; it contains 500 units per ml.
19. True.
20. True.

CHAPTER 25

Thyroid and antithyroid agents

OBJECTIVES   After studying this chapter, the reader should be able to:
  1. Explain the functions of the thyroid gland and the thyroid hormones.
  2. Describe the physiologic effects of insufficient and excess hormone levels and identify pharmacologic interventions.
  3. Describe the pharmacokinetics, pharmacodynamics, and pharmacotherapeutics of thyroid and antithyroid agents.
  4. Identify the major drug interactions and adverse reactions for the major classes of thyroid and antithyroid agents.
  5. Describe the nursing implications of thyroid and antithyroid therapy.

OVERVIEW OF CONCEPTS   Located just below the larynx and anterior to the trachea, the thyroid gland secretes two significant hormones: triiodothyronine (T_3) and thyroxine (T_4). Thyroid hormones regulate growth and development, produce heat by increasing the metabolic rate of body tissues, stimulate the cardiovascular system, and increase protein, lipid, and carbohydrate metabolism. The thyroid gland also secretes calcitonin, which helps regulate calcium.

Thyroid hormone secretion is controlled primarily by thyroid-stimulating hormone (TSH) secreted by the anterior pituitary gland. TSH in turn is stimulated by thyrotropin-releasing hormone (TRH) from the hypothalamus. Circulating levels of thyroid hormone act as a feedback mechanism, telling the body to increase or decrease the hormone secretion rate.

Iodine, a major component of T_3 and T_4, must be present for thyroid hormone synthesis to occur. The daily iodine requirement for adults is 150 to 300 mg. After thyroid hormone synthesis is complete, the hormone may be released or stored in thyroglobulin molecules for up to several months.

Thyroid agents are used as replacement therapy in patients with hypothyroidism (thyroid hormone deficiency) and antithyroid agents are used to treat hyperthyroidism (thyroid hormone excess). (For a

SELECTED MAJOR DRUGS

Thyroid and antithyroid agents

This chart summarizes the drugs most commonly used in treating hypothyroidism and hyperthyroidism.

DRUG	MAJOR INDICATIONS	USUAL ADULT DOSAGES
Thyroid agents		
thyroid USP	Mild hypothyroidism	Initially, 60 mg P.O. daily, increased until desired response is achieved
	Adult myxedema	16 mg P.O. daily; may double dosage every 2 weeks up to a maximum of 120 mg daily
levothyroxine	Mild hypothyroidism	Initially, 50 mcg P.O. daily, increased by 25 to 50 mcg every 2 to 4 weeks; for maintenance, 100 to 400 mcg P.O. daily
	Myxedema coma	Initially, 400 mcg I.V. in a concentration of 100 mcg/ml, increased by 100 to 300 mcg or more, as needed
Antithyroid agents		
propylthiouracil	Hyperthyroidism, adjunct preparation before thyroid surgery or radioactive iodine therapy, thyroid crisis	100 to 200 mg P.O. t.i.d., increased to 1,200 mg P.O. daily for thyroid crisis, as needed; for maintenance, 50 to 200 mg P.O. daily
iodine	Adjunct preparation before thyroid surgery	3 to 5 drops of Lugol's solution P.O. t.i.d. or 1 to 5 drops of SSKI P.O. t.i.d. for 10 to 14 days before surgery
	Thyroid crisis	1 g I.V. of sodium iodide or 10 drops of SSKI every 8 hours, or 30 drops of Lugol's solution P.O. or by nasogastric tube daily
	Hyperthyroidism	3 to 5 drops of Lugol's solution P.O. t.i.d. or 1 drop of SSKI P.O. t.i.d.

summary of representative drugs, see Selected Major Drugs: *Thyroid and antithyroid agents.*)

Thyroid agents Thyroid agents may be natural or synthetic and may contain T_3, T_4, or both. Natural thyroid agents, which are derived from animal thyroid, includes thyroid USP (desiccated) and thyroglobulin (Proloid). Both contain T_3 and T_4. Synthetic thyroid agents are sodium salts of the L-isomers of the hormones. These agents include levothyroxine sodium (Levothroid, Synthroid), which contains T_4; liothyronine sodium (Cytomel), which contains T_3; and liotrix (Euthroid, Thyrolar), which contains T_3 and T_4. All of these agents are used for the exogenous replacement of thyroid hormones.

Pharmacokinetics
Natural and synthetic thyroid agents are absorbed variably from the gastrointestinal (GI) tract. Absorption may increase with fasting and decrease with malabsorption states. These drugs are distributed in plas-

ma bound to serum proteins. They are metabolized through deiodination, primarily in the liver, and excreted unchanged in the feces.

The fastest-acting thyroid agent is liothyronine. Maximum effects occur 24 to 72 hours after oral therapy is begun. The drug continues to work for up to 72 hours after its discontinuation. Its half-life is only 1 to 2 days. Levothyroxine has a much slower onset of action and longer duration of action: its maximum effects occur in 1 to 3 weeks. Liotrix and thyroglobulin are intermediate-acting agents.

Pharmacodynamics

Natural and synthetic thyroid agents act as essential hormones. Their principal pharmacologic effect is an increased metabolic rate in body tissue. They affect protein and carbohydrate metabolism and stimulate protein synthesis. They promote gluconeogenesis (carbohydrate formation from protein or lipid molecules) and increase the use of glycogen stores. By decreasing cholesterol concentrations, thyroid hormones affect lipid metabolism. They stimulate the heart and increase cardiac output. They may increase the heart's sensitivity to catecholamines and increase the number of myocardial beta-adrenergic receptors. Thyroid hormones also may increase renal blood flow and glomerular filtration rates in hypothyroid patients, producing diuresis within 24 hours of administration.

Pharmacotherapeutics

Thyroid agents act as replacement or substitute hormones to treat primary hypothyroidism (caused by thyroid gland malfunction due to reduced functional thyroid mass or impaired hormone synthesis or release), secondary hypothyroidism (caused by pituitary dysfunction or insufficiency that results in insufficient TSH secretion), or tertiary hypothyroidism (caused by hypothalamic dysfunction).

Thyroid agents also may be used with antithyroid agents to prevent goiter formation and hypothyroidism. In diagnostic testing, these agents help differentiate between primary and secondary hypothyroidism. Thyroid carcinoma also may be treated with thyroid agents.

Levothyroxine is the drug of choice for thyroid replacement and TSH suppression therapy because it can be given orally, intravenously, or intramuscularly, and its effects are predictable. Liothyronine is recommended for short-term TSH suppression therapy because of its rapid onset and short duration of action.

Initially, the thyroid agent dosage should be relatively low. Subsequently, the dosage may be increased at weekly to monthly intervals to achieve the desired response. Maintenance dosages must be individualized. Geriatric patients generally need lower dosages than younger adults. Dosages for children age 1 and over may approach the adult dosage because children metabolize thyroid hormone more quickly than adults. Treatment for myxedema, the most severe form of hypothyroidism, may require high parenteral dosages.

DRUG INTERACTIONS

Thyroid and antithyroid agents

Although all thyroid agents can interact with several common drugs, the antithyroid agents produce only one clinically significant interaction.

DRUG	INTERACTING DRUGS	POSSIBLE EFFECTS
Thyroid agents		
levothyroxine, liothyronine, liotrix, thyroglobulin, thyroid USP	oral anticoagulants	Increased risk of bleeding
	cholestyramine, colestipol	Reduced hormone absorption and recirculation
	phenytoin	Increased thyroid hormone metabolism, increased T_4 levels
	cardiac glycosides	Decreased serum digitoxin or digoxin level; increased risk of arrhythmias
	carbamazepine	Increased thyroid hormone metabolism
	theophylline	Decreased serum theophylline level
Antithyroid agents		
stable iodine, radioactive iodine	lithium	Hypothyroidism

Drug interactions

Thyroid agents interact with several common medications. (For details, see Drug interactions: *Thyroid and antithyroid agents*.)

Adverse drug reactions

Most adverse reactions to thyroid agents result from toxicity. Common GI signs and symptoms of thyroid toxicity include diarrhea, abdominal cramps, weight loss, and increased appetite. Cardiovascular signs and symptoms include palpitations, diaphoresis, tachycardia, increased blood pressure, angina pectoris, and arrhythmias. Other manifestations of toxicity include headache, tremor, insomnia, nervousness, fever, heat intolerance, and menstrual irregularities. These effects usually subside when the drug is discontinued. When the regimen is restarted, the dosage must be decreased.

Hypersensitivity reactions may occur and depend on the drug's components. In a patient with adrenal insufficiency, thyroid agents can precipitate an acute adrenal crisis because they increase tissue demand for adrenal hormones. In a geriatric patient, the cardiostimulatory effects of a thyroid agent may produce angina pectoris or a myocardial infarction if coronary artery disease is present.

Other thyroid agents Also known as thyroid-stimulating hormone or TSH, thyrotropin (Thytropar) aids in the differential diagnosis of primary and secondary hypothyroidism. It is administered parenterally 1 to 3 days before serum T_3 and T_4 measurements.

A synthetic form of thyrotropin-releasing hormone or TRH, protirelin (Relefact TRH, Thypinone) also is used in differential diagnosis of secondary and tertiary hypothyroidism. It is administered intravenously after blood is drawn for a baseline TSH level. Blood samples are drawn 30 and 60 minutes after protirelin administration to evaluate TSH levels. Complications of this test may include transient hypotension or hypertension.

Antithyroid agents

A number of antithyroid agents, or thyroid antagonists, are used to treat hyperthyroidism (thyrotoxicosis). These agents include the thionamides—propylthiouracil [PTU] (Propyl-Thyracil) and methimazole [thiamazole] (Tapazole)—and the iodides—stable iodine (potassium iodide solution, USP [SSKI]; sodium iodide, USP; strong iodine solution, USP [Lugol's solution]) and radioactive iodine (^{131}I).

Pharmacokinetics

The thionamides and iodides are absorbed through the GI tract, concentrated in the thyroid gland, metabolized in the liver, and excreted in the urine. Because the thionamides inhibit the synthesis, rather than the release of hormones, their onset of action may take 3 to 4 weeks. However, iodides can decrease symptoms in 2 to 7 days.

Pharmacodynamics

Thionamides inhibit thyroid hormone synthesis by reducing the combination of iodide and tyrosine. Propylthiouracil inhibits the peripheral conversion of T_4 to T_3. All thionamides act as immunosuppressants, which may help decrease the concentrations of thyroid-stimulating antibodies acting on thyroid cells.

Stable iodine also inhibits hormone synthesis, but it does so through the Wolff-Chaikoff effect, in which above-critical concentrations of intracellular iodide seem to deter hormone synthesis. Radioactive iodine limits hormone secretion by destroying thyroid tissue, which usually begins 3 to 10 days after drug administration.

Pharmacotherapeutics

Antithyroid agents are used to treat the most common form of hyperthyroidism, Grave's disease, which is an autoimmune disorder that affects only the thyroid gland. The goal of treatment is to produce a temporary euthyroid state that will allow the autoimmune response to recede spontaneously or as a result of the drug's immunosuppressive properties. Propylthiouracil is the drug of choice in pregnancy because it is safer for the fetus. Because methimazole has a longer duration of action, it is used for once-daily therapy in patients with mild to moderate hyperthyroidism. Therapy may continue for 12 to 24 months before remission occurs.

Stable iodine is used for rapid treatment of hyperthyroidism because it produces effects in 3 days. It also may be used to prepare the thyroid gland before surgery or to control symptoms of hyperthyroidism until radiation therapy takes effect. (Methimazole and propylthiouracil also may be used for these indications.) Radioactive iodine exposes only the thyroid tissue to radiation, eliminates the problems of surgery (especially for geriatric patients or those with cardiac disease), and allows for outpatient treatment. It is the treatment of choice when hyperthyroidism persists after thyroidectomy or when drug therapy has not produced remission.

Drug interactions
Iodide preparations may interact with lithium. (For details, see Drug interactions: *Thyroid and antithyroid agents,* page 355.)

Adverse drug reactions
The most serious adverse reaction to thionamide therapy is potentially fatal granulocytopenia. It typically appears after 4 to 8 weeks of treatment and usually produces a precipitous drop in the white blood cell count and such early signs as sore throat or fever.

The iodides can cause iodism (chronic toxicity related to iodine therapy), which is dose-dependent. Iodism can produce an unpleasant, brassy taste and burning sensation in the mouth, increased salivation, swelling of the parotid and submaxillary glands, headache, rhinitis, conjunctivitis, gastric irritation, bloody diarrhea, anorexia, and depression. These reactions should resolve a few days after discontinuation of iodide therapy.

Potassium iodide can cause tooth discoloration. Thionamides can cause hypersensitivity reactions, such as pruritus, rash, or fever, in the first 3 weeks of treatment. Although rare, the iodides can cause more acute hypersensitivity reactions than thionamides. Thyroid crisis may occur after an acute hypersensitivity reaction, abrupt propylthiouracil withdrawal, or administration of iodine or iodinated contrast dye.

Nursing implications When caring for a patient who is receiving a thyroid or antithyroid agent, the nurse should be aware of the following implications.
• Develop appropriate nursing diagnoses for the patient. (For examples, see Sample Nursing Diagnoses: *Thyroid and antithyroid agents,* page 358.)
• Do not administer a thyroid or antithyroid agent to a patient with a condition that contraindicates its use.
• Administer a thyroid or antithyroid agent cautiously to a patient at risk because of a preexisting condition.
• Monitor the patient closely for adverse reactions or signs of drug interactions.
• Notify the physician if adverse reactions or drug interactions occur.
• Evaluate the patient's response to therapy regularly.

SAMPLE NURSING DIAGNOSES

Thyroid and antithyroid agents

The following nursing diagnoses address representative problems and etiologies that a nurse may encounter when caring for a patient who is receiving a thyroid or antithyroid agent.

- Altered health maintenance related to thyroid disturbances caused by a thyroid or antithyroid agent
- Altered nutrition: less than body requirements, related to thyroid agent-induced weight loss
- Altered protection related to thionamide-induced granulocytopenia
- Altered thought processes related to iodide-induced depression
- Decreased cardiac output related to thyroid agent-induced arrhythmias
- Diarrhea related to the adverse gastrointestinal effects of a thyroid or antithyroid agent
- High risk for infection related to antithyroid agent-induced infection
- High risk for injury related to acute adrenal crisis precipitated by thyroid agent use in a patient with adrenal insufficiency
- High risk for injury related to adverse drug reactions
- High risk for injury related to a preexisting condition that contraindicates the use of a thyroid of antithyroid agent
- High risk for injury related to a preexisting condition that requires cautious use of a thyroid or antithyroid agent
- High risk for injury related to drug interactions
- Hyperthermia related to fever caused by a thyroid agent or thionamide antithyroid agent
- Knowledge deficit related to the prescribed thyroid or antithyroid agent
- Noncompliance related to long-term use of a thyroid or antithyroid agent
- Pain related to angina pectoris or myocardial infarction caused by a thyroid agent
- Sensory or perceptual alterations (gustatory) related to iodide-induced taste disturbances
- Sleep pattern disturbance related to thyroid agent-induced insomnia

---

- Evaluate thyroid function test results carefully because a thyroid or antithyroid agent can affect results.
- Teach the patient and family the name, dose, frequency, action, and adverse effects of the prescribed drug.
- Stress the importance of returning for routine thyroid studies, as prescribed, to assess drug effectiveness and to detect toxicity.
- Remind the patient to store the thyroid or antithyroid agent in a tightly capped, light-resistant container at 59° to 86° F (15° to 30° C) to prevent deterioration.
- Instruct the patient that drug therapy may be needed for months or years.
- Monitor for compliance with drug regimen. Notify the physician if noncompliance occurs.

Thyroid agents

- Assess for a history of pork sensitivity before administering thyroid USP or thyroglobulin, lactose sensitivity before administering levothyroxine, and aspirin sensitivity before administering Euthroid or Synthroid. If the patient has a history of sensitivity, consult the physician about using a different thyroid preparation.

- Monitor the patient's prothrombin time and partial thromboplastin time, and adjust anticoagulant dosages, as prescribed. Instruct the patient to report any unusual bleeding or bruising.
- Ensure that a patient with adrenal insufficiency receives corticosteroid therapy, as prescribed, to correct insufficiency before beginning thyroid therapy.
- Reconstitute levothyroxine for injection immediately before administration. Do not add it to other I.V. fluids. Discard any unused portions.
- Monitor for chest pain or other indications of cardiac problems if the patient is elderly or has a history of cardiac disease.
- Do not withdraw a thyroid agent abruptly in a patient with myxedema because it may precipitate myxedema coma. This medical emergency commonly results from untreated hypothyroidism or abrupt withdrawal of thyroid medication. Its signs and symptoms include lethargy, stupor, or decreased level of consciousness; decreased cardiac output, bradycardia, and hypotension; progressive cerebral hypoxia; hypothermia; and hypoglycemia.
- Teach the patient to recognize and report the signs and symptoms of hyperthyroidism, such as fatigue, breathlessness, and heat intolerance. Also instruct the patient to report any symptoms of thyroid hormone overdose, such as headache, palpitations, or nervousness.
- Remind the patient to take a thyroid agent in the morning to help prevent insomnia and to mimic normal hormone release.
- Teach the patient that different brands of thyroid agents may vary slightly in concentration and that the drug should be prescribed by brand name and dispensed as written.

Antithyroid agents
- Monitor the patient receiving an iodide for signs and symptoms of iodism. Expect to discontinue the drug if iodism occurs.
- Monitor the patient for signs and symptoms of thyroid crisis after administering iodine or iodinated contrast dye or discontinuing propylthiouracil. Be prepared to begin emergency treatment if needed.
- Monitor the patient for signs of toxicity, such as thyroid gland enlargement, and for signs of hypothyroidism, such as depression, cold intolerance, and nonpitting edema.
- Take full radiation precautions for 24 hours after a patient receives a dose of radioactive iodine for hyperthyroidism. Urine and saliva will be slightly radioactive for 24 hours; vomitus will be highly radioactive for 6 to 8 hours.
- Isolate a patient who receives a dose of radioactive iodine for thyroid cancer because urine, saliva, and perspiration will be radioactive for 3 days.
- Instruct the patient receiving a thionamide to call the physician immediately if a sore throat or fever develops. Explain that the patient may need blood tests and a throat culture.

- Advise the patient to take an antithyroid agent with meals to prevent adverse GI reactions. Instruct the patient to dilute potassium iodide with water, milk, or fruit juice to mask its salty taste, and to drink it through a straw to avoid tooth discoloration.
- Advise the patient to consult the physician before eating iodized salt and iodine-rich foods, such as shellfish, and before using over-the-counter cough medications (which may contain iodine) during treatment with an antithyroid agent.
- Instruct the patient that thyroid crisis or thyroid storm may be triggered by excess intake of thyroid hormones, abrupt withdrawal of an antithyroid agent, radioactive iodine therapy, infection, trauma, severe stress, and thyroidectomy (if antithyroid agent is not given preoperatively).
- Teach the patient to recognize the signs and symptoms of a hypersensitivity reaction, such as pruritus and a rash. Explain that such reactions may be treated by switching medications or administering an antihistamine.
- Review radiation precautions with the patient receiving radioactive iodine for hyperthyroidism.
- Recommend that the patient wait several months after radiation therapy before getting pregnant or fathering a child.

STUDY ACTIVITIES

Fill in the blank

1. Thyroid hormone secretion is controlled by _____, which is produced by the _____ gland.

2. The two major hormones produced by the thyroid gland are _____ and _____.

3. Calcitonin, also secreted by the thyroid, helps regulate _____.

4. Thyroid hormone synthesis requires dietary intake of _____.

5. Thyroid hormones _____ metabolic functions throughout the body.

6. Thyroid agents are used as _____ when the body's thyroid hormone level is inadequate.

7. Thionamide antithyroid agents inhibit the _____ of thyroid hormones.

8. Radioactive iodine limits hormone secretion by destroying _____ tissue.

Multiple choice

9. Linda Barnet, age 26, has just begun propylthiouracil (PTU) therapy for hyperthyroidism. After 2 weeks of treatment, Ms. Barnet reports that she still feels weak and has not regained any weight. How should the nurse respond?

    A. "Double the prescribed propylthiouracil dosage."
    B. "The drug may take several weeks to produce effects."
    C. "You need to return to the office for tests for anemia."
    D. "Avoid taking the drug with food to improve absorption."

10. After taking PTU for 2 months, Ms. Barnet stops taking it because her home pregnancy test is positive. Abrupt discontinuation of this drug may cause which problem?

    A. Thyroid crisis
    B. Granulocytopenia
    C. Hyperthyroidism
    D. Cerebral hypoxia

11. Marian Blume, age 67, must take methimazole for several weeks before having a thyroidectomy. Which statement indicates the need for more patient teaching?

    A. "I'll report any rash or itching."
    B. "Fever could mean I'm allergic to the medicine."
    C. "I'll need a blood count if I develop a fever."
    D. "A sore throat is no problem, as long as I don't have a fever."

12. Because Ms. Blume's hyperthyroidism persists after thyroidectomy, the physician prescribes radioactive iodine 4 mCi P.O. For how long after drug administration should the nurse take radiation precautions?

    A. 12 hours
    B. 24 hours
    C. 48 hours
    D. 72 hours

13. The nurse teaches Ms. Blume that she could develop hypothyroidism. Which signs and symptoms suggest this disorder?

    A. Headache and diarrhea
    B. Tachycardia and weight gain
    C. Depression and cold intolerance
    D. Edema and thyroid gland enlargement

14. Susan Jenks, age 58, has hyperthyroidism and takes a maintenance dosage of levothyroxine. The nurse monitors her regularly for adverse reactions. Which ones are most likely to occur?

    A. Nausea, bradycardia, and cold intolerance
    B. Diarrhea, tachycardia, and nervousness
    C. Vomiting, dry skin, and paresthesia
    D. Anorexia, hypotension, and sedation

15. Ms. Jenks also takes the cardiac glycoside digoxin for atrial fibrillation. Concomitant use of levothyroxine and digoxin is likely to produce which drug interaction?
   A. Angina pectoris
   B. Thyroid crisis
   C. Myxedema coma
   D. Arrhythmias

16. Edward Gaines, age 71, is rushed to the emergency department with myxedema coma. The physician orders levothyroxine 400 mcg I.V. Sensitivity to which substance could contraindicate levothyroxine use?
   A. Pork
   B. Lactose
   C. Aspirin
   D. Shellfish

17. Considering Mr. Gaines's age, what is the major risk of giving him high doses of levothyroxine?
   A. Causing angina pectoris or myocardial infarction
   B. Triggering an acute hyperthyroid state
   C. Precipitating an adrenal crisis
   D. Inducing acute hyperglycemia

True or false

18. Basically, different brands of thyroid agents all contain the same hormone concentration.
   ☐ True   ☐ False

19. Iodides can cause iodism, which produces a brassy taste and burning sensation in the mouth.
   ☐ True   ☐ False

20. The nurse should encourage a patient to consume plenty of iodine-rich foods during antithyroid therapy.
   ☐ True   ☐ False

21. Discontinuation of propylthiouracil can cause thyroid crisis.
   ☐ True   ☐ False

ANSWERS   **Fill in the blank**
   1. Thyroid-stimulating hormone (TSH), anterior pituitary
   2. Triiodothyronine (T_3), thyroxine (T_4)
   3. Calcium
   4. Iodine
   5. Increase
   6. Replacements
   7. Synthesis
   8. Release

Multiple choice

9. B. Because the thionamides inhibit the synthesis, rather than the release of hormones, their onset of action may take 3 to 4 weeks.

10. A. Thyroid crisis may occur after an acute hypersensitivity reactions, abrupt propylthiouracil withdrawal, or administration of iodine or iodinated contrast dye.

11. D. The patient may need a throat culture and blood tests if a fever or sore throat develops because they may be early signs of potentially fatal granulocytopenia.

12. B. The nurse should take full radiation precautions for 24 hours because urine and saliva will be slightly radioactive for 24 hours; vomitus will be highly radioactive for 6 to 8 hours.

13. C. Signs and symptoms of hypothyroidism include depression, cold intolerance, and nonpitting edema.

14. B. Common adverse reactions include diarrhea, increased appetite, diaphoresis, tachycardia, increased blood pressure, heat intolerance, nervousness, and insomnia.

15. D. This drug interaction may decrease digoxin levels and increase the risk of arrhythmias.

16. B. A history of pork sensitivity may contraindicate thyroid USP or thyroglobulin use; lactose sensitivity, levothyroxine use; and aspirin sensitivity, Euthroid or Synthroid use.

17. A. In a geriatric patient, the cardiostimulatory effects of a thyroid agent may produce angina pectoris or a myocardial infarction if coronary artery disease is present.

True or false

18. False. Different brands of thyroid agents may vary slightly in concentration. Therefore, the drug should be prescribed by brand name and dispensed as written.

19. True.

20. False. The patient should consult the physician before eating iodized salt and iodine-rich foods, such as shellfish, during treatment with an antithyroid agent.

21. True.

CHAPTER 26

Pituitary agents

OBJECTIVES   After studying this chapter, the reader should be able to:
   1. Identify the hormones secreted by the pituitary gland.
   2. Describe several diagnostic and therapeutic uses of the anterior pituitary agents corticotropin, cosyntropin, and somatrem.
   3. Explain why the patient must be monitored carefully for adverse reactions during corticotropin therapy.
   4. Identify the uses of the posterior pituitary agents.
   5. Describe the interactions between posterior pituitary agents and other drugs.
   6. Discuss common adverse reactions to posterior pituitary agents.
   7. Describe the nursing implications of pituitary agent therapy.

OVERVIEW OF   Also called the master gland, the pituitary gland is about $\frac{1}{2}''$ (1.25 cm)
CONCEPTS   in diameter and lies in the sella turcica. It consists of an anterior lobe (adenohypophysis) and a posterior lobe (neurohypophysis). Pituitary gland secretions are controlled by neurohormones produced by the hypothalamus.
   The anterior pituitary gland secretes six major hormones: growth hormone (GH), corticotropin (also known as adrenocorticotropic hormone or ACTH), thyroid-stimulating hormone (TSH), follicle-stimulating hormone (FSH), luteinizing hormone (LH), and prolactin. GH acts on muscles and adipose tissue, stimulating growth and protein synthesis. Corticotropin affects the adrenal cortex, stimulating growth, triggering cortisol secretion, and increasing protein, fat, and carbohydrate metabolism. TSH regulates thyroid hormone synthesis and secretion from the thyroid gland. FSH and LH are necessary for ovulation, spermatogenesis, and estrogen, testosterone, and progesterone production. Prolactin stimulates lactation.
   The posterior pituitary gland produces two hormones: antidiuretic hormone (ADH) and oxytocin. ADH is secreted in response to hypovolemia and increased serum osmolality; it regulates fluid balance in the body. Oxytocin is secreted in response to estrogen and nipple stimulation, and stimulates uterine contractions during labor and milk ejection during lactation.

Pituitary hormone drugs may be derived from animal proteins or created synthetically. Because the animal-protein agents may precipitate hypersensitivity reactions, synthetic agents are preferred, except when the synthetic agent does not produce exactly the same action as the natural hormone it is replacing. (For a summary of representative drugs, see Selected Major Drugs: *Pituitary agents,* page 366.)

Anterior pituitary agents Commonly used anterior pituitary hormone drugs include corticotropin (Acthar), corticotropin repository (ACTH Gel, Cortigel, Cortrophin Gel), corticotropin zinc hydroxide (Cortrophin-Zinc), cosyntropin (Cortrosyn), and somatrem (Protropin).

Pharmacokinetics
Because enzymes in the gastrointestinal (GI) tract can destroy pituitary hormones, oral administration of these agents is ineffective. Therefore, these agents must be administered parenterally or topically. Generally, the hormones are absorbed and distributed rapidly and are metabolized in the liver and kidneys and excreted in the urine.

After parenteral administration, corticotropin is absorbed rapidly, acts within 5 minutes, and has a duration of 2 to 4 hours. When combined with zinc (corticotropin zinc hydroxide) or gelatin (corticotropin repository), it is absorbed slowly, acts in 6 hours, and has a duration of 18 to 72 hours. Cosyntropin acts in 5 minutes and produces effects for 2 to 4 hours. Somatrem acts immediately and produces effects for several days.

Pharmacodynamics
Anterior pituitary agents profoundly affect growth and development. Under neurohormonal control, they alter the functions of their target tissues. Their concentration in blood helps determine hormone production rate. Increased concentrations inhibit production; decreased concentrations raise production and secretion.

Pharmacotherapeutics
Corticotropin, corticotropin repository, and corticotropin zinc hydroxide are used to test adrenocortical function and to treat adrenal insufficiency. They also are used as anti-inflammatory and immunosuppressant agents (like glucocorticoids), and for their effects on the hematopoietic and lymphatic systems. These characteristics make the corticotropins useful for treating dermatologic, allergic, ophthalmic, respiratory, edematous, hematologic, and GI diseases. Corticotropin also is used to treat the symptoms of multiple sclerosis and to increase muscle strength in patients with myasthenia gravis. It also may be used to treat collagen diseases, rheumatoid arthritis, and acute rheumatic fever.

Cosyntropin, a synthetic form of corticotropin, is used only to differentiate primary (caused by adrenal gland malfunction) from secondary (caused by pituitary gland malfunction) adrenal insufficiency.

Pituitary agents

The following chart summarizes the major pituitary agents currently in clinical use.

DRUG	MAJOR INDICATIONS	USUAL ADULT DOSAGES
Anterior pituitary hormones		
corticotropin	Diagnostic testing of adrenal function	Up to 80 units in a single I.M. or S.C. injection; 10 to 25 units I.V. (aqueous form) in 500 ml dextrose 5% in water infused over 8 hours
	Adrenal insufficiency	20 units I.M. or S.C. q.i.d.; 40 to 80 units repository preparation I.M. or S.C. q 24 to 72 hours; or 40 units zinc hydroxide preparation I.M. q 12 to 24 hours
cosyntropin	Diagnostic testing of adrenal function	0.25 to 0.75 mg I.M. or 0.25 mg I.V. infused over 4 to 8 hr
Posterior pituitary hormones		
vasopressin	Diabetes insipidus	5 to 10 units S.C. or I.M. b.i.d. to t.i.d.
oxytocin	Labor induction	Initially, 1 to 2 mU/minute I.V., increased gradually up to a maximum of 20 mU/minute, as needed

Somatrem is used in children to treat growth hormone deficiency before epiphyseal closure occurs.

Drug interactions
Each anterior pituitary agent can interact with different drugs. (For details, see Drug Interactions: *Pituitary agents.*)

Adverse drug reactions
The major adverse reactions to all anterior pituitary hormone drugs are hypersensitivity reactions. These reactions are most likely to occur with hormones derived from natural sources. Corticotropin also commonly causes the following dose-related adverse reactions: sodium and water retention, impaired wound healing, dizziness, seizures, and euphoria. Less commonly, hypokalemia, hypertension, ketosis, immunosuppression, skin hyperpigmentation, or mood elevation can occur. Long-term corticotropin use can produce Cushing's syndrome. Cosyntropin can cause pruritus and flushing; somatrem, glucose intolerance and hypothyroidism.

Posterior pituitary agents
Commonly used posterior pituitary hormones include all forms of ADH, such as desmopressin acetate (DDAVP), lypressin (Diapid), and vasopressin (Pitressin). They also include the oxytocic agents oxytocin (Pitocin, Syntocinon), and oxytocin citrate (Pitocin Citrate).

DRUG INTERACTIONS

Pituitary agents

Drug interactions with anterior pituitary agents may reduce the effectiveness of therapy or create additional abnormalities. Interactions with posterior pituitary agents can be antagonistic, synergistic, or potentiating.

DRUG	INTERACTING DRUGS	POSSIBLE EFFECTS
Anterior pituitary agents		
corticotropin	immunosuppressants	Neurologic complications
	aspirin	Decreased salicylate levels
	diuretics	Electrolyte losses
	barbiturates, phenytoin, rifampin	Decreased corticotropin effects
	estrogens	Increased corticotropin effects
cosyntropin	amphetamines, estrogens, lithium	Altered test results
somatrem	thyroid agents and androgens (concurrently)	Precipitation of epiphyseal closure
	corticosteroids	Diminished growth response; decreased hyperglycemia and insulin sensitivity
Posterior pituitary agents		
desmopressin, lypressin, vasopressin	alcohol, demeclocycline, lithium	Decreased antidiuretic hormone (ADH) activity
	chlorpropamide, clofibrate, carbamazepine, cyclophosphamide	Increased ADH activity
	barbiturate or cyclopropane anesthetics	Coronary insufficiency or cardiac arrhythmias
oxytocin	cyclophosphamide	Increased oxytocic effects
	vasopressors (anesthetics, ephedrine, methoxamine)	Increased risk of hypertensive crisis and postpartum rupture of cerebral blood vessels

Pharmacokinetics

Like the anterior pituitary agents, posterior pituitary agents are ineffective when administered orally. Therefore, these hormone preparations are given by injection or topical intranasal spray. Desmopressin and lypressin are absorbed effectively after intranasal administration. These agents, vasopressin, and oxytocin are distributed throughout the extracellular fluid, metabolized in the liver and kidneys, and excreted in the urine.

Desmopressin, lypressin, and subcutaneous (S.C.) vasopressin act within 1 hour. Intravenous (I.V.) vasopressin and oxytocin act within 1 minute. The duration of action of these agents ranges from 2 to 20 hours, depending on the agent and administration route used.

Pharmacodynamics

Under neurohormonal control, the posterior pituitary agents affect smooth muscle contraction in the uterus, bladder, and GI tract; fluid balance via renal reabsorption of water; and blood pressure via stimulation of arterial wall muscles.

Pharmacotherapeutics

All forms of ADH are used to control the symptoms of diabetes insipidus, relieve postoperative intestinal distention, and increase the Factor VIII level in patients with hemophilia S or B or Type I von Willebrand's disease. The oxytocics are used to treat uterine inertia, induce labor, and treat patients with preeclampsia, eclampsia, or premature rupture of membranes. Oxytocin also may be used to control postpartum hemorrhage and uterine atony, and to complete inevitable abortions.

Drug interactions

ADH and oxytocic agents interact with different drugs. (For details, see Drug Interactions: *Pituitary agents,* page 367.)

Adverse drug reactions

Hypersensitivity reactions are the most common adverse reactions to ADH drugs and oxytocics, especially those derived from natural sources. Common dose-related reactions to ADH drugs include headache, nausea, nasal congestion, rhinitis, flushing, abdominal or uterine cramps, vulvar pain, and increased blood pressure. Other reactions may include tinnitus, anxiety, hyponatremia, albuminuria, increased GI motility, mydriasis, and transient edema. Nasal preparations can cause irritation, rhinorrhea, and mucosal ulceration.

In the pregnant patient, oxytocic agents may cause postpartum hemorrhage, arrhythmias, GI disturbances, diaphoresis, headache, dizziness, tinnitus, and water intoxication. Uterine hypertonicity, tetany, or uterine rupture may result from hypersensitivity or large doses.

Nursing implications

When caring for a patient who is receiving a pituitary agent, the nurse should be aware of the following implications.
- Develop appropriate nursing diagnoses for the patient. (For examples, see Sample Nursing Diagnoses: *Pituitary agents.*)
- Do not administer a pituitary agent to a patient with a condition that contraindicates its use.
- Administer a pituitary agent cautiously to a patient at risk because of a preexisting condition.
- Monitor the patient frequently for hypersensitivity reactions and other adverse reactions.
- Be prepared to deliver emergency treatment, as prescribed. For example, keep epinephrine 1:1,000 readily available for treating a hypersensitivity reaction to an anterior pituitary agent.
- Monitor the patient for signs of drug interactions.
- Evaluate the effectiveness of the prescribed agent. For example, monitor for decreased urine output when ADH is used to treat diabetes in-

SAMPLE NURSING DIAGNOSES

Pituitary agents

The following nursing diagnoses address representative problems and etiologies that a nurse may encounter when caring for a patient who is receiving a pituitary agent.

- Altered health maintenance related to iatrogenic Cushing's syndrome caused by long-term corticotropin use
- Altered health maintenance related to ineffectiveness of the prescribed pituitary agent
- Altered health maintenance related to oxytocin-induced uterine problems and hypertensive disorders
- Altered health maintenance related to somatrem-induced endocrine imbalances
- Altered protection related to the adverse effects of corticotropin on wound healing
- Anxiety related to the adverse central nervous system effects of a natural antidiuretic hormone
- Body image disturbance related to corticotropin-induced hyperpigmentation
- Decreased cardiac output related to oxytocin-induced arrhythmias
- Diarrhea related to increased gastrointestinal (GI) motility caused by an antidiuretic hormone
- Fluid volume excess related to sodium and water retention caused by a pituitary agent
- Fluid volume excess related to water intoxication caused by oxytocin
- High risk for fluid volume deficit related to the adverse GI effects of a posterior pituitary agent
- High risk for infection related to corticotropin-induced immunosuppression
- High risk for injury related to adverse drug reactions
- High risk for injury related to a hypersensitivity reaction to the pituitary agent
- High risk for injury related to a preexisting condition that contraindicates the use of a pituitary agent
- High risk for injury related to a preexisting condition that requires cautious use of a pituitary agent
- High risk for injury related to drug interactions
- High risk for trauma related to oxytocin-induced uterine rupture
- Impaired tissue integrity related to mucosal ulcerations caused by nasal administration of a posterior pituitary agent
- Knowledge deficit related to the prescribed pituitary agent
- Pain related to abdominal and uterine cramps caused by a posterior pituitary agent

---

sipidus and for return of peristalsis when it is given for abdominal distention.
- Notify the physician if adverse reactions and drug interactions occur or if the drug is ineffective.
- Teach the patient and family the name, dose, frequency, action, and adverse effects of the prescribed pituitary agent.
- Teach the patient to recognize and report adverse reactions. Also instruct the patient to notify the physician if the drug is ineffective.

Anterior pituitary agents
- Perform a hypersensitivity skin test before administering an anterior pituitary hormone. Inform the patient that this skin test must be per-

formed before drug administration. Begin therapy only if the result is negative.

- Observe the patient closely for hypersensitivity reactions during the first 15 minutes of I.V. administration or immediately after intramuscular (I.M.) or S.C. injection.
- Check the urinary and plasma corticosteroid values, as prescribed, to measure the adrenal response before and after administering corticotropin to test adrenal function.
- Match the preparation with the administration route. I.V. infusions of corticotropin require aqueous solutions; I.M. and S.C. injections require suspensions and gelatin solutions.
- Reconstitute all preparations according to the manufacturer's directions.
- Shake corticotropin zinc hydroxide or corticotropin repository before injecting into the gluteal muscle.
- Protect corticotropin solutions from heat, freezing, and agitation to avoid denaturing the protein molecules in the drug.
- Avoid sudden discontinuation of corticotropin to prevent adrenocorticotropic hypofunction.
- Monitor the patient for signs of fluid retention, such as ankle swelling, sudden weight gain of 2 lb (.9 kg), jugular vein distention, and crackles in the lungs, during corticotropin therapy.
- Provide a high-protein, high-potassium, or low-sodium diet and restrict fluids, as prescribed, during corticotropin therapy.
- Monitor the patient's blood pressure and fluid intake and output during corticotropin therapy. Also assess for poor wound healing.
- Refrigerate the anterior pituitary agent for storage but avoid freezing. Use the contents of reconstituted vials within 1 week.
- Monitor the patient's thyroid function and blood glucose level during somatrem administration.
- Inform the patient that a skin test must be performed before drug administration to assess for hypersensitivity reactions.
- Instruct the patient to report immediately any signs of hypersensitivity, such as hives or pruritus.
- Instruct the patient to return for regular laboratory tests, as prescribed.
- Warn the patient that corticotropin injections are painful.
- Inform the patient that wound healing may be delayed during corticotropin therapy.

Posterior pituitary agents
- Obtain a prescription for an antiemetic or antidiarrheal agent, as needed.
- Monitor the patient's blood pressure and heart rate and rhythm to detect adverse cardiovascular reactions.
- Expect to reduce the dosage if the patient develops adverse reactions, such as headache, abdominal cramping, and vulvar pain.

- Inspect the patient's nasal passages for irritation, ulcerations, or rhinorrhea during nasal spray therapy.
- Ensure that a physician is present during parenteral administration of oxytocin.
- Keep magnesium sulfate available during I.M. administration of oxytocin to produce uterine relaxation, if needed.
- Dilute oxytocin for I.V. use in dextrose 5% in water or other prescribed solution. Always administer the drug with an infusion pump, and never administer it by more than one route at a time.
- Discontinue the oxytocin infusion, administer oxygen, and notify physician if contractions become more frequent than every 2 minutes, last longer than 60 seconds, or become excessively strong (exceeding 50 mm Hg) or if the fetal heart rate indicates bradycardia, tachycardia, or irregular rhythm.
- Monitor the patient for signs and symptoms of hypertensive crisis, such as sudden, severe increase in blood pressure above 200/120 mm Hg, severe headache, vision disturbances, and epistaxis, if local or regional anesthesia is administered during oxytocin therapy,
- Monitor the patient for early signs of water intoxication, such as decreased level of consciousness, headache, and vomiting.
- Instruct the patient to clear the nasal passages before administering a nasal preparation, to hold the bottle upright, and to spray into the nostril while sitting or standing with the head vertical.
- Teach the patient how to measure fluid intake and output and to interpret these measurements during ADH therapy.
- Instruct the patient not to increase the number of intranasal vasopressin sprays without consulting the physician.
- Explain the purpose and expected outcome of I.V. oxytocin administration to the patient.

STUDY ACTIVITIES Fill in the blank

1. The hypothalamus produces _____, which control pituitary gland secretions.

2. The anterior lobe of the pituitary gland is known as the

_____; the posterior lobe is known as the _____.

3. _____ hormone regulates the fluid balance in the body.

4. The most common adverse effects of natural pituitary hormone drugs are _____ reactions.

5. Anterior pituitary hormone drugs are used for _____ and treatment of adrenal insufficiency.

Multiple choice

6. Janet Howe, age 52, is admitted for Addison's disease testing. She must receive 40 units of ACTH I.V. over 8 hours. The nurse should expect to use which corticotropin preparation?
  A. Corticotropin zinc hydroxide
  B. Corticotropin repository
  C. Corticotropin aqueous
  D. Corticotropin gel

7. After the I.V. infusion begins, the nurse should perform which intervention?
  A. Perform a hypersensitivity skin test.
  B. Observe for a hypersensitivity reaction.
  C. Keep the patient on bed rest to prevent dizziness.
  D. Restrict sodium and potassium to prevent electrolyte imbalances.

8. Betty Adams, age 38, is treated with corticotropin for exacerbation of the symptoms of multiple sclerosis. Ms. Adams complains that the injections are painful and asks why she can't take the medication orally. How should the nurse respond?
  A. "The hormone is destroyed by GI enzymes."
  B. "The effects of an injection last much longer."
  C. "Oral administration causes more adverse reactions."
  D. "Rotating the injection sites can reduce the pain."

9. The nurse monitors Ms. Adams's response to treatment. Which symptom suggests an adverse reaction to corticotropin?
  A. Depression
  B. Paresthesia
  C. Ankle edema
  D. Frequent falls

10. Ericka Blaine, age 5, begins somatrem therapy for GH deficiency. The nurse teaches Ericka's parents the drug's therapeutic and adverse effects. What is the most common dose-related adverse reaction to somatrem therapy?
  A. Delayed epiphyseal closure
  B. Altered protein synthesis
  C. Electrolyte imbalance
  D. Glucose intolerance

11. Alan Harrison, age 43, has just been diagnosed with diabetes insipidus. He receives a prescription for desmopressin acetate (DDAVP) 0.2 ml intranasally b.i.d. After a patient-teaching session, which statement by Mr. Harrison indicates the need for more instruction?

    A. "My urine output should be about half of my fluid intake."
    B. "I can increase the number of nasal sprays, as needed."
    C. "I won't use my nasal spray while lying down."
    D. "I'll weigh myself every day and record it."

12. Desmopressin can cause which adverse reactions?

    A. Hypotension and tachycardia
    B. Hypernatremia and hyperkalemia
    C. Transient edema and hypertension
    D. Increased thirst and diaphoresis

13. The nurse double checks Mr. Harrison's medication history. Use of which drug could interact with desmopressin?

    A. Methoxamine
    B. Phenytoin
    C. Aspirin
    D. Alcohol

14. Karen Hanna, age 25, has insulin-dependent diabetes mellitus. She is admitted to the hospital in labor. Her physician enhances labor with an oxytocin drip. After 1 hour, which occurrence should cause the nurse to discontinue the oxytocin and notify the physician?

    A. Cervical dilation
    B. Flushing and diaphoresis
    C. Amniotic fluid gush from the vagina
    D. Strong contractions that last 90 seconds

15. After giving birth, Ms. Hanna develops postpartum uterine bleeding, for which she receives a onetime dose of oxytocin 10 units I.M. Which nursing intervention is most appropriate at this time?

    A. Increase Ms. Hanna's fluid intake.
    B. Monitor for early signs of water intoxication.
    C. Keep epinephrine available for emergency treatment.
    D. Administer a vasopressor to enhance oxytocin's effects.

Matching related elements

Match the pituitary hormone on the left with an interacting drug (or drugs) on the right.

16. ___ Corticotropin   **A.** Thyroid agents and androgens

17. ___ Cosyntropin   **B.** Aspirin

18. ___ Somatrem   **C.** Ephedrine

19. ___ Vasopressin   **D.** Carbamazepine

20. ___ Oxytocin   **E.** Amphetamines

ANSWERS

Fill in the blank
1. Neurohormones
2. Adenohypophysis, neurohypophysis
3. Antidiuretic
4. Hypersensitivity
5. Diagnosis

Multiple choice
6. C. Corticotropin aqueous is used for I.V. administration.
7. B. The nurse should observe the patient for hypersensitivity reactions during the first 15 minutes of I.V. administration.
8. A. Because enzymes in the GI tract can destroy pituitary hormones, oral administration of these agents is ineffective.
9. C. Corticotropin commonly causes dose-related sodium and water retention, which can cause edema, crackles, and jugular vein distention.
10. D. Somatrem may cause glucose intolerance and hypothyroidism.
11. A. The nurse should teach the patient how to monitor fluid intake and output, which should be equal.
12. C. Dose-related reactions to ADH drugs, such as desmopressin, include flushing, increased blood pressure, hyponatremia, albuminuria, and transient edema.
13. D. Alcohol may decrease desmopressin's activity.
14. D. The nurse should discontinue the oxytocin infusion, administer oxygen, and notify physician if contractions become more frequent than every 2 minutes, last longer than 60 seconds, or become excessively strong.
15. B. The nurse should monitor for early signs of water intoxication, keep magnesium sulfate readily available, and avoid the use of vasopressors because concomitant use can lead to hypertensive crisis.

Matching related elements
16. B
17. E
18. A
19. D
20. C

CHAPTER 27

Antihistaminic agents

OBJECTIVES After studying this chapter, the reader should be able to:
1. Describe the sequence of physiologic events in a type I hypersensitivity reaction.
2. Explain the mechanism of action of histamine$_1$ (H$_1$)-receptor antagonists and explain how they relieve allergy symptoms.
3. Describe the interactions between H$_1$-receptor antagonists and other drugs.
4. Discuss the major adverse reactions to the H$_1$-receptor antagonists.
5. Describe the nursing implications of antihistaminic therapy.

OVERVIEW OF CONCEPTS Antihistamines primarily act to block histamine effects that occur in a type I, or immediate, hypersensitivity reaction, commonly called an allergic reaction. To understand the action of antihistaminic agents, the nurse must understand the immunologic sequence and the antigen–antibody reaction.

The human immune system reacts to agents that it recognizes as foreign to the host (self). These foreign substances (antigens) stimulate the production of antibodies that help defend the body against bacterial, viral, or other types of invasion. An allergy occurs when an individual has an antigen response to an ordinary substance in the environment. Most people with allergies have inherited an immune system deficiency that makes them more vulnerable than others to foreign substances.

Type I hypersensitivity develops after the first exposure to a protein or other substance that the host recognizes as foreign. This antigen, or allergen, stimulates production of unusual amounts of immunoglobulin E (IgE) antibodies, which normally are present in very small quantities. These antibodies sensitize mast cells (connective tissue cells that contain histamine) and basophils (a type of leukocyte) by attaching to their surfaces. Later, when sensitized cells are reexposed to the antigen, a reaction occurs between the antigen and the IgE antibodies. This antigen-antibody reaction stimulates the sensitized cells to release chemical mediators, including histamine, bradykinin, prostaglandin, chemotactic factors (substances that produce cell movement), and slow-reacting substance of anaphylaxis (SRS-A). The body responds to these mediators by dilating the veins and arteries, increasing capillary permeability, constricting smooth muscles (except arterioles), and increasing the secretions of exocrine glands, such as parietal cells and lacrimal glands.

Histamine is the major chemical mediator in this reaction and is responsible for producing most allergy symptoms. When histamine binds to H_1 receptors on effector tissues (tissues that contract or secrete substances in response to nerve impulses), it produces a wide range of effects. Oronasopharyngeal effects include rhinorrhea, sneezing, and itching in the nose and throat. In the skin, the mediators can produce itching, angioedema, flushing, and wheals. In the respiratory system, they can cause bronchial smooth muscle contraction, bronchial constriction accompanied by bronchospasm, increased mucus production, and decreased vital capacity. They also affect the cardiovascular system, increasing the heart rate, vasodilation, and capillary permeability, and decreasing blood pressure. In the gastrointestinal (GI) system, chemical mediators may increase smooth muscle contraction and parietal cell secretion. In the endocrine system, they may increase the release of epinephrine and norepinephrine.

Antihistamines work to block histamine binding to H_1-receptors. By doing this, they diminish most histamine effects and relieve the symptoms of a type I hypersensitivity reaction. These agent are available alone or in combination products, by prescription or over the counter. (For a summary of representative drugs, see Selected Major Drugs: *Antihistaminic agents.*)

H_1-receptor antagonists

The term antihistamine refers to drugs that act as H_1-receptor antagonists. Drugs that antagonize H_2 receptors are not considered antihistamines and are discussed separately. (For details, see Chapter 21, Peptic ulcer agents.) Based on chemical structure, antihistamines are categorized into six major classes:

- ethanolamines, which include clemastine fumarate (Tavist), dimenhydrinate (Dimentabs, Dramamine), diphenhydramine hydrochloride (Benadryl, Benylin, Compoz, Nytol with DPH, Sominex Formula 2), and phenyltoloxamine citrate (Naldecon)
- ethylenediamines, which include pyrilamine maleate (Nisaval) and tripelennamine (PBZ)
- phenothiazines, which include methdilazine hydrochloride (Tacaryl), promethazine hydrochloride (Pentazine, Phenergan), and trimeprazine tartrate (Temaril)
- piperazines, which include cyclizine lactate (Marezine), hydroxyzine hydrochloride (Atarax), hydroxyzine pamoate (Vistaril), and meclizine hydrochloride (Antivert, Bonine)
- propylamines (alkylamines), which include brompheniramine (Bromphen, Dimetane), chlorpheniramine maleate (Chlor-Trimeton,

SELECTED MAJOR DRUGS

Antihistaminic agents

This chart summarizes the major antihistamines currently in clinical use.

DRUG	MAJOR INDICATIONS	USUAL ADULT DOSAGES
Ethanolamines		
dimenhydrinate	Nausea, vomiting, and vertigo associated with motion sickness; vestibular system disease	50 to 100 mg P.O. every 4 to 6 hours, p.r.n., not to exceed 400 mg/day; 50 to 100 mg I.M. every 4 hours, p.r.n.; or 50 mg I.V. in 10 ml of 0.9% sodium chloride solution injected over 2 minutes every 4 hours
diphenhydramine	Motion sickness; rhinitis and other allergy symptoms	25 to 50 mg P.O. t.i.d. or q.i.d., or 10 to 50 mg I.V. or deep I.M. injection
	Dyskinesias, Parkinson's disease	50 mg P.O. once daily to t.i.d., or 25 to 50 mg I.V. or deep I.M. injection
	Hypnotic effects	25 to 50 mg P.O. h.s.
Ethylenediamines		
tripelennamine	Allergy symptoms	37.5 to 75 mg of tripelennamine citrate P.O. every 4 to 6 hours, not to exceed 900 mg/day; 25 to 50 mg of tripelennamine hydrochloride P.O. every 4 to 6 hours, not to exceed 600 mg/day; or 100 mg of sustained-release tripelennamine hydrochloride P.O. b.i.d. or t.i.d.
Propylamines		
brompheniramine	Allergy symptoms; seasonal and perennial allergic rhinitis	4 mg P.O. every 4 to 6 hours, not to exceed 24 mg/day; 8 to 12 mg of sustained-release tablets P.O. every 8 to 12 hours; or 10 mg I.V., I.M., or S.C. every 6 to 12 hours, p.r.n., not to exceed 40 mg/day
chlorpheniramine	Allergy symptoms	4 mg P.O. every 4 to 6 hours, not to exceed 24 mg/day; or 8 to 12 mg of sustained-release tablets P.O. b.i.d.
	Uncomplicated allergic reactions	5 to 20 mg I.V. or I.M.
	Anaphylactic reactions	10 to 20 mg I.V. or I.M.
Miscellaneous antihistamines		
astemizole	Allergic rhinitis	10 mg P.O. daily
terfenadine	Allergic rhinitis	60 mg P.O. b.i.d.

Teldrin), dexchlorpheniramine maleate (Polaramine), and triprolidine hydrochloride (Actidil)
- miscellaneous antihistamines, which include astemizole (Hismanal), azatadine maleate (Optimine), cyproheptadine hydrochloride (Periactin), phenindamine tartrate (Nolahist), and terfenadine (Seldane).

All antihistamines can halt the progress of a type I hypersensitivity reaction. Some also can counteract motion sickness, vertigo, nausea, and vomiting. Astemizole and terfenadine are longer-acting and produce fewer central nervous system (CNS) effects than other antihistamines.

Pharmacokinetics

After oral or parenteral administration, H_1-receptor antagonists are absorbed well, distributed widely throughout the body, metabolized by the liver, and excreted in the urine almost entirely as degradation products of metabolism. Unlike the other antihistamines, astemizole and terfenadine do not penetrate the CNS.

Their onset of action ranges from 15 to 60 minutes with oral administration and from 20 to 30 minutes with parenteral administration. The peak concentration level usually occurs 1 to 2 hours after administration. (Although terfenadine achieves a peak concentration in 2 hours, it does not reach peak effects for 3 to 4 hours.) For most antihistamines, the duration varies from 4 to 8 hours. For astemizole and terfenadine, the duration is up to 12 hours.

Pharmacodynamics

All antihistamines competitively block the binding of histamine to H_1-receptor sites on effector cells in the small blood vessels, smooth muscles, peripheral nerves, adrenal medulla, exocrine glands, and brain. This blocking action can halt the progression of a type I hypersensitivity reaction but cannot reverse effects that already are present.

Pharmacotherapeutics

Antihistamines are used to treat the symptoms of type I hypersensitivity reactions, such as allergic rhinitis, vasomotor rhinitis, allergic conjunctivitis, urticaria (hives), and angioedema (submucosal swelling in the hands, face, and feet). They also are used as adjuncts in treating anaphylactic reactions after acute manifestations are controlled.

Several antihistamines have a high affinity for H_1 receptors in the brain and are used for their CNS effects in treating nausea, vomiting, motion sickness, and vertigo. Because most antihistamines (especially the ethanolamines) cause CNS depression, they may be used for preoperative sedation or in other situations as sedative or hypnotic agents. In addition, diphenhydramine can help treat Parkinson's disease and drug-induced extrapyramidal reactions, such as dyskinesias.

Drug interactions

When given with other drugs, antihistamines may cause many different interactions. (For details, see Drug Interactions: *Antihistaminic agents.*)

Adverse drug reactions

Used as antiallergy agents, antihistamines produce many predictable adverse reactions, especially CNS depression. Because a predictable adverse reaction may be a desired therapeutic response or a dose-related reaction, the nurse must consider the goal of antihistaminic treatment before determining that an adverse reaction is undesirable.

DRUG INTERACTIONS

Antihistaminic agents

Antihistamines can increase the anticholinergic effects of anticholinergic drugs and the sedative effects of central nervous system (CNS) depressants. The combination of these drugs with antihistamines can cause life-threatening consequences.

DRUG	INTERACTING DRUGS	POSSIBLE EFFECTS
clemastine, dimenhydrinate, diphenhydramine, phenyltoloxamine, pyrilamine, tripelennamine, brompheniramine, chlorpheniramine, dexchlorpheniramine, triprolidine, methdilazine, promethazine, trimeprazine, cyclizine, hydroxyzine, meclizine, azatadine, cyproheptadine, phenindamine, astemizole	CNS depressants, including barbiturates, tranquilizers, alcohol, and opiates	Additive CNS depression
	anticholinergic drugs, including tricyclic antidepressants, phenothiazines, and antiparkinsonian agents	Additive anticholinergic effects
	ototoxic drugs, including aminoglycosides and salicylates	Masked signs and symptoms of ototoxicity
	epinephrine	Vasodilation, increased heart rate, decreased blood pressure

The most common adverse reaction to antihistamines is CNS depression, which can produce sedation and other symptoms. Other CNS reactions may include dizziness, lassitude, impaired coordination, and muscle weakness. Less common reactions include CNS excitation, restlessness, insomnia, palpitations, and seizures.

The next most common adverse reactions are GI effects, which include epigastric distress, loss of appetite, nausea, vomiting, and constipation or diarrhea. Taking the drug with meals or milk may reduce these symptoms.

The third most common reactions are anticholinergic ones, which occur especially with ethanolamines. Dryness of the mouth, nose, and throat and thickening of bronchial secretions commonly occur. Although these effects may be desired, they may lead to airway obstruction in a patient with asthma or chronic obstructive pulmonary disease. Such a patient should use antihistamines cautiously and only under a physician's direction. Other anticholinergic effects include urine retention and dysuria; vertigo, tinnitus, and labyrinthitis; vision disturbances, such as diplopia and blurred vision; and cardiovascular effects, such as hypotension or hypertension, tachycardia, and extrasystole.

Sensitivity reactions to antihistamines occur much less commonly but may include hypersensitivity, drug fever, hematologic complications, and teratogenic effects (effects that interfere with fetal development).

Acute poisoning may occur, especially in children, causing such signs and symptoms as hallucinations, excitement, ataxia, athetosis, involuntary movements, seizures, fever, and fixed, dilated pupils.

SAMPLE NURSING DIAGNOSES

Antihistaminic agents

The following nursing diagnoses address representative problems and etiologies that a nurse may encounter when caring for a patient who is receiving an antihistaminic agent.
- Altered health maintenance related to ineffectiveness of the prescribed antihistamine
- Constipation related to the adverse gastrointestinal (GI) effects of an antihistamine
- Diarrhea related to the adverse GI effects of an antihistamine
- High risk for injury related to adverse drug reactions
- High risk for injury related to a preexisting condition that contraindicates the use of an anti-histamine
- High risk for injury related to a preexisting condition that requires cautious use of an anti-histamine
- High risk for injury related to drug interactions
- High risk for poisoning related to the use of an antihistamine
- High risk for trauma related to the sedative effects of an antihistamine
- Hyperthermia related to antihistamine-induced drug fever
- Ineffective airway clearance related to thickening of bronchial secretions caused by an anti-histamine
- Knowledge deficit related to the prescribed antihistamine
- Noncompliance related to long-term use of an antihistamine
- Sensory or perceptual alterations (auditory, visual) related to the adverse sensory effects of an antihistamine
- Sleep pattern disturbance related to antihistamine-induced insomnia or sedation
- Urinary retention related to the anticholinergic effects of an antihistamine

Nursing implications

When caring for a patient receiving an antihistaminic agent, the nurse should be aware of the following implications.
- Develop appropriate nursing diagnoses for the patient. (For examples, see Sample Nursing Diagnoses: *Antihistaminic agents.*)
- Do not administer an antihistamine to a patient with a condition that contraindicates its use.
- Administer an antihistamine cautiously to a patient at risk because of a preexisting condition.
- Monitor the patient for adverse reactions and signs of drug interactions.
- Assess the effectiveness of the prescribed antihistamine.
- Monitor the patient—especially a pediatric patient—for signs of acute poisoning. Discontinue therapy immediately if they occur.
- Take safety precautions if patient develops sedation, vision disturbances, dizziness, vertigo, lassitude, impaired coordination, or muscle weakness.
- Monitor the patient's vital signs frequently for signs of anticholinergic effects, such as changes in blood pressure, heart rate or rhythm, or respiratory rate or rhythm.
- Take seizure precautions, especially in a patient with history of seizures.

- Administer a parenteral antihistamine by deep intramuscular injection, using the Z-track method to prevent subcutaneous irritation.
- Notify the physician if adverse reactions or drug interactions occur or if the prescribed antihistamine is ineffective.
- Teach the patient and family the name, dose, frequency, action, and adverse effects of the prescribed antihistamine.
- Advise the patient with a severe allergy to carry medical identification that lists the type of allergy, the usual treatment, and the physician's name.
- Review adverse CNS, anticholinergic, and GI reactions with the patient.
- Explain that antihistamines can produce drowsiness and reduce alertness, and that these effects may diminish in 2 to 3 days. Advise the patient not to drive or engage in activities that require mental alertness until the reaction to the drug is known.
- Inform the patient that combining an antihistamine with alcohol or another CNS depressant adds to the sedative effects of the drugs. Advise the patient to consult the physician before taking any CNS depressants, such as narcotics, sedatives, barbiturates, over-the-counter sleep aids, tranquilizers, tricyclic antidepressants, muscle relaxants, anesthetics, or alcohol.
- Remind the patient to keep the drug out of the reach of children and to seek help immediately if signs of acute poisoning occur.
- Instruct the patient to drink fluids, chew sugarless gum, or suck on sugarless candy if the antihistamine causes dry mouth.
- Teach the patient to take an oral antihistamine with food or milk to prevent adverse GI reactions.
- Instruct the patient to take an antihistamine prescribed for motion sickness at least 30 minutes—preferably 1 to 2 hours—before traveling.

STUDY ACTIVITIES   **Fill in the blanks**

1. The major chemical mediator in type I hypersensitivity or allergic reaction is _____.

2. Foreign substances that stimulate antibody production are known as _____.

3. In an allergic reaction, the body responds to chemical mediators by _____ the veins, _____ capillary permeability, _____ smooth muscles (except arterioles), and _____ exocrine gland secretions.

Matching related elements
Match the drug on the left with its subclass on the right.

4. ___ Dimenhydri-   **A.** Miscellaneous
nate

5. ___ Chlorphenir-   **B.** Piperazine
amine

6. ___ Cyclizine   **C.** Propylamine

7. ___ Pyrilamine   **D.** Phenothiazine

8. ___ Terfenadine   **E.** Ethylenediamine

9. ___ Promethazine   **F.** Ethanolamine

Multiple choice

10. Ann Kleinman, age 32, is admitted to the emergency department with a wasp sting that has caused a type I hypersensitivity reaction with skin flushing, hives, and itching. The physician prescribes diphenhydramine (Benadryl) 50 mg P.O. for Ms. Kleinman. How does diphenhydramine exerts its therapeutic effect?
  A. By reversing the effects of histamine
  B. By desensitizing mast cells and basophils
  C. By competitively blocking histamine binding
  D. By noncompetitively blocking histamine binding

11. Ms. Kleinman's condition stabilizes and she leaves the hospital with a prescription for diphenhydramine 50 mg P.O. q 4 hours p.r.n. for discomfort. Ms. Kleinman is *most* likely to experience which adverse reaction to diphenhydramine?
  A. Dizziness
  B. Dry mouth
  C. Drowsiness
  D. Drug fever

12. The nurse teaches Ms. Kleinman how to manage adverse reactions to diphenhydramine. Which action would help control a common adverse anticholinergic reaction?
  A. Take the drug with food.
  B. Take the drug with milk.
  C. Restrict fluid intake.
  D. Chew sugarless gum.

13. The nurse also advises Ms. Kleinman to avoid drugs that could interact with diphenhydramine. Which type of drug is *most* likely to cause an interaction?
  A. Oral contraceptive
  B. Antihypertensive
  C. Loop diuretic
  D. Barbiturate

True of false

14. Sedation may be a therapeutic or adverse effect of an antihistamine.
☐ True   ☐ False

15. Diphenhydramine may be used to treat motion sickness and Parkinson's disease as well as allergy symptoms.
☐ True   ☐ False

ANSWERS

Fill in the blanks
1. Histamine
2. Antigens
3. Dilating, increasing, constricting, increasing

Matching related elements
4. F
5. C
6. B
7. E
8. A
9. D

Multiple choice
10. C. All antihistamines competitively block the binding of histamine to H_1-receptor sites on effector cells.
11. A. The most common adverse reaction to antihistamines is CNS depression, which can produce sedation, dizziness, lassitude, and muscle weakness.
12. D. The nurse should instruct the patient to drink fluids, chew sugarless gum, or suck on sugarless candy if the antihistamine produces the anticholinergic effect of dry mouth.
13. D. All antihistamines can interact with CNS depressants, including barbiturates, tranquilizers, alcohol, and opiates.

True or false
14. True.
15. True.

CHAPTER 28

Corticosteroids and other immunosuppressant agents

OBJECTIVES   After studying this chapter, the reader should be able to:

1. Discuss the mechanisms of action for corticosteroid and other immunosuppressant agents.

2. Identify common clinical uses of corticosteroid and other immunosuppressant agents.

3. Identify drugs that are likely to interact with specific corticosteroid and other immunosuppressant agents.

4. Describe the most common adverse reactions to specific corticosteroid and other immunosuppressant agents.

5. Describe the nursing implications of corticosteroid and immunosuppressant therapy.

OVERVIEW OF CONCEPTS   The adrenal glands, which lie atop each kidney, secrete epinephrine, norepinephrine, and three types of adrenocortical hormones (glucocorticoids, mineralocorticoids, and androgens). Hydrocortisone (also known as cortisol) is the primary glucocorticoid. Like the other glucocorticoids, its production increases with stress. Aldosterone is the major mineralocorticoid. Its secretion is stimulated by sodium depletion in the circulatory system. Although androgens are secreted by the adrenal glands, they are not considered corticosteroids.

Besides their primary uses as anti-inflammatory and immunosuppressant agents, glucocorticoids and mineralocorticoids are used to replace hormones in patients with adrenal insufficiency and to suppress adrenocortical hyperfunction in patients with adrenogenital syndrome. The noncorticosteroid immunosuppressants are used primarily to prevent rejection of transplanted organs. (For a summary of representative drugs, see Selected Major Drugs: *Corticosteroid and other immunosuppressant agents*.)

Systemic glucocorticoids   Drugs in this class include beclomethasone dipropionate (Beclovent, Vanceril), betamethasone (Celestone), cortisone acetate (Cortone Acetate), dexamethasone (Decadron, Hexadrol), dexamethasone acetate

SELECTED MAJOR DRUGS

Corticosteroid and other immunosuppressant agents

This chart summarizes the major corticosteroids and other immunosuppressants currently in clinical use.

DRUG	MAJOR INDICATIONS	USUAL ADULT DOSAGES
Systemic glucocorticoids		
cortisone	Adrenocortical insufficiency, anti-inflammatory conditions	25 to 300 mg P.O. daily or 20 to 300 mg I.M. daily
dexamethasone sodium phosphate	Cerebral edema	Initially, 10 mg I.V., then 4 to 6 mg I.M. every 6 hours for 2 to 4 days, then tapered off
methylprednisolone	Inflammatory conditions, immunosuppression	Initially, 2 to 60 mg P.O. daily; further therapy must be individualized
prednisone	Inflammatory conditions, immunosuppression	Initially, 5 to 60 mg P.O. daily; further therapy must be individualized
Topical glucocorticoids		
betamethasone valerate	Inflammatory conditions, such as corticosteroid-responsive dermatoses	0.1% cream, ointment, or lotion applied b.i.d. or t.i.d.
fluocinolone	Inflammatory conditions, such as corticosteroid-responsive dermatoses	0.01% to 0.2% cream, 0.025% ointment, or 0.01% solution applied b.i.d. to q.i.d.
triamcinolone acetonide	Inflammatory conditions, such as corticosteroid-responsive dermatoses	0.025% or 0.5% cream, ointment, or lotion applied b.i.d. to q.i.d.
Mineralocorticoids		
fludrocortisone	Adrenocortical insufficiency, salt-losing adrenogenital syndrome	0.1 to 0.2 mg P.O. daily with 10 to 37.5 mg cortisone P.O. daily or with 10 to 30 mg hydrocortisone P.O. daily in three or four divided doses
Immunosuppressants		
azathioprine	Prevention of kidney allograft rejection	3 to 5 mg/kg P.O. daily, starting on the day of transplantation or 1 to 3 days before; after transplantation, the same dosage I.V. until the patient can tolerate oral dosing
lymphocyte immune globulin, antithymocyte globulin (ATG)	Prevention or delay of allograft rejection	15 mg/kg I.V. daily for 14 days, followed by alternate-day therapy with the same dosage for 14 more days
	Prevention of graft-versus-host disease after bone marrow allograft transplantation	7 to 10 mg/kg I.V. every other day for six doses
	Management of acute allograft rejection	10 to 15 mg/kg I.V. daily for 14 days, followed by alternate-day therapy with the same dosage for up to 14 more days
muromonab-CD3	Treatment or "rescue" of allograft rejection unresponsive to other therapies, prevention of allograft rejection	5 mg I.V. daily for 10 to 14 days

(Decadron-LA), dexamethasone sodium phosphate (Decadron Phosphate, Hexadrol Phosphate), hydrocortisone (Cortef, Hydrocortone), hydrocortisone acetate (Hydrocortone Acetate), hydrocortisone sodium phosphate (Hydrocortone Phosphate), hydrocortisone sodium succinate (A-hydroCort, Solu-Cortef), methylprednisolone (Medrol), methylprednisolone acetate (Depo-Medrol, Medrol Enpak), methylprednisolone sodium succinate (Solu-Medrol), paramethasone acetate (Haldrone), prednisolone (Delta-Cortef), prednisolone acetate (Key-Pred, Predcor), prednisolone sodium phosphate (Hydeltrasol), prednisolone tebutate (Hydeltra-TBA), prednisone (Deltasone, Orasone), triamcinolone (Aristocort, Kenacort), triamcinolone diacetate (Amcort, Aristocort Forte). The main active ingredients in all of these drugs is prednisone.

Pharmacokinetics

After oral administration, most systemic glucocorticoids are absorbed well and quickly from the gastrointestinal (GI) tract. After parenteral administration (except for the intravenous [I.V.] route), absorption varies. Bound to plasma proteins, glucocorticoids are distributed throughout the body. They are metabolized in the liver and excreted by the kidneys. Their onset and duration of action varies with the dose, administration route, concentration, and patient characteristics.

Glucocorticoids may be short-acting (with a half-life of 8 to 12 hours), intermediate-acting (with a half-life of 18 to 36 hours), or long-acting (with a half-life of 36 to 54 hours). However, their pharmacologic effects can last days, weeks, or longer.

Pharmacodynamics

The action of glucocorticoids is not understood clearly. They may inhibit hypersensitivity and immune responses by suppressing or preventing cell-mediated immune responses. This action also may account for their anti-inflammatory effects and their ability to mask the signs and symptoms of serious concomitant infections. These drugs also affect protein, lipid, and carbohydrate metabolism and enhance sodium retention and calcium excretion.

Pharmacotherapeutics

Clinically, systemic glucocorticoids are used for their anti-inflammatory and immunosuppressant properties. They also are used as replacement therapy in patients with adrenocortical insufficiency and as treatment for vitamin D intoxication, multiple myeloma, and hypercalcemia in patients with cancer that has metastasized to bone. Depending on the indication, glucocorticoids may be administered by inhalation or by the oral, intramuscular (I.M.), I.V., rectal, topical, or intra-articular route.

Drug interactions

Systemic glucocorticoids interact with many drugs and can cause serious effects for the patient. (For details, see Drug Interactions: *Corticosteroid and other immunosuppressant agents,* pages 388 and 389.)

Adverse drug reactions

Systemic glucocorticoids can cause widespread adverse reactions, especially with long-term therapy. (For details, see *Adverse reactions to systemic corticosteroids,* page 390.) Prolonged therapy also can produce cushingoid signs and symptoms, such as acne, moon face, hirsutism and masculinization, cervicodorsal fat (buffalo hump), protruding abdomen, girdle obesity, amenorrhea, purplish abdominal striae, edema, thinning and atrophy of the arms and legs, muscle weakness or atrophy, hypertension, hyperglycemia, glycosuria, renal disorders, mental changes, and lowered resistance to infection.

Topical glucocorticoids

Topical glucocorticoid preparations are available as creams, ointments, gels, aerosols, lotions, solutions, or drug-impregnated tape. Drugs in these preparations include amcinonide (Cyclocort), betamethasone dipropionate (Diprolene, Diprosone), betamethasone valerate (Betatrex, Valisone), clobetasol propionate (Temovate), clocortolone pivalate (Cloderm), desonide (DesOwen, Tridesilon), desoximetasone (Topicort), dexamethasone (Aeroseb-Dex, Decaderm, Decaspray), diflorasone diacetate (Florone, Maxiflor), fluocinolone acetonide (Fluonid, Synalar, Synemol), fluocinonide (Lidex), flurandrenolide (Cordran), halcinonide (Halog), hydrocortisone (Aerseb-HC, Cort-Dome, Dermacort), methylprednisolone acetate (Medrol), and triamcinolone acetonide (Aristocort, Kenalog).

Pharmacokinetics

The topical glucocorticoids are absorbed through the skin in varying degrees and enter the circulation. Then they are metabolized in the liver and excreted by the kidneys.

Pharmacodynamics

The anti-inflammatory effects of the topical glucocorticoids may result from vasoconstriction, interference with polymorphonuclear leukocyte migration, and other actions. These drugs may produce antiproliferative effects on epidermal cells and dermal fibroblasts by reducing ribonucleic acid (RNA) transcription, which decreases deoxyribonucleic acid (DNA) synthesis.

Pharmacotherapeutics

All topical glucocorticoids are used to treat acute and chronic inflammatory dermatoses, psoriasis, atopic eczema, pruritus ani, neurodermatitis, contact dermatitis, seborrheic dermatitis, and exfoliative dermatitis. Because glucocorticoid creams evaporate, they are used on acute, wet lesions. Because glucocorticoid ointments moisturize, they are used on chronic, dry, scaly lesions.

Drug interactions

Topical glucocorticoids cause no significant drug interactions. However, ethylenediamine (a stabilizer in some glucocorticoid prepara-

DRUG INTERACTIONS

Corticosteroid and other immunosuppressant agents

Systemic glucocorticoids and mineralocorticoids produce the same drug interactions, which typically affect electrolyte levels and medication dosages. Topical glucocorticoids interact with few drugs and cause relatively minor problems. Immunosuppressants can interact with various drugs, increasing the patient's risk of infection or causing other problems.

DRUG	INTERACTING DRUGS	POSSIBLE EFFECTS
Corticosteroids		
systemic glucocorticoids, mineralocorticoids	barbiturates, phenytoin, rifampin, aminoglutethimide	Decreased corticosteroid effects
	amphotericin B, chlorthalidone, ethacrynic acid, furosemide, thiazide diuretics	Increased incidence or severity of hypokalemia
	erythromycin, troleandomycin	Decreased corticosteroid metabolism
	salicylates	Increased risk of gastrointestinal ulceration; decreased plasma concentration and effects of salicylates
	nonsteroidal anti-inflammatory drugs	Increased risk of peptic ulcer
	vaccines, toxoids	Decreased response to vaccines and toxoids; increased replication of attenuated viruses
	estrogen, oral contraceptives that contain estrogen	Increased corticosteroid effects
	hypoglycemic agents	Increased blood glucose level in patients with diabetes mellitus
	cholestyramine	Decreased corticosteroid absorption
	isoniazid	Decreased effects of isoniazid; decreased metabolism and increased effects of corticosteroid
	antihypertensives	Decreased antihypertensive effects
Topical glucocorticoids		
preparations that contain the stabilizer ethylenediamine	aminophylline, antazoline, antazoline hydrochloride ophthalmic solution, ophthalmic solutions that contain the preservative edetate disodium	Allergic contact dermatitis, urticaria, systemic eczematous contact-type dermatitis
Immunosuppressants		
azathioprine	allopurinol	Increased blood level of azathioprine
cyclosporine	acyclovir, aminoglycosides, amphotericin B	Increased risk of nephrotoxicity
	other immunosuppressants (except corticosteroids)	Increased risk of infection and lymphoma
	barbiturates, rifampin, phenytoin, sulfonamides, trimethoprim	Decreased plasma cyclosporine concentration
	calcium channel blockers, cimetidine	Increased plasma cyclosporine concentration

DRUG INTERACTIONS

Corticosteroid and other immunosuppressant agents *(continued)*

DRUG	INTERACTING DRUGS	POSSIBLE EFFECTS
Immunosuppressants *(continued)*		
cyclosporine *(continued)*	anabolic steroids, oral contraceptives, erythromycin, metoclopramide, ketoconazole	Increased serum cyclosporine concentration
	digoxin	Increased serum digoxin concentration
lymphocyte immune globulin, (antithymocyte globulin, ATG)	other immunosuppressants	Increased risk of infection and lymphoma
muromonab-CD3	other immunosuppressants	Increased immunosuppressant effects

tions) can interact with some drugs. (For details, see Drug Interactions: *Corticosteroid and other immunosuppressant agents.*)

Adverse drug reactions
Long-term use of topical glucocorticoids may cause striae, telangiectasia, subcutaneous fat or muscle wasting, ecchymosis, and increased skin fragility. Other adverse reactions may include skin reddening, papulopustular lesions, and facial skin eruptions. All adverse reactions are more severe when fluorinated preparations (fluocinolone, fluocinonide, or flurandrenolide) are used or when any glucocorticoid is used under an occlusive dressing. Indiscriminate use of a topical glucocorticoid in or around the eyes may result in periorbital swelling, glaucoma, or cataracts. Percutaneous absorption of these drugs may cause the same adverse reactions as the systemic glucocorticoids.

Mineralocorticoids
The mineralocorticoid drug, fludrocortisone acetate (Florinef), is a synthetic analogue of hormones secreted by the adrenal glands.

Pharmacokinetics
Fludrocortisone is administered orally, absorbed well, distributed throughout the body, metabolized by the liver and other tissues, and excreted by the kidneys. Its onset of action occurs 30 minutes after administration and lasts 1 to 2 days.

Pharmacodynamics
Fludrocortisone affects fluid and electrolyte balance by acting on the distal renal tubule to enhance sodium reabsorption and potassium and hydrogen secretion. The net effect usually is sodium retention.

Adverse reactions to systemic corticosteroids

Systemic corticosteroids—the systemic glucocorticoids and mineralocorticoids—affect almost all body systems, so they can cause widespread adverse reactions. The list below presents the most common of these reactions by body system.

Central nervous system
- Behavioral changes, ranging from mood alterations to psychosis and suicidal behavior
- Insomnia
- Increased intracranial pressure
- Seizures
- Cerebral edema
- Blunted sensorium

Endocrine system (and metabolic functions)
- Diabetes mellitus
- Hyperlipidemia
- Adrenal atrophy
- Hypothalamic-pituitary axis suppression
- Dysmenorrhea
- Altered protein, fat, and carbohydrate metabolism and protein catabolism
- Cushingoid signs and symptoms
- Increased serum cholesterol level
- Inhibited protein synthesis

Urinary system
- Increased sodium and water retention
- Increased potassium excretion

Immune system
- Suppressed immune response
- Suppressed inflammation
- Increased susceptibility to infection
- Suppressed signs and symptoms of infection

Musculoskeletal system
- Osteoporosis
- Aseptic necrosis of bone
- Increased susceptibility to fractures
- Muscle wasting
- Myopathy
- Arthralgia

Gastrointestinal system
- Intestinal perforation
- Peptic ulcer
- Pancreatitis

Cardiovascular system
- Hypertension
- Edema
- Hypercoagulability
- Thrombophlebitis
- Embolism
- Atherosclerosis
- Polycythemia

Integumentary system
- Impaired wound healing
- Hirsutism
- Ecchymoses
- Acne
- Striae
- Thin, fragile skin

Ophthalmic system
- Glaucoma
- Posterior subcapsular cataracts

Pharmacotherapeutics
This mineralocorticoid is used to replace hormones in patients with adrenocortical insufficiency and to treat salt-losing congenital adrenogenital syndrome after the electrolyte balance has been restored.

Drug interactions
Drug interactions associated with mineralocorticoids are similar to those associated with systemic glucocorticoids. (For details, see Drug Interactions: *Corticosteroid and other immunosuppressant agents,* pages 388 and 389.)

Adverse drug reactions

Fludrocortisone causes the same adverse reactions as the glucocorticoids. (For details, see *Adverse reactions to systemic corticosteroids.*) Chemicals used in fludrocortisone preparations may cause hypersensitivity reactions.

Immunosuppressants

Immunosuppressant drugs include azathioprine (Imuran); cyclosporine (Sandimmune); lymphocyte immune globulin, which also is known as antithymocyte globulin (equine) or ATG (Atgam); and muromonab-CD3 (Orthoclone OKT3).

Pharmacokinetics

Because these drugs vary in structure, their pharmacokinetics also vary greatly. Azathioprine is absorbed readily from the GI tract, bound partially to serum protein, metabolized in the liver, and excreted in the urine. It reaches a peak concentration in 2 hours and has a half-life of 5 hours.

Cyclosporine's absorption is varied and incomplete. Because about 90% of a dose is protein-bound, the drug is distributed widely throughout the body. Cyclosporine is metabolized in the liver and excreted in the bile. It achieves a peak concentration in 3.5 hours; its half-life ranges from 10 to 27 hours.

After I.V. administration, ATG's distribution and metabolism are unknown. The drug is excreted in the urine. Its peak concentration varies; its half-life ranges from 1.5 to 12 days.

After I.V. administration, muromonab-CD3 is distributed throughout the body and consumed by T cells. The drug produces an onset of action within minutes of I.V. administration. Little is known about its other pharmacokinetic properties.

Pharmacodynamics

Azathioprine may act by inhibiting RNA and DNA synthesis or altering RNA and DNA. It suppresses cell-mediated immune responses and alters the production of various antibodies. Cyclosporine may act by inhibiting helper T cells and suppressor T cells. ATG may inhibit the immune response by altering T cell function, eliminating antigen-reactive T cells, or both. As a monoclonal antibody, muromonab-CD3 acts by blocking T-cell function.

Pharmacotherapeutics

Immunosuppressants are used primarily to prevent organ or graft rejection after transplantation. Used in combination with corticosteroids, radiation, and cytotoxic agents, azathioprine helps prevent rejection of kidney allografts. It also is used to treat rheumatoid arthritis that does not respond to conventional therapies. Cyclosporine, which always is given with corticosteroids, is used to prevent organ or bone marrow rejection after transplantation. ATG may be used to prevent or treat the rejection of kidney, heart, skin, and bone marrow grafts. It also may be used to treat aplastic anemia. Muromonab-CD3 is used as first-line therapy or to "rescue" allograft rejection that has not responded to other therapies.

Drug interactions

Immunosuppressants interact with other immunosuppressant and anti-inflammatory drugs as well as with antimicrobial drugs. (For details, see Drug Interactions: *Corticosteroid and other immunosuppressant agents,* pages 388 and 389.)

Adverse drug reactions

Because immunosuppressants can produce multisystemic toxic reactions (including hypersensitivity reactions), they should be administered only under close supervision. The primary adverse reaction to azathioprine is bone marrow depression, which leads to leukopenia, macrocytic anemia, pancytopenia, and thrombocytopenia. Azathioprine also may cause esophagitis, mouth ulcers, hepatic dysfunction, alopecia, arthralgia, retinopathy, pulmonary edema, Raynaud's disease, and hemorrhage.

The most severe adverse reaction to cyclosporine is nephrotoxicity, which usually elevates blood urea nitrogen and serum creatinine levels. More common reactions may include hyperkalemia, hyperuricemia, decreased serum bicarbonate level, hypertension, tremor, gingival hyperplasia, hirsutism, nausea, vomiting, diarrhea, abdominal pain, hiccups, and peptic ulcers. Less common reactions include flushing, paresthesia, headache, leukopenia, thrombocytopenia, anemia, hematuria, psychiatric disorders, sinusitis, gynecomastia, conjunctivitis, tinnitus, hearing loss, hyperglycemia, fever, chills, edema, and muscle pain.

The most common adverse reactions to ATG are fever, chills, leukopenia, and thrombocytopenia. Other reactions include nausea, vomiting, infection, diarrhea, stomatitis, hiccups, epigastric pain, abdominal distention, dermatologic problems, hypotension or hypertension, tachycardia, and edema.

Fever and chills are the most common adverse reactions to muromonab-CD3. Dyspnea, chest pain, wheezing, nausea, vomiting, diarrhea, tremor, pulmonary edema, and infection also may occur.

Nursing implications   When caring for a patient who is receiving a corticosteroid or other immunosuppressant agent, the nurse should be aware of the following implications.
- Develop appropriate nursing diagnoses for the patient. (For examples, see Sample Nursing Diagnoses: *Corticosteroid and other immunosuppressant agents,* page 394.)
- Do not administer a corticosteroid or other immunosuppressant to a patient with a condition that contraindicates its use.
- Administer a corticosteroid or other immunosuppressant cautiously to a patient at risk because of a preexisting condition.

- Monitor the patient for adverse reactions and signs of drug interactions.
- Assess the effectiveness of therapy.
- Notify the physician if adverse reactions or drug interactions occur or if therapy is ineffective.
- Teach the patient and family the name, dose, frequency, action, and adverse effects of the prescribed corticosteroid or other immunosuppressant.
- Advise the patient to report adverse reactions to the physician.

Systemic glucocorticoids

- Observe the patient closely for an anaphylactic reaction after drug administration. Keep standard emergency equipment nearby.
- Obtain baseline data, such as chest and spinal X-rays, electrocardiogram, glucose tolerance test, and body weight and blood pressure measurements, before a patient begins long-term glucocorticoid therapy.
- Administer the daily dosage in four equally divided doses or in one single dose in the early morning for short-term oral therapy. (Early-morning administration mimics the natural circadian rhythm of corticosteroid secretion.)
- Monitor the patient's serum glucose level, body weight, blood pressure, complete blood cell count, blood chemistries (particularly electrolytes), and ocular pressure.
- Monitor the patient closely for signs of infection, such as delayed wound healing. Handle all wounds, sites, tubes, and catheters with meticulous care to reduce the risk of infection.
- Observe for and report any emotional changes. Take suicide precautions, as needed.
- Inject an I.M. glucocorticoid deeply into the gluteal muscle and rotate the injection sites.
- Encourage the patient to consume a diet that is high in protein, potassium, and calcium and low in sodium.
- Advise the patient to take the drug exactly as prescribed and never to double the dose or take doses erratically.
- Instruct the patient not to stop taking the drug abruptly. The dosage must be tapered off gradually.
- Instruct the patient to carry medical identification that states the patient is a prednisone user.
- Teach the patient how to reduce the risk of infection. For example, the patient should avoid people with infections.
- Teach the patient the correct way to use the beclomethasone oral inhaler.
- Advise the patient to take an oral glucocorticoid with food or milk to decrease GI upset.
- Instruct the patient to avoid caffeine, alcohol, cigarettes, and products that contain aspirin.

SAMPLE NURSING DIAGNOSES

Corticosteroid and other immunosuppressant agents

The following nursing diagnoses address representative problems and etiologies that a nurse may encounter when caring for a patient who is receiving a corticosteroid or other immunosuppressant agent.

- Altered oral mucous membrane related to immunosuppressant-induced mouth ulcers, gingival hyperplasia, or stomatitis
- Altered protection related to immunosuppression caused by long-term corticosteroid or other immunosuppressant therapy
- Body image disturbance related to the adverse dermatologic effects or abnormal fat distribution caused by long-term corticosteroid therapy
- Diarrhea related to the adverse gastrointestinal effects of an immunosuppressant
- Fluid volume excess related to sodium and water retention caused by a corticosteroid or other immunosuppressant
- High risk for activity intolerance related to muscle weakness or atrophy caused by prolonged corticosteroid therapy
- High risk for injury related to adverse drug reactions
- High risk for injury related to altered metabolism caused by prolonged corticosteroid therapy
- High risk for injury related to an electrolyte imbalance or hematologic disorder caused by a corticosteroid or other immunosuppressant
- High risk for injury related to a preexisting condition that contraindicates the use of a corticosteroid or other immunosuppressant
- High risk for injury related to a preexisting condition that requires cautious use of a corticosteroid or other immunosuppressant
- High risk for injury related to drug interactions
- High risk for trauma related to the adverse dermatologic effects of a corticosteroid
- Hyperthermia related to immunosuppressant-induced fever
- Impaired skin integrity related to adverse dermatologic reactions to a topical glucocorticoid
- Knowledge deficit related to the prescribed corticosteroid or other immunosuppressant
- Noncompliance related to long-term therapy with a corticosteroid or other immunosuppressant
- Pain related to corticosteroid-induced headache
- Sensory or perceptual alterations (auditory, tactile) related to cyclosporine-induced tinnitus, hearing loss, or paresthesia
- Sensory or perceptual alterations (visual) related to indiscriminate use of a topical glucocorticoid in or around the eye

Topical glucocorticoids

- Wash the patient's skin before applying the medication.
- Apply the drug in the smallest amount and the lowest concentration possible. Do not apply a high-potency glucocorticoid to the patient's face, axilla, or groin area and do not use a solution on dry lesions, except as prescribed.
- Administer an aerosol preparation by spraying at least 6″ above the site for 1 to 2 seconds; prevent inhalation by protecting the patient's nose and mouth as well as those of others in the immediate area.

- Apply an occlusive dressing, as prescribed. Remove the dressing and notify the physician if the patient's body temperature rises after an occlusive dressing is used.
- Do not cover clobetasol with an occlusive dressing. This action prevents percutaneous absorption of the drug.
- Apply a topical glucocorticoid cautiously to areas of thin or broken skin, such as around the patient's eyes.
- Inform the patient that the topical glucocorticoid is for external use only and that overuse may cause adverse reactions.
- Teach the patient to apply the drug properly and to use it only as prescribed.

Mineralocorticoids

- Monitor the patient regularly for signs of fluid and electrolyte imbalances, such as weight gain, edema, arrhythmias, mental changes, irritability, and muscle weakness.
- Provide a high-potassium, low-sodium diet for the patient, as prescribed. Also limit fluid intake to 64 oz (2 liters) daily, unless otherwise prescribed.
- Teach the patient the importance of having serum electrolyte and blood pressure evaluations done periodically.
- Advise the patient to control salt intake and to monitor weight daily. Teach the patient to recognize and report signs of edema, such as swollen ankles and feet.

Immunosuppressants

- Monitor the patient closely for hypersensitivity reactions. Keep standard emergency equipment nearby.
- Perform an intradermal test, as prescribed, before administering ATG to assess the patient's risk for severe systemic adverse reactions.
- Document that the patient starting muromonab-CD3 therapy has had a chest X-ray 24 hours before receiving the first dose; the chest must be clear of fluid.
- Monitor the patient's vital signs frequently and monitor laboratory test results, as prescribed.
- Take bleeding precautions if the patient's platelet level falls below normal.
- Administer oral azathioprine in divided doses after meals to reduce the risk of adverse GI reactions. Give I.V. azathioprine as a bolus or diluted in 0.9% sodium chloride solution or dextrose 5% in water (D_5W) and infuse over 30 to 60 minutes.
- Mix oral cyclosporine in a glass container with juice or milk to improve its taste. For I.V. administration, dilute each milliliter of cyclosporine with 20 to 100 ml of 0.9% sodium chloride solution or D_5W immediately before administration and infuse over 2 to 6 hours.
- Refrigerate the ATG solution after preparation. If refrigeration time plus infusion time exceeds 12 hours, discard the solution.

- Monitor the patient for signs of infection. Because the classic signs of infection may be masked, be sure to check the white blood cell count.
- Take infection control measures, such as reverse isolation, as needed.
- Urge the patient to postpone immunizations until after immunosuppressant therapy has been discontinued.
- Urge a female patient to avoid conception during immunosuppressant therapy and for up to 4 months afterward.

STUDY ACTIVITIES

True or false

1. Cyclosporine may act by inhibiting helper T cells and suppressor T cells.
   ☐ True   ☐ False

2. The nurse should apply clobetasol in a thin layer and cover it with an occlusive dressing.
   ☐ True   ☐ False

3. Glaucoma or cataracts may result from indiscriminate use of a topical glucocorticoid in or around the eyes.
   ☐ True   ☐ False

4. The nurse and patient should avoid inhaling the spray of an aerosol topical glucocorticoid.
   ☐ True   ☐ False

5. Mineralocorticoids affect fluid and electrolyte balance by enhancing potassium and hydrogen retention.
   ☐ True   ☐ False

Fill in the blank

6. The adrenal glands secrete three types of adrenocortical hormones:

   _____, _____, and _____.

7. Hydrocortisone (cortisol) secretion increases in response to

   _____; aldosterone secretion is stimulated by _____ depletion in the circulatory system.

8. Systemic glucocorticoids may produce their effects by inhibiting

   _____ immune responses.

9. Clinically, systemic glucocorticoids are used for their _____

   and _____ properties.

10. Immunosuppressants are used primarily to prevent _____.

Multiple choice

11. After undergoing a hypophysectomy to remove a pituitary tumor, Tom Johnson, age 46, develops adrenocortical insufficiency. The physician prescribes cortisone acetate (Cortone Acetate) 25 mg P.O. daily. Which statement by Mr. Johnson suggests that he needs additional teaching about his therapy?

    A. "I'll need to limit how much salt I eat."
    B. "I'll have to avoid people who have colds."
    C. "I'll include plenty of protein, potassium, and calcium in my diet."
    D. "If I forget to take a dose one day, I'll double the dose the next day."

12. The nurse instructs Mr. Johnson to avoid using salicylates, such as aspirin, and other drugs during cortisone therapy. Concomitant use of aspirin and cortisone could cause which interaction?

    A. Increased cortisone absorption rate
    B. Increased risk of photosensitivity
    C. Increased risk of GI ulceration
    D. Decreased cortisone metabolism

13. The nurse also teaches Mr. Johnson about the adverse reactions to cortisone. Which of the following are common adverse reactions to prolonged glucocorticoid therapy?

    A. Moon face, hirsutism, and glycosuria
    B. Ecchymosis, purple striae, and muscle building
    C. Impaired healing, dehydration, and hypotension
    D. Mood swings, protein anabolism, and menorrhagia

14. Amy Downes, age 27, has just received a kidney transplant. During the postoperative period, she receives ATG to prevent organ rejection. Which nursing intervention is essential during ATG therapy?

    A. Preventing infection and bleeding
    B. Monitoring electrolyte levels
    C. Providing a low-sodium diet
    D. Immunizing the patient

15 Marjorie Glenn, age 49, has just received a kidney transplant. To prevent transplant rejection, her physician prescribes a regimen that includes cyclosporine, azathioprine, and prednisone. When caring for Ms. Glenn, the nurse should assess for which primary adverse reaction to azathioprine?

    A. Peptic ulcer
    B. Renal failure
    C. Severe pulmonary edema
    D. Bone marrow depression

ANSWERS

True or false

1. True.

2. False. Clobetasol should not be covered with an occlusive dressing; this action prevents percutaneous absorption of the drug.

3. True.

4. True.

5. False. Mineralocorticoids affect fluid and electrolyte balance by enhancing sodium reabsorption and potassium and hydrogen secretion.

Fill in the blanks

6. Glucocorticoids, mineralocorticoids, androgens

7. Stress, sodium

8. Cell-mediated

9. Anti-inflammatory, immunosuppressant

10. Organ or graft rejection after transplantation

Multiple choice

11. D. As with all systemic glucocorticoids, cortisone should be taken exactly as prescribed. Doses should never be doubled or taken erratically.

12. C. Concomitant use of salicylates and systemic glucocorticoids increases the risk of GI ulceration and decreases the plasma concentration and effects of salicylates.

13. A. Prolonged glucocorticoid therapy may cause cushingoid signs and symptoms, such as moon face, hirsutism, glycosuria, purple striae, muscle weakness, lowered resistance to infection, edema, hypertension, mental changes, and amenorrhea.

14. A. Because ATG commonly causes leukopenia and thrombocytopenia, the nurse should take infection control measures and bleeding precautions for a patient who is receiving this drug.

15. D. The primary adverse reaction to azathioprine is bone marrow depression, which leads to leukopenia, macrocytic anemia, pancytopenia, and thrombocytopenia.

CHAPTER 29

Antibacterial agents

OBJECTIVES

After studying this chapter, the reader should be able to:

1. Identify the classes of antibacterial agents used to treat systemic bacterial infections.

2. Compare the mechanisms of action for the different classes of antibacterial agents.

3. Discuss the clinical uses of the various antibacterial agents.

4. Identify drugs that may interact with specific antibacterial agents.

5. Describe the adverse reactions to the different classes of antibacterial agents.

6. Describe the nursing implications of antibacterial therapy.

OVERVIEW OF CONCEPTS

This chapter describes drugs used to treat systemic bacterial infections. The antibacterial classes discussed include aminoglycosides, penicillins, cephalosporins, tetracyclines, chloramphenicol, clindamycin and lincomycin, erythromycin, vancomycin, carbapenems, and monobactams. (For a summary of representative drugs, see Selected Major Drugs: *Antibacterial agents,* page 400.)

The antibacterial drugs vary in their effectiveness against different microorganisms. A drug's spectrum of activity refers to the number and type of organisms vulnerable to its action. Broad-spectrum antibacterials affect a wide variety of pathogens, and narrow-spectrum drugs affect a few. Antibacterials tend to affect pathogens with similar biochemical characteristics.

Selecting an appropriate antibacterial agent involves isolating and identifying the causative microorganism, and then determining its susceptibility to various drugs. Because culture and sensitivity test results take 48 hours, treatment usually is initiated upon clinical assessment and then reevaluated when test results are complete.

Aminoglycosides

Currently used aminoglycosides include amikacin sulfate (Amikin), gentamicin sulfate (Garamycin), kanamycin sulfate (Kantrex), neomycin sulfate (Mycifradin), netilmicin sulfate (Netromycin), paromomycin sulfate (Humatin), streptomycin sulfate, and tobramycin sulfate (Nebcin).

SELECTED MAJOR DRUGS

Antibacterial agents

The following chart summarizes the major antibacterial agents currently in clinical use.

DRUG	MAJOR INDICATIONS	USUAL ADULT DOSAGES
Aminoglycosides		
gentamicin	Infections caused by sensitive *Pseudomonas aeruginosa*, *Escherichia coli*, indole-positive and indole-negative *Proteus*, *Providencia*, *Klebsiella*, *Serratia*, *Enterobacter*, *Citrobacter*, *Staphylococcus*, and other gram-negative aerobic bacteria	1 to 1.75 mg/kg I.V. or I.M. every 8 hours; dosage adjusted for patients with renal impairment
Penicillins		
ampicillin	Respiratory tract infections	250 to 500 mg P.O. every 6 hours, or 1 to 3 g I.M. or I.V. every 6 hours
penicillin G aqueous	Infections, such as meningitis, septicemia, pericarditis, endocarditis, severe pneumonia, and other serious infections	600,000 to 5 million units I.V. or I.M. every 4 to 6 hours
ticarcillin	Uncomplicated urinary tract infections	1 g I.M. or I.V. every 6 hours
	Complicated urinary tract infections	3 g I.V. every 4 to 6 hours
	Septicemia	3 g I.V. every 3 to 6 hours
Cephalosporins		
ceftizoxime	Infections caused by gram-negative aerobic organisms (except *P. aeruginosa)* and gram-positive organisms (except enterococci) and anaerobes (such as *Bacteroides fragilis*)	1 to 2 g I.V. or I.M. every 8 to 12 hours
cefaclor	Respiratory tract infections, otitis media	250 to 500 mg P.O. every 8 hours
Tetracyclines		
minocycline	Infections caused by sensitive gram-negative and gram-positive organisms, *Chlamydia trachomatis*, or amebiasis	Initially, 200 mg P.O. or I.V., then 100 mg every 12 hours or 50 mg P.O. every 6 hours
	Meningococcal carrier state	100 to 200 mg P.O. every 12 hours for 5 days
	Uncomplicated urethral, endocervical, or rectal infection caused by *C. trachomatis* or *Ureaplasma urealyticum*	100 mg P.O. b.i.d. for at least 7 days
	Uncomplicated gonococcal urethritis in males	100 mg P.O. b.i.d. for 7 days
tetracycline	Infections caused by sensitive gram-negative and gram-positive organisms, *Rickettsia*, or *Mycoplasma*	250 to 500 mg P.O. every 6 hours, 250 mg I.M. daily, 150 mg I.M. every 12 hours, or 250 to 500 mg I.V. every 8 to 12 hours (use only hydrochloride salt form in I.M. or I.V. administration)

SELECTED MAJOR DRUGS

Antibacterial agents *(continued)*

DRUG	MAJOR INDICATIONS	USUAL ADULT DOSAGES
Tetracyclines *(continued)*		
tetracycline *(continued)*	Uncomplicated urethral, endocervical, or rectal infections caused by *C. trachomatis*	500 mg P.O. every 6 hours for at least 7 days
	Brucellosis	500 mg P.O. every 6 hours for 3 weeks with 1 g streptomycin I.M. every 12 hours in week 1 and daily in week 2
	Syphilis in a patient hypersensitive to penicillin	30 to 50 g (total) P.O. in equally divided doses over 10 to 15 days
	Acne	Initially, 250 mg P.O. every 6 hours, then 125 to 500 mg P.O. daily or every other day
	Lyme disease	500 mg P.O. b.i.d. for 10 to 30 days
Chloramphenicol		
chloramphenicol	Serious infections caused by many gram-positive and gram-negative aerobic organisms and some anaerobic organisms	50 to 100 mg/kg P.O. daily in divided doses every 6 hours
Clindamycin and lincomycin		
clindamycin	Serious infections caused by aerobic gram-positive cocci and anaerobes	300 to 600 mg I.V. or I.M. every 6 to 8 hours
Macrolides		
erythromycin	Infections caused by many gram-positive and gram-negative bacteria, including *Acinetobacter, Mycobacterium, Treponema, Mycoplasma, Rickettsia,* and *Chlamydia*	250 mg P.O. every 6 hours
Vancomycin		
vancomycin hydrochloride	Serious staphylococcal infections when other antibacterials are ineffective or contraindicated	500 mg I.V. every 6 hours, or 1 g I.V. every 12 hours; daily dosage not to exceed 2 g
Carbapenems		
imipenem-cilastatin	Infections caused by gram-positive, gram-negative, and anaerobic organisms	250 mg imipenem and 250 mg cilastatin I.V. via intermittent infusion; for more serious infections, 500 mg imipenem and 500 mg cilastatin I.V. via intermittent infusion
Monobactams		
aztreonam	Urinary tract infections	500 to 1,000 mg I.M. or I.V. every 8 to 12 hours
	Moderate to severe systemic infections caused by a wide range of gram-negative aerobic organisms, including *P. aeruginosa*	1 to 2 g I.M. or I.V. every 8 to 12 hours
	Severe systemic or life-threatening infections	2 g I.V. every 6 to 8 hours

Serum aminoglycoside levels

Periodic assessment of aminoglycoside serum peak and trough concentration levels is needed to assess therapeutic efficacy and toxicity. The goal is to obtain a peak serum concentration between 4 and 8 mcg/ml for gentamicin or tobramycin, 4 and 10 mcg/ml for netilmicin, or 15 and 30 mcg/ml for kanamycin or amikacin; and to obtain serum trough concentrations for gentamicin, tobramycin, and netilmicin of less than 2 mcg/ml; for amikacin and kanamycin, of less than 5 mcg/ml. High trough concentrations correlate with nephrotoxicity; high peak concentrations, with ototoxicity and nephrotoxicity.

Blood for serum aminoglycoside trough concentrations should be obtained within 30 minutes before the next dose. Blood for peak concentrations should be obtained 1 hour after the administration of an I.M. dose and 30 minutes after the end of a 30-minute infusion. Each specimen must be dated and timed.

Pharmacokinetics

Aminoglycosides are absorbed poorly after oral administration but completely and rapidly after intravenous (I.V.) or intramuscular (I.M.) administration. (Because of its ototoxicity, neomycin is never given intravenously or intramuscularly.) These drugs are distributed widely in extracellular fluid, are not metabolized, and are excreted in the urine. After I.M. administration, the drug concentration peaks in 30 minutes to 2 hours; after I.V. administration, it peaks in 30 minutes.

Pharmacodynamics

As bactericidal agents, aminoglycosides cross the pathogen's cell membrane to bind with its ribosomes, which process genetically coded information. This inhibits protein synthesis, which is necessary to the pathogen's structure and metabolic activity.

Pharmacotherapeutics

Aminoglycosides are most useful in treating infections caused by aerobic gram-negative bacilli. They also are valuable in treating serious nosocomial infections, such as gram-negative bacteremia, peritonitis, and pneumonia, in critically ill patients. Against gram-positive organisms, aminoglycosides are used as synergistic combinations with penicillins to treat staphylococcal infections. Aminoglycosides are inactive against anaerobic bacteria. Bacterial resistance to aminoglycosides and potential toxicity limit the usefulness of these drugs. Toxic and therapeutic effects can be monitored by assessing the aminoglycoside level. (For details, see *Serum aminoglycoside levels*.) Because the susceptibility of organisms to particular aminoglycosides varies with time and clinical setting, a culture and sensitivity test should be performed before and periodically during therapy.

Drug interactions

Various drugs can interact with aminoglycosides. (For details, see Drug Interactions: *Antibacterial agents*.)

DRUG INTERACTIONS

Antibacterial agents

This chart summarizes significant interactions between antibacterial agents and other drugs. The nurse should be familiar with these interactions before initiating antibacterial therapy.

DRUG	INTERACTING DRUGS	POSSIBLE EFFECTS
Aminoglycosides		
all aminoglycosides	antihistamines	Masking of ototoxicity
	loop diuretics	Increased ototoxicity
	methoxyflurane	Increased nephrotoxicity and neurotoxicity
amikacin, gentamicin, kanamy-cin, neomycin, netilmicin, strep-tomycin, tobramycin	neuromuscular blockers	Increased neuromuscular blockade
	carbenicillin, ticarcillin, azlocillin, mezlocillin, piperacillin	Decreased effects of the aminoglycoside
gentamicin, tobramycin	amphotericin B, cephalosporins, acyclovir, cyclosporine	Increased nephrotoxicity
Penicillins		
all penicillins	probenecid	Increased plasma penicillin concentration
	methotrexate	Increased methotrexate action and toxicity
	tetracyclines, chloramphenicol	Decreased bactericidal action of penicillin
penicillin G (high doses) and ex-tended-spectrum penicillins (azlocillin, carbenicillin,mezlo-cillin piperacillin, ticarcillin)	aminoglycosides	Decreased effects of the aminoglycoside
penicillin V	neomycin	Decreased absorption of penicillin V
penicillin V, ampicillin	oral contraceptives	Decreased contraceptive efficacy, breakthrough bleeding
Cephalosporins		
cefamandole, cefoperazone, moxalactam	alcohol	Disulfiram (Antabuse) reaction (headache, flushing, dizziness, nausea, vomiting, and abdominal cramps)
all cephalosporins	imipenem-cilastatin	Reduced antibacterial activity of cephalosporins
	probenecid	Prolonged plasma cephalosporin concentration
Tetracyclines		
chlortetracycline, demeclocy-cline, doxycycline, minocycline, oxytetracycline, tetracycline	antacids containing divalent or trivalent cations, such as aluminum and magnesium	Decreased absorption of oral tetracycline
	methoxyflurane	Nephrotoxicity
doxycycline, methacycline, oxy-tetracycline, tetracycline	iron salts, bismuth subsalicylate, zinc sulfate	Decreased gastrointestinal absorption of tetracycline
doxycycline	barbiturates, carbamazepine, phenytoin	Increased doxycycline metabolism

(continued)

Antibacterial agents (continued)

DRUG	INTERACTING DRUGS	POSSIBLE EFFECTS
Tetracyclines (continued)		
tetracycline	oral contraceptives	Decreased contraceptive efficacy, breakthrough bleeding
all tetracyclines	penicillin	Decreased bactericidal action of penicillin
Chloramphenicol		
chloramphenicol	oral hypoglycemic agents	Hypoglycemia
	phenytoin	Phenytoin toxicity
	oral anticoagulants	Hemorrhage
	other drugs that cause bone marrow suppression	Increased bone marrow suppression
Clindamycin and lincomycin		
clindamycin, lincomycin	neuromuscular blockers	Increased neuromuscular blockade
clindamycin phosphate solution	ampicillin, aminophylline, calcium gluconate, magnesium sulfate	Solution incompatibility
lincomycin	kaolin and pectin preparations	Decreased lincomycin absorption
Erythromycin		
all erythromycins, azithromycin, clarithromycin	theophylline (high doses)	Decreased theophylline clearance, increased theophylline concentrations
erythromycin, azithromycin, clarithromycin	chloramphenicol, clindamycin, lincomycin	Decreased antibacterial activity
clarithromycin	carbamazepine	Increased carbamazepine level
erythromycin lactobionate	vitamins B complex and C, cephalothin, tetracycline, heparin, chloramphenicol	Precipitation and ineffectiveness of both drugs
Vancomycin		
vancomycin	other nephrotoxic or ototoxic drugs, such as aminoglycosides, amphotericin B, cisplatin, bacitracin, colistin, and polymyxin B sulfate	Increased nephrotoxicity or ototoxicity
Carbapenems		
imipenem-cilastatin	probenecid	Higher and prolonged serum carbapenem concentration
	aminoglycosides	Increased effectiveness against *Streptococcus faecalis*, ineffectiveness against most strains of *Pseudomonas aeruginosa*
	chloramphenicol	Decreased carbapenem activity against *Klebsiella pneumoniae*

DRUG INTERACTIONS

Antibacterial agents *(continued)*

DRUG	INTERACTING DRUGS	POSSIBLE EFFECTS
Monobactams		
aztreonam	probenecid	Decreased aztreonam effects
	aminoglycosides, other beta-lactam antibiotics, such as azlocillin and clindamycin	Increased effects of both drugs
	cefoxitin, imipenem-cilastatin	Inactivation of aztreonam
	chloramphenicol	Decreased aztreonam effects
	clavulanic acid	Increased or decreased effects (depending on organism involved)
	furosemide	Increased serum aztreonam concentration

Adverse drug reactions

The most notable adverse reactions to aminoglycosides are ototoxicity (with irreversible eighth cranial nerve damage) and nephrotoxicity. These reactions most commonly occur in geriatric patients, dehydrated patients, those with renal impairment, and those receiving concomitant therapy with an ototoxic or nephrotoxic drug. Aminoglycoside therapy can cause renal tubular necrosis, resulting in elevated serum creatinine and blood urea nitrogen (BUN) levels. Renal tubular damage usually is reversible after drug discontinuation. The most common adverse reactions to oral aminoglycosides are nausea, vomiting, and diarrhea. Aminoglycosides also can produce neuromuscular reactions that range from peripheral nerve toxicity to neuromuscular blockade.

Penicillins The penicillins can be divided into natural penicillins, penicillinase-resistant penicillins, aminopenicillins, and extended-spectrum penicillins. (For a list, see *Penicillins,* page 406.)

Pharmacokinetics

After oral administration, penicillins are absorbed mainly in the duodenum and upper jejunum. The extent of absorption of oral preparations varies and depends on such factors as the particular penicillin, the patient's gastric and intestinal pH, and the presence of food in the gastrointestinal (GI) tract. For example, penicillin G is inactivated rapidly in the stomach's acidic environment, but penicillin V resists acid hydrolysis and is absorbed after oral administration. Azlocillin, carbenicillin, mezlocillin, piperacillin, and ticarcillin are not absorbed well from the GI tract and must be given parenterally.

Penicillins are distributed widely to most areas of the body. The highest concentrations occur in the plasma, where most of a dose is

Penicillins

Natural or semisynthetic derivatives of the *Penicillium* fungus, penicillins are prepared by chemically modifying a natural penicillin. The resulting drugs are classified by antimicrobial spectrum of activity.

Natural penicillins
- penicillin G aqueous
- penicillin G benzathine (Bicillin, Bicillin L-A)
- penicillin G potassium (Pentids)
- penicillin G procaine (Wycillin)
- penicillin V
- penicillin V potassium [phenoxymethylpenicillin potassium] (Pen Vee K, V-Cillin K)

Penicillinase-resistant penicillins
- cloxacillin sodium (Tegopen)
- dicloxacillin sodium (Dynapen)
- methicillin sodium (Staphcillin)
- nafcillin sodium (Unipen)
- oxacillin sodium (Prostaphlin)

Aminopenicillins
- amoxicillin/clavulanate potassium (Augmentin)
- amoxicillin trihydrate (Amoxil)
- ampicillin (Omnipen)
- ampicillin sodium/sulbactam sodium (Unasyn)
- bacampicillin hydrochloride (Spectrobid)

Extended-spectrum penicillins
- azlocillin sodium (Azlin)
- carbenicillin disodium (Geopen)
- carbenicillin indanyl sodium (Geocillin)
- mezlocillin sodium (Mezlin)
- piperacillin sodium (Pipracil)
- ticarcillin disodium (Ticar)
- ticarcillin disodium/clavulanate potassium (Timentin)

bound reversibly to plasma albumin. Penicillins undergo limited metabolism in the liver. Most are excreted via the kidneys; nafcillin is excreted via the biliary route. The half-life of penicillins is short, ranging from 30 to 72 minutes.

Pharmacodynamics
Penicillins usually are bactericidal in action. Although their exact mechanism of action is not understood, research has shown that penicillins bind reversibly to several enzymes outside the bacterial cytoplasmic membrane. These enzymes are involved in cell wall synthesis and cell division. Interference with these processes increases internal osmotic pressure and ruptures the cell.

Pharmacotherapeutics
No other class of antibacterial agents provides as wide a spectrum of antimicrobial activity as the penicillins. Natural penicillins and their derivatives are used to treat common infections. Their low incidence of serious toxicity and their relatively low cost make penicillins the drugs of choice for eradicating susceptible organisms in nonallergic patients. Concurrent administration of probenecid increases the penicillin serum concentration by 50% to 100%, making probenecid-penicillin therapy useful in treating bacterial endocarditis and acute gonorrhea.

Cephalosporins

The following list shows the specific drugs in each cephalosporin generation.

First-generation
- cefadroxil monohydrate (Duricef, Ultracef)
- cefazolin sodium (Ancef, Kefzol)
- cephalexin monohydrate (Keflex)
- cephalothin sodium (Keflin)
- cephapirin sodium (Cefadyl)
- cephradine (Anspor, Velosef)
- loracarbef (Lorabid)

Second-generation
- cefaclor (Ceclor)
- cefamandole nafate (Mandol)
- cefmetazole sodium (Zefazone)
- cefonicid sodium (Monocid)
- ceforanide (Precef)

- cefoxitin sodium (Mefoxin)
- cefprozil (Cefzil)
- cefuroxime axetil (Ceftin)
- cefuroxime sodium (Zinacef)

Third-generation
- cefixime (Suprax)
- cefoperazone sodium (Cefobid)
- cefotaxime sodium (Claforan)
- cefotetan disodium (Cefotan)
- ceftazidime (Fortaz, Tazicef, Tazidime)
- ceftizoxime sodium (Cefizox)
- ceftriaxone sodium (Rocephin)
- moxalactam disodium (Moxam)

Drug interactions
Penicillins can interact with other antibacterial agents as well as some other drugs. (For details, see Drug Interactions: *Antibacterial agents,* pages 403 to 405.)

Adverse drug reactions
Hypersensitivity reactions, including anaphylactic reactions, serum sickness, drug fever, and skin rashes, are the major adverse reactions to penicillins. Large doses, prolonged therapy, and parenteral therapy can increase the risk of allergic reactions.

Other adverse reactions may include neurotoxicity (seizures, coma), nephrotoxicity (renal failure and interstitial nephritis), hypernatremia and hyperkalemia (when disodium salt forms are administered), hematologic reactions (hemolytic anemia and platelet dysfunction), hepatotoxicity, and anaphylactic shock.

Cephalosporins
Cephalosporins are classified into generations based on their antibacterial spectra of activity. (For a listing, see *Cephalosporins.*)

Pharmacokinetics
A few cephalosporins are administered orally. Those that are not absorbed from the GI tract must be administered parenterally; I.M. injections may be painful. After absorption, cephalosporins are distributed widely to tissues, although not to the central nervous system (CNS). Many cephalosporins are not metabolized at all. All are excreted primarily unchanged in the urine, except for cefoperazone and ceftriaxone, which are excreted in the feces.

Pharmacodynamics

Like the penicillins, these beta-lactam antibacterials interfere with cell wall synthesis. Rapidly growing organisms are most susceptible to these antibacterials.

Pharmacotherapeutics

Cephalosporins are among the most prescribed antibacterials because they are effective and tolerated well. Their major disadvantages are their cost and the emergence of gram-negative bacterial resistance.

All cephalosporins are ineffective against enterococci (such as *Streptococcus faecalis*), methicillin-resistant staphylococci, and beta-hemolytic streptococci. However, they are the drugs of choice to treat serious *Klebsiella* infections. They also are used widely in surgical prophylaxis. Cephalosporins are used to treat infections involving the respiratory tract, skin, soft tissues, bones, joints, and urinary tract.

First-generation cephalosporins can be used as alternative therapy in patients allergic to penicillin. They also are used to treat staphylococcal and streptococcal infections, including pneumonia, cellulitis, and osteomyelitis. Second-generation cephalosporins are used to treat polymicrobial infections, such as foot ulcers in patients with diabetes, nosocomial aspiration pneumonias, and pelvic and intra-abdominal infections. Third-generation cephalosporins are the drugs of choice for infections caused by *Acinetobacter* and anaerobic organisms.

Drug interactions

Cephalosporins can interact with alcohol and other drugs. (For details, see Drug interactions: *Antibacterial agents,* pages 403 to 405.)

Adverse drug reactions

Cephalosporins are relatively safe. However, adverse reactions increase from first-generation to third-generation drugs. Hypersensitivity reactions are the most common systemic adverse reactions to cephalosporins. Because of structural similarities between penicillins and cephalosporins, a 5% to 10% cross-sensitivity exists.

I.M. administration may cause pain, induration, and tenderness at the injection site; I.V. administration can cause thrombophlebitis. Oral cephalosporins commonly cause nausea, vomiting, and diarrhea, which may be alleviated by administering the drug with food.

Cephalosporins may produce nephrotoxicity. High dosages can lead to acute tubular necrosis; usual dosages can be nephrotoxic in patients with renal disease. Cephalosporin use also may lead to superinfection, producing such problems as diarrhea, sore mouth (oral thrush), and vaginal itching.

Tetracyclines Short-acting tetracyclines include chlortetracycline hydrochloride (Aureomycin 3%), oxytetracycline hydrochloride (Terramycin), and tetracycline hydrochloride (Achromycin, Sumycin). One intermediate-acting compound is demeclocycline hydrochloride (Declomycin).

Long-acting tetracyclines include doxycycline hyclate (Vibramycin) and minocycline hydrochloride (Minocin).

Pharmacokinetics
After oral administration, tetracyclines are absorbed from the duodenum. Absorption is impaired by intake of dairy products; it also is reduced drastically by the concomitant use of iron preparations or antacids that contain calcium, magnesium, or aluminum salts. Doxycycline and minocycline should be taken with food to minimize GI irritation. Other tetracyclines should be taken on an empty stomach because food can adversely affect their absorption.

The tetracyclines are distributed widely into body tissues and fluids, undergo little or no metabolism, and (except for doxycycline and minocycline) are excreted primarily by the kidneys. Oral drug administration results in detectable serum concentrations in 30 minutes; peak concentrations are reached in 1 to 4 hours.

Pharmacodynamics
Tetracyclines are primarily bacteriostatic. Like the aminoglycosides, they interfere with protein synthesis in the bacteria.

Pharmacotherapeutics
Tetracyclines provide a broad spectrum of activity against gram-positive, gram-negative, aerobic, and anaerobic bacteria as well as spirochetes, mycoplasmas, rickettsiae, chlamydiae, and some protozoa. Doxycycline and minocycline typically are effective against more bacteria than other tetracyclines.

Although tetracyclines are among the most commonly prescribed antibacterials in the world, tetracyclines rarely are considered the drugs of choice for most common bacterial infections. Overuse of tetracyclines has led to the emergence of tetracycline-resistant bacteria.

Drug interactions
Tetracyclines may interact with numerous drugs. (For details, see Drug Interactions: *Antibacterial agents,* pages 403 to 405.) Except for doxycycline and minocycline, they also may interact with milk and milk products, which bind with these drugs and prevent their absorption.

Adverse drug reactions
Tetracyclines produce many of the same adverse reactions as other antibacterials, such as superinfection (overgrowth of tetracycline-resistant organisms) and GI disturbances. Because these drugs can discolor tooth enamel and disrupt bone growth, they are not recommended for children under age 8 or for pregnant patients. Other adverse reactions may include photosensitivity, hepatotoxicity, and nephrotoxicity in patients with renal failure.

Chloramphenicol

Drugs in this class include chloramphenicol (Chloromycetin), chloramphenicol palmitate (Chloromycetin Palmitate), and chloramphenicol sodium succinate (Chloromycetin Sodium Succinate).

Pharmacokinetics
Chloramphenicol is available for oral, I.V., or topical administration. When administered orally, the drug is absorbed rapidly and completely from the GI tract; its absorption is not impaired by the presence of food or antacids. It is distributed widely throughout the body, metabolized primarily by the liver, and excreted in the urine. Serum concentration peaks 2 to 3 hours after oral administration.

Pharmacodynamics
Chloramphenicol usually is bacteriostatic and may be bactericidal against some organisms. It inhibits protein synthesis in susceptible organisms and in cells that proliferate rapidly, such as bone marrow cells. This inhibition can lead to bone marrow suppression.

Pharmacotherapeutics
Chloramphenicol usually is reserved for treating serious infections and infections caused by ampicillin-resistant *Haemophilus influenzae*. Chloramphenicol is extremely effective against anaerobic bacteria and is the drug of choice for treating ampicillin-resistant typhoid fever and systemic *Salmonella* infections. Topical chloramphenicol is used to treat eye and external ear infections.

Drug interactions
Chloramphenicol may interact with oral hypoglycemic agents, phenytoin, and other drugs. (For details, see Drug Interactions: *Antibacterial agents,* pages 403 to 405.)

Adverse drug reactions
The use of chloramphenicol is limited by its potential toxicities. Bone marrow suppression, the most toxic reaction, produces reversible granulocytopenia, reticulocytopenia, anemia, leukopenia, and thrombocytopenia. Other adverse reactions include GI distress, aplastic anemia (which usually is irreversible), and hypersensitivity reactions. Gray syndrome, a potentially fatal adverse reaction, is most common in neonates. This syndrome causes abdominal distention, vomiting, anorexia, tachypnea, cyanosis, green stools, lethargy, and an ashen color. These reactions are followed by circulatory collapse and death.

Clindamycin and lincomycin

Clindamycin hydrochloride (Cleocin HCl), clindamycin palmitate hydrochloride (Cleocin Pediatric), clindamycin phosphate (Cleocin Phosphate), and lincomycin hydrochloride (Lincocin) comprise this drug class.

Pharmacokinetics
These drugs can be administered by the oral, I.M., or I.V. routes. After oral administration, clindamycin is absorbed well and distributed wide-

ly in the body. Lincomycin absorption is slower and less extensive, especially if food is present in the GI tract. Both drugs are metabolized in the liver before undergoing renal and biliary excretion. Oral clindamycin's peak concentration is reached earlier and is at least twice as high as that of lincomycin.

Pharmacodynamics
Clindamycin and lincomycin inhibit bacterial protein synthesis. They may compete for the same binding sites on bacterial ribosomes.

Pharmacotherapeutics
Because of its greater activity, enhanced absorption properties, and smaller potential for toxicity, clindamycin is preferred over lincomycin. However, because of its potential for serious toxicity and for pseudomembranous colitis, clindamycin's use is limited to a few clinical indications where safer, alternative antibacterials are not available, such as anaerobic intra-abdominal or pleuropulmonary infections caused by *Bacteroides fragilis.*

Drug interactions
Clindamycin and lincomycin may interact with various drugs. (For details, see Drug Interactions: *Antibacterial agents,* pages 403 to 405.)

Adverse drug reactions
Severe and even fatal reactions to clindamycin and lincomycin can occur. During clindamycin therapy, diarrhea occurs in about 80% of patients. It may begin a few days after initiation of therapy or days to weeks after the drug is discontinued, and it can be severe. Pseudomembranous colitis and hypersensitivity reactions also may occur in patients receiving clindamycin or lincomycin.

Macrolides Drugs in this class include erythromycin derivatives, such as erythromycin (E-Mycin, Ery-Tab), erythromycin estolate (Ilosone), erythromycin ethylsuccinate (E.E.S., Pediamycin), erythromycin glucceptate (Ilotycin), erythromycin lactobionate (Erythrocin Lactobionate), and erythromycin stearate (Erythrocin), and two new macrolides, azithromycin (Zithromax) and clarithromycin (Biaxin).

Pharmacokinetics
Because gastric acid destroys erythromycin, oral preparations are made with an acid-resistant coating that delays drug dissolution until it reaches the small intestine. Erythromycin is distributed well to most tissues and body fluids, metabolized by the liver, and excreted in the bile in high concentrations. The mean peak serum concentration occurs 2 to 4 hours after a single 250-mg dose in a fasting patient.

After oral administration, azithromycin and clarithromycin are absorbed rapidly from the GI tract and are distributed widely. Their metabolism is not known fully. Azithromycin is excreted unchanged in the bile with a small amount excreted in the urine. Clarithromycin and its active metabolite are excreted by the kidneys.

Pharmacodynamics

Macrolides act on the organism's ribosomal subunit to inhibit RNA-dependent protein synthesis.

Pharmacotherapeutics

Erythromycin provides a broad spectrum of antimicrobial activity against gram-positive and gram-negative bacteria. In patients who are allergic to penicillin, erythromycin is effective for infections caused by group A beta-hemolytic streptococci or *Streptococcus pneumoniae.* Because this highly effective drug is considered one of the safest antibiotics, its clinical indications continue to increase.

Azithromycin provides a broad spectrum of antimicrobial activity against gram-positive and gram-negative bacteria, including *Mycobacterium, Treponema, Mycoplasma,* and *Chlamydia.* It also is effective against pneumococci and groups C, F, and G *Streptococcus* and may be used to treat *Staphylococcus aureus* and *H. influenzae.*

Clarithromycin is a broad-spectrum antibacterial agent that has been shown to be active against gram-positive aerobes, such as *Staphylococcus aureus, Streptococcus pneumonia,* and *Streptococcus pyogenes;* gram-negative aerobes, such as *H. influenzae* and *Moraxella catarrhalis;* and other aerobes, such as *Mycoplasma pneumoniae.*

Drug interactions

Concurrent use of erythromycin with various other drugs can produce a wide range of interactions. (For details, see Drug Interactions: *Antibacterial agents,* pages 403 to 405.)

Adverse drug reactions

Few adverse reactions are associated with erythromycin. Dose-related GI reactions (epigastric distress, nausea, vomiting, and diarrhea) are the most common. Allergic reactions, including rash, fever, and anaphylaxis, can occur.

Azithromycin and clarithromycin cause fewer adverse GI reactions than erythromycin. Less common adverse reactions to azithromycin include palpitations, chest pain, vaginal moniliasis, nephritis, CNS disturbances, fatigue, rash, photosensitivity, angioedema, and cholestatic jaundice. Less common reactions to clarithromycin include abnormal taste and headache.

Vancomycin Vancomycin may take one of two forms: vancomycin hydrochloride (Vancocin) and vancomycin hydrochloride pulvules.

Pharmacokinetics

Because vancomycin is absorbed poorly from the GI tract, it usually is administered by intermittent I.V. infusions over 30 to 60 minutes to treat systemic infections. (Rapid or bolus administration is dangerous and can cause flushing and anaphylactic reactions.) Vancomycin diffuses well into pleural, pericardial, synovial, and ascitic fluids. Its metabolism is unknown. About 85% of a dose is excreted unchanged in the urine within 24 hours.

Peak serum concentrations of vancomycin occur 1 to 2 hours after I.V. administration. Because high and potentially toxic serum concentrations of vancomycin can occur in patients with renal insufficiency, dosage adjustments must be made.

Pharmacodynamics
Vancomycin has a narrow spectrum of antibacterial activity. It inhibits the synthesis of peptidoglycan, the major structural component of the bacterial cell wall. After the cell wall is damaged, the body's natural defenses can attack the organism.

Pharmacotherapeutics
Vancomycin is active against gram-positive organisms. When used with an aminoglycoside, it is the treatment of choice for enterococcal endocarditis in patients who are allergic to penicillin. I.V. vancomycin is the treatment of choice for patients with serious staphylococcal infections; infections caused by methicillin-, oxacillin-, nafcillin-, or cephalosporin-resistant organisms; or intolerance to those drugs.

Drug interactions
When administered with other nephrotoxic or ototoxic drugs, vancomycin increases the risk of toxicity. (For details, see Drug Interactions: *Antibacterial agents,* pages 403 to 405.)

Adverse drug reactions
Ototoxicity is the most serious reaction to parenteral vancomycin. It is most likely to affect patients with renal impairment and those receiving long-term, high-dose therapy. Tinnitus may precede deafness and necessitates drug discontinuation.

Parenteral vancomycin must be administered intravenously only. Pain and thrombophlebitis may result from I.V. administration. Hypotensive reactions may be caused by rapid infusion and may be accompanied by a maculopapular or erythematous rash. Hypersensitivity reactions occur in 5% to 10% of patients receiving vancomycin.

Carbapenems
Imipenem-cilastatin sodium (Primaxin) is the first of a new class of beta-lactam antibacterials called carbapenems.

Pharmacokinetics
After parenteral administration, imipenem-cilastatin is absorbed well and distributed widely. It is metabolized by several mechanisms and excreted primarily in the urine. With I.V. administration, the drug's half-life is about 1 hour; with I.M. administration, it is about 2 to 3 hours. In patients with decreased renal function, the serum half-life increases.

Therefore, the drug dose should be reduced when the patient's creatinine clearance falls below 30 ml/minute.

Pharmacodynamics
Imipenem-cilastatin usually is bactericidal. It inhibits mucopeptide synthesis in the bacterial cell wall.

Pharmacotherapeutics
This combination drug's spectrum of activity is broader than that of any other antibacterial studied to date and includes gram-positive, gram-negative, and anaerobic organisms. It may be used to treat mixed aerobic and anaerobic infections, serious nosocomial infections, and infections in immunocompromised patients.

Drug interactions
Imipenem-cilastatin produces a few significant drug interactions. (For details, see Drug Interactions: *Antibacterial agents,* pages 403 to 405.)

Adverse drug reactions
Adverse reactions to imipenem-cilastatin are neither common nor particularly serious. The most common adverse reactions include nausea, vomiting, and diarrhea.

Monobactams

Aztreonam (Azactam) is the first member of a new class of monobactam antibiotics, which have a unique monocyclic beta-lactam ring.

Pharmacokinetics
After parenteral administration, aztreonam is absorbed completely, distributed widely, metabolized partially, and excreted primarily in the urine. Serum concentrations usually peak within 1 hour after an I.M. injection.

Pharmacodynamics
Aztreonam binds to the penicillin-binding protein of susceptible gram-negative bacteria. This inhibits cell wall division and causes lysis.

Pharmacotherapeutics
Aztreonam has a narrow spectrum of activity that includes many gram-negative aerobic bacteria. It is used to treat a variety of complicated and uncomplicated infections. It should not be used alone for empiric therapy in seriously ill patients if the infection may be caused by gram-positive or mixed aerobic-anaerobic bacteria.

Drug interactions
Several drugs may interact with aztreonam. (For details, see Drug Interactions: *Antibacterial agents,* pages 403 to 405.)

Adverse drug reactions
Adverse reactions to aztreonam are similar to those of other beta-lactam antibiotics. The drug usually is tolerated well. The most common GI reactions include diarrhea, nausea, and vomiting. Hematologic

reactions range from leukopenia to anemia. Although aztreonam does not appear to be nephrotoxic, it can cause a transient increase in the BUN or serum creatinine level. The drug also may cause various cardiovascular, CNS, dermatologic, and hypersensitivity reactions.

Nursing implications When caring for a patient who is receiving an antibacterial agent, the nurse should be aware of the following implications.

- Develop appropriate nursing diagnoses for the patient. (For examples, see Sample Nursing Diagnoses: *Antibacterial agents,* page 416.)
- Do not administer an antibacterial agent to a patient with a condition that contraindicates its use.
- Administer an antibacterial agent cautiously to a patient at risk because of a preexisting condition.
- Monitor the patient closely for adverse reactions—including hypersensitivity reactions—and signs of drug interactions during antibacterial therapy.
- Keep standard emergency equipment nearby when administering an antibacterial agent that can cause a hypersensitivity reaction.
- Notify the physician if adverse reactions or drug interactions occur.
- Obtain blood, urine, sputum, or wound specimens, as prescribed, for culture and sensitivity testing before administering an antibacterial agent.
- Teach the patient and family the name, dose, frequency, action, and adverse effects of the prescribed antibacterial agent.
- Instruct the patient to take the antibacterial agent for the full amount of time prescribed.
- Teach the patient to recognize and report signs of superinfection, such as diarrhea, sore mouth (oral thrush), and vaginal itching.
- Advise the patient to consume yogurt or buttermilk, which replenishes normal GI flora, to prevent intestinal superinfection; a patient taking an oral antibacterial agent should do so at least 2 hours after taking a dose.
- Stress the importance of keeping follow-up appointments and having laboratory tests done, as prescribed, to evaluate drug effectiveness or detect adverse reactions.
- Monitor I.V. sites routinely for signs of thrombophlebitis, such as localized redness, swelling, and pain.
- Instruct the patient to notify the physician if adverse reactions occur or if the condition persists or worsens.

Aminoglycosides

- Monitor the patient's serum aminoglycoside level regularly. Notify the physician if the peak or trough serum level does not fall within the expected range.
- Monitor the patient's serum creatinine level to help detect changes in renal function.

SAMPLE NURSING DIAGNOSES

Antibacterial agents

The following nursing diagnoses address representative problems and etiologies that a nurse may encounter when caring for a patient who is receiving an antibacterial agent.
- Altered health maintenance related to ineffectiveness of the prescribed antibacterial agent
- Altered protection related to the adverse hematologic effects or development of super-infection caused by an antibacterial agent
- Altered protection related to chloramphenicol-induced bone marrow suppression
- Altered thought processes related to penicillin-induced coma
- Body image disturbance related to tooth discoloration caused by tetracycline use during tooth formation
- Decreased tissue perfusion (systemic) related to hypotension caused by rapid intravenous (I.V.) administration of vancomycin
- Diarrhea related to the adverse gastrointestinal (GI) effects of an antibacterial agent
- Fluid volume excess related to administration of the disodium salt form of a penicillin
- High risk for fluid volume deficit related to the adverse GI effects of an antibacterial agent
- High risk for injury related to adverse drug reactions
- High risk for injury related to a preexisting condition that contraindicates the use of an antibacterial agent
- High risk for injury related to a preexisting condition that requires cautious use of an antibacterial agent
- High risk for injury related to chloramphenicol-induced Gray syndrome
- High risk for injury related to drug interactions
- High risk for injury related to hypersensitivity reactions to an antibacterial agent
- High risk for injury related to the adverse hepatic effects of an antibacterial agent
- High risk for trauma related to the adverse central nervous system effects of an antibacterial agent
- Impaired physical mobility related to aminoglycoside-induced neuromuscular blockade
- Impaired tissue integrity related to pseudomembranous colitis caused by an antibacterial agent
- Impaired tissue integrity related to thrombophlebitis caused by I.V. administration of an antibacterial agent
- Knowledge deficit related to the prescribed antibacterial agent
- Noncompliance related to the adverse reactions caused by an antibacterial agent
- Pain related to parenteral administration of an antibacterial agent
- Sensory or perceptual alterations (auditory) related to ototoxicity caused by an antibacterial agent
- Sensory or perceptual alterations (visual) related to photosensitivity caused by a tetracycline

- Monitor the patient's respiratory rate and heart rhythm to detect neuromuscular blockade.
- Monitor for symptoms of ototoxicity, such as tinnitus, dizziness, and high-frequency hearing loss, especially if the patient is elderly or dehydrated, has a hearing impairment, or is receiving concomitant therapy with another ototoxic drug.
- Refrigerate prepared I.V. aminoglycoside solution until use; infuse the drug over at least 30 minutes.

- Administer an aminoglycoside and an extended-spectrum penicillin or cephalosporin at least 2 hours apart to prevent a decrease in the aminoglycoside level and half-life in a patient with normal renal function.
- Advise the patient to notify the physician immediately if breathing difficulty, irregular heartbeat, or hearing changes occur.

Penicillins
- Obtain a complete patient history to assess the risk of allergic reaction whenever penicillin therapy is considered.
- Discontinue the prescribed penicillin immediately if the patient develops anaphylactic shock (exhibited by rapidly developing dyspnea and hypotension). Notify the physician and prepare to administer immediate emergency treatment, such as epinephrine and antihistamines, as prescribed.
- Monitor the patient for skin rash, fever, decreased level of consciousness, seizures, abnormal bleeding, or signs of renal failure. Discontinue the prescribed medication and notify the physician if any of these reactions occur.
- Administer oral penicillin 1 hour before or 2 hours after meals to ensure an optimal serum concentration.
- Review the signs and symptoms of allergic reactions with the patient. Instruct the patient to withhold the drug and notify the physician if such a reaction occurs. Instruct the family to seek emergency help immediately if an anaphylactic reaction occurs.

Cephalosporins
- Infuse all I.V. cephalosporins over 30 minutes to prevent pain and irritation.
- Administer an oral cephalosporin with food to prevent or minimize GI distress.
- Monitor closely for signs of superinfection, such as diarrhea, sore mouth, and vaginal itching, and for signs of pseudomembranous colitis, such as abdominal pain and diarrhea.

Tetracyclines
- Administer doxycycline or minocycline with food to minimize GI irritation. Administer any other tetracycline on an empty stomach, 1 hour before or 2 hours after meals.
- Do not administer a tetracycline (except doxycycline or minocycline) with milk, milk products, or drugs that contain calcium, magnesium, aluminum, or iron because they can prevent drug absorption.
- Check any prescription for I.M. injection because I.M. administration usually is not recommended. If an I.M. injection must be administered, inject the drug deeply into a large muscle.
- Advise the patient to avoid direct sunlight, cover exposed skin, or use a sunscreen with a sun protective factor of 15 or higher during tetracycline therapy.

• Advise the female patient taking an oral contraceptive to use an alternative means of contraception during tetracycline therapy and for 1 week after therapy is discontinued.

Chloramphenicol

• Screen the patient for a history of chloramphenicol hypersensitivity before initiating therapy and monitor the patient closely for hypersensitivity reactions during therapy.
• Monitor the patient's serum chloramphenicol concentration regularly for values that exceed 25 mcg/ml. If the concentration exceeds this amount, institute bleeding precautions and infection control measures (because of the risk of bone marrow suppression) and consult the physician about decreasing the dosage or substituting another antibacterial agent.

Clindamycin and lincomycin

• Do not refrigerate reconstituted oral clindamycin palmitate hydrochloride solution because it thickens and becomes difficult to measure accurately. The solution remains stable for 2 weeks at room temperature.
• Inspect the I.V. infusion site regularly for signs and symptoms of thrombophlebitis. If thrombophlebitis occurs, switch the infusion to another site.

Macrolides

• Monitor for hearing changes in a patient receiving I.V. erythromycin lactobionate, especially a geriatric patient or one with renal insufficiency.
• Do not mix I.V. erythromycin with vitamin B complex, vitamin C, cephalothin, tetracycline, heparin, or chloramphenicol because they are incompatible.
• Do not administer erythromycin stearate with food. Administer azithromycin at least 1 hour before or 2 hours after a meal.
• Do not administer erythromycin by I.M. injection; the injection is painful and may cause abscess or local tissue necrosis.
• Monitor the patient for hepatic dysfunction. Teach the patient on long-term therapy the importance of having routine liver function studies, as prescribed.

Vancomycin

• Assess the patient's renal status before beginning vancomycin therapy. Monitor the serum vancomycin concentration (peak and trough levels) and the serum creatinine level if the patient is receiving another ototoxic or nephrotoxic drug concurrently.
• Monitor the patient periodically for ototoxicity, nephrotoxicity, hypersensitivity reactions, and eosinophilia or neutropenia.
• Do not administer vancomycin by I.M. injection because it is painful and can produce tissue necrosis.

- Do not administer vancomycin by rapid I.V. infusion. It should be infused slowly over 30 to 60 minutes in a large volume of fluid to avoid a hypotensive reaction.
- Instruct the patient to report tinnitus or hearing loss.

Carbapenems
- Do not mix imipenem-cilastatin with, or add it to, other antibiotics.
- Take seizure precautions during therapy. Be especially alert for seizure activity in a geriatric patient or one with a history of previous seizure activity, underlying CNS disease, or renal insufficiency.

Monobactams
- Take seizure precautions throughout aztreonam therapy.
- Notify the physician if adverse hematologic or hepatic reactions occur. If the reaction becomes severe, expect to discontinue aztreonam therapy.
- Warn the patient receiving I.M. aztreonam that pain may occur at the infusion site and that it should be reported immediately.
- Inspect the patient's mouth regularly for ulcers. Provide symptomatic relief, such as warm-water rinses and a soft-food diet, if ulcers occur.
- Teach the patient the importance of having blood studies done, as prescribed, to detect adverse hematologic or hepatic reactions.
- Instruct the patient with thrombocytopenia to take bleeding precautions, such as avoiding cuts and bruises and using soft a toothbrush and electric razor.

STUDY ACTIVITIES

Multiple choice

1. After undergoing emergency surgery for a ruptured appendix, Alvin Keifer, age 65, is admitted to the surgical floor. His physician prescribes the aminoglycoside gentamicin sulfate (Garamycin) 80 mg I.V. every 8 hours. How should the nurse infuse this drug?
- **A.** By I.V. push
- **B.** Over 15 minutes
- **C.** Over at least 30 minutes
- **D.** Over at least 60 minutes

2. During aminoglycoside therapy, the nurse should review the results of which laboratory study?
- **A.** Serum sodium
- **B.** Serum potassium
- **C.** Prothrombin time
- **D.** Serum creatinine

3. The nurse also should monitor Mr. Keifer for which adverse reaction?

    A. Wheezing

    B. Tinnitus

    C. Sleep disturbance

    D. Circular rash on the legs

4. By checking the serum aminoglycoside peak and trough levels, the nurse can assess for which adverse reaction?

    A. Nephrotoxicity

    B. Hepatotoxicity

    C. Cardiotoxicity

    D. Neurotoxicity

5. Aaron Smith, age 22, seeks care for an upper respiratory infection. Until the results of Mr. Smith's sputum culture are known, his care is likely to include which medication(s)?

    A. An antipyretic

    B. Antibiotic therapy based on his signs and symptoms

    C. Over-the-counter drugs to prevent the infection from worsening

    D. No medications until culture and sensitivity test results are known

6. Nellie Granger, age 61, develops a systemic infection, for which her physician prescribes amoxicillin 250 mg P.O. every 8 hours. Before administering any penicillin, what should the nurse do?

    A. Plan for additional nutritional support.

    B. Obtain a baseline serum creatinine level.

    C. Evaluate the patient for a history of penicillin allergy.

    D. Determine the patient's religious beliefs. (Many products are bovine-based.)

7. Priscilla Cole, age 16, is taking tetracycline 250 mg P.O. once daily to treat acne. Why is this drug not recommended in children under age 8?

    A. The drug is absorbed poorly from the immature GI tract.

    B. The drug decreases hearing acuity, especially in children.

    C. The drug may darken permanent teeth and disrupt bone growth.

    D. The drug poses an increased risk of hypersensitivity reactions in pediatric patients.

8. When teaching Priscilla about tetracycline therapy, the nurse should include which instruction?

    A. Limit sodium intake during therapy.

    B. Eat plenty of foods rich in vitamins A and D.

    C. Avoid taking the drug with milk or milk products.

    D. Take an antacid with the medication if GI upset occurs.

True or false

9. The nurse should instruct the patient to discontinue any antibacterial agent as soon as the symptoms subside.
☐ True ☐ False

10. The patient should take an antacid during antibacterial therapy to replenish normal GI flora.
☐ True ☐ False

11. Hepatotoxicity is a serious adverse reaction that limits the use of chloramphenicol.
☐ True ☐ False

12. The I.M. route is preferred for administering erythromycin.
☐ True ☐ False

13. The nurse should take seizure precautions during imipenem-cilastatin therapy.
☐ True ☐ False

14. The nurse should advise the female patient to avoid taking oral contraceptives during tetracycline therapy.
☐ True ☐ False

Fill in the blank

15. _____-generation cephalosporins are most likely to cause adverse reactions.

16. A ___% to ___% cross-sensitivity exists between cephalosporins and penicillins.

17. Because clindamycin can cause serious toxicity and _____, its use is limited to a few clinical indications where safer, alternative antibacterials are not available.

18. I.V. vancomycin should be administered over _____ to _____ minutes to avoid a _____ reaction.

19. Imipenem-cilastatin should not be mixed with, or added to, _____.

20. Aztreonam has a narrow spectrum of activity that includes many _____ bacteria.

ANSWERS **Multiple choice**
1. C. The nurse should administer an I.V. aminoglycoside over at least 30 minutes; the drug reaches its peak concentration in 30 minutes.
2. D. The nurse should monitor the patient's serum creatinine level to detect changes in renal function caused by aminoglycoside therapy.
3. B. The nurse should monitor for symptoms of ototoxicity, such as tinnitus, dizziness, and high-frequency hearing loss.

4. A. High trough aminoglycoside concentrations correlate with nephrotoxicity; high peak concentrations, with ototoxicity and nephrotoxicity.

5. B. Because culture and sensitivity test results take 48 hours, treatment usually is initiated upon clinical assessment and then reevaluated when test results are complete.

6. C. The nurse should obtain a complete patient history to assess the risk of allergic reaction because anaphylactic reactions to penicillin may occur.

7. C. Because tetracyclines discolor tooth enamel and disrupt bone growth, they are not recommended for children under age 8 or for pregnant patients.

8. C. The patient should avoid taking a tetracycline with milk, milk products, or drugs that contain calcium, magnesium, aluminum, or iron because they prevent drug absorption.

True or false

9. False. The patient should take the antibacterial agent for the full amount of time prescribed (unless a serious adverse reaction occurs) to eradicate the causative organism.

10. False. The patient should consume yogurt or buttermilk, which replenishes normal GI flora, to prevent intestinal superinfection.

11. False. The use of chloramphenicol primarily is limited by potentially toxic bone marrow suppression.

12. False. Erythromycin is not administered by I.M. injection because it is painful and may cause abscess or local tissue necrosis.

13. True.

14. True.

Fill in the blank

15. Third

16. 5, 10

17. Pseudomembranous colitis

18. 30, 60, hypotensive

19. Other antibiotics

20. Gram-negative aerobic

CHAPTER 30

Antiviral agents

OBJECTIVES

After studying this chapter, the reader should be able to:

1. Compare the pharmacokinetics and pharmacodynamics of selected antiviral agents.

2. Identify the major indications for the antiviral agents.

3. Discuss the adverse reactions associated with the antiviral agents.

4. Describe the difficulties and dangers of administering parenteral antiviral agents.

5. Describe the nursing implications of antiviral therapy.

OVERVIEW OF CONCEPTS

Antiviral agents are drugs that are used to prevent or treat viral infections. They usually work by interfering with viral replication. Unlike other invading organisms, viruses are intracellular parasites that survive and multiply through the metabolic processes of the invaded cell. Thus, any agent that kills the virus also may destroy the cells that harbor it. In fact, many experimental antiviral compounds are too toxic for human use. However, six major antiviral agents currently are in clinical use. This chapter will focus primarily on systemic therapy with these agents. (For a summary of representative drugs, see Selected Major Drugs: *Antiviral agents,* page 424.)

Acyclovir and ganciclovir

Acyclovir sodium (Zovirax) and its derivative, ganciclovir (Cytovene), are potent antiviral agents.

Pharmacokinetics

Acyclovir may be administered orally, intravenously, or topically. Although the drug undergoes slow and incomplete gastrointestinal (GI) absorption, it is distributed throughout the body and reaches therapeutic serum concentrations. Acyclovir is metabolized in the liver and in infected cells and is excreted primarily in the urine. It reaches a peak concentration 1.5 to 2.5 hours after oral administration and immediately after intravenous (I.V.) administration.

Ganciclovir must be administered intravenously because it is absorbed poorly from the GI tract. Its distribution is not known fully. The

SELECTED MAJOR DRUGS

Antiviral agents

The following chart summarizes the major antiviral agents currently in clinical use.

DRUG	MAJOR INDICATIONS	USUAL ADULT DOSAGES
acyclovir	Primary genital herpes simplex virus (HSV) infection	200 mg P.O. every 4 hours while awake, five times a day for 10 days; 5 mg/kg I.V. every 8 hours for 5 to 7 days in patients with creatinine clearance greater than 50 ml/minute
	Recurrent genital HSV infection	200 mg P.O. five times a day for 5 days
	Varicella-zoster infection	5 to 10 mg/kg I.V. every 8 hours for at least 10 days
ganciclovir	Cytomegalovirus retinitis in immunocompromised patients, including those with acquired immunodeficiency syndrome (AIDS)	5 mg/kg I.V. infused over 1 hour every 12 hours for 14 to 21 days, followed by a maintenance dosage of 5 mg/kg I.V. infused over 1 hour once daily or 6 mg/kg I.V. once daily for 5 out of 7 days a week
vidarabine	Herpes simplex encephalitis	15 mg/kg I.V. daily, infused over 12 to 24 hours for 10 days
	Varicella-zoster infection	10 mg/kg I.V. daily, infused over 12 to 24 hours for 5 days
	Varicella-zoster infection in immunocompromised patients	10 mg/kg I.V. daily, infused over 12 to 24 hours for 5 days or more
zidovudine	Patients with AIDS or AIDS-related complex (ARC) who have a history of *Pneumocystis carinii* pneumonia or a T lymphocyte count below 200/mm^3	200 mg P.O. every 4 hours around the clock

kidneys excrete more than 90% of the drug unchanged. Peak concentration of ganciclovir occurs immediately after I.V. administration.

Pharmacodynamics

Acyclovir and ganciclovir are metabolized to their active form in cells infected by the herpesvirus. (Metabolism in uninfected cells is so slow and limited that it does not cause significant toxicity to uninfected cells.) Within the infected cells, acyclovir disrupts viral replication by inhibiting an enzyme necessary for viral growth. Ganciclovir inhibits viral deoxyribonucleic acid (DNA) synthesis.

Pharmacotherapeutics

Acyclovir is effective against herpes simplex virus 1 (HSV-1), herpes simplex virus 2 (HSV-2), and the varicella-zoster virus. The oral form is used to treat initial and recurrent genital HSV infection. Long-term use of oral acyclovir significantly decreases recurrence in patients with genital herpes infections, but all patients experience recurrent infection if acyclovir is discontinued. Parenteral acyclovir is used to treat severe infections and infections in immunocompromised patients. It prevents new vesicle formation, but does not seem to reduce the frequency of genital herpes lesions. Use of parenteral acyclovir in treating self-limiting, acute genital HSV infections reduces viral shedding, shortens healing time, and limits the duration of symptoms.

Ganciclovir is used to treat cytomegalovirus retinitis in immunocompromised patients, including those with acquired immunodeficiency syndrome (AIDS). Patients with renal dysfunction require dosage adjustments during therapy with acyclovir or ganciclovir.

Drug interactions

Acyclovir and ganciclovir can interact with various drugs. (For details, see Drug Interactions: *Antiviral agents,* page 426.)

Adverse drug reactions

Although adverse reactions to oral and parenteral acyclovir usually are minimal, reactions that do occur are significant. Local reactions at the injection site (irritation, phlebitis, inflammation, and pain), particularly with inadvertent extravasation, are the most common problems with parenteral acyclovir. Reversible renal impairment may occur, especially in patients who receive too-rapid I.V. infusion (less than 60 minutes) or who are dehydrated or have low urine output. Headache and GI distress are common with oral acyclovir. Other reactions include vertigo, blood dyscrasias, and rash.

About one-third of patients who receive ganciclovir develop a significant reaction that requires discontinuation or interruption of therapy. The most common adverse reactions are granulocytopenia and thrombocytopenia. Anemia, fever, rash, and abnormal liver function test results also may occur. Less common reactions include pruritus, arrhythmias, headache, dizziness, and other central nervous system (CNS) and GI effects. Ganciclovir has displayed mutagenic and carcinogenic effects in animals.

Vidarabine

Vidarabine monohydrate (Vira-A) was the first important anti-herpesvirus drug clinically available for parenteral use.

Pharmacokinetics

After I.V. administration, vidarabine and its active metabolite are distributed widely and excreted primarily by the kidneys. The half-life of vidarabine is 1.5 hours; its metabolite, 3.3 hours.

Pharmacodynamics

Vidarabine's exact mechanism of action is unknown. Vidarabine and its metabolite may halt viral DNA synthesis by inhibiting viral DNA polymerase.

Pharmacotherapeutics

Vidarabine is active against HSV-1, HSV-2, and varicella-zoster virus. It is indicated primarily to treat herpes simplex encephalitis and herpes zoster infection (shingles) caused by reactivated varicella-zoster infections in immunocompromised adults and children. Although vidara-

DRUG INTERACTIONS

Antiviral agents

Drug interactions with acyclovir and ganciclovir therapy are potentially serious. Less severe drug interactions may occur with most of the other antiviral agents.

DRUG	INTERACTING DRUGS	POSSIBLE EFFECTS
acyclovir, ganciclovir	probenecid, other drugs that inhibit renal tubular secretion or reabsorption	Decreased renal clearance and increased plasma concentration of acyclovir or ganciclovir
acyclovir	nephrotoxic agents	Increased risk of renal dysfunction
ganciclovir	cytotoxic drugs, such as amphotericin B, dapsone, doxorubicin, flucytosine, pentamidine, trimethoprim-sulfa combinations, vinblastine, and vincristine	Inhibited replication of rapidly dividing cells in bone marrow, gastrointestinal (GI) tract, skin, and spermatogonia; increased toxicity
	imipenem-cilastatin	Increased frequency of seizures
	zidovudine	Granulocytopenia
vidarabine	allopurinol	Decreased vidarabine metabolism, tremor, anemia, nausea, pain, pruritus
amantadine	anticholinergic agents	Increased anticholinergic effects
ribavirin	zidovudine	Decreased antiviral effects of zidovudine
	cardiac glycosides	Cardiac glycoside intoxication (GI distress, central nervous system abnormalities, and arrhythmias)
zidovudine	dapsone, doxorubicin, flucytosine, ganciclovir, interferons, pentamidine, vinblastine, vincristine	Increased nephrotoxic and cytotoxic effects
	acetaminophen, aspirin, cimetidine, indomethacin, lorazepam, probenecid	Decreased zidovudine metabolism, increased risk of toxicity
	acyclovir	Profound drowsiness and lethargy
didanosine	tetracyclines	Decreased tetracycline absorption
	drugs whose absorption is pH-dependent, such as ketoconazole and dapsone	Altered absorption of pH-dependent drugs
didanosine formulations that contain magnesium or aluminum	quinilone antibiotics	Decreased plasma concentration of some quinilone antibiotics
didanosine, zalcitabine	amphotericin B, foscarnet, aminoglycosides, chloramphenicol, cisplatin, dapsone, disulfiram, ethionamide, glutethimide, gold salts, hydralazine, metronidazole, nitrofurantoin, phenytoin, ribavirin, vincristine	Increased risk of peripheral neuropathy or nephropathy
	pentamidine isethionate	Increased risk of fulminant pancreatitis

bine decreases mortality from herpes simplex encephalitis, it does not decrease the neurologic aftereffects of the disease. Vidarabine also is used to treat varicella infections (chicken pox) in immunocompromised patients.

Drug interactions
Allopurinol can interact with vidarabine. (For details, see Drug Interactions: *Antiviral agents.*)

Adverse drug reactions
The primary adverse reactions to vidarabine affect the GI tract (nausea, vomiting, diarrhea, anorexia, and weight loss) and the CNS (weakness, tremor, ataxia, hallucinations, malaise, and confusion). These reactions are more common in patients who receive more than 10 mg/kg daily or have decreased renal function. The reactions usually subside after therapy is discontinued. Hypersensitivity reactions, including rash and pruritus, also may occur during vidarabine therapy.

Amantadine

Amantadine hydrochloride (Symmetrel) was the first oral antiviral drug available for clinical use.

Pharmacokinetics
After oral administration, amantadine is absorbed well from the GI tract and distributed only to saliva, cerebrospinal fluid, nasal secretions, breast milk, and lung tissue. Amantadine is not metabolized, but is eliminated primarily in the urine. It reaches a peak concentration 1 to 4 hours after oral administration.

Pharmacodynamics
Although its exact mechanism of action is unknown, amantadine appears to inhibit an early stage of viral replication, such as prevention of virus penetration into the host cell.

Pharmacotherapeutics
Amantadine is used to prevent or treat influenza A infections. Its effectiveness depends on the concentration of the drug and varies with the viral strain. The drug reduces the severity and duration of fever and other symptoms of influenza A infections. It is particularly useful because it can be administered to patients undergoing immunization and can protect them during the 2 weeks needed to develop immunity. It also is useful for patients who cannot take the influenza vaccine because of hypersensitivity. This drug requires dosage reductions in patients with renal impairment or a history of seizure disorders. Amantadine also is used to treat parkinsonism and drug-induced extrapyramidal reactions. (For more information, see Chapter 7, Antiparkinsonian agents.)

Drug interactions
Amantadine interacts with anticholinergic drugs. (For details, see Drug Interactions: *Antiviral agents.*)

Adverse drug reactions

Amantadine usually is tolerated well. The most common reactions are nausea, anorexia, nervousness, fatigue, depression, irritability, insomnia, psychosis, anxiety, confusion, forgetfulness, and hallucinations. Patients with seizure disorders are more prone to seizures while receiving amantadine. Other reactions may include headache, dizziness, congestive heart failure (CHF), orthostatic hypotension, and rash.

Ribavirin

Ribavirin (Virazole) is an aerosol antiviral agent.

Pharmacokinetics

Upon nasal or oral inhalation, ribavirin is absorbed well. It has a limited, specific distribution, with the highest concentration found in the pulmonary tract and red blood cells (RBCs). Ribavirin is metabolized in the liver and in RBCs and is excreted in the urine and feces. Onset of action and peak concentration of ribavirin occur immediately after inhalation.

Pharmacodynamics

The mechanism of action of ribavirin is not known completely, but the drug probably becomes effective after it is converted to metabolites that inhibit viral DNA and ribonucleic acid (RNA) synthesis.

Pharmacotherapeutics

Ribavirin currently is available only to treat respiratory syncytial virus (RSV) infections in children. It also has been used experimentally to treat respiratory infections caused by influenza viruses A and B in geriatric patients.

Drug interactions

Ribavirin can interact with zidovudine and cardiac glycosides. (For details, see Drug Interactions: *Antiviral agents,* page 426.)

Adverse drug reactions

Adverse reactions to ribavirin therapy are infrequent, but may include worsening of respiratory function, ventilator dependence, pneumothorax, apnea, cardiac arrest, and hypotension. Reticulosis, rash, and conjunctivitis also may occur.

Zidovudine, didanosine, and zalcitabine

Also known as azidothymidine (AZT), zidovudine (Retrovir) is used to treat AIDS and AIDS-related complex (ARC). Didanosine and zalcitabine are used to treat advanced human immunodeficiency virus (HIV) infections.

Pharmacokinetics

After oral administration, zidovudine is absorbed well from the GI tract and distributed widely. It undergoes rapid hepatic metabolism and is excreted by the kidneys. The drug reaches a peak concentration in 0.5 to 1.5 hours and has a duration of action of 4 hours.

Didanosine tablets and powder contain a buffering agent to prevent rapid drug degradation at gastric pH. Although didanosine's metabolism is not known fully, about 50% of a dose is excreted in the urine. The average plasma half-life is 1.6 hours.

Oral zalcitabine is absorbed well from the GI tract when administered on an empty stomach. It penetrates the blood-brain barrier, probably undergoes little metabolism in the liver, and is excreted primarily by the kidneys. The drug's half-life ranges from 1 to 3 hours.

Pharmacodynamics

All three drugs are converted by cellular enzymes to active metabolites. Zidovudine's metabolite prevents viral DNA replication; didanosine's and zalcitabine's metabolites block HIV replication.

Pharmacotherapeutics

Zidovudine is used to treat patients with AIDS and ARC who have a history of *Pneumocystis carinii* pneumonia or a T lymphocyte count lower than $200/\text{mm}^3$. The drug also reduces the incidence and severity of opportunistic infections. Didanosine is used to treat advanced HIV infection in adults and children (over age 6 months) who cannot tolerate zidovudine or who have demonstrated significant clinical or immunologic deterioration during zidovudine therapy. Zalcitabine is used in combination with zidovudine to treat advanced HIV infection (a CD4 cell count less than $200/\text{mm}^3$) in adults who have significant clinical or immunologic deterioration.

Drug interactions

Zidovudine can interact with a variety of drugs. (For details, see Drug Interactions: *Antiviral agents,* page 426.)

Adverse drug reactions

The most common adverse reactions to zidovudine are hematologic. Significant anemia occurs 4 to 6 weeks after therapy begins; granulocytopenia appears within 6 to 8 weeks. When reductions in RBC and white blood cell (WBC) counts occur, the dosage usually is adjusted or stopped, immediately reversing the abnormal blood counts. The drug also may cause headache, dizziness, and other mild adverse CNS reactions, GI distress, fever, and rash.

Adverse reactions to didanosine include a wide range of GI disturbances, pancreatitis, headache, peripheral neuropathy, CNS depression and other neurological reactions, dermatomucosal reactions, myalgia, and arthritis. Adverse reactions to zalcitabine include peripheral neuropathy, mouth ulcers, nausea, rash, headache, myalgia, and fatigue.

Nursing implications   When caring for a patient who is receiving an antiviral agent, the nurse should be aware of the following implications.
• Develop appropriate nursing diagnoses for the patient. (For examples, see Sample Nursing Diagnoses: *Antiviral agents,* page 430.)

- Do not administer an antiviral agent to a patient with a condition that contraindicates its use.
- Administer an antiviral agent cautiously to a patient at risk because of a preexisting condition.
- Monitor the patient closely for adverse reactions and signs of drug interactions.
- Monitor the patient's complete blood count regularly during therapy with all antiviral agents except amantadine.
- Take safety precautions if the patient experiences adverse CNS reactions. For example, place the bed in a low position, keep the side rails up, and supervise the patient's activities. Also teach the patient how to minimize CNS reactions.
- Administer a mild analgesic, as prescribed, for headache, which may accompany therapy with any antiviral agent, except vidarabine and ribavirin.
- Notify the physician if adverse reactions or drug interactions occur. Also notify the physician of any abnormal laboratory test results.
- Teach the patient and family the name, dose, frequency, action, and adverse effects of the prescribed antiviral agent.

- Teach the patient the importance of returning for regular blood tests, as prescribed.
- Instruct the patient to report pruritus or rash.

Acyclovir and ganciclovir

- Monitor the patient's renal function—especially the serum creatinine level—closely during parenteral therapy. Expect to decrease the dosage, as prescribed, for a patient with decreased renal function.
- Monitor the neutrophil and platelet counts every 2 days during twice-daily ganciclovir therapy and at least weekly thereafter. Institute infection control measures until the patient's WBC count returns to normal.
- Administer an I.V. infusion slowly (over 60 minutes or as prescribed) to prevent drug crystals from precipitating in renal tubules. Keep the patient well hydrated during parenteral therapy to ensure good urine output.
- Inspect the I.V. infusion site regularly for signs of irritation, phlebitis, inflammation, and extravasation. Ask the patient about pain at the I.V. site. Rotate the I.V. infusion sites regularly.
- Avoid inhalation or direct skin contact because of ganciclovir's carcinogenic potential.
- Monitor closely for signs of bleeding, such as spontaneous epistaxis and easy bruising, if the patient develops thrombocytopenia. Test urine, feces, and emesis for occult blood. Take bleeding precautions until the patient's thrombocyte level returns to normal.
- Advise a patient of childbearing age to use effective contraception during ganciclovir therapy and for at least 90 days after it is discontinued.
- Advise the female patient to discontinue breast-feeding and not to resume it for at least 72 hours after the last ganciclovir dose.

Vidarabine

- Ensure that the I.V. solution is clear before infusion. Use an in-line 0.45-micron (or smaller) filter for the infusion. Do not exceed the maximum of 450 mg of vidarabine in a liter of I.V. solution. Inspect and rotate I.V. infusion sites regularly.
- Monitor the patient for signs of fluid volume excess (such as crackles, jugular vein distention, sudden weight gain, and ankle swelling), especially if the patient has a cardiac disorder, because vidarabine must be diluted in large volumes of fluid for I.V. administration and can cause fluid overload.

Amantadine

- Administer amantadine after meals for maximum absorption. If insomnia occurs, administer the drug several hours before bedtime.
- Administer the drug cautiously to a patient who also is receiving an anticholinergic agent.

- Monitor the patient with a history of CHF closely for exacerbation or recurrence of CHF, as evidenced by shortness of breath, tachycardia, jugular vein distention, or crackles.
- Expect to reduce the dosage, as prescribed, in a patient with renal impairment or a history of seizures.

Ribavirin

- Use sterile water for injection, not bacteriostatic water, for reconstituting ribavirin powder. Store reconstituted solutions at room temperature for up to 24 hours.
- Administer ribavirin with a small particle aerosol generator. Do not use any other aerosol-generating device.
- Perform a complete respiratory assessment every hour throughout ribavirin therapy. Monitor arterial blood gases and be prepared to support the patient's ventilation if respiratory condition worsens. Notify the physician immediately of any change in the patient's respiratory status.
- Monitor the patient's cardiac status throughout therapy. Report hypotension or cardiac dysfunction. Keep standard emergency equipment nearby and be prepared to begin cardiopulmonary resuscitation if cardiac arrest occurs.

Zidovudine, didanosine, and zalcitabine

- Monitor the patient's temperature for fever.
- Monitor the patient closely for pancreatitis and peripheral neuropathy when administering didanosine or zalcitabine. Be aware that pancreatitis may be fatal. If pancreatitis is suspected, expect to discontinue didanosine or zalcitabine immediately.
- Administer didanosine and zalcitabine on an empty stomach.
- Expect to decrease the dose or discontinue the drug, as prescribed, if reductions in blood counts occur.
- Instruct the patient to take the drug every 4 hours around the clock, even though it means interrupting sleep.
- Inform the patient that zidovudine does not reduce the risk of transmitting the virus to others through sexual contact or blood contamination.
- Caution the patient to avoid over-the-counter medications without first consulting the physician, pharmacist, or nurse.

STUDY ACTIVITIES   **Fill in the blanks**

1. Viral infections are difficult to treat because viruses are

_____ parasites.

2. _____ was the first oral antiviral drug available for clinical use.

3. _____ is used to treat AIDS and ARC.

Multiple choice

4. While receiving ganciclovir, Susan Smithers, age 25, develops leukopenia. For this patient, which nursing intervention is most important?
    A. Preventing infection
    B. Limiting fluid intake
    C. Administering zidovudine
    D. Increasing the drug dosage

5. Dave Keller, age 42, receives parenteral acyclovir to treat an acute genital HSV-1 infection. This drug produces which therapeutic effect?
    A. It reduces cell lysis.
    B. It shortens healing time.
    C. It increases viral shedding.
    D. It reduces the frequency of recurrence.

6. Which patient is most likely to experience adverse reactions to acyclovir?
    A. One receiving a 90-minute infusion of the drug
    B. One with a history of chicken pox
    C. One with a low urine output
    D. One who is fully hydrated

7. A herpes zoster infection is reactivated in Evelyn Shoemaker, age 90. Because she is immunocompromised, the physician is most likely to prescribe which drug?
    A. Acyclovir
    B. Ribavirin
    C. Vidarabine
    D. Zidovudine

8. Betsy Callan, age 8, needs inhalation treatment with ribavirin for an RSV infection. For Betsy, which nursing intervention is appropriate?
    A. Using bacteriostatic water to reconstitute ribavirin
    B. Refrigerating reconstituted ribavirin for up to 72 hours
    C. Giving ribavirin with any fine-aerosol generating device
    D. Assessing respiratory status every hour during treatment

9. The nurse should monitor Betsy for which adverse reaction?
    A. Anemia
    B. Hypotension
    C. Thrombocytopenia
    D. Renal impairment

10. Alan Kremens, age 37, is beginning zidovudine therapy. What is the primary effect of this antiviral agent?
    A. Prevention of AIDS in patients with ARC
    B. Reduced incidence and severity of opportunistic infections
    C. Decreased T lymphocyte count in patients with ARC
    D. Cure of *P. carinii* pneumonia

11. What is zidovudine's primary mechanism of action?
  A. It inhibits infected cell metabolism.
  B. It disrupts viral enzyme activity.
  C. It increases DNA and RNA synthesis.
  D. It prevents viral DNA replication.

12. Megan Hurst, age 29, must take vidarabine for a varicella-zoster virus infection. Before giving vidarabine, what should the nurse do?
  A. Check the patient's history for malabsorption syndromes.
  B. Dilute the drug in a small amount of diluent.
  C. Install an in-line filter for the infusion.
  D. Put the patient in protective isolation.

ANSWERS

Fill in the blank
  1. Intracellular
  2. Amantadine
  3. Zidovudine

Multiple choice
  4. A. The nurse should take infection control measures until the patient's WBC count returns to normal.
  5. B. Use of parenteral acyclovir in self-limiting, acute genital HSV infections reduces viral shedding, shortens healing time, and limits the duration of symptoms.
  6. C. Acyclovir may cause reversible renal impairment, especially in patients who receive too-rapid infusion (less than 60 minutes) or who are dehydrated or have low urine output.
  7. C. Vidarabine is indicated primarily to treat herpes simplex encephalitis and herpes zoster (shingles) caused by reactivated varicella-zoster infections in immunocompromised adults and children.
  8. D. The nurse should use sterile water to reconstitute ribavirin, store reconstituted solution at room temperature for up to 24 hours, administer it with a small particle aerosol generator, and perform a respiratory assessment every hour during ribavirin therapy.
  9. B. Adverse reactions to ribavirin include worsening of respiratory function, apnea, hypotension, and cardiac arrest.
  10. B. In patients with AIDS and ARC who have a history of *P. carinii* pneumonia or a decreased T lymphocyte count, zidovudine reduces the incidence and severity of opportunistic infections.
  11. D. Zidovudine is converted by cellular enzymes to an active metabolite that prevents viral DNA replication.
  12. C. Before administering vidarabine, the nurse should ensure that the I.V. solution is clear and should use an in-line 0.45-micron (or smaller) filter for the infusion.

CHAPTER 31

Antimycotic (antifungal) agents

OBJECTIVES

After studying this chapter, the reader should be able to:

1. Compare the pharmacokinetics of systemic and topical antimycotic agents.

2. Describe the antimycotic agents used to treat systemic and topical fungal infections.

3. Explain how certain antimycotic agents can be used together for synergistic effects.

4. Identify significant interactions between the antimycotic agents and other drugs.

5. Identify the adverse reactions to the antimycotic agents, and describe how to prevent or treat them.

6. Describe the nursing implications of antimycotic therapy.

OVERVIEW OF CONCEPTS

Antimycotic, or antifungal, agents include many drugs that are used to treat fungal infections. Two general types of fungal infections exist: topical (superficial) infections, which affect the skin and mucous membranes; and systemic infections, which affect such areas as the lungs, central nervous system (CNS), and blood.

Of the two types, topical infections of the skin and mucous membrane are more common and include candidiasis and infections caused by dermatophytes (various skin fungi). Most these infections respond well to topical therapy. However, infected nail beds require long-term systemic treatment.

Systemic fungal infections are caused by pathogenic fungi or opportunistic fungi (those that are normally nonpathogenic, but become pathogenic under certain circumstances, such as a decreased immune response). Pathogenic fungi usually enter the host by the respiratory tract; opportunistic fungi may enter through various routes, including the GI tract and intravenous (I.V.) lines.

Treatment of a topical or systemic infection requires an antimycotic agent chosen according to the site and severity of the infection. (For a summary of representative drugs, see Selected Major Drugs: *Antimycotic agents,* page 436.)

SELECTED MAJOR DRUGS

Antimycotic agents

The following chart summarizes the major antimycotic agents currently in clinical use.

DRUG	MAJOR INDICATIONS	USUAL ADULT DOSAGES
amphotericin B	Life-threatening systemic fungal infections and meningitis	0.25 to 1.5 mg/kg I.V. daily infused over 4 to 6 hours
	Candidal infection of the bladder	50 mg in 1 liter sterile water continuously or intermittently instilled into the bladder
	Coccidioidal meningitis, cryptococcal meningitis	0.025 to 1 mg intrathecally two to three times weekly
nystatin	Oral or esophageal candidiasis	500,000 units oral suspension, gargled and then swallowed, or 500,000 units of oral tablets, dissolved in the mouth, t.i.d. or q.i.d. for 10 days or until 48 hours after overt symptoms have subsided
	Vaginal candidiasis	100,000 units inserted vaginally once or twice daily for 14 days or longer
	Intestinal candidiasis	500,000 to 1 million units of oral tablets t.i.d. or q.i.d.
ketoconazole	Systemic, subcutaneous, and superficial fungal infections	200 to 400 mg P.O. daily for 1 week to 12 months, depending on the organism and the infection site
flucytosine	Fungal infections caused by *Candida* or *Cryptococcus*	50 to 150 mg/kg P.O. daily divided in four equal doses and administered every 6 hours
fluconazole	Oropharyngeal candidiasis	200 mg P.O. or I.V. on the first day, followed by 100 mg P.O. or I.V. daily for 2 weeks
	Esophageal candidiasis	200 mg P.O. or I.V. on the first day, followed by 100 mg P.O. or I.V. daily for a minimum of 3 weeks and for at least 2 weeks after resolution of symptoms
	Systemic candidiasis	400 mg P.O. or I.V. on the first day, followed by 200 mg P.O. or I.V. daily for a minimum of 4 weeks
	Cryptococcal meningitis	400 mg P.O. or I.V. on the first day, followed by 200 mg P.O. or I.V. daily for 10 to 12 weeks after the cerebrospinal fluid culture becomes negative

Amphotericin B   A polyene antimycotic, amphotericin B (Fungizone) is the most widely used agent for treating severe systemic fungal infections.

Pharmacokinetics
After I.V. administration, amphotericin B is distributed throughout the body and excreted by the kidneys. Its exact metabolic fate is unknown. In a patient with normal renal function, the drug's half-life is 24 hours. As therapy continues, the half-life lengthens and may reach 15 days with long-term administration.

Pharmacodynamics

Amphotericin B binds irreversibly to sterols in the membranes of amphotericin B–sensitive fungal cells. This seems to produce pores or channels that increase cell membrane permeability, which prevents the cell membrane from functioning normally as a barrier.

Pharmacotherapeutics

Amphotericin B is used to treat life-threatening systemic fungal infections and meningitis caused by fungi sensitive to the drug. Amphotericin B therapy usually begins with a test dose that is increased daily until the desired dosage is reached. Duration of therapy depends on the maturity and severity of the infection. Some patients may need months of therapy with a total dosage that ranges from 300 to 4,000 mg.

Drug interactions

Amphotericin B can cause significant interactions with many drugs. (For details, see Drug Interactions: *Antimycotic agents,* page 438.)

Adverse drug reactions

Amphotericin B may be the most toxic antibiotic in use. Almost all patients receiving I.V. amphotericin B experience chills, fever, nausea, vomiting, anorexia, muscle and joint pain, headache, abdominal pain, weight loss, and dyspepsia, especially at the beginning of therapy with low doses. Most patients also develop normochromic or normocytic anemia that significantly decreases the hematocrit.

Up to 80% of patients receiving amphotericin B develop nephrotoxicity, which usually disappears within 3 months after the drug is discontinued, but sometimes leads to permanent renal impairment. Up to 25% of patients develop hypokalemia, which can be severe and lead to extreme muscle weakness and electrocardiogram changes. Other adverse reactions to amphotericin include phlebitis and thrombophlebitis (with I.V. administration), hypersensitivity, and electrolyte imbalances.

Nystatin Like amphotericin B, nystatin (Mycostatin, Nilstat) is a polyene antimycotic. Unlike amphotericin B, it is used only topically or orally to treat local infections because it is extremely toxic when administered parenterally.

Pharmacokinetics

Oral nystatin undergoes little or no absorption, distribution, or metabolism. It is excreted as unchanged drug in the feces. Topical nystatin is not absorbed through the skin or mucous membranes.

Pharmacodynamics

Nystatin binds to sterols in fungal cell membranes, altering membrane permeability and leading to loss of essential cell components.

DRUG INTERACTIONS

Antimycotic agents

Among the major antimycotic agents, only amphotericin B, ketoconazole, and fluconazole cause significant drug interactions.

DRUG	INTERACTING DRUGS	POSSIBLE EFFECTS
amphotericin B	aminoglycosides, cyclosporine, acyclovir	Increased nephrotoxicity
	corticosteroids	Increased hypokalemia, cardiac dysfunction
	extended-spectrum penicillins	Increased hypokalemia
	cardiac glycosides	Increased hypokalemia, digitalis toxicity
	nondepolarizing skeletal muscle relaxants	Increased muscle relaxant effects
	electrolyte solutions	Inactivation of amphotericin B colloid
ketoconazole	antacids, anticholinergic agents, cimetidine, famotidine, ranitidine, other drugs that decrease gastric acidity	Decreased absorption and antimycotic effects of ketoconazole
	phenytoin	Altered metabolism and blood levels of both drugs
	theophylline	Decreased serum theophylline level,
	hepatotoxic drugs	Increased risk of hepatotoxicity
	cyclosporine	Increased cyclosporine level, increased serum creatinine level
	oral anticoagulants	Increased anticoagulant effects, hemorrhage
fluconazole	warfarin	Increased prothrombin time
	phenytoin, cyclosporine	Increased phenytoin or cyclosporine level
	glyburide, glipizide	Decreased glyburide or glipizide metabolism (increased blood level), hypoglycemia
	rifampin	Increased fluconazole metabolism

Pharmacotherapeutics
Nystatin is used primarily to treat fungal skin infections, especially candidal infections. It is available in different forms to treat different types of infections.

Drug interactions
No significant drug interactions occur with nystatin use.

Adverse drug reactions
Reactions to nystatin, which rarely occur, are mild. Oral preparations may cause adverse GI reactions; topical preparations may cause skin irritation. Both preparations can produce hypersensitivity reactions.

Flucytosine   An antimetabolite antimycotic, flucytosine (Ancobon) is used primarily with another antimycotic agent to treat systemic fungal infections.

Pharmacokinetics

After oral administration, flucytosine is absorbed rapidly and well from the GI tract. Although the presence of food in the stomach slows the rate of absorption, it does not affect its extent. The drug is distributed widely, undergoes little metabolism, and is excreted primarily by the kidneys. In patients with normal renal function, flucytosine usually reaches a peak concentration 2 to 4 hours after administration, and its half-life ranges from 2.5 to 8 hours.

Pharmacodynamics

Flucytosine penetrates fungal cells and then undergoes conversion to its active metabolic fluorouracil, a metabolic antagonist. Fluorouracil alters protein synthesis in fungal cells, causing cell death.

Pharmacotherapeutics

Because some fungal species and strains are not susceptible to flucytosine, susceptibility tests should be done before the drug is used. Flucytosine is administered orally with another antimycotic agent, such as amphotericin B, because some fungi can develop a resistance to flucytosine when it is given alone. However, flucytosine can be used alone to treat certain urinary tract infections because the drug reaches a high concentration in the urine.

Drug interactions

Flucytosine does not cause any significant drug interactions.

Adverse drug reactions

Adverse reactions to flucytosine predominantly involve rapidly proliferating cells in the bone marrow and GI tract. Bone marrow depression typically occurs when serum flucytosine concentration exceeds 100 mcg/ml and may lead to leukopenia, thrombocytopenia, anemia, pancytopenia, or granulocytopenia. This adverse reaction most commonly affects patients with renal failure who also are taking amphotericin B or who are receiving large doses of flucytosine.

Adverse GI reactions may be severe and may include nausea, vomiting, diarrhea, abdominal distention, anorexia, and hepatotoxicity. Adverse urinary reactions may include azotemia, elevated blood urea nitrogen (BUN) and creatinine levels, crystalluria, and renal failure. Unpredictable reactions to flucytosine include vertigo, hallucinations, dyspnea, and skin rash.

Ketoconazole An imidazole antimycotic agent, ketoconazole (Nizoral) is the first effective oral antimycotic agent that has a broad spectrum of activity.

Pharmacokinetics

After oral administration, ketoconazole is absorbed well from the GI tract. The drug is absorbed best when the pH of the GI tract is acidic, as when the stomach is empty. The drug is distributed widely, and its protein-binding ranges from 84% to 99%. It undergoes metabolism in the liver and is excreted primarily in the feces. When administered 30 to 60 minutes after meals, ketoconazole reaches a peak concentration in 1 to 4 hours.

Pharmacodynamics
Ketoconazole interferes with sterol synthesis in fungal cells, damaging the cell membrane and increasing its permeability. This leads to a loss of essential intracellular elements and inhibits cell growth.

Pharmacotherapeutics
This oral antimycotic agent is used to treat topical and systemic infections caused by susceptible fungi, which include dermatophytes and most other fungi. Ketoconazole also may be used to treat pulmonary and disseminated blastomycosis, chromomycosis, coccidioidomycosis, histoplasmosis, candidiasis, and paracoccidioidomycosis.

Drug interactions
Ketoconazole can interact with various drugs. (For details, see Drug Interactions: *Antimycotic agents,* page 438.)

Adverse drug reactions
Although ketoconazole appears to be safer than amphotericin B, it can produce adverse reactions that primarily affect the CNS, GI tract, and skin. The most common reactions to ketoconazole are nausea and vomiting. Although rare, hepatotoxicity can occur.

Fluconazole   A bistriazole derivative, fluconazole (Diflucan) is a synthetic broad-spectrum antimycotic agent.

Pharmacokinetics
Fluconazole may be administered intravenously or orally. After oral administration, the drug is about 90% absorbed, distributed to all body fluids, and excreted primarily unchanged in the urine. Elimination may be reduced in patients with decreased renal function. It reaches a peak concentration 1 to 2 hours after administration.

Pharmacodynamics
This antimycotic agent causes fungal cells to lose normal sterol, thereby promoting cell death.

Pharmacotherapeutics
Fluconazole is used primarily to treat oropharyngeal and esophageal candidiasis and serious systemic candidal infections. It also is used to treat cryptococcal meningitis. The recommended oral and I.V. doses are similar because the oral product is absorbed well.

Drug interactions
Fluconazole can interact significantly with several drugs. (For details, see Drug Interactions: *Antimycotic agents,* page 438.)

Adverse drug reactions

In clinical trials, 5% to 7% of patients receiving fluconazole experienced transient elevations in aspartate aminotransferase (AST [formerly SGOT]), alanine aminotransferase (ALT [formerly SGPT]), alkaline phosphatase, and bilirubin levels. Fewer patients developed dizziness, nausea, vomiting, abdominal pain, diarrhea, skin rash, headache, hypokalemia, and increased BUN and creatinine levels. Adverse reactions occur more commonly in patients infected with the human immunodeficiency virus.

Other antimycotic agents

Several other antimycotic agents offer alternative forms of treatment for topical fungal infections. Clotrimazole (Gyne-Lotrimin, Mycelex) is used topically to treat infections caused by dermatophytes or *Candida albicans* infections, orally to treat oral candidiasis, and vaginally to treat vaginal candidiasis. Adverse reactions may include elevated liver function test results, nausea, vomiting, and adverse dermatologic reactions.

Griseofulvin (Fulvicin-U/F, Grifulvin V, Grisactin Ultra) is an oral preparation used to treat fungal infections of the skin, nails, and scalp. To prevent a relapse, griseofulvin therapy must continue until the fungus is eradicated completely and the infected skin or nails are replaced. When adverse reactions occur, they usually include nausea, vomiting, diarrhea, fatigue, confusion, and headache.

Miconazole (Monistat I.V.) and miconazole nitrate (Micatin, Monistat 3, Monistat 7) are used to treat systemic fungal infections, such as coccidioidomycosis, paracoccidioidomycosis, cryptococcosis, and candidiasis. They also are useful in treating local fungal infections, such as vulvovaginal candidiasis, and topical fungal infections, such as chronic mucocutaneous candidiasis. Adverse reactions to I.V. miconazole include phlebitis, pruritus, nausea, fever, chills, rash, hyperlipidemia, arrhythmias, tachypnea, and cardiopulmonary arrest.

Nursing implications

When caring for a patient who is receiving an antimycotic agent, the nurse should be aware of the following implications.
• Develop appropriate nursing diagnoses for the patient. (For examples, see Sample Nursing Diagnoses: *Antimycotic agents,* page 443.)
• Do not administer an antimycotic agent to a patient with a condition that contraindicates its use.
• Administer an antimycotic agent cautiously to a patient at risk because of a preexisting condition.
• Monitor the patient regularly for adverse reactions to the prescribed antimycotic agent. For a patient with a serious disorder, such as leukemia, cancer, or acquired immunodeficiency syndrome, monitor more frequently.
• Monitor the patient for signs of drug interactions during amphotericin B, ketoconazole, or fluconazole therapy.

- Notify the physician if adverse reactions or drug interactions occur.
- Teach the patient and family the name, dose, frequency, action, and adverse effects of the prescribed antimycotic agent.
- Emphasize the importance of compliance with drug therapy.
- Teach the patient how to apply a topical antimycotic agent.

Amphotericin B

- Monitor the patient's BUN and serum creatinine levels before therapy begins, every other day during initiation of therapy, and once a week after the optimal dosage is reached. Expect to administer a reduced dosage or to use alternate-day therapy, as prescribed, if the serum creatinine level approaches 3 mg/dl.
- Monitor the patient for signs of an immediate hypersensitivity reaction, including dyspnea, wheezing, urticaria, pruritus, laryngeal edema, hypotension, and tachycardia.
- Dilute amphotericin B for infusion or injection in a dextrose 5% in water solution with a pH greater than 4.2 or in sterile water. This drug is not compatible with any electrolyte solution.
- Observe the I.V. site for phlebitis and rotate sites regularly. Expect to use alternate-day therapy if phlebitis becomes severe.
- Monitor the patient's serum electrolyte levels. Also watch for muscle weakness, cramping, and fatigue, which may be the first signs of hypokalemia.
- Inform the patient receiving I.V. amphotericin B that chills, fever, GI upset, muscle and joint pain, headache, abdominal pain, weight loss, and dyspepsia probably will occur, but that these reactions should subside with continued therapy.

Nystatin

- Instruct the patient to avoid using occlusive dressings during therapy with nystatin ointment or cream because they provide a favorable environment for fungal growth.
- Instruct the patient with oral candidiasis to dissolve—not chew—the nystatin tablet in the mouth.

Flucytosine

- Monitor the patient's hematologic values, liver function test results, and BUN and creatinine levels.
- Monitor the patient for signs of infection, such as sore throat, fever, and productive cough, if leukopenia occurs. Take infection control measures, such as keeping the patient away from others with infections, until the white blood cell count returns to normal.
- Monitor for signs of bone marrow suppression, such as easy bruising, bleeding, unusual fatigue or weakness, and for other adverse reactions, such as severe nausea, vomiting, and skin rash.
- Monitor the patient's fluid intake and output. Notify the physician if the patient develops signs of renal failure, such as azotemia, crystalluria, or decreased urine output.

SAMPLE NURSING DIAGNOSES

Antimycotic agents

The following nursing diagnoses address representative problems and etiologies that a nurse may encounter when caring for a patient who is receiving an antimycotic agent.

- Altered health maintenance related to hepatotoxicity caused by flucytosine or ketoconazole
- Altered health maintenance related to ineffectiveness of the prescribed antimycotic agent
- Altered nutrition: less than body requirements, related to the adverse gastrointestinal (GI) effects of an antimycotic agent
- Altered protection related to hematologic abnormalities caused by an antimycotic agent
- Altered thought processes related to the adverse central nervous system effects of an antimycotic agent
- Altered urinary elimination related to amphotericin B-induced nephrotoxicity
- Diarrhea related to the adverse GI effects of an antimycotic agent
- High risk for impaired skin integrity related to the adverse dermatologic effects of a topical antimycotic agent
- High risk for infection related to flucytosine-induced leukopenia
- High risk for injury related to adverse drug reactions
- High risk for injury related to a preexisting condition that contraindicates the use of an antimycotic agent
- High risk for injury related to a preexisting condition that requires cautious use of an antimycotic agent
- High risk for injury related to drug interactions
- Hyperthermia related to fever caused by an antimycotic agent
- Impaired physical mobility related to extreme muscle weakness caused by amphotericin B-induced hypokalemia
- Impaired tissue integrity related to phlebitis caused by intravenous administration of amphotericin B
- Knowledge deficit related to the prescribed antimycotic agent
- Noncompliance related to adverse reactions to the prescribed antimycotic agent
- Pain related to headache caused by an antimycotic agent

- Monitor the serum flucytosine level regularly during long-term therapy; therapeutic serum concentrations range from 25 to 120 mcg/ml.
- Instruct the patient to take a missed dose as soon as possible, but not to take a double dose. Explain that missing a dose is safer than overmedicating with a double dose.

Ketoconazole

- Monitor the patient's liver function test results. Expect to discontinue the drug if test results show persistent elevations. Monitor for signs of hepatotoxicity, such as unusual fatigue, dark or amber-colored urine, pale stools, jaundice, or right upper quadrant abdominal pain.
- Administer ketoconazole on an empty stomach, if possible, to promote absorption. If the patient experiences GI distress, however, administer the drug with food.
- Do not administer ketoconazole with drugs that decrease gastric acidity, such as antacids and anticholinergic agents. If these drugs must

be used, administer ketoconazole at least 2 hours before administering the other drugs.

Fluconazole

• Monitor laboratory test results to detect elevations in AST, ALT, alkaline phosphatase, bilirubin, BUN, and creatinine levels.
• Adjust the dosage of one or both drugs, as prescribed, if the patient displays abnormal laboratory test results during concomitant administration of drugs known to interact with fluconazole.
• Expect to administer a low dose of fluconazole, as prescribed, to a patient with renal dysfunction.
• Do not administer fluconazole by continuous I.V. infusion at a rate greater than 200 mg/hr.
• Instruct the patient to take bleeding precautions during concomitant therapy with warfarin, which may increase the prothrombin time.
• Instruct the patient with diabetes to monitor the blood glucose level regularly and to watch for signs of hypoglycemia (profuse sweating, nervousness, irritability, and headache) when taking glyburide or glipizide concomitantly with fluconazole.

STUDY ACTIVITIES   Fill in the blanks

1. An antimycotic agent is selected based on the _____ and _____ of the fungal infection.

2. The two general types of fungal infections are _____ and _____ infections.

3. _____ fungal infections are caused by pathogenic or opportunistic fungi.

4. Fluconazole may _____ the prothrombin time when administered concomitantly with warfarin.

5. _____ is the most widely used agent for treating severe systemic fungal infections.

Multiple choice

6. Elise Dormand, age 48, is receiving amphotericin B. Which statement accurately characterizes this antimycotic agent?
  A. It is relatively safe even in high doses.
  B. It is one of the most toxic antibiotics in use today.
  C. It is useful for treating a variety of topical infections.
  D. It can be inactivated by drugs that decrease gastric acidity.

7. The nurse should monitor Ms. Dormand's BUN and serum creatinine levels to detect which adverse reaction to amphotericin B?
- **A.** Blood dyscrasias
- **B.** Hypersensitivity
- **C.** Nephrotoxicity
- **D.** Hepatotoxicity

8. During amphotericin B therapy, Ms. Dormand develops hyponatremia. To correct this imbalance, the physician prescribes an I.V. of 0.9% sodium chloride solution. What should the nurse do?
- **A.** Ask the pharmacy to prepare an amphotericin–0.9% sodium chloride solution mixture.
- **B.** Mix amphotericin with 0.9% sodium chloride solution using sterile technique.
- **C.** Check the patient's sodium level to determine the proper ratio of amphotericin B to 0.9% sodium chloride solution.
- **D.** Infuse 0.9% sodium chloride solution via a separate I.V. line because it is not compatible with amphotericin B.

9. Daniel Shelby, age 23, has a fungal infection of the groin. Nystatin ointment is to be applied to the groin area b.i.d. for 14 days. When teaching Mr. Shelby about his therapy, the nurse should include which instruction?
- **A.** Remove loose fungal growth with a damp washcloth before drug application.
- **B.** Do not cover the area with an occlusive dressing after drug application.
- **C.** Report signs of bleeding, a common adverse reaction to nystatin.
- **D.** Avoid over-the-counter products that contain aspirin.

10. Dana Adams, age 36, will be taking flucytosine for a systemic infection. Dana asks the nurse what to do if she misses a dose of the medication. How should the nurse respond?
- **A.** "Take the missed dose as soon as possible, but don't double it."
- **B.** "Begin the medication regimen all over again."
- **C.** "Double the next two doses."
- **D.** "Double the next dose."

11. Vernon Glaser, age 62, must take ketoconazole for a fungal infection. The nurse should instruct Mr. Glaser to contact the physician if he experiences which adverse reaction to ketoconazole?
- **A.** Pale stools
- **B.** Clear urine
- **C.** Hair loss
- **D.** Dysuria

True or false

12. Amphotericin B usually is given in conjunction with ketoconazole.

☐ True   ☐ False

13. Griseofulvin is less effective against nail infections than skin infections.

☐ True   ☐ False

14. Miconazole can be used to treat systemic, local, and topical fungal infections.

☐ True   ☐ False

ANSWERS

Fill in the blank

1. Site, severity

2. Systemic, topical

3. Systemic

4. Increase

5. Amphotericin B

Multiple choice

6. B. Because amphotericin B is a highly toxic antibiotic, its use must be limited to patients with a definitive diagnosis of systemic life-threatening infection.

7. C. Up to 80% of patients receiving amphotericin B develop nephrotoxicity, which can be detected by changes in BUN and serum creatinine levels.

8. D. Concomitant use of amphotericin B with any electrolyte solution causes precipitation and inactivation of the drug.

9. B. The nurse should instruct the patient to avoid using occlusive dressings during therapy with nystatin ointment or cream because they provide a favorable environment for fungal growth.

10. A. The patient should take a missed dose as soon as possible, but should not take a double dose because missing a dose is safer than over-medicating with a double dose.

11. A. Ketoconazole can cause hepatotoxicity, which causes such effects as unusual fatigue, dark or amber colored urine, pale stools, jaundice, or right upper quadrant abdominal pain.

True or false

12. False. Amphotericin B commonly is administered with flucytosine because fungi can develop a resistance to flucytosine when flucytosine is administered alone.

13. True.

14. True.

CHAPTER 32

Antineoplastic agents

OBJECTIVES After studying this chapter, the reader should be able to:

1. Discuss the cell cycle and its importance in antineoplastic therapy.

2. Compare the mechanisms and sites of action for selected antineoplastic agents.

3. Describe how to handle and administer antineoplastic agents safely.

4. Identify common adverse reactions to antineoplastic agents.

5. Identify drugs that belong to each class of antineoplastic agent.

6. Compare the therapeutic and adverse effects of the alkylating, antimetabolite, antibiotic, hormonal, and other antineoplastic agents.

7. Describe the nursing implications of antineoplastic therapy.

OVERVIEW OF CONCEPTS Antineoplastic agents may be used to cure, prevent, or relieve cancer symptoms. For patients with systemic cancer, such as leukemia, chemotherapy may be given as a curative treatment. In other patients, it may be given as an adjuvant treatment based on the premise that micrometastases, although undetectable, exist. In patients with advanced neoplastic disorders, chemotherapy may be palliative, reducing tumor size or relieving pain and other symptoms. Chemotherapy commonly is combined with other cancer treatments. For example, it may be given preoperatively to reduce tumor size and allow less radical surgery.

Cell cycle To understand the pharmacodynamics of antineoplastic agents, the nurse must know about the cell cycle. All animal cells follow a series of basic steps as they undergo division and replication. This series of steps is called the cell cycle; each step is a phase. During each phase, biochemical events that are necessary for cell division occur. (For a summary of these phases, see *Cell cycle,* page 448.)

In the first phase, G_1 (G stands for gap), the cell manufactures the enzymes needed for deoxyribonucleic acid (DNA) synthesis. The time a cell spends in G1 varies greatly, but averages about 18 hours.

Next the cell enters the S phase (S stands for synthesis). In this phase, DNA replication occurs in preparation for mitosis (cell division). This phase lasts from 10 to 20 hours.

Cell cycle

Every cell progresses through a series of phases to replicate itself. During each phase, the cell is vulnerable to certain drugs that can interfere with its replication. This concept is the basis of antineoplastic therapy.

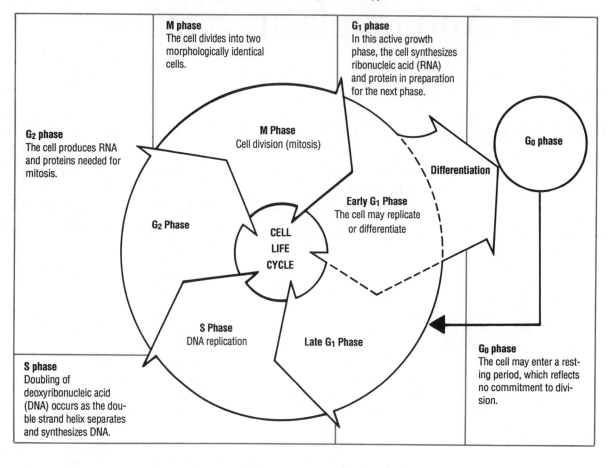

M phase
The cell divides into two morphologically identical cells.

G₁ phase
In this active growth phase, the cell synthesizes ribonucleic acid (RNA) and protein in preparation for the next phase.

G₂ phase
The cell produces RNA and proteins needed for mitosis.

G₀ phase
The cell may enter a resting period, which reflects no commitment to division.

S phase
Doubling of deoxyribonucleic acid (DNA) occurs as the double strand helix separates and synthesizes DNA.

Then the cell enters the G2 phase, when specialized DNA proteins and ribonucleic acid (RNA) are synthesized for later mitosis. This phase lasts about 3 hours.

Finally, the cell is ready to divide and enters the M phase (M stands for mitosis). During mitosis, the cell progresses through four subphases: *prophase,* when the chromosomes aggregate or clump; *metaphase,* when the chromosomes line up in the middle of the cell; *anaphase,* when the chromosomes segregate; and *telophase,* when the cell divides, producing two morphologically identical cells. The entire M phase lasts only 1 hour.

From the M phase, the cell may follow one of three paths. It may differentiate into a functional cell, enter the G0 (resting) phase, or begin the cycle again by entering the G_1 phase. Resting cells in the G_0 phase may enter the G_1 phase and progress through the cell cycle.

In different phases of the cycle, cells are susceptible to different drugs because the drugs interfere with specific biochemical events that occur in these phases.

Mechanisms of action

Although not understood completely, cancer seems to occur when one cell undergoes a malignant transformation and produces an abnormal cell. Antineoplastic agents interfere with cell reproduction, leading to tumor destruction. (For details, see *Mechanisms and sites of action of selected antineoplastic agents,* page 450.)

During administration of an antineoplastic agents, a fixed percentage of cells die. After treatment, the remaining cells reproduce, and resting cells in the G_0 phase may return to a reproducing phase. (Cells in the G_0 phase are less sensitive to chemotherapy because they are not synthesizing DNA actively.) Total eradication of cancer cells, therefore, depends on repeated administration of the antineoplastic agent. An interval between treatments permits healthy cells to recover.

Because cancer cells are at various phases in the cell cycle, therapy commonly combines drugs that act on cells in different phases or that have different sites of action.

Although an antineoplastic agent kills cells as soon as they pass through a specific cell cycle, this action produces no immediate clinical response. Most patients need at least three treatments before a clinical response can be evaluated by physical examination, X-ray, computed tomography, magnetic resonance imaging, or biological marker determination.

Tumor regression depends on several factors, such as the percentage of cells killed, the rate of regrowth, and the development of resistant cells. Evaluation of chemotherapy is difficult, however, because the cancer may be undetected clinically but may be present. Therefore, treatments may continue for a while after the disease no longer is detectable.

Tumor resistance

Combination drug regimens may be used for patients with tumor resistance. Tumor cell populations are heterogenous; some cells are sensitive to antineoplastic agents while others are not. When an antineoplastic agent is administered, it kills drug-sensitive cells initially. Repeated administration kills more drug-sensitive cells. Over time, however, tumor cells that are not drug-sensitive remain and replicate, producing a drug-resistant tumor. If these resistant cells also are resistant to other drugs, they will be even more difficult to kill.

Drug resistance may develop by one or more of the following mechanisms: decreased drug entry into tumor cells, decreased drug-activating enzymes, increased drug-deactivating enzymes, increased levels of target enzymes, decreased target enzyme affinity for the drug, in-

Mechanisms and sites of action of selected antineoplastic agents

During various phases in the cell cycle, antineoplastic agents act to halt cell growth or destroy it. Knowing where in the cycle these agents can act will help the nurse understand the basic principles of chemotherapy.

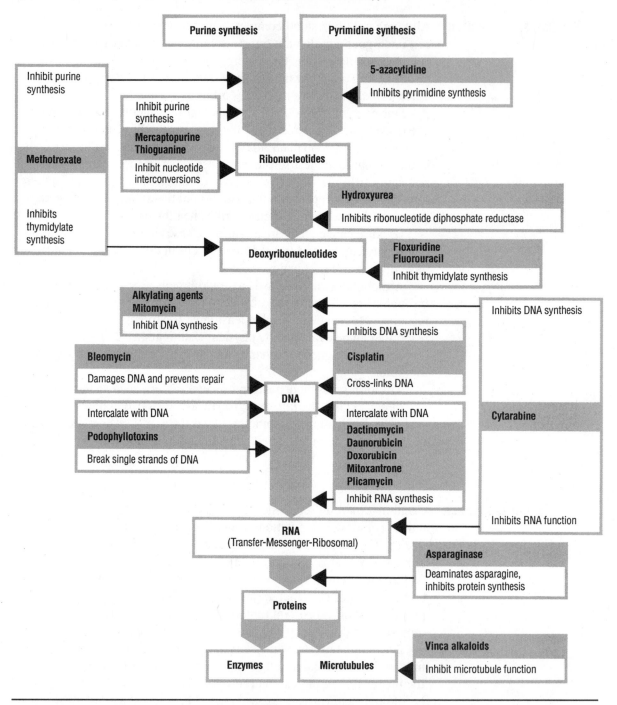

creased DNA repair, or development of alternate pathways that circumvent the drug's action.

General nursing implications

When caring for a patient who is receiving an antineoplastic agent, the nurse must handle and administer these drugs properly and must provide care related to adverse reactions and other aspects of drug therapy. All care should be based on appropriate nursing diagnoses for the patient. (For examples, see Sample Nursing Diagnoses: *Antineoplastic agents,* page 452.)

Handling antineoplastic agents

Although safe handling of antineoplastic agents remains controversial, most experts recommend conservative, protective methods. For maximum safety, the nurse should use the following techniques when handling antineoplastic agents.
- Mix antineoplastic agents in a Class II biological safety cabinet only.
- Wear powder-free, disposable, latex surgical gloves and a protective barrier garment with a closed front and long, cuffed sleeves to protect the body when mixing or administering antineoplastic agents. Some clinicians recommend wearing double gloves.
- Reconstitute and administer antineoplastic agents in syringes or intravenous (I.V.) sets with luer-lock connections.
- Use a closed delivery technique when administering these agents.
- Do not prime I.V. lines and syringes into a sink or wastebasket; use sterile 2″ × 2″ gauze pads or alcohol wipes instead.
- Dispose of any waste in a leakproof, punctureproof container labeled "hazardous waste." Such containers must be disposed of by incineration or burial at a hazardous chemical waste site.
- Clean up any spill by following the health care facility's policy for cleaning up hazardous materials.

Administering antineoplastic agents

Administration of antineoplastic agents requires these special nursing actions.
- Review information about the benefits and risks of treatment that the patient received from the physician. Provide additional information to a patient who consents to investigational chemotherapy. Throughout the patient's therapy, continue to teach and reinforce this information to promote patient safety and compliance.
- Select an appropriate site and vein for drug therapy. Begin with a distal spot, such as the hand, and proceed to proximal areas, such as the upper forearm.
- Consider drug compatibilities before administering the prescribed antineoplastic agent. As a rule, antineoplastic agents should not be mixed with any other medications because of the nature and toxicity of antineoplastic agents.

SAMPLE NURSING DIAGNOSES

Antineoplastic agents

The following nursing diagnoses address representative problems and etiologies that a nurse may encounter when caring for a patient who is receiving an antineoplastic agent.

- Altered health maintenance related to endocrine and metabolic imbalances caused by a hormonal antineoplastic agent
- Altered health maintenance related to flulike syndrome caused by an antineoplastic agent
- Altered health maintenance related to ineffectiveness of the prescribed antineoplastic agent
- Altered health maintenance related to severe hypertension caused by procarbazine–tyramine interaction
- Altered health maintenance related to the adverse central nervous system (CNS) effects of methotrexate
- Altered nutrition: less than body requirements, related to stomatitis or other adverse gastrointestinal (GI) effects of an antineoplastic agent
- Altered oral mucous membrane related to stomatitis caused by an antineoplastic agent
- Altered protection related to an acute hypersensitivity reaction to an antineoplastic agent
- Altered protection related to thrombocytopenia caused by an antineoplastic agent
- Altered protection related to plicamycin-induced hemorrhagic diathesis
- Altered thought processes related to the adverse CNS effects of an antineoplastic agent
- Anxiety related to the adverse effects of flutamide
- Body image disturbance related to alopecia caused by an antineoplastic agent
- Body image disturbance related to virilization in a female patient caused by a hormonal antineoplastic agent
- Decreased cardiac output related to cardiomyopathy caused by daunorubicin, doxorubicin, or mitoxantrone
- Fatigue related to anemia caused by an antineoplastic agent
- Fluid volume excess related to congestive heart failure caused by interferons, daunorubicin, doxorubicin, or mitoxantrone
- Fluid volume excess related to fluid retention caused by a hormonal antineoplastic agent
- High risk for activity intolerance related to anemia caused by an antineoplastic agent
- High risk for fluid volume deficit related to the adverse GI effects of an antineoplastic agent
- High risk for infection related to leukopenia caused by an antineoplastic agent
- High risk for injury related to adverse drug reactions
- High risk for injury related to a preexisting condition that contraindicates the use of an antineoplastic agent
- High risk for injury related to a preexisting condition that requires cautious use of an antineoplastic agent
- Hyperthermia related to fever caused by an antineoplastic agent
- Impaired cerebral, peripheral, or pulmonary tissue perfusion related to a thromboembolism caused by a hormonal antineoplastic agent
- Impaired gas exchange related to the adverse pulmonary effects of an antineoplastic agent
- Impaired tissue integrity related to extravasation of an antineoplastic agent
- Impaired tissue integrity related to hemorrhagic cystitis caused by cyclophosphamide or ifosfamide
- Knowledge deficit related to the prescribed antineoplastic agent
- Pain related to administration of an antineoplastic agent
- Pain related to tumor flare caused by an antineoplastic agent
- Sexual dysfunction related to the adverse genitourinary effects of a hormonal antineoplastic agent

Classification of antineoplastic agents

To administer an antineoplastic agent safely, the nurse needs to know whether it is a vesicant (capable of producing blisters), an irritant (capable of producing undue sensitivity), or a nonvesicant drug.

Vesicants
- dacarbazine
- dactinomycin
- daunorubicin
- doxorubicin
- mitomycin
- mitoxantrone
- nitrogen mustards
- plicamycin
- vinblastine
- vincristine
- vindesine

Irritants
- carmustine
- etoposide
- streptozocin

Nonvesicant drugs
- asparaginase
- bleomycin
- carboplatin
- cisplatin
- cyclophosphamide
- cytarabine
- floxuridine
- fluorouracil
- ifosfamide

- Choose the proper drug sequencing and delivery technique by determining the drug's potential to act as a vesicant. (For details, see *Classification of antineoplastic agents.*) For intermittent therapy, administer a vesicant agent by direct push or delivery into the side port of an infusing I.V. line. For continuous infusion, administer a vesicant only via a central line or vascular access device. Give nonvesicant agents (including irritants) by direct I.V. push (through the side port of an infusing I.V. line) or by continuous infusion. Some facilities require administration of the vesicant first because vein integrity decreases over time; others require administration of the vesicant last because it may increase vein fragility.
- Administer the drug exactly as prescribed. Check dosages closely because even a minute dosage calculation error may cause severe problems.
- Reduce patient discomfort by administering a vesicant via a venous access device that removes the necessity for multiple I.V. insertions.
- Assess the infusion site regularly during I.V. antineoplastic administration. Ensure patency of the vein by eliciting a blood return before, during, and after drug administration.
- Prevent extravasation by using a splint to stabilize the needle and checking frequently for blood return.
- Treat extravasation by discontinuing the infusion, aspirating any residual drug from the tubing and needle, instilling an I.V. antidote, and removing the needle. After administering an antidote, apply cold compresses and elevate the affected limb, as needed. To decrease tissue damage, instill hydrocortisone, as prescribed, into the affected site

via an I.V. catheter, subcutaneous injection, or as indicated by health care facility protocol.

Understanding adverse reactions

The adverse reactions to antineoplastic agents result from the systemic effects of these drugs. Some reactions can be life-threatening, requiring modification of the drug dosage or treatment regimen. Others are less severe but may be stressful to the patient. (For a summary, see *Common adverse reactions and associated nursing implications*.)

Nausea and vomiting are common adverse reactions. Chemotherapy can cause nausea and vomiting by three basic mechanisms. Orally administered drugs can irritate the gastric mucosa directly, causing nausea and vomiting that is less severe than that caused by the other two mechanisms.

Other antineoplastic agents can stimulate the chemoreceptor trigger zone. The incidence of nausea and vomiting from this mechanism depends on the inherent emetic potential of the drug:

- Drugs with a high emetic potential (greater than 50% incidence) include azacytidine, carmustine, cisplatin, cyclophosphamide, dacarbazine, dactinomycin, daunorubicin, doxorubicin, mechlorethamine, mithramycin, and streptozocin.
- Drugs with a moderate emetic potential (25% to 50% incidence) include 5-azacytidine, cytarabine, etoposide, interferons, procarbazine, thiotepa, and vinblastine.
- Drugs with a low emetic potential (less than 25% incidence) include asparaginase, bleomycin, busulfan, carboplatin, chlorambucil, fluorouracil, hydroxyurea, mercaptopurine, methotrexate, plicamycin, thioguanine, and vincristine.

Finally, chemotherapy can cause psychogenic nausea and vomiting, which originates in the cerebral cortex. Known as anticipatory emesis, this reaction can be disabling. A patient who remembers the unpleasantness of previous chemotherapy may feel nauseated or may vomit just by thinking about future treatments. This reaction may become so severe that sights, sounds, and smells associated with treatment may induce emesis, no matter how far removed the patient is from the actual treatment setting.

Chemotherapy-induced nausea and vomiting is of great concern because it can cause fluid and electrolyte imbalances, noncompliance with the treatment regimen, Mallory-Weiss syndrome (tears at the esophageal-gastric junction, leading to massive bleeding), wound dehiscence, and pathological fractures. It also can cause distress by limiting the patient's ability and motivation to take an active role in life.

To combat nausea and vomiting caused by chemotherapy, nurses commonly administer antiemetic drugs, such as metoclopramide, lorazepam, dexamethasone, prochlorperazine, diphenhydramine, droperidol, and dronabinol. Usually, an antiemetic drug is given with several other antiemetics that act by different mechanisms. A combina-

Common adverse reactions and associated nursing implications

The antineoplastic agents share many of the same adverse reactions and require similar nursing interventions. To provide quality patient care, the nurse must be aware of the following reactions and implications.

ADVERSE REACTIONS	NURSING IMPLICATIONS
Bone marrow suppression	
Bone marrow suppression is the most common and potentially serious adverse reaction to the antineoplastic agents.	• Check the patient's complete blood count and platelet count before administering the initial antineoplastic dose and after each subsequent dose, as prescribed. • Watch for the blood count nadir because that is when the patient is at greatest risk for the complications of leukopenia, thrombocytopenia, and anemia. • Plan a patient-teaching program about bone marrow suppression, including information about blood counts, potential sites of infection, and personal hygiene.
Leukopenia. This reaction increases the patient's risk of infection, especially if the granulocyte count is under 1,000/mm^3	• Monitor the patient for signs and symptoms of infection, such as fever, chills, cough, malaise, and sore throat if leukopenia occurs. Keep in mind that a patient with leukopenia is subject to infections. • Take infection control measures until the patient's white blood cell count returns to normal. • Provide information about good hygiene. • Teach the patient to recognize and report the signs and symptoms of infection. • Teach the patient how to take a temperature. • Teach the patient infection control measures to use, as needed. For example, caution the patient to avoid crowds and people with colds or the flu during the nadir. • Remember that the inflammatory response may be decreased and the complications of leukopenia more difficult to detect if the patient is receiving a corticosteroid.
Thrombocytopenia. This reaction accompanies leukopenia. When the platelet count is under 50,000/mm^3, the patient is at risk for bleeding. When it is under 20,000/mm^3, the patient is at severe risk and may require a platelet transfusion.	• Monitor the patient for signs and symptoms of bleeding, such as spontaneous epistaxis, bleeding gums, easy bruising, petechiae, hypermenorrhea, tarry stools, hematuria, and coffee-ground vomitus, if thrombocytopenia occurs. • Take bleeding precautions until the patient's platelet count returns to normal. Avoid all intramuscular (I.M.) injections and venipunctures when the platelet count is low. When a venipuncture must be done, apply firm pressure to the site for at least 5 minutes afterward. • Teach the patient bleeding precautions to use, as needed. For example, advise the patient to avoid cuts and bruises and to use a soft toothbrush and an electric razor. • Instruct the patient to report sudden headaches, which could indicate potentially fatal intracranial bleeding. • Instruct the patient to use a stool softener, as prescribed, to prevent colonic irritation and bleeding. • Instruct the patient to avoid using a rectal thermometer and receiving I.M. injections, to prevent bleeding.
Anemia. This reaction develops slowly over several courses of treatment.	• Take energy conservation measures if anemia occurs. For example, stagger the patient's activities and provide frequent rest periods. • Assess the patient for dizziness, fatigue, pallor, and shortness of breath on minimal exertion. • Monitor the patient's hematocrit, hemoglobin level, and red blood cell count. Remember that a patient dehydrated from nausea, vomiting, or anorexia may exhibit a false-normal hematocrit. Once this patient is rehydrated, the hematocrit will decrease. • Be prepared to administer a blood transfusion to a symptomatic patient, as prescribed. • Teach the patient energy conservation measures to use, as needed. For example, instruct the patient to rest more frequently • Instruct the patient to increase the dietary intake of iron-rich foods. Advise the patient to take a multivitamin with iron, as prescribed.

(continued)

Common adverse reactions and associated nursing implications *(continued)*

ADVERSE REACTIONS	NURSING IMPLICATIONS
Nausea and vomiting	
These reactions can result from gastric mucosal irritation, chemical irritation of the central nervous system, or psychogenic factors that may be activated by sensations, suggestions, or anxiety.	• Control chemical irritation by administering combinations of antiemetics, as prescribed. • Monitor the patient for signs and symptoms of aspiration because most antiemetics also sedate the patient. • Control psychogenic factors by helping the patient perform relaxation techniques before chemotherapy to minimize feelings of isolation and anxiety. • Monitor hydration if the patient experiences nausea or vomiting. Maintain intravenous hydration, as prescribed, until the patient can tolerate adequate oral intake. • Encourage the patient to express feelings of anxiety. • Encourage the patient to listen to music or engage in relaxation exercises, meditation, or hypnosis to promote feelings of control and well-being. • Adjust the drug administration time to meet the patient's needs. Some patients prefer treatments in the evening when they find sedation comfortable. Patients who are employed may prefer their treatments on their days off.
Stomatitis	
Although epithelial tissue damage can affect any mucous membrane, the most common site is the oral mucosa. Stomatitis is temporary and can range from mild and barely noticeable to severe and debilitating. (Debilitation may result from poor nutritional intake during acute stomatitis.)	• Initiate preventive mouth care before chemotherapy to provide comfort and to decrease the severity of stomatitis. • Provide oral care at least twice daily during chemotherapy until a special program is required; then after each meal and at bedtime; for severe stomatitis, every 2 hours. • Use appropriate aids, such as a soft toothbrush or a foam toothbrush (Toothette), lip moisturizer, and an oral irrigating device. • Inspect the patient's oral cavity regularly for signs of stomatitis, such as redness, ulceration, or bleeding of the oral mucous membrane. If stomatitis is present, provide symptomatic care. • Relieve mouth pain with dyclonine hydrochloride (Dyclone), lidocaine (Xylocaine 2% Viscous Solution), or Benadryl and Maalox as a swish; or administer a systemic analgesic for severe pain, as prescribed. • Apply a topical antibiotic, as prescribed. • Teach the patient how to manage stomatitis at home. • Advise the patient to rinse mouth with an isotonic solution of 0.9% sodium chloride and sodium bicarbonate—not hydrogen peroxide or any mouthwash that contains alcohol.
Alopecia	
To the patient, alopecia may be the most distressing adverse reaction.	• Prepare the patient for alopecia. Inform the patient that hair loss usually is gradual and is reversible after treatment ends. • Inform the patient that alopecia may be partial or complete and that it affects men and women. • Inform the patient that alopecia may affect the scalp, eyebrows, eyelashes, and body hair. • Consult the physician before initiating scalp hypothermia to decrease alopecia because the procedure is not appropriate for every patient.

tion regimen is more effective than a single drug, especially for a strong emetic agent, such as cisplatin. The nurse also can help control psychogenic factors related to nausea and vomiting by teaching the patient relaxation techniques that can help minimize feelings of isolation and anxiety, encouraging the patient to express anxieties, and helping the patient use relaxation techniques during chemotherapy.

Providing additional care

The nurse must provide care based on the patient's specific needs and specific drug regimen. However, the following general nursing interventions commonly apply to antineoplastic therapy.

- Do not administer an antineoplastic agent to a patient with a condition that contraindicates its use.
- Administer an antineoplastic agent cautiously to a patient at risk because of a preexisting condition.
- Monitor all infusion sites for signs of extravasation, such as pain and swelling at the insertion site. Change infusion sites according to health care facility protocol and as needed.
- Monitor the patient for signs and symptoms of neurotoxicity, such as sensory or motor peripheral neuropathies, loss of proprioception or taste, intestinal ileus, tinnitus, and hearing loss.
- Take safety precautions if the antineoplastic agent produces adverse central nervous system (CNS) reactions. For example, keep the bed in the low position, raise the side rails, and advise the patient not to perform activities that require mental alertness until the drug's adverse CNS effects are known.
- Monitor the patient for adverse reactions and signs of drug interactions.
- Monitor urinalysis, blood urea nitrogen level, and creatinine level, as prescribed, for abnormalities that indicate nephrotoxicity and renal failure. Keep in mind that mild proteinuria is an early sign of nephrotoxicity.
- Monitor the patient's liver function studies, as prescribed. If abnormalities occur, expect to lower the antineoplastic dose or change to a different agent, as prescribed.
- Notify the physician if adverse reactions or drug interactions occur.
- Teach the patient and family the name, dose, frequency, action, and adverse effects of the prescribed antineoplastic agent.

Alkylating agents   The alkylating agents fall into one of six classes: nitrogen mustards, alkyl sulfonates, nitrosoureas, triazines, ethylenimines, and alkylating-like agents. (For a list of the specific drugs in each class, see *Antineoplastic agents by class,* page 458.)

With the exception of the triazine dacarbazine, the alkylating agents have the same mechanisms of action. These highly reactive drugs enter the cell by active transport. Then they form covalent bonds with DNA molecules in a chemical reaction known as alkylation. Al-

Antineoplastic agents by class

This chart lists the different classes of antineoplastic agents as well as specific drugs in each class.

ALKYLATING AGENTS
Nitrogen mustards
- chlorambucil (Leukeran)
- cyclophosphamide (Cytoxan)
- estramustine phosphate sodium (Emcyt)
- ifosfamide (Ifex)
- mechlorethamine hydrochloride (Mustargen)
- melphalan (Alkeran)
- uracil mustard (Uracil Mustard Capsules)

Alkyl sulfonates
- busulfan (Myleran)

Nitrosoureas
- carmustine [BCNU] (BiCNU)
- lomustine [CCNU] (CeeNU)
- semustine [methyl CCNU] (investigational drug)
- streptozocin (Zanosar)

Triazines
- dacarbazine [DTIC] (DTIC-Dome)

Ethylenimines
- thiotepa (Thiotepa)

Alkylating-like agents
- carboplatin (Paraplatin)
- cisplatin [cis-platinum] (Platinol)

ANTIMETABOLITE AGENTS
Folic acid analogues
- methotrexate sodium (Folex, Mexate)

Pyrimidine analogues
- 5-azacytidine (investigational drug)
- cytarabine [ARA-C or cytosine arabinoside] (Cytosar-U)
- floxuridine (FUDR)
- fluorouracil [5-fluorouracil or 5-FU] (Adrucil, Efudex)

Purine analogues
- fludarabine phosphate (Fludara)
- mercaptopurine [6-MP or 6-mercaptopurine] (Purinethol)
- thioguanine [6-thioguanine]

ANTIBIOTIC ANTINEOPLASTIC AGENTS
Microbial tumoricidal agents
- bleomycin sulfate (Blenoxane)
- dactinomycin [actinomycin D] (Cosmegen)
- daunorubicin hydrochloride [DNR] (Cerubidine)
- doxorubicin hydrochloride (Adriamycin)
- idarubicin hydrochloride (Idamycin)
- mitomycin [mitomycin-C] (Mutamycin)
- mitoxantrone (Novantrone)
- plicamycin [mithramycin] (Mithracin)

HORMONAL ANTINEOPLASTIC AGENTS
Estrogens
- chlorotrianisene (TACE)
- conjugated estrogens (Premarin)
- diethylstilbestrol (DES)
- diethylstilbestrol diphosphate (Stilphostrol)
- ethinyl estradiol (Estinyl)

Antiestrogens
- tamoxifen citrate (Nolvadex)

Androgens
- fluoxymesterone (Halotestin)
- testolactone (Teslac)
- testosterone enanthate (Delatestryl)
- testosterone propionate (Testex)

Antiandrogens
- flutamide (Eulexin)

Adrenocortical suppressants
- aminoglutethimide (Cytadren)

Progestins
- hydroxyprogesterone caproate (Duralutin)
- medroxyprogesterone acetate (Depo-Provera)
- megestrol acetate (Megace)

Corticosteroids
- dexamethasone (Decadron)
- hydrocortisone (Cortef)
- methylprednisolone sodium succinate (Medrol, Solu-Medrol)
- prednisolone (Delta-Cortef)
- prednisone (Deltasone)

Gonadotropin-releasing hormone analogues
- goserelin acetate (Zoladex)
- leuprolide acetate (Lupron)

OTHER ANTINEOPLASTIC AGENTS
Vinca alkaloids
- vinblastine sulfate [VLB](Velban)
- vincristine sulfate (Oncovin)
- vindesine sulfate (investigational drug)

Podophyllotoxins
- etoposide [VP-16] (VePesid)
- teniposide [VM-26] (investigational drug)

Asparaginase
- asparaginase [L-asparaginase] (Elspar)

Procarbazine
- procarbazine hydrochloride (Matulane)

Hydroxyurea
- hydroxyurea (Hydrea)

Interferons
- interferon alpha-2a, recombinant (Roferon-A)
- interferon alpha-2b, recombinant (Intron A)
- interferon alpha-n3 (Alferon N)
- interferon gamma-1b (Actimmune)

kylated cells cannot reproduce properly, resulting in cell death. These drugs exert cytotoxic activity in a cell-cycle-nonspecific manner but may act more effectively in the late G_1 phase and S phase. (Dacarbazine acts primarily on RNA synthesis.) Interference with normal cell division in rapidly proliferating tissue explains the therapeutic and adverse effects of alkylating agents.

Alkylating agents, given alone or with other drugs, effectively act against various malignant neoplasms. Nitrogen mustards are indicated for Hodgkin's disease, certain leukemias, and many solid tumors. The alkyl sulfonate busulfan is used to treat chronic leukemia and other myeloproliferative disorders. Nitrosoureas are effective against brain tumors and meningeal leukemias. The triazine dacarbazine is used to treat malignant melanoma. Of the alkylating agents, carboplatin is used to treat ovarian cancer, and cisplatin is used primarily to treat metastatic ovarian and testicular cancers. The ethylenimine derivative thiotepa is prescribed for bladder cancer, ovarian or breast cancer, or lymphomas.

The most common and potentially harmful adverse reaction to the alkylating agents is bone marrow suppression, resulting in leukopenia and thrombocytopenia. Other major adverse reactions include nausea, vomiting, alopecia, and damage to epithelial tissue. The severity of the adverse reactions depends on many variables, including drug dosage, prior chemotherapy, the patient's physical condition, and psychological factors. Adverse reactions, which usually are reversible, may occur early or later in the therapeutic regimen.

Cyclophosphamide and ifosfamide also may cause hemorrhagic cystitis. To help prevent this adverse reaction, the nurse should increase the patient's fluid intake, administer the drug early in the day to prevent prolonged contact with the bladder during sleep, and administer mesna with ifosfamide 4 to 8 hours after treatment to help prevent hemorrhagic cystitis.

After long-term therapy (1 to 3 years), busulfan may cause irreversible interstitial pulmonary fibrosis (busulfan lung). To help prevent this adverse reaction, the nurse should monitor pulmonary function studies, perform regular respiratory assessments, and notify the physician if respiratory abnormalities occur.

Antimetabolite agents   The antimetabolite agents are structural analogues of natural metabolites essential to cellular functioning. They are divided into three classes: folic acid analogues, pyrimidine analogues, and purine analogues. (For a list of the specific drugs in each class, see *Antineoplastic agents by class.*)

These drugs produce their antineoplastic effects by replacing a metabolite in the molecule, competing with a metabolite for a particular site of an enzyme, or competing with a metabolite that regulates enzymes; all of these mechanisms alter the catalytic rate. This interferes with nucleic acid and protein synthesis. Because antimetabolites are cell-cycle-specific and primarily affect cells that actively synthesize DNA, they are called S-phase-specific. These drugs affect normal cells that are reproducing actively, as well as cancer cells. To help protect normal cells during treatment with the folic acid analogue methotrexate, the physician may prescribe leucovorin. (For details, see *Leucovorin rescue.*)

Malignancies that respond to the action of antimetabolites include acute leukemia, breast cancer, adenocarcinoma of the gastrointestinal (GI) tract, malignant lymphomas, and squamous cell carcinoma of the head, neck, and cervix.

Adverse reactions usually are dose-related and reversible, and many patients may not experience any of these reactions. The most common adverse reactions to antimetabolites include bone marrow suppression and stomatitis. During antimetabolite therapy, oral care can minimize injury to the mucosa, which is a first-line defense against infection. Other adverse reactions can include pulmonary or CNS toxicity with methotrexate, mild to severe skin reactions with fluorouracil, bile duct sclerosis with floxuridine, fever and flulike symptoms with 5-azacytidine and cytarabine, and cholestatic jaundice with any pyrimidine analogue.

Antibiotic antineoplastic agents

Antibiotic antineoplastic agents are antimicrobial products that produce tumoricidal effects by binding with DNA. These drugs inhibit the cellular processes of normal and malignant cells and are cell-cycle-nonspecific, except for bleomycin, which is G_2-phase-specific. The seven antibiotic antineoplastic agents form one class, the microbial tumoricidal agents. (For a list of the specific drugs in this class, see *Antineoplastic agents by class,* page 458.)

With the exception of mitomycin, the antibiotic antineoplastic agents intercalate, or insert themselves, between adjacent base pairs of a DNA molecule, physically separating them. When the DNA chain replicates, an extra base is inserted opposite the intercalated antibiotic, resulting in a mutant DNA molecule. The overall effect is cell death. Mitomycin is activated within the cell to an alkylating agent that produces single-strand breakage of DNA.

The antibiotic antineoplastic agents are products of microbial fermentation that exhibit antimicrobial activity. Their cytotoxic effects, however, preclude their antimicrobial use. These agents act against many tumors, including Hodgkin's disease and malignant lymphomas; testicular carcinoma; squamous cell carcinoma of the head, neck, and cervix; Wilms' tumor, osteogenic sarcoma, and rhabdomyosarcoma; Ewing's sarcoma and other soft-tissue sarcomas; breast, ovarian, bladder, and bronchogenic carcinomas; acute leukemias; melanoma; carcinomas of the GI tract; and choriocarcinoma. They also are used to treat hypercalcemia.

Leucovorin rescue

Methotrexate interferes with cell division in the S phase of the cell cycle by inhibiting dihydrofolate reductase (DHFR), an enzyme involved in deoxyribonucleic acid (DNA) synthesis. High-dose methotrexate is most effective against cells that have a high metabolic rate, such as leukemia cells. Used alone, high-dose methotrexate eventually will affect normal cells as well, producing toxicity.

To protect normal cells, methotrexate commonly is prescribed with leucovorin (folinic acid). Leucovorin rescues cells by bypassing the S phase, which methotrexate inhibits, as this diagram illustrates. It also acts by other mechanisms that are not understood completely. Leucovorin must be administered exactly on time, as prescribed, for the drug to work efficiently. When administered properly, leucovorin rescues cells before they begin active growth and division. Although leucovorin is considered a vitamin, doses must not be skipped because this drug plays an important role in preventing severe methotrexate toxicity.

Because leucovorin cannot prevent methotrexate toxicity completely, the nurse should closely monitor any patient on high-dose methotrexate therapy for bone marrow suppression, stomatitis, pulmonary complications, and renal damage (from drug precipitation in tubules). The nurse also should maintain urine alkalinity to avoid precipitation in tubules and monitor the urine output closely.

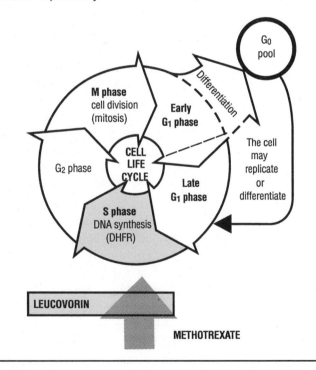

The antibiotic antineoplastics produce many of the same reactions as other antineoplastic agents. The most common adverse reactions are bone marrow suppression, alopecia, nausea, and vomiting. Except for bleomycin, all antibiotic antineoplastics can cause severe tissue damage if extravasated. Daunorubicin, doxorubicin, and mitoxantrone may cause adverse cardiovascular reactions, such as congestive heart failure; bleomycin may produce pulmonary fibrosis; plicamycin can cause hemorrhagic diathesis. Mitomycin causes delayed myelosuppression that requires 6 to 8 weeks for the bone marrow to recover.

Hormonal antineoplastic agents

The hormonal antineoplastic agents fall into eight classes: estrogens, antiestrogens, androgens, antiandrogens, adrenocortical suppressants, progestins, corticosteroids, and gonadotropin-releasing hormone analogues. (For a list of the specific drugs in each class, see *Antineoplastic agents by class,* page 458.)

The mechanisms of action of these drugs are not understood completely. Although not cytotoxic, the hormonal antineoplastic agents can be cytostatic and inhibit malignant neoplasm growth by altering the hormonal environment of the tumor. Most hormonal antineoplastic agents have a slow onset of action and require a therapeutic trial of 2 to 3 months.

These agents are prescribed to alter the growth of malignant neoplasms or to manage and treat their physiologic effects. They prove effective against hormone-dependent tumors. For example, estrogens are prescribed as palliative therapy for metastatic breast cancer in postmenopausal women and for metastatic prostate cancer. The antiestrogen tamoxifen is the drug of choice for treating advanced breast cancer of estrogen receptor-positive tumors in postmenopausal women. Androgens prove effective in treating breast cancer in men and advanced breast cancer in women. The antiandrogen flutamide is used in combination with a gonadotropin-releasing hormone analogue to treat advanced prostate cancer. The adrenocortical suppressant aminoglutethimide is as effective as surgical adrenalectomy in treating advanced breast cancer. Progestins are used as palliative treatment of advanced endometrial, breast, and renal cancers. Because of their lympholytic potential, corticosteroids usually are used to treat lymphocytic leukemias, myeloma, and malignant lymphomas. They also are prescribed for edema resulting from metastatic cancer because of their anti-inflammatory effects. Gonadotropin-releasing hormone analogues treat advanced prostate cancer by decreasing testosterone levels.

Most adverse reactions to hormonal antineoplastic agents are extensions of their natural hormonal activities. For example, estrogens can cause feminization (gynecomastia and impotence) in men and decreased libido and breast tenderness in women. Androgens can produce virilization in females as well as fluid retention. The most common reactions to the antiandrogen flutamide include hot flashes, decreased libido, impotence, and gynecomastia.

Many hormonal antineoplastics can produce nausea and vomiting. Estrogens also can cause adverse cardiovascular, endocrine, and metabolic reactions. Although tamoxifen is relatively nontoxic, it can cause hot flashes and tumor flare. Androgen therapy is associated with fluid retention, jaundice, and hypercalcemia. Besides its adverse hormonal effects, flutamide can cause adverse CNS reactions, such as confusion, depression, and anxiety. About 50% of the patients taking aminoglutethimide experience rash, hypotension, fatigue, drowsiness, and dizziness. Progestins can produce fluid retention, thromboembolism, and liver function abnormalities. Patients taking corticosteroids may experience fluid and sodium retention, behavioral changes, immunosuppression, and cushingoid symptoms. The gonadotropin-releasing hormone analogues commonly cause hot flashes, impotence, decreased libido, and tumor flare.

The nurse should instruct the patient that hormonal antineoplastic therapy may extend over many weeks or months. Also, the nurse should monitor for compliance with drug regimen.

Other antineoplastic agents

Additional antineoplastic agents include natural products (the vinca alkaloids and podophyllotoxins) and other drugs that do not belong in existing classifications (asparaginase, procarbazine, hydroxyurea, and interferons). (For a list of the specific drugs in each class, see *Antineoplastic agents by class,* page 458.)

The vinca alkaloids are cell-cycle-specific for the M phase. They may disrupt the normal function of the microtubules, inhibiting mitosis and causing cell death. They are used to treat Hodgkin's disease, malignant lymphomas, testicular cancer, Kaposi's sarcoma, neuroblastoma, choriocarcinoma, breast cancer, acute lymphocytic leukemia (ALL), rhabdomyosarcoma, and Wilms' tumor. At low concentrations, podophyllotoxins block cells at the late S or G_2 phase; at higher concentrations, they arrest cells in the G_2 phase. These drugs are used to treat various tumors, including lymphomas, leukemias, small-cell lung carcinoma, and testicular carcinoma.

Asparaginase is a cell-cycle-specific enzyme that acts in the G_1 phase. Because it hydrolyzes asparagine, which leukemic cells need for survival, it is used primarily to induce remission in ALL. Procarbazine acts by causing chromosome damage, producing antimitotic activity, and inhibiting DNA, RNA, and protein synthesis. It is given with other drugs to treat Hodgkin's disease and CNS tumors. Hydroxyurea may act as a DNA-selective antimetabolite in the S and G_1 phases, interfering with DNA synthesis. It is used primarily in combination therapy to manage myeloproliferative disorders, such as acute refractory and chronic granulocytic leukemia. Interferons are naturally occurring molecules that inhibit viral replication, suppress cell proliferation, enhance macrophage activity, and increase lymphocyte cytotoxicity. They are used to treat hairy-cell leukemia, Kaposi's sarcoma caused by acquired immunodeficiency syndrome (AIDS), and condylomata acuminata.

Most vinca alkaloids and podophyllotoxins can produce bone marrow suppression, nausea, vomiting, and stomatitis. The vinca alkaloids also can cause severe local necrosis (with extravasation) and neuromuscular abnormalities; vinblastine may produce tumor pain. Acute hypotension may result if a podophyllotoxin is infused too rapidly.

Because asparaginase increases the patient's risk of anaphylaxis, it should be administered with a physician present. This drug also may cause adverse GI reactions, hepatotoxicity, hypersensitivity reactions, orthostatic hypotension, and CNS toxicity. Procarbazine can interact with tyramine, causing severe hypertension. Therefore, a patient taking procarbazine should avoid eating tyramine-rich foods. (For information about these foods, see *Foods that may interact with MAO inhibitors,* page 165.) Procarbazine also may cause nausea, vomiting, flulike syndrome, and CNS toxicity. Common reactions to hydroxyurea include bone marrow suppression, drowsiness, headache, nausea, vomiting, and anorexia. Patients taking hydroxyurea may need to take allopurinol to prevent uric acid nephropathy and renal damage. The most common adverse reaction to interferons is a flulike syndrome, which can be minimized by administering the drug in the evening or premedicating the patient with acetaminophen. Interferons also may cause adverse hematologic and GI reactions, CNS disturbances, and cardiopulmonary reactions, such as hypotension, coughing, dyspnea, and congestive heart failure.

STUDY ACTIVITIES

Matching related elements
Match the drug on the left with its class on the right.

1. ___ Cisplatin	**A.** Ethylenimine
2. ___ Methotrexate	**B.** Pyrimidine analogue
3. ___ Thiotepa	**C.** Microbial tumoricidal agent
4. ___ Daunorubicin	**D.** Alkylating-like agent
5. ___ Tamoxifen	**E.** Adrenocortical suppressant
6. ___ Etoposide	**F.** Folic acid analogue
7. ___ Fluorouracil	**G.** Podophyllotoxin
8. ___ Aminoglutethimide	**H.** Antiestrogen

Fill in the blank
9. During the early _____ phase of the cell cycle, the cell may replicate or differentiate.

10. The _____ phase of the cell cycle also is known as the resting phase.

11. Most alkylating agents form covalent bonds with _____ in a chemical reaction known as alkylation.

12. Because the antimetabolite agents primarily affect cells that actively synthesize DNA, they are called _____-phase specific.

13. The antibiotic antineoplastic agents _____ between adjacent _____ of a DNA molecule, physically separating them.

14. Although not cytotoxic, the hormonal antineoplastic agents can be _____ and prevent _____ growth.

15. Vinca alkaloids may disrupt the normal function of the _____, inhibiting _____ and causing cell death.

True or false

16. Before administering an I.V. antineoplastic, the nurse should prime the I.V. line carefully into a sink.
☐ True   ☐ False

17. After administering the drug, the nurse should dispose of any waste in a leakproof, punctureproof container labeled "hazardous waste."
☐ True   ☐ False

18. When selecting an I.V. site for antineoplastic administration, the nurse should begin with a proximal spot and proceed to a distal area.
☐ True   ☐ False

19. For continuous infusion, a vesicant should be administered through the side port of an infusing I.V. line.
☐ True   ☐ False

20. Bone marrow suppression is the most common and potentially serious adverse reaction to the antineoplastic agents.
☐ True   ☐ False

Multiple choice

21. John Bowes, age 35, is receiving busulfan (Myleran) for chronic myelogenous leukemia. The nurse assess Mr. Bowes regularly for adverse reactions. Which adverse reaction is associated with long-term busulfan therapy?
　A. Hemorrhagic cystitis
　B. Cushingoid syndrome
　C. Pulmonary fibrosis
　D. Infertility

22. Ellen Sugarman, age 56, has bladder cancer. For this patient, the physician is most likely to prescribe which alkylating agent?
　A. Dacarbazine
　B. Carboplatin
　C. Cisplatin
　D. Thiotepa

23. To maintain a remission of ALL, Robert Larson, age 27, receives a high dosage of methotrexate sodium (Folex). To protect normal cells, he also should receive which drug?
  A. Leucovorin
  B. Prednisone
  C. Lomustine
  D. Mitomycin

24. Mr. Larson develops stomatitis. To help minimize this adverse reaction to methotrexate, the nurse should provide which instruction?
  A. Limit oral care to once a day to avoid irritation.
  B. Brush the teeth vigorously with a hard toothbrush.
  C. Rinse regularly with 0.9% sodium chloride solution and sodium bicarbonate.
  D. Use a mouthwash that is a mixture of alcohol and mineral oil.

25. Shirley Allen, age 47, is scheduled to begin therapy with bleomycin, plicamycin, and doxorubicin for breast cancer. The nurse administers doxorubicin with extreme caution because it is a vesicant. Nevertheless, extravasation occurs. What should the nurse do?
  A. Stop the infusion immediately and apply cold compresses.
  B. Stop the infusion immediately and lower the limb.
  D. Decrease the flow and administer the antidote.
  C. Decrease the flow and apply heat.

26. During antineoplastic therapy, Ms. Allen's granulocyte count drops below 1,000/mm^3. At this point, the nurse should teach her to report which signs and symptoms?
  A. Dizziness, fatigue, and pallor
  B. Fever, cough, and sore throat
  C. Easy bruising and tarry stools
  D. Sudden headaches or seizures

27. Sam Reeves, age 48, has lung cancer that has metastasized to the brain. The physician is most likely to prescribe which type of drug to reduce edema resulting from intracranial metastasis?
  A. Androgen
  B. Estrogen
  C. Antiandrogen
  D. Corticosteroid

ANSWERS **Matching related elements**
  1. D
  2. F
  3. A
  4. C
  5. H
  6. G

7. B
8. E

Fill in the blank

9. G_1
10. G_0
11. DNA molecules
12. S
13. Intercalate, base pairs
14. Cytostatic, malignant neoplasm
15. Microtubules, mitosis

True or false

16. False. The nurse should not prime I.V. lines and syringes into a sink or wastebasket. Instead, the nurse should use sterile $2'' \times 2''$ gauze pads or alcohol wipes.
17. True.
18. False. To select an appropriate I.V. site, the nurse should begin with a distal spot and proceed to proximal areas.
19. False. For continuous infusion, a vesicant should be administered only via a central line or vascular access device.
20. True.

Multiple choice

21. C. After long-term therapy (1 to 3 years), busulfan may cause irreversible interstitial pulmonary fibrosis (busulfan lung).
22. D. Thiotepa is prescribed to treat bladder cancer, ovarian or breast cancer, or lymphomas
23. A. To protect normal cells during high-dose therapy, methotrexate commonly is prescribed with leucovorin (folinic acid).
24. C. The nurse should recommend frequent oral care and use of an isotonic solution of 0.9% sodium chloride and sodium bicarbonate as a rinse.
25. A. The nurse should discontinue the infusion, aspirate residual drug from the tubing and needle, instill an I.V. antidote, remove the needle, apply cold compresses, and elevate the affected limb.
26. B. The nurse should teach the patient with leukopenia to recognize and report signs and symptoms of infection, such as fever, cough, sore throat, or a burning sensation on urination.
27. D. Because of their anti-inflammatory effects, corticosteroids are prescribed for edema resulting from metastatic cancer.

CHAPTER 33

Other major drugs

OBJECTIVES
After studying this chapter, the reader should be able to:

1. Differentiate between the nondepolarizing and depolarizing neuro-muscular blockers.
2. Distinguish between narcotic agonists and narcotic antagonists.
3. Differentiate among general, local, and topical anesthetics.
4. Discuss the clinical uses of the hematinic agents.
5. Describe how to administer and monitor therapy with anticoagulant and thrombolytic agents.
6. Compare the therapeutic uses of various vitamins and minerals.
7. Describe the nursing implications of electrolyte replacement therapy.
8. Discuss the therapeutic and adverse effects of alkalinizing and acidifying agents.
9. Describe the therapeutic and adverse effects of cation-exchange resins and ammonia-detoxicating agents.
10. Identify commonly used parathyroid agents.
11. Discuss the use and abuse of androgenic and anabolic steroid agents.
12. Contrast the uses of estrogens, progestins, and oral contraceptive agents.
13. Differentiate between antigout agents and gold salts.
14. Describe the therapeutic and adverse effects of the following anti-infective agents: antitubercular, antileprotic, anthelmintic, antimalarial, other antiprotozoal, and urinary antiseptic agents.
15. Describe how to administer ophthalmic and otic agents for appropriate eye and ear disorders.

OVERVIEW OF CONCEPTS
This chapter presents major drugs that are used infrequently, such as antileprotic agents; those used to treat unique conditions, such as antigout agents; or those that require advanced preparation to use, such as general anesthetic agents. For each drug class, it provides information about the drugs' mechanisms of action, clinical uses, adverse reactions, and related nursing considerations.

Neuromuscular blocking agents

Neuromuscular blockers are divided into two main classes: nondepolarizing and depolarizing blockers. They may be used to relax skeletal muscles for various procedures. Because these drugs do not cross the blood-brain barrier, the patient remains conscious and may experience anxiety and pain, but cannot communicate feelings.

Both types of neuromuscular blockers require similar nursing care. During administration, the nurse should monitor closely for adverse reactions; should keep endotracheal equipment, oxygen, suction equipment, and a mechanical ventilator available for respiratory support; and should be prepared to give emergency care. For a patient who is completely paralyzed and cannot communicate, the nurse should reduce anxiety by maintaining a calm environment, providing reassurance, and explaining all procedures and outcomes. The nurse should monitor respirations closely until the patient has recovered fully from neuromuscular blockade, as evidenced by tests of muscle strength (hand grip and ability to cough).

Nondepolarizing blocking agents

The nondepolarizing blockers, also called competitive or stabilizing agents, include atracurium besylate (Tracrium), gallamine triethiodide (Flaxedil), metocurine iodide (Metubine), pancuronium bromide (Pavulon), pipecuronium bromide (Arduan), tubocurarine chloride (Tubarine), and vecuronium bromide (Norcuron).

After intravenous (I.V.) administration, these agents compete with acetylcholine at cholinergic receptor sites in the skeletal muscle membrane. This prevents the muscle membrane from depolarizing. The initial muscle weakness produced by the drugs quickly changes to a flaccid paralysis that affects the muscles in a specific sequence. The first muscles to exhibit flaccid paralysis are those innervated by the motor portions of the cranial nerves and small, rapidly moving muscles in the eyes, face, and neck. Next, the limb, abdomen, and trunk muscles become flaccid. Finally, the intercostal muscles and diaphragm are paralyzed. Recovery usually occurs in the reverse order.

Nondepolarizing blockers are used for intermediate or prolonged muscle relaxation. They facilitate endotracheal intubation and are used during surgery to decrease the amount of anesthetic required and to facilitate manipulations. They also are used to paralyze patients who need ventilatory support but who fight the endotracheal tube and ventilator. Some nondepolarizing blockers also prevent muscle injury during electroconvulsive therapy (ECT) by reducing the intensity of muscle spasms. Because plasma levels of the nondepolarizing blockers are difficult to predict, nerve stimulators are used to assess the drug's effect on the patient.

Inhalation anesthetics, aminoglycosides, clindamycin, polymyxin B sulfate, calcium channel blockers, magnesium salts, and potassium-depleting drugs can increase neuromuscular blockade when administered with a nondepolarizing blocker. Cholinesterase inhibitors, such as neostigmine or pyridostigmine, can decrease the blockade, which makes them effective as antidotes.

Apnea is the most serious adverse reaction to the nondepolarizing blockers. Adverse cardiovascular, respiratory, and dermatologic reactions also may occur. Specific nursing interventions include keeping an antidote readily available; monitoring the patient's fluid intake and output; and turning the patient, providing chest physiotherapy, and suctioning.

Depolarizing blocking agents

Succinylcholine (Anectine, Quelicin, Sucostrin) is the only therapeutic depolarizing blocker. After I.V. or intramuscular (I.M.) administration, it produces a biphasic effect. Phase I blockade produces brief periods of repetitive excitation—manifested by muscle fasciculations—followed by muscle paralysis and flaccidity. Phase II blockade, which normally occurs only with a high drug concentration or repeated doses, causes prolonged neuromuscular blockade.

Succinylcholine is the drug of choice for short-term muscle relaxation, such as during intubation and ECT. Anesthetics, antibiotics, and cholinesterase inhibitors can increase its neuromuscular blockade. Its primary adverse reactions are prolonged apnea and cardiovascular alterations. Patients also commonly experience muscle pain, myoglobulinemia, myoglobinuria, increased serum potassium level, and transient elevation of intraocular pressure. To determine a patient's sensitivity to succinylcholine, an initial test dose of 10 mg may be administered.

Narcotic agonist and antagonist agents

Narcotic agonists (analgesics) reduce pain without causing loss of consciousness. Most also possess antitussive and antidiarrheal actions and can cause serious adverse effects. Narcotic antagonists block the therapeutic and adverse effects of narcotic agonists. Mixed narcotic agonist-antagonists display properties of both types of drugs. They relieve pain and decrease the risk of toxicity and drug dependence.

Narcotic agonists

Narcotic agonists are classified according to their abuse potential. Schedule II drugs include codeine, fentanyl citrate (Sublimaze), hydrocodone bitartrate and acetaminophen (Vicodin), hydromorphone hydrochloride (Dilaudid), levorphanol tartrate (Levo-Dromoran), meperidine hydrochloride (Demerol), methadone hydrochloride (Dolophine), morphine sulfate (Duramorph PF), morphine sulfate sustained-release tablets (MS Contin, Roxanol SR), morphine sulfate intensified oral solution (Roxanol), oxycodone hydrochloride (Roxicodone), oxycodone hydrochloride with acetaminophen (Percocet, Tylox), oxycodone hydrochloride with aspirin (Percodan), and oxymorphone hydrochloride (Numorphan). Hydrocodone bitartrate and chlorpheniramine maleate (Tussionex) is classified as a Schedule III drug as are codeine preparations in combination with aspirin or acetaminophen. Schedule IV drugs include propoxyphene hydrochloride (Darvon) and propoxyphene napsylate (Darvon-N).

These drugs may be administered by the oral, I.V., I.M., subcutaneous (S.C.), epidural, intrathecal, sublingual, transdermal, and rectal routes. After administration, they bind to opiate receptors in the central and peripheral nervous systems and activate the endogenous pain-relief system.

Narcotic agonists are used to relieve pain in acute, chronic, and terminal illnesses, to decrease preanesthesia anxiety, and to relieve diarrhea and cough. Morphine also reduces the dyspnea of pulmonary edema and left ventricular failure. Narcotic agonists are contraindicated in patients with head injuries or increased intracranial pressure because they can mask changes in level of consciousness.

An equianalgesic dose of any narcotic drug is a dose that produces the same level of analgesia as an agent and dose selected as a standard, usually 10 mg of morphine I.M. When a patient must be changed from one narcotic to another, using an equianalgesic dose decreases the risk of toxicity and inadequate pain relief. (For more information, see *Narcotic agonists: Equianalgesic doses*, page 472.)

The use of narcotic agonists with other drugs that decrease respiration increases the patient's risk of severe respiratory depression. Concomitant use of tricyclic antidepressants, phenothiazines, or anticholinergic agents may cause severe constipation and urine retention.

Common adverse reactions to the narcotic agonists include dose-dependent respiratory depression and adverse gastrointestinal (GI) reactions, such as nausea, vomiting, biliary colic, and constipation. Flushing, orthostatic hypotension, urine retention, and pupillary constriction also may occur. Long-term use produces physical dependence. Therefore, sudden discontinuation will cause withdrawal symptoms, including increased sensory perceptions, especially pain and touch, tactile hallucinations, increased GI secretions, diarrhea, dilated pupils, and photophobia.

Before and after administering a narcotic agonist, the nurse should monitor the patient's pain level and respiratory rate, depth, and rhythm. Inadequate pain relief or requests for increased drug administration suggest tolerance to the drug's effects. A respiratory rate of 8 to 10 breaths/minute or less indicates the need to withhold the dose and consult the physician. Throughout therapy, the nurse should monitor for adverse reactions and provide symptomatic relief, as needed. Patient-teaching points should include avoidance of central nervous system (CNS) depressants and techniques to minimize adverse reactions.

Mixed narcotic agonist-antagonists

Three mixed narcotic agonist-antagonists are Schedule IV drugs: pentazocine hydrochloride, pentazocine lactate (Talwin), and buprenorphine hydrochloride (Buprenex). The others—butorphanol tartrate (Stadol), dezocine (Dalgan), and nalbuphine hydrochloride (Nubain)—

Narcotic agonists: Equianalgesic doses

The so-called standard narcotic agonist dose, 10 mg of morphine sulfate I.M., is used to calculate equally effective (equianalgesic) doses of the various narcotic agonists. This method is particularly useful when a patient must be switched from one narcotic agonist to another with no change in dose effectiveness. In this chart, which lists equianalgesic doses of selected narcotic agonists, all doses are I.M. except for codeine, which is administered orally.

NARCOTIC AGONIST	EQUIANALGESIC DOSE
codeine	120 mg
fentanyl	0.1 to 0.2 mg
hydromorphone	1.5 mg
levorphanol	2 mg
meperidine	75 to 100 mg
methadone	8 to 10 mg
morphine	10 mg
oxymorphone	1.0 to 1.5 mg

have a low abuse potential and are not controlled drugs. After oral, I.V., I.M., or S.C. administration, these drugs occupy opiate receptors, but their exact mechanism of action is unknown.

Mixed narcotic agonist-antagonists are prescribed primarily for the relief of moderate to severe pain, for obstetric analgesia in selected cases, and for preoperative medication to reduce anxiety and pain perception. They sometimes are preferred over narcotic agonists because they pose a lower risk of drug dependence and respiratory depression.

Concomitant use of a mixed narcotic agonist-antagonist with a narcotic agonist can cause withdrawal symptoms; concomitant use with a CNS depressant can cause increased CNS depression and decreased respiratory rate and depth.

The mixed narcotic agonist-antagonists cause fewer adverse reactions than the narcotic agonists. They commonly cause nausea, vomiting, light-headedness, sedation, and euphoria. Other adverse reactions include hypertension, anticholinergic effects (such as dry mouth, blurred vision, constipation, and urine retention), and hypersensitivity reactions.

The nurse should not administer a mixed narcotic agonist-antagonist to a narcotic-dependent patient; it may precipitate withdrawal symptoms. The nurse also should question any prescription for S.C. pentazocine because it may cause severe tissue damage when administered by this route. Before and after drug administration, the nurse should assess the patient's pain level and monitor the respiratory rate, depth, and rhythm. During therapy, the nurse should monitor for drug interactions and adverse reactions and should intervene, as needed. If an overdose occurs, the nurse should provide emergency care, as prescribed.

Narcotic antagonists

The pure narcotic antagonists naloxone hydrochloride (Narcan) and naltrexone hydrochloride (Trexan) act by competitive inhibition. They occupy opiate receptor sites, displace narcotic molecules already present, and block further narcotic binding at these sites. This prevents narcotics from producing their effects.

Usually administered intramuscularly or intravenously, naloxone is the drug of choice for treating narcotic overdose. It rapidly reverses narcotic-induced respiratory depression, sedation, and analgesia. If the patient does not improve after receiving 3 doses or 10 mg, supportive measures, such as mechanical ventilation, should be used. Naloxone produces no significant drug interactions, but may cause nausea, vomiting, hypertension, and tachycardia. An unconscious patient returned to consciousness abruptly after naloxone administration may hyperventilate and experience tremors.

Orally administered naltrexone is used only as an adjunct to psychotherapy for former narcotic users who wish to remain drug-free. Naltrexone will cause withdrawal symptoms if given to a patient receiving a narcotic agonist or to a narcotic addict. It also can produce adverse cardiopulmonary, CNS, GI, genitourinary, eye, ear, nose, throat, and skin reactions.

Before and after administering a narcotic antagonist, the nurse should monitor the patient's respiratory rate, depth, and rhythm. If respiratory depression recurs, the nurse should prepare to administer additional doses of naloxone and perform other emergency care, such as mechanical ventilation. During therapy, the nurse should observe the patient for adverse reactions and notify the physician, as needed.

Anesthetic agents

Anesthesia can be produced by general, local, and topical anesthetic agents. General anesthetics are volatile liquids or gases vaporized in oxygen and administered by inhalation or nonvolatile solutions administered by injection. Commonly used inhalation anesthetics include enflurane (Ethrane), halothane (Fluothane), isoflurane (Forane), and nitrous oxide. Methoxyflurane (Penthrane), another inhalation agent, has limited application because it produces renal toxicity at high doses. Four agents are used solely as injection anesthetics: droperidol (Inapsine), etomidate (Amidate), ketamine hydrochloride (Ketalar), and propofol (Diprivan). The rest belong to other chemical categories, such as benzodiazepines (diazepam [Valium], lorazepam [Ativan], and midazolam hydrochloride [Versed]), opiates (meperidine hydrochloride [Demerol] and morphine sulfate [Astramorph]), barbiturates (methohexital sodium [Brevital Sodium], thiamylal sodium [Surital], and thiopental sodium [Pentothal Sodium]), and other classes (alfentanil hydrochloride [Alfenta], fentanyl citrate [Sublimaze], and sufentanil citrate [Sufenta]). General anesthesia usually is achieved by using a combination of drugs, which may be administered by injection or inhalation.

Local anesthetics include amide and ester agents. Amide agents include bupivacaine hydrochloride (Marcaine), etidocaine hydrochloride (Duranest), lidocaine hydrochloride (Xylocaine), mepivacaine hydrochloride (Carbocaine, Isocaine), and prilocaine hydrochloride (Citanest Plain). Ester agents include chloroprocaine hydrochloride (Nesacaine), procaine hydrochloride (Novocain), and tetracaine hydrochloride (Pontocaine). Local anesthetics cause temporary loss of sensation in a limited the area of the body; they are injected directly into the area.

Common topical anesthetics include: benzocaine (Americaine), benzyl alcohol, butacaine sulfate, butamben picrate (Butesin Picrate), clove oil, cocaine hydrochloride, dibucaine hydrochloride (Nupercainal), dyclonine hydrochloride (Dyclone), ethyl chloride, lidocaine (Xylocaine), menthol, pramoxine hydrochloride (Tronothane), and tetracaine (Pontocaine Eye). Like local anesthetics, topical anesthetics cause a temporary loss of sensation in a limited area of the body. They are applied directly to the skin or mucous membranes.

General anesthetics depress the CNS, thereby producing loss of consciousness, loss of response to sensory stimulation, and muscle relaxation. Local and topical anesthetics control pain by blocking nerve impulses, causing a temporary loss of sensation to the area. When a local anesthetic blocks large nerves, it produces a wide field of anesthesia.

Isoflurane is the most widely used general (inhalation) anesthetic because of its lack of serious toxicity. It also produces the greatest degree of skeletal muscle relaxation. Halothane, another inhalation anesthetic, relaxes bronchial smooth muscle, making it useful for anesthesia during surgery on patients with asthma. It is the primary anesthetic for children. Nitrous oxide is the least potent, fastest-acting inhalation anesthetic and it produces the fewest adverse reactions. The injection anesthetics usually are used in situations that require a short duration of anesthesia, such as outpatient surgery. They also are used to promote rapid induction of anesthesia and to supplement inhalation anesthetics.

Local anesthetics prevent and relieve pain from medical procedures, disease, and injuries. They are used for severe pain that topical anesthetics and analgesics cannot relieve. They usually are preferred for minor surgical or dental procedure and for surgery in a debilitated or geriatric patient or one who cannot tolerate a general anesthetic. For some procedures, a local anesthetic is combined with a vasoconstrictor, such as epinephrine. Epinephrine helps delay anesthetic absorption and reduces bleeding at the site.

Topical anesthetics are used to relieve pain—especially minor burn pain—itching, and irritation. They also are used to anesthetize an area before an injection is given and to numb mucosal surfaces before a tube, such as a cystoscope, is inserted. Sometimes they are used in combination with other drugs.

Most adverse reactions to general anesthetics are extensions of their therapeutic effects. These include adverse CNS reactions, bradycardia, nausea, vomiting, shivering, hypothermia, and depressed respirations. The inhalation anesthetics also can cause malignant hyperthermia (sudden and often lethal increase in body temperature). Methoxyflurane may cause dose-related nephrotoxicity.

Adverse reactions to local anesthetics usually result from overdose, improper injection technique, or hypersensitivity. An overdose may cause CNS and cardiovascular reactions. Because local anesthetics rapidly cross the placenta, they may produce similar adverse reactions in the fetus. When injected, they can cause a temporary burning sensation. They also may cause hypersensitivity reactions, including anaphylaxis.

Adverse reactions to topical anesthetics vary with the individual drug, but may include CNS and cardiovascular symptoms. Benzyl alcohol may cause topical reactions, such as skin irritation; ethyl chloride and other refrigerants may produce frostbite in the area. Any topical anesthetic may cause a hypersensitivity reaction, such as rash, pruritus, or throat swelling.

General anesthetics can enhance the depressant effects of CNS, cardiac, or respiratory depressants, requiring the nurse to monitor the patient's vital signs, airway, and level of consciousness closely. Before a general anesthetic is used, the nurse can expect to administer other drugs to reduce anxiety (neuroleptics), produce sedation (opiates and sedatives), and decrease bronchial secretions (anticholinergics and antihistamines). Also, the nurse should advise the patient not to eat for at least 8 hours before surgery to prevent aspiration during surgery. After general anesthesia, the nurse can expect to administer atropine, naloxone, and other drugs, as prescribed, to reverse the effects of drugs given before or during surgery. Also, the nurse should advise the patient not to drink alcohol or use any other CNS depressants for at least 24 hours.

Nursing interventions for a patient receiving a local anesthetic include positioning the patient as directed for a spinal block to ensure proper anesthetic distribution and instructing the patient to remain supine after spinal anesthesia to prevent postanesthesia headache. Also, the nurse should teach the patient to protect numb areas until sensation returns.

When caring for a patient receiving a topical anesthetic, the nurse should monitor for topical irritation and localized frostbite. The nurse should teach the patient and family how to apply a topical anesthetic, as directed, and to avoid contact with the eyes. For a patient whose oropharyngeal mucosa has been anesthetized, the nurse should advise the patient to delay eating until sensation returns.

Hematinic agents   The major hematinic agents include iron, vitamin B_{12}, and folic acid. These agents promote the normal production of red blood cells (RBCs) by providing essential elements for erythropoiesis (RBC production). Normally, these elements are present in a well-balanced diet. A deficiency in one or more of these elements can lead to anemia.

General nursing interventions related to hematinic therapy include observing for drug interactions and adverse reactions; monitoring laboratory tests, such as hematocrit and reticulocyte count, to determine effectiveness of therapy; assessing the patient's dietary habits; and teaching the patient to consume a well-balanced diet that includes the deficient nutrients.

Iron

Iron preparations include ferrous fumarate (Feostat), ferrous gluconate (Fergon), ferrous sulfate (Feosol), and iron dextran (Imferon). After administration, iron is distributed to all body tissues. In the bone marrow, erythroblasts use it to synthesize hemoglobin.

Iron is prescribed to prevent and treat iron deficiency anemia. In most individuals, oral drug therapy is effective. Parenteral therapy is used for patients who cannot absorb oral preparations, do not comply with oral therapy, or have a bowel disorder, such as ulcerative colitis. The average length of iron therapy for anemia is 6 months.

Antacids, coffee, tea, eggs, and milk may decrease iron absorption. Iron may interfere with the absorption of tetracyclines, penicillamine, and methyldopa. The major adverse reactions to iron are GI disturbances. Other reactions include stool darkening; tooth staining (with liquid preparations); hypersensitivity reactions; soreness, inflammation, and discoloration at the I.M. injection site (with iron dextran); and lymphadenopathy, phlebitis at the infusion site, and peripheral vascular reddening (with rapid I.V. administration).

For a patient receiving iron therapy, the nurse should administer oral preparations between meals and at least 2 hours before or after giving an antacid, infuse iron dextran I.V. at a rate of 1 ml/minute, or administer iron dextran I.M. by the Z-track method to avoid subcutaneous leakage. For I.V. administration, the nurse should use only single-dose vials and should not administer a single dose of more than 100 mg intravenously. Also, the nurse should teach the patient to avoid drinking coffee or tea for at least 1 hour after an iron dose, to take liquid preparations with a straw to prevent stained teeth, to eat iron-rich foods (such as meat, eggs, greens, and dried fruits), and to take measures to prevent adverse reactions.

Vitamin B$_{12}$

Vitamin B$_{12}$ drugs include cyanocobalamin (Betalin 12, Rubramin) and hydroxocobalamin (Alphamine, alphaRedisol). They are used to replace the vitamin B$_{12}$ that the body normally would absorb from meat, seafood, milk, eggs, liver, and legumes.

Cyanocobalamin and hydroxocobalamin are used to treat vitamin B$_{12}$ deficiency anemia. They usually are administered by the I.M. route, because the deficiency usually is caused by an inability to absorb dietary sources. However, cyanocobalamin may be administered orally.

Vitamin B$_{12}$ causes no significant drug interactions. However, parenteral forms sometimes cause adverse reactions, such as potentially fatal hypersensitivity reactions, cardiovascular reactions (pulmonary edema, congestive heart failure, and peripheral vascular thrombosis), and adverse hematologic, dermatologic, and GI reactions.

During vitamin B$_{12}$ therapy, the nurse should monitor compliance by reviewing the results of appropriate laboratory tests. The nurse also should teach the patient to store the parenteral form of the drug in a light-resistant container at room temperature and should demonstrate how to administer it.

Folic acid

Common folic acid preparations include folic acid (Folvite), which also is known as folate or vitamin B$_9$, and leucovorin calcium (Wellcovorin). Dietary sources of folic acid include fresh green vegetables, meat, and eggs.

Folic acid is administered orally to treat folic acid deficiency or to prevent this deficiency in a patient who is pregnant or undergoing treatment for liver disease, hemolytic anemia, alcoholism, skin disease, or renal failure. Folic acid is administered parenterally to reverse the effect of antifolates during cancer chemotherapy.

Folic acid may counteract the therapeutic effects of anticonvulsants and pyrimethamine. Glutethimide, isoniazid, cycloserine, and oral contraceptives may decrease folic acid absorption. Methotrexate, antimalarial agents, triamterene, pentamidine, and trimethoprim may cause a deficiency of active folate compounds.

Folic acid may produce allergic responses, such as erythema, rash, and itching. In a patient with vitamin B$_{12}$ deficiency anemia, it may worsen neurologic symptoms.

In addition to following the general nursing considerations, the nurse should take seizure precautions for a patient receiving large doses of folic acid during concomitant anticonvulsant therapy. Also, the nurse should monitor for recurrence of megaloblastic anemia if the patient takes drugs that interfere with folic acid absorption.

Other hematinic agents

Epoetin alfa is a hematinic agent that stimulates RBC production. It is used to treat patients with normocytic anemia caused by chronic renal failure. Epoetin alfa produces its therapeutic effects by replacing erythropoietin, which normally is formed in the kidneys in response to hypoxia and anemia and stimulates erythropoiesis. No known drug interactions exist. Hypertension is the most common adverse reaction.

Anticoagulant and thrombolytic agents

Anticoagulant agents, such as heparin, oral anticoagulants, and antiplatelet drugs, are prescribed to reduce clotting and prevent further coagulation in patients with diseases that cause a tendency toward clotting. Thrombolytic agents are used to dissolve newly formed clots, especially in patients with coronary artery thrombus, pulmonary embolus, or deep vein thrombosis.

Most nursing interventions for a patient receiving an anticoagulant or thrombolytic agent relate to bleeding and clotting. For example, the nurse should monitor the patient's vital signs, hemoglobin level, hematocrit, and other test results frequently. The nurse also should assess regularly for signs of bleeding, such as epistaxis, hematuria, and oozing from wounds, drainage tubes, and I.V. sites. During patient-teaching sessions, the nurse should emphasize using an electric razor and a soft toothbrush, returning for laboratory tests, reporting signs of bleeding, avoiding drugs (unless the physician is consulted first), and wearing a medical identification tag or bracelet.

Heparin

Heparin sodium (Liquaemin Sodium) impairs blood coagulation, but does not affect synthesis of clotting factors. Thus, it prevents clots from enlarging, but cannot dissolve them. Heparin also reduces the triglyceride level in the plasma, has anticomplement properties, exerts a slight antihistamine effect, and inhibits hypersensitivity reactions.

Heparin is the drug of choice to treat acute thromboembolism and to prevent clot formation because of its immediate anticoagulant effect after I.V. administration. It also is used to manage patients whose blood must circulate outside the body through a machine, to treat disseminated intravascular coagulation and arterial clotting in patients with atrial fibrillation, and to prevent venous thromboembolism after orthopedic surgery.

Heparin's anticoagulant effects are measured by the activated partial thromboplastin time (APTT) test and partial thromboplastin time (PTT) test. These effects can be reversed easily by protamine sulfate. One milligram of protamine sulfate can neutralize about 100 units of heparin and should be administered by I.V. infusion over 1 to 3 minutes.

Concomitant use of heparin and other anticoagulants increases the risk of bleeding. Concomitant use with cardiac glycosides, nitroglycerin, certain antibiotics, and other drugs can decrease heparin's effects. Bleeding is the most common adverse reaction to heparin. The drug also may cause thrombocytopenia; hypersensitivity reactions; and alopecia, osteoporosis, and spontaneous bone fractures (with long-term therapy).

To administer S.C. heparin, the nurse should inject the drug into the abdominal wall fold above the iliac crest and 2″ or more from the umbilicus to avoid risk of bleeding. After S.C. administration, the nurse should avoid aspirating and massaging the site to prevent subcutaneous bleeding. During therapy, the nurse should have the antidote protamine sulfate available in case of bleeding and should avoid all I.M. injections.

Oral anticoagulants

The oral anticoagulants are dicumarol and warfarin sodium (Coumadin). These drugs alter the synthesis of vitamin K-dependent clotting factors, including prothrombin. Their anticoagulant effects occur when circulating clotting factors are depleted; thus, optimal prothrombin time (PT) response is achieved in 1 to 4 days.

Oral anticoagulants are used to treat thromboembolism after initial treatment with heparin. They are the drugs of choice to prevent clotting in patients with deep vein thrombosis, prosthetic heart valves, or diseased mitral valves. Because these drugs can cross the placenta and damage the fetus, they should not be administered to pregnant patients. (Heparin, which does not cross the placenta, is the anticoagulant of choice during pregnancy.)

Vitamin K–rich foods and such drugs as barbiturates can interact with oral anticoagulants, increasing the risk of clotting; salicylates, phenylbutazone, and other drugs can increasing the risk of bleeding. Bleeding is the most common adverse reaction to the oral anticoagulants.

During oral anticoagulant therapy, the nurse should monitor the PT daily. Although a therapeutic PT ratio is 1.2 to 1.5 times the control, bleeding can occur even when the PT falls within the therapeutic range. If minor bleeding occurs, the nurse can expect to reduce the dosage; if frank bleeding occurs, to administer 5 to 50 mg of phytonadione (vitamin K_1) parenterally; if severe bleeding occurs, to administer 250 to 500 ml of fresh frozen plasma or commercial Factor IX complex. In addition to assessing for adverse reactions, the nurse should teach the patient when and how to take the medication.

Antiplatelet drugs

The major antiplatelet drugs include aspirin, dipyridamole (Persantine), and sulfinpyrazone (Anturane). Dextrans, clofibrate, indomethacin, and other drugs also show some antiplatelet activity. Antiplatelet drugs may work by interfering with platelet aggregation in atherosclerotic plaque development.

Low dosages of aspirin effectively prevent aortocoronary bypass shunt thrombosis, reduce clot formation in arteriovenous shunts, and reduce the risk of transient ischemic attacks. Aspirin also may help prevent reinfarction and sudden death in men with acute myocardial infarction (MI) and postoperative venous thrombosis in patients who undergo hip and knee surgery. When used with warfarin, dipyridamole may help prevent thromboembolism in patients with prosthetic heart valves. When used with aspirin, the drug may be effective in patients with cerebral ischemic attacks and those who undergo coronary bypass graft surgery. Sulfinpyrazone is used in cardiovascular disorders, including angina, MI, transient cerebral ischemic attacks, peripheral arterial atherosclerosis, and deep vein and recurrent venous thrombosis. It also may be ordered for patients with arteriovenous dialysis shunts or prosthetic mitral valves. Bleeding time and platelet aggregation studies measure the effectiveness of these agents.

The antiplatelet drugs, especially aspirin, interact with other anticoagulants, increasing the risk of bleeding. Aspirin also may interact with sulfinpyrazone, methotrexate, and valproic acid.

In the dosage prescribed to prevent arterial clotting, aspirin most commonly produces GI disturbances. Larger dosages may cause salicylism, which is characterized by dizziness, tinnitus, difficulty hearing, nausea, vomiting, diarrhea, confusion, and lethargy. Aspirin overdose may result in respiratory alkalosis. Dipyridamole produces minimal adverse reactions: headache, dizziness, nausea, and mild GI distress. Sulfinpyrazone primarily causes epigastric discomfort, which may aggravate or reactivate peptic ulcer disease. Less commonly, it may produce reversible renal dysfunction. Hypersensitivity reactions to the antiplatelet drugs—including bronchospasm, asthma-like symptoms, and anaphylaxis—can occur.

The nurse should administer aspirin or sulfinpyrazone with food, milk, or an antacid to reduce GI distress. If distress persists during aspirin therapy, the nurse should ask the physician to prescribe enteric-coated tablets. The nurse should administer dipyridamole 1 hour before meals with 8 oz (240 ml) of water. Throughout drug therapy, the nurse should monitor for adverse reactions, especially salicylism and breathing difficulty.

Thrombolytic agents

Thrombolytic agents include alteplase (Activase), anistreplase (Eminase), streptokinase (Kabikinase, Streptase), and urokinase (Abbokinase). These drugs act in various ways to convert plasminogen to the enzyme plasmin, which lyses (dissolves) thrombi, fibrinogen, and other plasma proteins.

These agents are used to treat certain thromboembolic disorders and to dissolve thrombi in arteriovenous cannulas. They are the drugs of choice to break down newly formed thrombi. They are most effective when administered immediately after thrombosis and up to 6 hours after onset of symptoms. When emboli are dissolved quickly, blood flow is reestablished to distal tissues, minimizing or preventing necrosis.

Thrombolytic agents interact with anticoagulants, antiplatelet drugs, and nonsteroidal anti-inflammatory drugs (NSAIDs), thereby increasing the risk of bleeding. Heparin or oral anticoagulant therapy often is begun after thrombolytic therapy ends, but not until the patient's thrombin time is less than twice the control.

The major adverse reactions to thrombolytic agents are bleeding and allergic responses. When administered by intracoronary catheter, streptokinase may cause hemorrhagic infarction at the site of myocardial necrosis as well as reperfusion arrhythmias. Anistreplase may produce conduction disorders, hypotension, and cardiopulmonary and CNS reactions.

For a patient receiving a thrombolytic agent, the nurse should monitor coagulation studies before and for at least 4 hours after drug administration. If severe bleeding occurs, the nurse should stop the infusion; administer fresh whole blood, packed RBCs, or fresh frozen plasma; and prepare to administer aminocaproic acid (Amicar) as an antidote. Throughout therapy, the nurse should assess for adverse reactions and should not administer I.M. injections or insert new arterial lines.

After intracoronary thrombolytic therapy, the nurse should leave arterial or venous sheaths in place for 24 hours. The nurse should immobilize the patient's leg for 24 hours to prevent bleeding and should monitor the patient's color, temperature, and femoral and pedal pulses every 15 minutes for 1 hour, and then every 30 minutes for 8 hours.

Vitamins and minerals

Vitamins are organic compounds that are needed in small amounts and are essential for life. They are divided into two classes: fat-soluble and water-soluble. (For a list of specific vitamins, see *Fat-soluble and water-soluble vitamins,* page 482.) Minerals are inorganic chemicals that are components of all living tissues. Because the body cannot synthesize most vitamins and all minerals, it must obtain them from dietary sources or nutritional supplements.

Vitamins

Fat-soluble vitamins include vitamins A, D, E, and K. Vitamin A is necessary for vision in dim light, healthy skin and mucous membranes, and normal growth and reproduction. Vitamin D regulates calcium and phosphorus balance. Vitamin E acts as an antioxidant and enzyme cofactor. Vitamin K stimulates the synthesis of clotting factors by the liver.

Water-soluble vitamins include B-complex vitamins and vitamin C. Except for vitamin C, the water-soluble vitamins function as coenzymes in various cellular metabolic functions. Vitamin C may participate in many oxidation biochemical reactions in the body and is involved in the synthesis of intracellular substances.

The primary clinical indication for vitamins is dietary supplementation to compensate for low levels of the vitamin, which may result from inadequate intake, decreased absorption, or increased excretion.

Fat-soluble and water-soluble vitamins

The following list provides the generic and brand names of commonly used fat-soluble and water-soluble vitamins.

FAT-SOLUBLE VITAMINS
Vitamin A
- beta carotene (Solatene)
- isotretinoin (Accutane)
- retinol, retinyl acetate (Aquasol A), or retinyl palmitate

Vitamin D
- cholecalciferol or vitamin D_3 (Delta-D)
- ergocalciferol or vitamin D_2 (Calciferol)

Vitamin E
- vitamin E (Aquasol E)

Vitamin K
- menadiol sodium diphosphate (Synkayvite)
- phytonadione (AquaMEPHYTON, Konakion, Mephyton)

WATER-SOLUBLE VITAMINS
Vitamin B_1
- thiamine (Betalin S)

Vitamin B_2
- riboflavin

Vitamin B_3
- niacin or nicotinic acid (Nicobid, Nicolar)
- niacinamide or nicotinamide

Vitamin B_6
- pyridoxine (Beesix, Hexa-Betalin)

Vitamin C
- ascorbic acid (Cecon, Cebid, Ce-Vi-Sol)

Vitamin D also is used to treat calcium and phosphorus imbalances; vitamin K has been used to treat hypoprothrombinemia caused by vitamin K deficiency.

Adverse reactions to fat-soluble vitamins vary; however, nausea and vomiting commonly occur with all of them. Vitamin A may produce skin and mucous membrane changes and congenital anomalies. Vitamin D may result in hypercalcemia. Vitamin E has been linked to increased serum cholesterol and triglyceride levels and decreased serum thyroxine and triiodothyronine levels. Severe hypersensitivity-like reactions and death have been noted after I.V. administration of vitamin K, which also may cause bleeding.

Although generally considered nontoxic, water-soluble vitamins can cause adverse reactions, including nausea, vomiting, diarrhea, transient flushing, rashes, and neuropathy. Dental erosion may occur with long-term use of chewable vitamin C.

During oral therapy, the nurse should instruct the patient to take the vitamin with food to prevent adverse GI reactions. During parenteral fat-soluble vitamin therapy, the nurse should keep emergency equipment nearby to manage hypersensitivity-like reactions. Because all fat-soluble vitamins can accumulate in the body, the nurse should monitor the patient for signs of toxicity and teach about potential hazards. Because water-soluble vitamins can be destroyed by heat and light and rapidly lose their potency, the nurse should teach the patient to store them in a cool, dark place for no more than 3 months. Also, the nurse should inform the patient of the recommended daily allowance (RDA) and food sources for the prescribed vitamin.

Minerals

Various minerals are used as nutritional supplements, including chromium (Chrometrace), copper (Coppertrace), fluoride (Luride, Pediaflor), iodine (Iodopen), manganese (Mangatrace), molybdenum (Molypen), selenium (Selenitrace), and zinc (Orazinc). Many minerals function as components of enzyme systems, regulating or enhancing enzyme reactions. Some act as building materials for cells, bones, and teeth. Others play a role in such essential body processes as nerve transmission, cellular respiration, glucose metabolism, or hormone functions.

The primary clinical indication for minerals is to treat deficiencies and to act as a nutritional supplement, particularly in patients receiving total parenteral nutrition. Because all minerals are stored by the body, mineral levels can become toxic. However, toxicity is not as common an adverse reaction as GI irritation.

The nurse should be aware of the signs and symptoms of toxic levels of minerals. Toxicity usually can be prevented by limiting the patient's intake of minerals to that prescribed. When administering parenteral minerals, the nurse must ensure that they are diluted well and administered via a central vein to prevent phlebitis. When administering oral minerals, the nurse should give them with food to prevent GI irritation. Also, the nurse should inform the patient of the RDA and food sources for the prescribed mineral.

Electrolyte replacement agents

Electrolyte replacement agents are mineral salts that increase deficient electrolyte levels; this helps maintain homeostasis. Potassium is the primary intracellular fluid (ICF) electrolyte; calcium is a major extracellular fluid (ECF) electrolyte. Magnesium and sodium are two other essential electrolytes.

During therapy with any electrolyte replacement agent, the nurse should monitor closely for adverse reactions and signs of drug interactions, particularly noting signs of electrolyte imbalances on electrocardiogram (ECG) tracings, vital sign measurements, and serum electrolyte levels. Also the nurse should attempt to determine the cause of the electrolyte deficiency. For example, the nurse may evaluate the patient's diet to detect inadequate dietary intake.

Potassium

Potassium replacement can be accomplished orally or intravenously with potassium salts: potassium bicarbonate (K-Lyte), potassium chloride (Kaochlor, Slow-K), potassium gluconate (Kaon), and potassium phosphate (Neutra-Phos-K).

The major cation in ICF, potassium moves quickly into ICF to restore depleted potassium levels and reestablish homeostasis. It is used to prevent or reverse hypokalemia, which may result from various causes. It also is used to decrease the toxic effects of cardiac glycosides.

Potassium may interact with potassium-sparing diuretics and angiotensin-converting enzyme (ACE) inhibitors, causing hyperkalemia. The most common adverse reaction to potassium is hyperkalemia, which may produce listlessness, confusion, flaccid paralysis, paresthesia, weakness, limb heaviness, ECG changes, decreased blood pressure, arrhythmias, heart block, and cardiac arrest. Oral potassium may cause GI distress; I.V. infusion may cause pain at the I.V. site and phlebitis.

Before infusing an I.V. potassium preparation, the nurse should dilute it as prescribed. During I.V. therapy, the nurse should assess regularly for signs and symptoms of phlebitis. If phlebitis occurs, the nurse should change the I.V. site. During oral therapy, the nurse should administer potassium with or after meals to minimize GI distress. Also, the nurse should direct the patient to dissolve the powder or tablets in at least 4 oz (120 ml) of water or fruit juice, and to sip the solution slowly over 5 to 10 minutes. Finally, the nurse should teach the patient to consume a potassium-rich diet.

Calcium

Calcium is a major cation in ECF. When dietary calcium intake is insufficient to meet metabolic needs, calcium stores in bone are reduced. Calcium may be replaced orally or intravenously with calcium salts: calcium carbonate (Os-Cal 500), calcium chloride, calcium citrate (Citracal), calcium glubionate (Neo-Calglucon), calcium gluconate (Kalcinate), and calcium lactate.

The major clinical indication for I.V. calcium is treatment of acute hypocalcemia. I.V. calcium also is used to prevent hypocalcemic reactions during exchange transfusions, to treat magnesium intoxication, and to strengthen myocardial tissue after defibrillation or after a poor response to epinephrine. Oral calcium commonly is used to supplement the diet, prevent osteoporosis, and treat chronic hypocalcemia.

When administered with a cardiac glycoside, calcium may precipitate arrhythmias. When given with a calcium channel blocker, it may reduce the response to that drug. Consumption of calcium with large amounts of spinach, rhubarb, bran, whole grain products, and fresh fruits and vegetables alters calcium absorption.

The major adverse reaction to calcium is hypercalcemia, which may cause drowsiness, lethargy, muscle weakness, headache, constipation, a metallic taste in the mouth, and ECG changes. Severe hypercalcemia can cause cardiac arrhythmias and arrest and, eventually, coma. Other adverse reactions may include renal calculi, venous irritation (with I.V. administration), and severe burning, necrosis, and tissue sloughing (with I.M. injection).

The nurse should infuse I.V. calcium slowly and keep the patient recumbent for 15 minutes to prevent cardiac arrhythmias and arrest. During concomitant therapy with calcium and a cardiac glycoside, the nurse should administer both drugs slowly and in small amounts. Throughout calcium therapy, the nurse should monitor the patient regularly for early signs of hypercalcemia and should keep emergency equipment nearby. The nurse also should assess the patient's diet. As indicated, the nurse should teach the patient to take calcium tablets 1 to 2 hours after eating foods that alter calcium absorption and to consume foods that contain calcium and vitamin D, which enhances calcium absorption.

Magnesium
Magnesium is the most common cation in ICF after potassium. The body stores magnesium in bone, plasma, interstitial fluid, and cells. However, these stores may be depleted by malabsorption, chronic diarrhea, prolonged therapy with diuretics or parenteral fluids that do not contain magnesium, nasogastric suctioning, and certain endocrine disorders.

Magnesium sulfate is the drug of choice for replacement therapy in magnesium deficiency. Severe cases can be treated using an I.V. infusion. Magnesium sulfate also is used to treat seizures, severe toxemia, and acute nephritis in children.

Sodium
Sodium is the major cation in ECF. It maintains the osmotic pressure and concentration of ECF, acid-base balance, and water balance. Sodium replacement is necessary in conditions that rapidly deplete it, such as excessive loss of GI fluids, excessive perspiration, use of diuretics or tap water enemas, trauma, wound drainage, and adrenal gland insufficiency.

Severe symptomatic sodium deficiency may be treated by I.V. infusion of 3% or 5% sodium chloride (NaCl) solution. Other I.V. solutions containing various concentrations of NaCl are used to prevent sodium depletion in conditions that predispose the patient to sodium loss. Injectable sodium salts (sodium bicarbonate and sodium lactate) also are used to treat metabolic acidosis.

Alkalinizing and acidifying agents

Alkalinizing and acidifying agents act to correct acid-base imbalances in the blood. Alkalinizing agents increase the pH (hydrogen ion concentration) of the blood; acidifying agents decrease it.

Alkalinizing agents
Four alkalinizing agents are used to increase blood pH: sodium bicarbonate, sodium citrate (Shohl's solution), sodium lactate, and tromethamine (Tham). Sodium bicarbonate and acetazolamide (Diamox) are used to increase urine pH. Except for acetazolamide, all alkalinizing agents act by decreasing hydrogen ion concentration and increasing blood pH. Acetazolamide paradoxically decreases blood pH and increases urine pH.

Alkalinizing agents commonly are used to treat metabolic acidosis. Other uses include alkalinizing the urine pH to help remove certain substances, such as barbiturates, salicylates, and lithium after an overdose.

Alkalinizing agents can interact with amphetamines, ketoconazole, lithium, methenamine mandelate, quinidine, salicylates, and pseudoephedrine, altering their pharmacokinetics or therapeutic effects.

These drugs also may cause severe adverse reactions, usually related to overdose. The most severe reaction is metabolic alkalosis, which may cause hyperirritability and tetany. In a patient with diabetic keto-acidosis (DKA), too-rapid administration of sodium bicarbonate may cause cerebral dysfunction, tissue hypoxia, and lactic acidosis. Sodium bicarbonate and sodium lactate also may cause water retention; edema; and tissue sloughing, ulceration, and necrosis (with I.V. extravasation). Oral alkalinizing agents may cause GI distress.

During alkalinizing agent therapy, the nurse should monitor the patient's serum pH, urine pH, and serum bicarbonate levels regularly to evaluate therapy and detect problems. The nurse also should inspect the I.V. site for localized adverse reactions and should monitor the patient closely for signs of an overdose. Finally, the nurse should advise the patient to report signs of fluid retention and other adverse reactions.

Before administering Shohl's solution, the nurse should dilute it with 2 to 3 oz (60 to 90 ml) of water and refrigerate it to improve the taste. To prevent its laxative effects, the nurse should administer it after meals. The nurse should administer sodium bicarbonate slowly to a patient with DKA to prevent adverse effects.

Acidifying agents

To acidify the blood, ammonium chloride, arginine hydrochloride, or hydrochloric acid may be used. To acidify the urine, ammonium chloride or ascorbic acid [vitamin C] (Ascorbicap, Cebid Timecelles) may be used. These agents produce acidification by increasing the hydrogen ion concentration.

Acidifying agents—especially oral or parenteral doses of ammonium chloride—commonly are used to treat metabolic alkalosis. Urine-acidifying agents may be prescribed to help treat urinary tract infections (UTIs) or drug overdose.

Although acidifying agents do not cause significant drug interactions, they usually produce mild adverse reactions, such as GI distress. An overdose may lead to acidosis. Large doses of ammonium chloride also may cause loss of electrolytes and ammonium toxicity, producing twitching and hyperreflexia. Too-rapid administration of arginine hydrochloride may cause adverse CNS and GI reactions, irritation at the infusion site, and hypersensitivity reactions. High doses of ascorbic acid may result in GI distress and CNS disturbances.

During therapy with an acidifying agent, the nurse should monitor the patient for signs of metabolic acidosis, ammonium toxicity, electrolyte imbalances, and other adverse reactions. For I.V. therapy, the nurse should infuse the agent slowly to prevent pain or irritation at the infusion site and other adverse reactions. For ascorbic acid or ammonium chloride therapy, the nurse should instruct the patient to take the agent exactly as prescribed, to report severe adverse GI reactions, and to monitor the urine pH regularly.

Cation-exchange resins and ammonia-detoxicating agents

These drugs decrease toxic levels of endogenous substances via the GI tract. A cation-exchange resin may be prescribed to reduce potassium levels; an ammonia-detoxicating agent, to reduce ammonia levels.

Cation-exchange resins

Sodium polystyrene sulfonate (Kayexalate, SPS) is the only commercially available drug that is effective as a cation-exchange resin. A nonabsorbable resin, it exchanges sodium ions for potassium ions in the GI tract, which makes it useful for treating hyperkalemia. Because sodium polystyrene sulfonate's onset of action is slow, the serum potassium level may not change for 2 to 24 hours after administration. Therefore, it should not be used in a patient with a life-threatening serum potassium level because it may not remove the excess potassium quickly enough.

After oral or rectal administration, sodium polystyrene sulfonate may absorb calcium, magnesium, and other electrolytes, causing imbalances. It also may release sufficient sodium to cause problems for a patient who cannot tolerate a high sodium load. The most common adverse reactions to this drug involve GI tract disturbances, such as nausea, vomiting, anorexia, and constipation. Because the drug tends to solidify in the GI tract, it can cause fecal impaction.

When caring for a patient receiving sodium polystyrene sulfonate, the nurse should administer to drug by enema (instilled at least 8″ [20 cm] into the colon and retained for 20 to 30 minutes) or by mouth (mixed with low-potassium fruit juice, water, syrup, or soft drink to increase its palatability). During cation-exchange resin therapy, the nurse should monitor the patient closely for signs and symptoms of fluid and electrolyte imbalances and should evaluate electrolyte levels regularly. To minimize constipation and prevent fecal impaction, the nurse may administer the drug in 70% sorbitol solution, which forms softer stools and helps excrete the resin.

Ammonia-detoxicating agents

The ammonia-detoxicating drugs lactulose (Cephulac, Chronulac) and neomycin (Mycifradin, Neo-fradin) commonly are used to lower blood ammonia concentration levels.

Lactulose, a synthetic derivative of lactose, is metabolized by colonic bacteria to lactic, acetic, and formic acid, thereby acidifying the colon contents. As the colon contents become more acidic, ammonia found within the bowel and diffused from the serum is trapped in the stool and excreted from the body. Neomycin, an aminoglycoside, acts in the GI tract to eliminate colonic bacteria that form ammonia from urea. Because of these actions, the drugs may be used as adjuncts to protein restriction and supportive therapy in patients with hepatic encephalopathy.

Effective lactulose therapy generally results in two to three soft stools per day. Diarrhea may result if large dosages are used to treat acute toxicity. Other adverse GI reactions to lactulose include gaseous abdominal distention, abdominal pain, belching, or flatulence. The drug also may cause hyperglycemia in patients with diabetes mellitus. Nausea, vomiting, and diarrhea probably are the most common adverse reactions to neomycin. Prolonged use of neomycin can lead to nephrotoxicity, ototoxicity, or neuromuscular blockade.

For a patient receiving an ammonia-detoxicating agent, the nurse can monitor the drug's effectiveness by assessing the patient's level of consciousness, asterixis, muscle coordination, and blood ammonia level. (These factors should improve as the blood ammonia level decreases.) To detect adverse reactions to lactulose, the nurse should inquire about GI distress and monitor the blood glucose level regularly in a diabetic patient receiving lactulose. To detect adverse reactions to neomycin, the nurse should instruct the patient to report hearing or equilibrium changes and should evaluate renal, auditory, and vestibular functions before, during, and after drug therapy. The nurse also should keep calcium gluconate and neostigmine on hand to counteract neomycin-induced neuromuscular blockade.

Parathyroid agents   Also known as calcium regulators, the major parathyroid agents include calcitonin-human (Cibacalcin), calcitonin-salmon (Calcimar), etidronate disodium (Didronel), and the vitamin D analogues calcifediol (Calderol), calcitriol (Rocaltrol), and dihydrotachysterol (DHT, Hytakerol).

Calcitonin and etidronate decrease the serum calcium concentration; the vitamin D analogues increase it. Calcitonin is used to treat hypercalcemia, vitamin D intoxication, postmenopausal osteoporosis, osteolytic bone metastases, hyperphosphatemia, and Paget's disease. A drug of choice for Paget's disease, etidronate also is used to treat heterotopic ossification after hip replacement or spinal cord injury. Uses of the vitamin D analogues vary with the specific agent and include metabolic bone disease, hypocalcemia, hypoparathyroidism, pseudohypoparathyroidism, and renal osteodystrophy.

Most adverse reactions to parathyroid agents are dose-dependent. Depending on the agent prescribed, toxicity can result in hypocalcemia or hypercalcemia. Calcitonin can cause a systemic allergic reaction.

When caring for a patient receiving a parathyroid agent, the nurse should monitor for allergic reactions, signs of hypocalcemia or hypercalcemia, and kidney dysfunction. The nurse also should teach the patient about taking the specific drug, following the prescribed diet, and avoiding over-the-counter products, especially those that contain calcium.

Androgenic and anabolic steroids

Androgenic steroids stimulate the growth of male accessory sex organs and produce masculinizing effects, such as facial hair growth and voice deepening. Anabolic steroids promote a positive nitrogen balance in the body, which stimulates tissue building and reverses tissue depletion.

No purely androgenic or anabolic steroids exist. All androgenic steroids provide some anabolic effects, and all anabolic steroids provide some androgenic effects. However, the distinction between androgenic and anabolic remains useful because one effect always predominates. Predominantly androgenic steroids include danazol (Danocrine), fluoxymesterone (Halotestin), methyltestosterone (Metandren), testosterone (Histerone, Testoject), testosterone cypionate (Andro-Cyp, Depo-Testosterone), testosterone enanthate (Android-T, Andryl), and testosterone propionate (Testex). Predominantly anabolic steroids include ethylestrenol (Maxibolin), nandrolone decanoate (Deca-Durabolin), nandrolone phenpropionate (Durabolin), oxandrolone (Anavar), oxymetholone (Anadrol-50), stanozolol (Winstrol), and testolactone (Teslac).

The steroid agents have many clinical uses. In androgen-deficient males, predominantly androgenic agents can correct hypogonadism and related disorders. In females, they can prevent postpartal breast engorgement and may be used to treat certain types of breast cancer and related disorders. Predominantly anabolic agents can promote weight gain in underweight patients affected by a catabolic disorder or drug. They also may be used to treat certain types of osteoporosis and anemia.

In females, long-term or high-dose use of steroids may cause masculinizing reactions, including voice deepening, menstrual irregularities, and clitoral enlargement. In males, steroids may cause increased libido and feminization (gynecomastia and testicular atrophy). In children, these drugs may cause premature closure of the growth plate in the long bones, thus retarding growth. Other adverse reactions include hepatic dysfunction that may lead to liver failure, increased cholesterol and calcium levels, and sodium and water retention.

Before androgenic and anabolic steroid therapy begins, the nurse should obtain baseline data against which the drug's effects can be measured. During therapy, the nurse should monitor the patient for signs of hepatotoxicity, hypercalcemia, and fluid imbalances. The nurse also should help the patient cope with drug-induced changes in the body or sexuality patterns. The nurse should advise a female patient to report masculinizing effects and a male patient to report feminizing effects. Finally, the nurse should warn all patients not to take an androgenic or anabolic steroid for bodybuilding or aphrodisiac effects because the risks outweigh the benefits.

Estrogens, progestins, and oral contraceptive agents

Estrogens, progestins, and oral contraceptives mimic the physiologic effects of the natural female sex hormones, the estrogens and progesterone. Estrogens and progestins commonly are used as contraceptives and as replacement therapy after menopause.

Estrogens and progestins

Estrogen primarily promotes the growth and development of the female reproductive system. It also is responsible for proliferation of the endometrium during each reproductive cycle and for the maintenance of pregnancy. Natural estrogens include conjugated estrogens (Premarin), estradiol (Estrace, Estrace Vaginal Cream), estradiol transdermal system (Estraderm), and estrone (Theelin Aqueous). Synthetic estrogens include chlorotrianisene (TACE), dienestrol (DV), diethylstilbestrol (DES), diethylstilbestrol diphosphate (Stilphostrol), esterified estrogens (Estratab, Estratest, Menest), estradiol cypionate (Depo-Estradiol, Dura-Estrin), estradiol valerate (Duragen, Estradiol L.A.), ethinyl estradiol (Estinyl, Feminone), and quinestrol (Estrovis).

Natural and synthetic progestins prepare the endometrium for pregnancy and the breasts for lactation. Progesterone (Femotrone, Progestaject) is a natural progestin. Synthetic progestins include hydroxyprogesterone caproate (Duralutin), medroxyprogesterone acetate (Amen, Depo-Provera), norethindrone (Norlutin), and norethindrone acetate (Aygestin, Norlutate).

Estrogens are used primarily for hormonal replacement therapy for postmenopausal women to relieve vasomotor symptoms and urogenital atrophy and to prevent osteoporosis. Less commonly, they are used for hormonal replacement therapy in patients with primary ovarian failure or female castration and in patients who have undergone surgical castration. Estrogens also are prescribed to prevent postpartal breast engorgement in women who do not breast-feed and palliatively to treat advanced, inoperable breast cancer in postmenopausal women and prostate cancer in men.

The primary clinical indications for progestin therapy are secondary amenorrhea, abnormal uterine bleeding, endometriosis, and premenstrual syndrome. Used alone and in combination with estrogens, progestins also are used as oral contraceptives.

The incidence of endometrial and breast cancer, gallbladder disease, hypertension, decreased glucose tolerance, fluid retention, and cholestatic jaundice increases with estrogen use. Thromboembolic disorders may occur in postmenopausal women, although they have not been linked directly with estrogen replacement therapy. Estrogens also may alter thyroid and liver function test results and increase serum lipoprotein levels. Adverse genitourinary and CNS reactions also may occur.

The most common adverse reactions to progestins are menstrual abnormalities. Other reactions include cervical erosions, vaginal candidiasis, edema, depression, cholestatic jaundice, melasma, and adverse CNS reactions.

During estrogen or progestin therapy, the nurse should monitor the patient regularly for adverse reactions, including signs of fluid retention. The nurse also should monitor the results of laboratory tests to detect drug-induced abnormalities. When caring for a postmenopausal patient receiving cyclic estrogen therapy, the nurse should explain that withdrawal bleeding may occur. The nurse also should instruct a patient with diabetes to monitor the blood glucose level regularly and adjust the insulin or oral hyperglycemic agent dosage, as prescribed. In addition, the nurse should instruct the patient to return for routine follow-up examinations.

Oral contraceptives

Most oral contraceptives contain estrogen and progestin. These agents include ethinyl estradiol-ethynodiol diacetate (Demulen 1/35), ethinyl estradiol-levonorgestrel (Levlen, Nordette), ethinyl estradiol-norethindrone (Brevicon, Ortho-Novum 1/35, Ovcon-35), ethinyl estradiol-norethindrone acetate (Loestrin 21 1/20, Norlestrin 21 1/50), ethinyl estradiol-norgestrel (Lo/Ovral, Ovral), mestranol-norethindrone (Genora 1/50, Nelova 1/50 M), and mestranol-norethynodrel (Enovid). The few progestin-only preparations are known as minipills. These include norethindrone (Micronor, Nor-Q.D.) and norgestrel (Ovrette).

Oral contraceptives act primarily by suppressing ovulation. Estrogens interfere with implantation of the fertilized ovum; progestins prevent sperm migration, slow ovum transport, and promote endometrial changes that make it unsuitable for ovum implantation.

Oral contraceptives are used primarily to prevent pregnancy. They also are used to treat hypermenorrhea, endometriosis, and dysmenorrhea and to promote cyclic withdrawal bleeding. Full contraceptive benefits do not occur until the agents have been taken for at least 10 days. Monophasic preparations provide fixed doses of estrogen and progestin throughout a 21-day cycle. Biphasic preparations deliver a constant amount of estrogen throughout a 21-day cycle but an increased amount of progestin during the last 11 days. The progestin dose in triphasic preparations varies every 7 days; the estrogen dose may remain fixed throughout the 21-day cycle or may vary every 7 days.

The most common adverse reactions to oral contraceptives are nausea and melasma. The most severe reactions include hypertension and increased risk of cerebrovascular accident, thromboembolism, MI, and possibly cervical cancer. Other reactions depend on whether the drug is estrogen-dominant or progestin-dominant.

Oral contraceptive patient-teaching tips

The nurse should see that the patient receives and reads the patient package insert before taking an oral contraceptive. The insert provides information about adverse reactions to oral contraceptives and explains which precautions to take while using them. The nurse also should provide the following instructions.

- Take the pills in the proper sequence. Begin taking the pills on day 5 of menstrual bleeding or on the first Sunday after menstrual bleeding begins, as prescribed.
- Take the pill at the same time each day and swallow it whole.
- Expect your period to begin while taking the last seven pills in a 28-pill pack, or a few days after taking the last pill in a 21-pill pack.
- If you miss one pill, take it as soon as you remember it. If you miss two pills in a row, take two pills daily for the next 2 days and use an alternative contraceptive method during the rest of the cycle. If you miss three or more pills in a row, discard the pill pack and use another contraceptive method until your period begins. Then start a new pack on the regular schedule.
- Stop taking the pills and contact the physician if pregnancy is suspected or confirmed.
- Wait 3 months after discontinuing oral contraceptives before trying to become pregnant because the endometrium may take that long to return to normal.

Patient-teaching is an important part of nursing care related to oral contraceptives. (For details, see *Oral contraceptive patient-teaching tips.*) The nurse also should advise the patient who smokes to stop because smoking increases the risk of thromboembolic events and cardiovascular problems.

Antigout agents and gold salts

Antigout agents and gold salts are used to treat joint inflammation associated with gout and rheumatoid arthritis, respectively. In gout, an inborn error in metabolism leads to hyperuricemia and deposition of monosodium urate crystals (tophi) in and around a joint, causing inflammation and pain. In rheumatoid arthritis, inflammation and destruction occur primarily in the peripheral joints, producing pain.

Antigout agents

The antigout agents include the uricosurics probenecid (Benemid) and sulfinpyrazone (Anturane) as well as allopurinol (Zyloprim) and colchicine (Colsalide). Indomethacin, naproxen, and phenylbutazone also are used to treat gout. (For more information about these drugs, see Chapter 9, Nonnarcotic analgesic, antipyretic, and nonsteroidal anti-inflammatory agents.)

The uricosurics act by increasing uric acid excretion in the urine. Allopurinol inhibits uric acid production, which lowers serum and urine uric acid levels. Colchicine's mechanism of action is not understood completely. Colchicine is used to treat an acute gout attack. The uricosurics and allopurinol are used to treat chronic gouty arthritis or hyperuricemia, which places the patient at risk for an acute gout attack.

Antigout agents commonly cause GI distress. Probenecid may cause blood dyscrasias; sulfinpyrazone may reactivate peptic ulcer disease. Allopurinol's most common adverse reaction is skin rash, which usually is maculopapular. Skin problems associated with colchicine include dermatitis, urticaria, and alopecia.

To minimize the number of acute gout attacks, the nurse should teach the patient to avoid alcohol and foods high in purines (such as kidney, liver, sardines, and anchovies), to drink ten to twelve 8-oz glasses (2.4 to 2.8 liters) of water daily, and to consume a high-vegetable diet to alkalinize the urine. To prevent GI upset, the nurse should administer antigout agents after meals. During antigout therapy, the nurse should monitor the patient closely for therapeutic and adverse effects, particularly noting the results of laboratory tests, such as the complete blood count (CBC), urinalysis, serum uric acid level, and liver and kidney function tests.

Gold salts

The oral gold salt is auranofin (Ridaura); the parenteral forms are aurothioglucose (Solganal), an oil-based form, and gold sodium thiomalate (Myochrysine), a water-based form of injectable gold.

Gold salts are remittive agents (drugs that block the inflammatory disease process); they do not reverse structural damage to the joint. Like the uricosurics, gold salts do not provide a direct analgesic action. Rather, they relieve pain through their anti-inflammatory and antiarthritic effects.

Gold salts are prescribed only for patients who have an established diagnosis of rheumatoid arthritis and display an insufficient therapeutic response to an adequate trial of one or more NSAIDs.

Gold salts produce numerous adverse reactions, especially during the first 6 months of therapy. The most common reactions to the oral preparation include GI distress and relatively minor mucocutaneous reactions (conjunctivitis, glossitis, and stomatitis). Parenteral gold salts can cause hypersensitivity reactions; gold sodium thiomalate can produce a vasomotor reaction characterized by flushing, dizziness, nausea, weakness, tachycardia, and syncope.

After gold salt administration, the nurse should monitor the patient for other adverse reactions. If a vasomotor reaction occurs, the patient should lie down during and for 10 minutes after administration and may need to be changed to aurothioglucose. To assess the patient's response to therapy, the nurse should compare the results of regular urinalyses, CBCs, and platelet counts to baseline data. Finally, the nurse should stress the importance of compliance with the drug regimen.

Antitubercular and antileprotic agents

Antitubercular and antileprotic agents are used to treat mycobacterial infections: tuberculosis, which is caused by *Mycobacterium tuberculosis,* and Hansen's disease (previously called leprosy), which is caused by

Mycobacterium leprae. These agents are not always curative. However, they can halt the progression of a mycobacterial infection.

Antitubercular agents

Ethambutol hydrochloride (Myambutol), isoniazid [INH] (Nydrazid, Laniazid), and rifampin (Rifadin, Rimactane) are the mainstays of tuberculosis therapy. Aminosalicylate sodium [para-aminosalicylic acid or PAS] (Tubasal), capreomycin sulfate (Capastat), cycloserine (Seromycin), ethionamide (Trecator-SC), pyrazinamide, and streptomycin sulfate are used only when hypersensitivity, intolerance, or bacterial resistance to a first-line drug exists. This section will focus on the primary antitubercular agents only.

At usual doses, ethambutol and INH are tuberculostatic, inhibiting growth of *M. tuberculosis* bacteria. Rifampin is tuberculocidal, destroying the bacteria.

INH is the most important drug for treating tuberculosis. However, it usually is used in combination with ethambutol, rifampin, or streptomycin. This is because combination therapy for tuberculosis and other mycobacterial infections can prevent or delay the development of bacterial resistance to the drug regimen.

Adverse reactions to antitubercular agents primarily occur in the GI tract, the peripheral nervous system, and the hepatic system. Optic neuritis is the only significant adverse reaction to ethambutol. Daily pyridoxine (vitamin B_6) administration may prevent peripheral neuritis caused by INH therapy. Rifampin may cause hypersensitivity reactions.

During antitubercular therapy, the nurse should instruct the patient that treatment may last for months or years and should monitor patient compliance with the drug regimen. At regular intervals, the nurse should monitor the patient's liver function tests, serum uric acid level, and white blood cell count, as prescribed. The nurse also should assess the patient frequently for adverse reactions. To prevent peripheral neuritis, the nurse should administer pyridoxine, as prescribed. For a patient taking rifampin, the nurse should explain that the drug may produce red-orange urine, tears, sputum, sweat, and feces that stain clothes, linen, and soft contact lenses.

Antileprotic agents

Clofazimine (Lamprene), dapsone (Dapsone 100), and rifampin (Rifadin, Rimactane) currently dominate the treatment of Hansen's disease, although ethionamide (Trecator-SC) also may be used. The antileprotic agents are used together to improve their effectiveness and reduce the likelihood of the development of bacterial resistance.

The mechanisms of action of clofazimine and dapsone are not understood completely. Clofazimine appears to bind to mycobacterial deoxyribonucleic acid (DNA) and inhibit replication and growth. Dapsone is bacteriostatic for *M. leprae,* possibly because of its ability to inhibit folic acid synthesis by bacteria. Rifampin inhibits ribonucleic acid

(RNA) synthesis in susceptible organisms. The drug is effective primarily in replicating bacteria.

Dapsone is the drug of choice for treating Hansen's disease because it is effective, inexpensive, and relatively nontoxic. It also is used to treat dermatitis herpetiformis. Clofazimine is used to treat lepromatous Hansen's disease, including the type that does not respond to dapsone and the type that is complicated by erythema nodosum leprosum. Rifampin usually is used with other drugs to treat Hansen's disease and is the drug of choice for treating dapsone-resistant Hansen's disease.

Skin discoloration, other dermatologic effects, and GI distress are the most common adverse reactions to clofazimine. Hemolytic anemia and methemoglobinemia are the most common dose-related reactions to dapsone. These reactions are particularly severe in a patient with glucose-6-phosphate dehydrogenase deficiency.

Because antileprotic therapy may extend over months or years, the nurse should monitor patient compliance with the drug regimen. During dapsone therapy, the nurse should monitor the patient for signs and symptoms of hemolytic anemia (pallor, fatigue, and dyspnea) or methemoglobinemia (cyanosis) and should instruct the patient to return for blood tests periodically, as prescribed. During clofazimine therapy, the nurse should inspect the patient's skin for changes and should advise the patient that discoloration of the skin, conjunctivae, tears, sweat, sputum, urine, and feces may take months or years to disappear.

Anthelmintic agents

Anthelmintic agents destroy helminths—parasitic worms that infect humans. They are classified according to the type of helminths they affect: antinematodes, which kill nematodes (roundworms); anticestodes, which kill cestodes (tapeworms); and antitrematodes, which kill trematodes (flukes). Because some anthelmintics are highly toxic, positive helminth identification is imperative before treatment begins.

Antinematode agents

Mebendazole (Vermox), piperazine citrate (Antepar), pyrantel pamoate (Antiminth), and thiabendazole (Mintezol) are the major antinematode agents. Although their exact mechanisms of action are unknown, these drugs may immobilize or kill roundworms by impairing their ability to use energy from available sources or by interfering with their nervous systems. Then the immobilized or dead worms are excreted via the GI tract.

Mebendazole is the drug of choice against whipworm, pinworm, hookworm, and giant intestinal roundworm infections. Piperazine is a secondary agent for all nematode infections, but primarily for large *Ascaris* infections that cause intestinal blockage. Pyrantel is used as an alternative therapy to treat hookworm, pinworm, and giant intestinal roundworm infections. Because thiabendazole is highly toxic, it is the drug of choice to treat threadworm infections and is used to treat other nematode infections only when the drug of choice clearly has failed.

Piperazine and pyrantel should not be administered together because their effects could cancel each other out. Because piperazine may lower the seizure threshold, it should not be used with phenothiazines or other drugs that have the same effect, particularly in patients with epilepsy. Almost all antinematode agents cause adverse GI reactions ranging from abdominal pain to nausea, vomiting, and diarrhea.

During antinematode therapy, the nurse should monitor for adverse reactions and must ensure that all family members are treated because nematode infections otherwise may recur. Also the nurse should instruct the patient to change and wash underclothes and bedding daily, wash the perianal area daily, and wash hands and fingernails after each bowel movement to reduce the incidence of reinfection. During mebendazole or thiabendazole therapy, the nurse should teach the patient to chew the tablets for optimum effect.

Anticestode agents

Mebendazole (Vermox), niclosamide (Niclocide), paromomycin sulfate (Humatin), and praziquantel (Biltricide) are effective anticestode agents. Each of these drugs immobilizes or kills tapeworms by a different mechanism of action.

Although mebendazole is primarily an antinematode agent, it also is used experimentally to treat hydatid disease caused by liver tapeworm. Niclosamide and praziquantel, the anticestode drugs of choice, are similarly effective against all intestinal tapeworm species. If the patient cannot tolerate these drugs, paromomycin is an alternative choice.

Adverse reactions to mebendazole and paromomycin primarily affect the GI tract. Adverse reactions to niclosamide are uncommon. Praziquantel causes transient dizziness, headache, malaise, abdominal pain or distention, and nausea in about 90% of patients. Drowsiness and fatigue also may occur.

In addition to monitoring the patient for adverse reactions and intervening as needed, the nurse should teach the patient about the prescribed anticestode agent. For example, the nurse should instruct the patient to chew niclosamide tablets thoroughly and then drink water, or to chew and rapidly swallow the bitter praziquantel tablets to prevent gagging or vomiting. The nurse also should teach the patient the importance of compliance with the drug regimen.

Antitrematode agents

Two drugs are available to treat trematode infections of the blood, liver, and lungs: oxamniquine (Vansil) and praziquantel (Biltricide). Oxamniquine induces adult blood flukes to migrate from the mesenteric veins into the liver, where they eventually die. Praziquantel causes spastic paralysis of the fluke's musculature, which eventually leads to disintegration. It is the drug of choice for all fluke infections. Oxamniquine is effective against only one variety of blood fluke.

Anticestode agents commonly cause adverse GI reactions and CNS disturbances. Oxamniquine causes orange-red urine that has no clinical significance. To prevent adverse GI reactions, the nurse should give oxamniquine as a single dose after meals or give praziquantel with meals. The nurse should tell the patient that CNS disturbances may occur, requiring curtailment of activities on the day of and the day after treatment.

Antimalarial and other antiprotozoal agents

Protozoal diseases, including malaria, have assumed critical importance in the United States because of the increased incidence of immune disorders, increased immigration from areas where protozoal diseases are endemic, and increased travel by Americans to those areas. Therefore, effective antimalarial and antiprotozoal drugs are needed.

Antimalarial agents

The major agents used to prevent and treat malaria are chloroquine hydrochloride (Aralen HCl), chloroquine phosphate (Aralen Phosphate), hydroxychloroquine sulfate (Plaquenil), mefloquine hydrochloride (Lariam), primaquine phosphate, pyrimethamine (Daraprim), quinine dihydrochloride, and quinine sulfate (Quinamm, Strema). Sulfonamides, sulfones, and tetracyclines also may be used with these agents.

The antimalarial agents seem to work in different ways to kill malarial parasites or inhibit their reproduction. Chloroquine is the drug of choice to prevent and treat all strains of malaria, except for chloroquine-resistant or multidrug-resistant strains of *Plasmodium falciparum.* Hydroxychloroquine serves as an alternative when chloroquine is not available.

For acute attacks of chloroquine-resistant or multidrug-resistant strains of *P. falciparum,* quinine is the drug of choice and is given with slower-acting antimalarial agents. Primaquine is the drug of choice to prevent *Plasmodium vivax* or *Plasmodium ovale* malaria relapse. Mefloquine is used for acute attacks of mild to moderate malaria caused by susceptible strains of *P. falciparum* and *P. vivax,* and also may be used to prevent malarial infection. Pyrimethamine-sulfadoxine (Fansidar) combination therapy should be used only with chloroquine prophylaxis for self-treatment of febrile illness when medical care is not immediately available. Fatalities have occurred with the use of this combination.

In the low dosages used to prevent or treat malaria, these agents usually produce few serious adverse reactions. Quinine commonly produces cinchonism (a toxic syndrome that includes tinnitus, headache, vertigo, fever, light-headedness, and vision disturbances). The other drugs typically produce adverse GI reactions, such as nausea, vomiting, and abdominal cramps. Adverse ocular and CNS reactions also may occur.

During antimalarial therapy, the nurse can monitor for adverse reactions by checking the patient's vital signs and assessing for visual or auditory changes regularly. If cinchonism occurs even after a single dose of quinine, the nurse should expect to discontinue the drug. To minimize adverse GI reactions, the nurse should administer chloroquine, primaquine, or quinine with food. To ensure patient safety, the nurse should take seizure precautions during chloroquine, hydroxychloroquine, mefloquine, or pyrimethamine therapy.

Other antiprotozoal agents

Common major antiprotozoal agents include atovaquone (Mepron), emetine hydrochloride, furazolidone (Furoxone), iodoquinol (Moebiquin, Yodoxin), metronidazole (Flagyl, Metryl), pentamidine isethionate (NebuPent, Pentam 300), and quinacrine hydrochloride (Atabrine).

Antiprotozoal agents act in different ways and many of their mechanisms of action are not understood well. They are used to treat a wide range of protozoal infections, including *Pneumocystis carinii* infections, amebiasis, giardiasis, trichomoniasis, toxoplasmosis, African trypanosomiasis, and leishmaniasis.

Drug interactions with antiprotozoal agents can be severe and unpredictable, and may lead to nephrotoxicity, acute psychosis, and increased drug toxicity. Several antiprotozoal agents can produce severe—even life-threatening—adverse reactions. All of them may cause adverse GI reactions. Other reactions vary with the drug used.

Because of the potential toxicity and drug interactions associated with these antiprotozoal agents, the nurse must supervise the patient closely during drug administration and monitor regularly for adverse reactions. Additional interventions include teaching the patient to take metronidazole with food to minimize GI distress, to refrain from sexual intercourse or use a condom during treatment for trichomoniasis, and to watch for a harmless discoloration of the urine during quinacrine therapy.

Urinary antiseptic agents

These agents inhibit the growth of many species of bacteria in the urine. Before therapy begins, however, a urine culture and sensitivity test is required to confirm the infection, identify the causative organism, and determine its drug sensitivity.

Common urinary antiseptics include the fluoroquinolones, sulfonamides, and nitrofurantoin. The fluoroquinolones used as urinary antiseptics include oral ciprofloxacin (Cipro), lomefloxacin hydrochloride (Maxaquin), norfloxacin (Noroxin), and ofloxacin (Floxin). The sulfonamides include co-trimoxazole (Bactrim, Septra), sulfadiazine (Microsulfon), sulfamethoxazole (Gantanol), and sulfisoxazole

(Gantrisin). Nitrofurantoin (Furadantin, Macrodantin) also is an orally administered urinary antiseptic. Less commonly used urinary antiseptics include cinoxacin (Cinobac), methenamine hippurate (Hiprex, Urex), methenamine mandelate (Mandelamine), nalidixic acid (Neg-Gram), and trimethoprim (Proloprim, Trimpex). This section will focus on the fluoroquinolones, sulfonamides, and nitrofurantoin, which are all used to treat UTIs.

The effectiveness of fluoroquinolones results from their affinity for enzymes in the bacterial cell; they interrupt DNA synthesis during bacterial replication. As bacteriostatic agents, the sulfonamides prevent microorganism growth by inhibiting folic acid synthesis, which is necessary for DNA, RNA, and protein synthesis. Nitrofurantoin's exact mechanism of action is unknown.

Among the fluoroquinolones, ciprofloxacin is used to treat infectious diarrhea and urinary tract, respiratory, skin, bone, or joint infections; norfloxacin is used to treat complicated and uncomplicated UTIs; and ofloxacin is used to treat UTIs, respiratory and skin infections, and such sexually transmitted diseases as gonorrhea and urethritis. Sulfonamides primarily are used to treat acute UTIs. However, the emergence of resistant strains of bacteria has limited the usefulness of sulfonamides. Nitrofurantoin is used to treat acute and chronic UTIs.

Urinary antiseptics commonly cause adverse GI reactions. Fluoroquinolones also may produce adverse CNS reactions. Sulfonamides may cause crystalluria and tubular deposits of sulfonamide crystals (with excessively high doses of less water-soluble forms), dermatologic reactions, photosensitivity, hypersensitivity, fever, and a reaction that resembles serum sickness. Nitrofurantoin may cause urine discoloration (dark yellow or brown), peripheral neuropathy, headache, dizziness, and hypersensitivity reactions (including anaphylaxis).

During urinary antiseptic therapy, the nurse should monitor the patient for adverse reactions and intervene as needed. For example, the nurse should monitor hydration if the patient experiences adverse GI reactions. When teaching the patient, the nurse should stress compliance with the drug regimen, recognition of adverse reactions, and physician notification if adverse reactions occur.

If the patient must take an antacid during fluoroquinolone therapy, the nurse should administer the antacid at least 2 hours after the fluoroquinolone dose to prevent decreased fluoroquinolone absorption. During sulfonamide therapy, the nurse should encourage sufficient fluid intake to maintain urine output at 1,500 ml (50 oz) or more daily to prevent crystal formation. The nurse also should caution the patient to avoid direct sunlight to prevent photosensitivity. When initiating nitrofurantoin therapy, the nurse should assess for hypersensitivity reactions, keep standard emergency equipment nearby, and withhold the drug and notify the physician if such reactions occur. If GI distress occurs, the nurse should administer nitrofurantoin with food or milk and monitor the patient's hydration status. If paresthesia or other signs of peripheral neuropathy occur, the nurse should withhold the drug and notify the physician.

Ophthalmic agents The ophthalmic agents in this section are instilled primarily as drops or applied as ointments. (For details, see *Administering ophthalmic agents.*) Mydriatics, cycloplegics, and miotics are the three groups of ophthalmic agents that most commonly are used. Other groups of ophthalmic agents include additional drugs that lower intraocular pressure, anesthetic agents, anti-inflammatory agents, and anti-infective preparations.

During ophthalmic agent therapy, the nurse should teach the patient and family how to instill the drug properly and how to minimize systemic absorption by applying pressure over the punctum at the inner canthus. The nurse also should advise the patient to avoid indiscriminate or prolonged use of an ophthalmic agent (unless specifically prescribed) and to have regular ophthalmic examinations to detect abnormalities during long-term ophthalmic agent therapy.

Mydriatics and cycloplegics

These agents include atropine sulfate (Atropisol, Isopto Atropine), cyclopentolate hydrochloride (Cyclogyl), dipivefrin (Propine), epinephrine bitartrate (Epitrate), epinephrine hydrochloride (Epifrin, Glaucon), epinephryl borate (Epinal, Eppy/N), homatropine hydrobromide (Homatrine, Isopto Homatropine), phenylephrine hydrochloride (Mydfrin, Neo-Synephrine), scopolamine hydrobromide (Isopto Hyoscine), and tropicamide (Mydriacyl).

Mydriatics act on the iris to dilate the pupil. They are used primarily to dilate pupils for intraocular examinations. Cycloplegics act on the ciliary body to paralyze the fine-focusing muscles, thereby preventing accommodation to near vision. They are essential for performing refraction in children; they also are used before and after ophthalmic surgery and as adjunct treatment for conditions involving the iris.

Local adverse reactions to mydriatics and cycloplegics can include irritation, blurred vision, and transient burning and stinging sensations. With prolonged use, some of these drugs can increase intraocular pressure and cause ocular congestion, conjunctivitis, contact dermatitis, and eye dryness. Systemic reactions include tachycardia, palpitations, flushing, dry skin, ataxia, and confusion.

The nurse should monitor the patient regularly to detect tachycardia and signs of adverse ocular reactions. The nurse also should instruct the patient to wear dark glasses after drug administration and avoid operating machinery until blurred vision disappears.

Miotics

Carbachol (Carbacel, Isopto Carbachol), pilocarpine hydrochloride (Isopto Carpine, Pilocar), and pilocarpine nitrate (P.V. Carpine

Administering ophthalmic agents

Many ophthalmic agents come in two forms: eye drops for instillation and ointments for application. The form of an agent determines how it is administered, as shown below. With either form, hand washing is essential before and after administration to prevent infection.

Eye ointment

Place the patient supine or in a sitting position with the neck hyperextended. Clean the eyelashes with saline solution and swabs to remove any secretions. Have the patient look upward; then pull down the lower lid with the finger. As the patient continues to look up, apply a thin ribbon of ointment (approximately 1/4") directly into the conjunctival sac, beginning at the inner canthus.

To avoid contamination, do not let the tube touch the eye or conjunctiva. At the outer canthus, rotate the tube to detach the ointment.

Instruct the patient to close the eye gently, but not to squeeze it.

Eye drops

Place the patient supine or in a sitting position with the neck hyperextended, looking toward the ceiling. With the finger, pull down firmly on the lower lid while the patient continues to look upward. This movement exposes the lower conjunctival sac by relaxing the upper tarsal plate as it is retracted into the orbit.

Instill 1 drop of medication into the lower conjunctival sac. Instruct the patient to close the eye gently. Wipe away excess tears with a cotton ball or tissue.

The eye can hold only 1 drop. When instilling more than 1 drop, wait 2 to 3 minutes between drops to avoid losing a drop from tearing or blinking.

After instilling drops, apply digital pressure over the punctum at the inner canthus for 2 to 3 minutes, and have the patient close the eyelids gently for 2 to 3 minutes to prevent drainage through the nasolacrimal duct. Stopping drainage through the nasolacrimal duct helps prevent systemic absorption. It also prevents the patient from tasting the drops.

To avoid contamination, do not allow the tip of the dropper to touch the lid or eyelashes. Discard discolored solutions or solutions with floating particles. Also, pay special attention during administration to prevent accidental instillation into the unaffected eye.

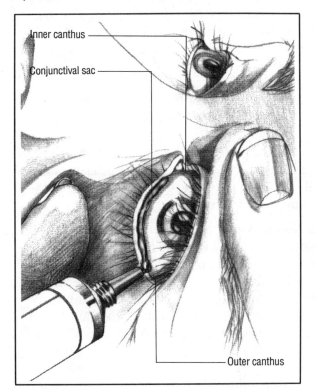

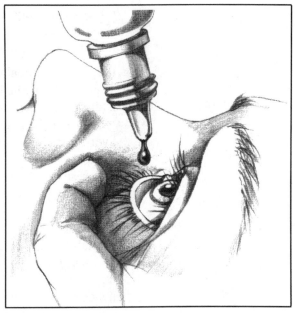

Liquifilm) are direct-acting cholinergic miotics. Physostigmine salicylate (Eserine Salicylate, Isopto-Eserine) and physostigmine sulfate (Eserine Sulfate) comprise the short-acting anticholinesterase miotics. Demecarium bromide (Humorsol), echothiophate iodide (Phospholine Iodide), and isoflurophate (Floropryl) are long-acting anticholinesterase miotics.

All miotics stimulate and contract the sphincter muscle of the iris, thereby constricting the pupil. This action is called miosis. Because of their action, miotics are used to treat chronic open-angle glaucoma, acute and chronic angle-closure glaucoma, and certain cases of secondary glaucoma resulting from disease- or injury-induced increases in intraocular pressure. Controlling intraocular pressure is the cornerstone of glaucoma therapy, and direct-acting miotics, such as pilocarpine, usually are the drugs of choice. Long-acting miotics such as isoflurophate, which can be toxic, are used only in patients who do not respond to direct- or short-acting agents.

Echothiophate, isoflurophate, and physostigmine may interact with succinylcholine, resulting in respiratory or cardiovascular collapse. Pilocarpine interacts with carbachol, causing additive effects, and with phenylephrine, decreasing phenylephrine-induced mydriasis. These interactions prohibit concomitant use of these drugs.

Miotics commonly cause blurred vision and eye and eyebrow pain. Reversible iris cysts, eyelid pain, photosensitivity, and cataract formation also may occur. Although uncommon, systemic absorption can lead to adverse GI reactions, bronchial constriction, pulmonary edema, and hypersensitivity reactions.

During miotic therapy, the nurse should monitor for signs of respiratory dysfunction and notify the physician if they occur. The nurse also should instruct the patient to instill the drops at bedtime to minimize problems caused by blurred vision.

Drugs that lower intraocular pressure

Topical adrenergic blockers, hyperosmotic agents, and carbonic anhydrase inhibitors are used to lower intraocular pressure. The adrenergic blockers include apraclonidine hydrochloride (Iopidine), betaxolol hydrochloride (Betoptic), levobunolol hydrochloride (Betagan), metipranolol (Opti-Pranolol), and timolol maleate (Timoptic). The hyperosmotic agents include anhydrous glycerin (Ophthalgan), glycerin (Osmoglyn), isosorbide (Ismotic), mannitol (Osmitrol), and urea (Ureaphil). The carbonic anhydrase inhibitors are acetazolamide (Ak-Zol, Diamox), acetazolamide sodium (Diamox Parenteral), dichlorphenamide (Daranide), and methazolamide (Neptazane).

The adrenergic blockers primarily may reduce aqueous humor production and slightly increase aqueous humor outflow. The hyperosmotic agents, which are reserved for emergencies, increase the absorption of water from the eye into the general circulation, thus lowering intraocular pressure. The carbonic anhydrase inhibitors inhibit the enzyme involved in aqueous humor production, which decreases aqueous production by 30% to 60% without affecting the aqueous outflow.

Apraclonidine is used to prevent or control elevated intraocular pressure after argon laser trabeculoplasty or iridotomy. Betaxolol, levobunolol, metipranolol, and timolol are used to treat chronic open-angle glaucoma. Timolol also is used to treat some secondary glaucoma. Hyperosmotic agents are used to treat acute angle-closure glaucoma; they also are used before and after ocular surgery. Carbonic anhydrase inhibitors are used to treat chronic open-angle glaucoma, episodes of acute angle-closure glaucoma, and secondary glaucoma.

Adrenergic blockers can reduce heart rate, causing headaches and fatigue; systemic timolol absorption may lead to bradycardia and bronchospasm. Apraclonidine may cause upper eyelid elevation, conjunctival blanching, and mydriasis. Hyperosmotic agents may cause stinging upon administration. Use of a topical anesthetic is recommended with glycerin administration. Carbonic anhydrase inhibitors may cause drowsiness, hypokalemia, nausea, and vomiting.

When a patient is taking a drug to lower intraocular pressure, the nurse should monitor for adverse reactions, such as bradycardia and wheezing, administer a bronchodilator as prescribed, and advise the patient to take a mild analgesic if headache occurs.

Ophthalmic anesthetic agents

Topical ophthalmic anesthetics include proparacaine hydrochloride (Alcaine, Ophthaine), tetracaine (Pontocaine Eye), and tetracaine hydrochloride (Pontocaine). Proparacaine and tetracaine act by interfering with cell activity. More drops may be required to anesthetize an inflamed eye because the dilated blood vessels carry the anesthetic away.

Besides anesthetizing the cornea to allow application of instruments for measuring intraocular pressure or removing foreign bodies, topical ophthalmic anesthetics are used for suture removal, conjunctival or corneal scraping, and lacrimal canal manipulation.

All three topical ophthalmic anesthetic agents can cause transient eye pain and redness. Prolonged use can cause keratitis, corneal opacities, scarring, loss of visual acuity, and delayed corneal healing.

When caring for a patient receiving an ophthalmic anesthetic agent, the nurse should assess for eye pain and redness and other adverse reactions. The nurse should advise the patient not to rub the eyes; corneal abrasion may occur because the usual pain signal is absent. If needed, the nurse should give the patient a protective eye patch to wear while the anesthetic effects of the drug last.

Ophthalmic anti-inflammatory agents

Topical ophthalmic anti-inflammatory agents include dexamethasone (Maxidex Ophthalmic Suspension), fluorometholone (Fluor-Op, FML,

FML Forte), medrysone (HMS Liquifilm Ophthalmic), prednisolone acetate (Econopred Ophthalmic, Pred-Forte, Pred Mild Ophthalmic), and prednisolone sodium phosphate (AK-Pred, Inflamase).

These drugs are corticosteroid solutions or suspensions that decrease leukocyte infiltration at the site of ocular inflammation. This reduces the exudative reaction of diseased tissue, leading to reduced edema, redness, and scarring. The corticosteroids are used to treat inflammatory disorders and hypersensitivity-related conditions of the cornea, iris, conjunctiva, sclera, and anterior uvea.

These drugs can increase intraocular pressure, cause corneal thinning or ulceration, interfere with corneal wound healing, and increase susceptibility to viral or fungal corneal infection. Long-term or excessive use can lead to exacerbation of glaucoma, cataracts, reduced visual acuity, and optic nerve damage. Excessive or long-term use of suspensions, which are absorbed more readily, can lead to adrenal suppression.

During anti-inflammatory therapy, the nurse should assess for signs of infection, corneal ulceration, or delayed corneal wound healing. During high-dose or long-term therapy, the nurse should teach the patient to recognize and report the signs and symptoms of adrenal suppression and should advise the patient to carry medical identification that describes this drug regimen.

Ophthalmic anti-infective agents

Ophthalmic anti-infective agents include antibacterial, antiseptic, and antiviral agents. Applied as solution or ointment, these drugs include bacitracin (AK-Tracin), boric acid (Blinx, Collyrium), chloramphenicol (Chloromycetin Ophthalmic), chlortetracycline hydrochloride (Aureomycin 3%), erythromycin (Ilotycin), gentamicin sulfate (Garamycin Ophthalmic Solution, Genoptic), idoxuridine (Herplex, Stoxil), natamycin (Natacyn), polymyxin B sulfate (Neosporin Ophthalmic), silver nitrate 1%, sulfacetamide sodium 10% (Bleph-10 Liquifilm Ophthalmic, Cetamide Ophthalmic), tetracycline hydrochloride (Achromycin), tobramycin (Tobrex), trifluridine (Viroptic Ophthalmic Solution 1%), and vidarabine (Vira-A Ophthalmic).

The anti-infective agents are chemical substances that inhibit the growth of or directly kill bacteria. To treat eye diseases, anti-infective agents may be injected beneath the conjunctiva, administered orally, or instilled into the eye.

Bacitracin is effective against infections with gram-positive organisms. Boric acid is used to irrigate the eye after ocular procedures and to soothe and cleanse the eye, especially in connection with contact lens use. Chloramphenicol and gentamicin are used to treat gram-positive and gram-negative bacterial infections. Chlortetracycline is prescribed for superficial ocular infections. Erythromycin is used to fight infections caused by gram-positive cocci and gram-positive bacilli. Idoxuridine is invaluable in treating herpes simplex of the cornea.

Natamycin is used to treat fungal infections. Polymyxin B is effective against infections caused by gram-negative organisms. Silver nitrate 1% is used to prevent gonorrheal ophthalmia neonatorum. Sulfacetamide provides a wide spectrum of activity against some gram-positive and gram-negative bacteria. Tetracycline is used to treat superficial ocular infections, inclusion conjunctivitis, and trachoma. Tobramycin is used to treat external ocular infections caused by susceptible gram-negative bacteria. Trifluridine is used to treat herpes simplex infections, keratoconjunctivitis, and recurrent epithelial keratitis. Vidarabine is used to treat corneal herpes simplex, particularly in the early stages.

Hypersensitivity reactions to sulfonamides may occur and may be severe. Secondary eye infections may occur with prolonged use of an ophthalmic anti-infective agent.

The nurse should keep standard emergency equipment nearby during sulfonamide therapy to manage hypersensitivity reactions. If a secondary eye infection occurs, the nurse should encourage the patient to see an ophthalmologist.

Otic agents

Otic agents fall into four major classes: anti-infective, anti-inflammatory, local anesthetic, and ceruminolytic agents. They may be administered via ear drops, ear irrigations, or ear wicks. (For more information, see *Administering ear drops,* page 506.)

Common nursing interventions for all otic agents include warming the drug to room temperature before instillation (to prevent CNS stimulation), showing the patient how to insert cotton moistened with the ear drops or a gauze wick into the ear canal, and instructing the patient to report adverse reactions to the physician.

Otic anti-infective agents

The otic anti-infective agents include the following antibiotics: acetic acid (Domeboro Otic, VoSol Otic), boric acid (Ear-Dry, Swim-Ear), chloramphenicol (Chloromycetin Otic), colistin sulfate (combined with neomycin, and hydrocortisone in Coly-Mycin S Otic), and polymyxin B sulfate.

These agents may be bactericidal or bacteriostatic. Boric acid and acetic acid possess weak bacteriostatic properties and also are fungistatic. Otic anti-infective agents are prescribed to treat otitis externa caused by various bacteria. Colistin and polymyxin B also prove effective in treating otitis media. Many combination products treat a wide range of microorganisms as well as ear pain and inflammation.

Superinfection sometimes occurs with the use of otic anti-infective agents, resulting in overgrowth of nonsusceptible organisms. Hypersensitivity reactions, such as ear pruritus or burning, urticaria, and vesicular or maculopapular dermatitis, may occur with any otic anti-infective agent.

Before administering an otic anti-infective solution or suspension, the nurse should clean and dry the ear canal. If the patient is sensitive

Administering ear drops

The nurse should administer ear drops properly for an adult or pediatric patient, as described below.

Adult patient

- Shake the bottle, as directed, and open it. Fill the dropper and place the bottle within reach.
- Tilt the patient's head so that the affected ear is up. Then gently pull the top of the ear up and back to straighten the ear canal.
- Position the dropper above but not touching the ear, and release the prescribed number of drops.
- Keep the patient's head tilted for 10 minutes. If desired, plug the ear with cotton moistened with the ear drops. Do not use dry cotton because it will absorb the drops.
- Repeat the procedure for the other ear, as prescribed.

Pediatric patient

- Lay the child on the side so that the affected ear is turned up.
- Gently pull the ear down and back, then slowly release the prescribed number of drops. (Note the difference in the direction the ear is moved for a child. This is because the child's ear cartilage is immature.)
- Notify the physician if the child experiences any pain after instillation.

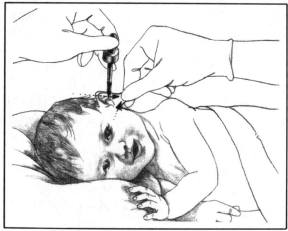

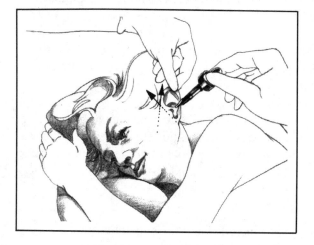

to other agents, the nurse also should perform a patch test to assess for allergic contact dermatitis. During therapy, the nurse must monitor the patient for adverse reactions, such as signs of superinfection.

Otic anti-inflammatory agents

These agents include dexamethasone sodium phosphate (AK-Dex, Decadron Phosphate cream), hydrocortisone (Acetasol HC, VoSol HC Otic), and hydrocortisone acetate. As corticosteroids, they inhibit edema, capillary dilation, fibrin deposition, and phagocyte and leukocyte migration. These anti-inflammatory, antipruritic, and vasoconstrictor effects account for the major clinical use of these agents: treatment of inflammatory conditions of the external ear canal.

Common adverse reactions to otic anti-inflammatory agents are transient, local stinging or burning sensations. These agents also may mask or exacerbate an underlying otic infection.

For a patient with allergic otitis externa, the nurse should not administer the otic anti-inflammatory agent with an otic anti-infective agent. For a patient with bacterial otitis externa, the nurse should expect to administer an otic anti-inflammatory agent and an otic anti-infective agent. Whenever an otic anti-inflammatory agent is prescribed, the nurse should administer it sparingly to prevent debris accumulation in the ear canal.

Otic anesthetic agents

The only local anesthetic approved for otic use is benzocaine (Americaine Otic, Tympagesic). After topical administration as a solution or gel, it blocks nerve conduction at and around the application site to produce an analgesic effect. Benzocaine is used for temporary relief of ear pain. It may be used in combination with an otic anti-infective agent if ear infection is present.

Benzocaine may cause ear irritation, pruritus, and edema. It may mask the symptoms of a fulminating middle ear infection, although hearing loss, dizziness, or a sensation of fullness in the ear may remain. It also may cause urticaria, a hypersensitivity reaction. The nurse should instruct the patient to avoid using benzocaine for a prolonged time and to contact the physician if the ear problem worsens.

Ceruminolytic agents

The ceruminolytic agents include carbamide peroxide (Debrox, Murine Ear) and triethanolamine polypeptide oleate-condensate (Cerumenex). These drugs remove hardened cerumen (ear wax) and prevent its accumulation by emulsifying and mechanically loosening it. Carbamide peroxide is combined with anhydrous glycerin to soften cerumen. Exposing the carbamide peroxide to moisture releases oxygen and hydrogen peroxide, which produces an effervescence that mechanically removes cerumen. The patient's ears should be irrigated after therapy to remove debris.

Adverse reactions to ceruminolytics usually are insignificant. Mild, localized erythema and pruritus may occur. Some patients using triethanolamine may experience hypersensitivity reactions, such as severe eczema.

Patient-teaching is a vital part of ceruminolytic therapy. The nurse should instruct the patient to let the ceruminolytic solution remain in the ear canal for at least 15 minutes, and to use carbamide peroxide for no more than 4 days or triethanolamine for no more than 30 minutes, unless otherwise directed by the physician. The nurse also should teach the patient to irrigate the affected ear gently with warm water after ceruminolytic administration and to lie on the affected side afterward to allow the solution to flow out.

STUDY ACTIVITIES

Matching related elements

Match the drug on the left with its clinical use on the right.

1. ___ Acetazolamide   **A.** To treat vitamin B_6 deficiency

2. ___ Cyanocobalamin   **B.** To treat Hansen's disease

3. ___ Pyridoxine   **C.** To decrease blood pH and increase urine pH

4. ___ Atracurium   **D.** To correct abnormal uterine bleeding

5. ___ Carbamide   **E.** To remove hardened ear wax

6. ___ Mebendazole   **F.** To correct hypogonadism

7. ___ Dapsone   **G.** To treat vitamin B_{12} deficiency anemia

8. ___ Danazol   **H.** To treat narcotic overdose

9. ___ Norethindrone   **I.** To produce prolonged muscle relaxation

10. ___ Naloxone   **J.** To treat glaucoma

11. ___ Pilocarpine   **K.** To treat roundworm infections

Fill in the blank

12. Topical anesthetics are applied directly to the _____ and _____.

13. Fat-soluble vitamins include vitamins _____, _____, _____, and _____; water-soluble vitamins include _____ vitamins and vitamin _____.

14. A cation-exchange resin exchanges _____ ions for _____ ions in the GI tract.

15. Gold salts are prescribed for patients who have an established diagnosis of _____ and display an insufficient response to _____ therapy.

16. _____ is a major ECF electrolyte; _____ is the primary ICF electrolyte.

17. _____ is the drug of choice to treat most strains of malaria; _____ is the drug of choice to treat acute attacks of chloroquine-resistant or multidrug-resistant strains of *P. falciparum.*

18. Fluoroquinolones, sulfonamides, and nitrofurantoin commonly are used to treat _____.

19. _____ agents are used to _____ the pupil for intraocular examinations.

True or false

20. Adverse reactions to local anesthetics usually result from overdose, improper injection technique, or hypersensitivity.
☐ True   ☐ False

21. Because minerals are not stored in the body, they must be obtained from dietary sources every day.
☐ True   ☐ False

22. Lactulose alkalinizes the colon contents.
☐ True   ☐ False

23. Oral contraceptives act primarily by suppressing ovulation.
☐ True   ☐ False

24. To maximize the therapeutic effects of warfarin, the nurse should encourage the patient to consume plenty of foods high in vitamin K.
☐ True   ☐ False

25. The only local anesthetic approved for otic use is hydrocortisone.
☐ True   ☐ False

Multiple choice

26. Amanda Davis, age 78, is admitted to the hospital with acute renal failure and hyperkalemia. The physician prescribes sodium polystyrene sulfonate (Kayexalate). To prevent constipation, the nurse can administer this drug with a solution that contains which substance?
A. Aluminum hydroxide
B. Calcium carbonate
C. Sorbitol
D. Neomycin

27. Joanna Reiser, age 57, is about to begin estrogen therapy to relieve her menopausal symptoms. Estrogen therapy can increase her risk of which type of cancer?
A. Skin
B. Liver
C. Ovarian
D. Endometrial

28. Andrew Thomas, age 64, has had periodic episodes of gout for the past 5 years. His physician prescribes colchicine for acute gout attacks. The nurse teaches Mr. Thomas about the therapeutic and adverse effects of colchicine. Which adverse reaction is the most common?
A. GI distress
B. Blood dyscrasias
C. Maculopapular skin rash
D. Mucocutaneous reactions

29. Carol Stuart, age 67, recently was diagnosed with pulmonary tuberculosis. Now her therapy includes INH, rifampin, and pyridoxine. The concomitant administration of INH and pyridoxine helps prevent which adverse reaction?

    A. Optic neuritis

    B. Drug resistance

    C. Hypersensitivity

    D. Peripheral neuritis

30. Fran Davis, age 59, has chronic open-angle glaucoma. Her physician prescribes carbachol (Isopto Carbachol) drops, which must be instilled every 8 hours. To prevent systemic drug absorption through the nasolacrimal duct, the nurse should give Ms. Davis which instruction?

    A. Apply digital pressure at the inner canthus for 2 to 3 minutes after instillation.

    B. Rub the eyes gently to distribute the drops after instillation.

    C. Keep the eyes open for at least 5 minutes after instillation.

    D. Hold the head back for 2 to 3 minutes after instillation.

ANSWERS

Matching related elements

1. C
2. G
3. A
4. I
5. E
6. K
7. B
8. F
9. D
10. H
11. J

Fill in the blanks

12. Skin, mucous membranes
13. A, D, E, K, B-complex, C
14. Sodium, potassium
15. Rheumatoid arthritis, NSAID
16. Calcium, potassium
17. Chloroquine, quinine
18. UTIs
19. Mydriatics, dilate

True or false

20. True.
21. False. Because all minerals are stored by the body, mineral levels can become toxic.
22. False. Lactulose is metabolized by colonic bacteria to lactic, acetic, and formic acid, thereby acidifying the colon contents.

23. True.
24. False. Vitamin K–rich foods can interact with oral anticoagulants, such as warfarin, and can increase the risk of clotting.
25. False. The only local anesthetic approved for otic use is benzocaine.

Multiple choice

26. C. To minimize constipation and prevent fecal impaction, the nurse may administer sodium polystyrene sulfonate in a 70% sorbitol solution, which forms softer stools and helps excrete the resin.
27. D. The incidence of endometrial and breast cancer, gallbladder disease, hypertension, decreased glucose tolerance, fluid retention, and cholestatic jaundice increases with estrogen use.
28. A. Colchicine and the other antigout agents commonly cause GI distress.
29. D. Daily pyridoxine (vitamin B_6) administration may prevent peripheral neuritis caused by INH therapy.
30. A. After instillation, digital pressure over the punctum at the inner canthus for 2 to 3 minutes helps prevent systemic absorption and the patient from tasting the drops.

Appendix 1: Commonly used abbreviations in drug therapy

In health care facilities that approve them, these abbreviations may be used in transcribing medication orders and documenting drug administration.

$\overline{aa}$	of each	Ⓛ	left
a.c.	before meals	L	liter
A.D.	right ear	LA	long acting
ad lib	as desired	lb or #	pound
A.M. or a.m.	morning	M$_x$ or ♏	minim
A.S.	left ear	mcg	microgram
A.U.	each ear	mEq	milliequivalent
b.i.d.	twice a day	mg	milligram
$\overline{c}$	with	ml	milliliter
caps	capsules	mm	millimeter
cc	cubic centimeter	N.P.O.	nothing by mouth
cm	centimeter	NR	no refills
comp	compound	NS or N/S	normal saline (0.9%)
/d	per day	¼NS	¼ normal saline (0.225%)
D/C or dc	discontinue	½NS	½ normal saline (0.45%)
disp	dispensary	O.D.	right eye
DS	double strength	os	mouth
D$_5$W	dextrose 5% in water	O.S.	left eye
EC	enteric coated	OTC	over the counter
elix	elixir	O.U.	each eye
ext	extract	$\overline{p}$	after
fl or fld	fluid	p.c.	after meals
g, gm, or GM	gram (quantity usually expressed in Arabic numerals)	per	by or through
		P.O. or p.o.	by mouth
gr	grain (quantity usually expressed in Roman numerals)	p.r.n.	as needed
		pt	pint
		q	every
gtt	drop	q a.m. or Q.M.	every morning
h or hr	hour	q.d.	every day
h.s.	at bedtime	q.h.	every hour
I.M.	intramuscular	q.i.d.	four times a day
in or "	inch	q3h, q4h, etc.	every 3 hours, every 4 hours, etc.
I.V.	intravenous		
IVPB	intravenous "piggyback"	q.o.d.	every other day
kg	kilogram	qt	quart

Appendix 1: Commonly used abbreviations in drug therapy *(continued)*

Ⓡ	right	**syr.**	syrup
R or PR	by rectum	**T, Tbs., or tbsp.**	tablespoon
Rx	treatment, prescription	**t or tsp.**	teaspoon
s̄	without	**tab**	tablet
s̄s̄	one-half	**t.i.d.**	three times a day
sat	saturated	**tinct or tr**	tincture
S.C. or SQ	subcutaneous	**U**	unit
sec	second	**ung.**	ointment
Sig.	write on label	**vag**	vaginal
SL or sl	sublingual	**VO**	verbal order
sp.	spirits	**x**	times, multiply
SR	sustained release	**f℈**	dram
stat	immediately	**f℥ or oz**	ounce
supp	suppository		

Appendix 2: NANDA taxonomy of nursing diagnoses

The currently accepted classification system for nursing diagnoses is that of the North American Nursing Diagnosis Association (NANDA) as shown in *NANDA nursing diagnoses: Definitions and classifications 1992-1993.* It is organized around nine human response patterns: exchanging, communicating, relating, valuing, choosing, moving, perceiving, knowing, and feeling.

The complete taxonomic structure is listed here. The series of numbers before each diagnosis is its classification number, used to determine the placement of the diagnosis within the taxonomy. The number of digits delineates the level of abstraction of the nursing diagnosis (more specific diagnoses are assigned longer numbers).

Pattern 1. Exchanging

1.1.2.1	Altered nutrition: More than body requirements
1.1.2.2	Altered nutrition: Less than body requirements
1.1.2.3	Altered nutrition: Potential for more than body requirements
1.2.1.1	High risk for infection
1.2.2.1	High risk for altered body temperature
1.2.2.2	Hypothermia
1.2.2.3	Hyperthermia
1.2.2.4	Ineffective thermoregulation
1.2.3.1	Dysreflexia
*1.3.1.1	Constipation
1.3.1.1.1	Perceived constipation
1.3.1.1.2	Colonic constipation
*1.3.1.2	Diarrhea
*1.3.1.3	Bowel incontinence
1.3.2	Altered urinary elimination
1.3.2.1.1	Stress incontinence
1.3.2.1.2	Reflex incontinence
1.3.2.1.3	Urge incontinence
1.3.2.1.4	Functional incontinence
1.3.2.1.5	Total incontinence
1.3.2.2	Urinary retention
*1.4.1.1	Altered (specify type) tissue perfusion (renal, cerebral, cardiopulmonary, gastrointestinal, peripheral)
1.4.1.2.1	Fluid volume excess
1.4.1.2.2.1	Fluid volume deficit
1.4.1.2.2.2	High risk for fluid volume deficit
*1.4.2.1	Decreased cardiac output
1.5.1.1	Impaired gas exchange

Appendix 2: NANDA taxonomy of nursing diagnoses *(continued)*

1.5.1.2	Ineffective airway clearance
1.5.1.3	Ineffective breathing pattern
#1.5.1.3.1	Inability to sustain spontaneous ventilation
#1.5.1.3.2	Dysfunctional ventilatory weaning response (DVWR)
1.6.1	High risk for injury
1.6.1.1	High risk for suffocation
1.6.1.2	High risk for poisoning
1.6.1.3	High risk for trauma
1.6.1.4	High risk for aspiration
1.6.1.5	High risk for disuse syndrome
1.6.2	Altered protection
1.6.2.1	Impaired tissue integrity
*1.6.2.1.1	Altered oral mucous membrane
1.6.2.1.2.1	Impaired skin integrity
1.6.2.1.2.2	High risk for impaired skin integrity

Pattern 2. Communicating

2.1.1.1	Impaired verbal communication

Pattern 3. Relating

3.1.1	Impaired social interaction
3.1.2	Social isolation
*3.2.1	Altered role performance
3.2.1.1.1	Altered parenting
3.2.1.1.2	High risk for altered parenting
3.2.1.2.1	Sexual dysfunction
3.2.2	Altered family processes
#3.2.2.1	Caregiver role strain
#3.2.2.2	High risk for caregiver role strain
3.2.3.1	Parental role conflict
3.3	Altered sexuality patterns

Pattern 4. Valuing

4.1.1	Spiritual distress (distress of the human spirit)

(continued)

Appendix 2: NANDA taxonomy of nursing diagnoses *(continued)*

Pattern 5. Choosing

5.1.1.1	Ineffective individual coping
5.1.1.1.1	Impaired adjustment
5.1.1.1.2	Defensive coping
5.1.1.1.3	Ineffective denial
5.1.2.1.1	Ineffective family coping: Disabling
5.1.2.1.2	Ineffective family coping: Compromised
5.1.2.2	Family coping: Potential for growth
#5.2.1	Ineffective management of therapeutic regimen (individual)
5.2.1.1	Noncompliance (specify)
5.3.1.1	Decisional conflict (specify)
5.4	Health-seeking behaviors (specify)

Pattern 6. Moving

6.1.1.1	Impaired physical mobility
#6.1.1.1.1	High risk for peripheral neurovascular dysfunction
6.1.1.2	Activity intolerance
6.1.1.2.1	Fatigue
6.1.1.3	High risk for activity intolerance
6.2.1	Sleep pattern disturbance
6.3.1.1	Diversional activity deficit
6.4.1.1	Impaired home maintenance management
6.4.2	Altered health maintenance
***6.5.1**	Feeding self-care deficit
6.5.1.1	Impaired swallowing
6.5.1.2	Ineffective breast-feeding
#6.5.1.2.1	Interrupted breast-feeding
6.5.1.3	Effective breast-feeding
#6.5.1.4	Ineffective infant feeding pattern
***6.5.2**	Bathing or hygiene self-care deficit
***6.5.3**	Dressing or grooming self-care deficit
***6.5.4**	Toileting self-care deficit
6.6	Altered growth and development
#6.7	Relocation stress syndrome

Appendix 2: NANDA taxonomy of nursing diagnoses *(continued)*

Pattern 7. Perceiving

*7.1.1	Body image disturbance
*7.1.2	Self-esteem disturbance
7.1.2.1	Chronic low self-esteem
7.1.2.2	Situational low self-esteem
*7.1.3	Personal identity disturbance
7.2	Sensory or perceptual alterations (specify visual, auditory, kinesthetic, gustatory, tactile, olfactory)
7.2.1.1	Unilateral neglect
7.3.1	Hopelessness
7.3.2	Powerlessness

Pattern 8. Knowing

8.1.1	Knowledge deficit (specify)
8.3	Altered thought processes

Pattern 9. Feeling

*9.1.1	Pain
9.1.1.1	Chronic pain
9.2.1.1	Dysfunctional grieving
9.2.1.2	Anticipatory grieving
9.2.2	High risk for violence: Self-directed or directed at others
#9.2.2.1	High risk for self-mutilation
9.2.3	Post-trauma response
9.2.3.1	Rape-trauma syndrome
9.2.3.1.1	Rape-trauma syndrome: Compound reaction
9.2.3.1.2	Rape-trauma syndrome: Silent reaction
9.3.1	Anxiety
9.3.2	Fear

New diagnostic categorieis in 1992
* Categories with modified label terminology

Selected References

AHFS drug informatiom 93. (1993). Bethesda, MD: American Society of Hospital Pharmacists.

Compendium of pharmaceuticals and specialties: The Canadian reference for health professionals. (1992). Toronto: CK Productions.

Drug facts and comparisons. (1993). St. Louis: Facts and Comparisons Division, Lippincott.

Drug interaction facts 1992. St. Louis: Facts and Comparisons Division, Lippincott.

Goodman and Gilman's the pharmacological basis of therapeutics (8th ed.) (1990). New York: McGraw-Hill.

Hansten, P., and Horn, J. (1989). *Drug interactions: Clinical significance of drug-drug interactions* (6th ed.). Philadelphia: Lea & Febiger.

North American Nursing Diagnosis Association (1992). *NANDA nursing diagnoses: Definitions and classifications 1992-1993.* Philadelphia: NANDA.

Nursing94 Drug Handbook. (1994). Springhouse, PA: Springhouse Corporation.

Physicians' Desk Reference. (47th ed., 1993). Montvale, NJ: Medical Economics Company.

Speight, T. (1987). *Avery's drug treatment: Principles and practice of clinical pharmacology and therapeutics* (3rd ed.). Baltimore: Williams & Wilkins.

USPDI. (1993). *Drug information for the health care professional* (Vol. I, 13th ed.). Rockville, MD: United States Pharmacopeial Convention.

USPDI. (1993). *Advice for the patient* (Vol. II, 13th ed.). Rockville, MD: United States Pharmacopeial Convention.

Index

i refers to an illustration; t refers to a table

i refers to an illustration; t refers to a table

i refers to an illustration; t refers to a table

i refers to an illustration; t refers to a table